Obstetrics and Gynecology
Fifth edition

National Medical Series for Independent Study Obstetrics and Gynecology

5th Edition

Editors

Mark Morgan, MD
University of Pennsylvania Medical Center
Philadelphia, Pennsylvania

Sam Siddighi, MD
Loma Linda Medical Center
Loma Linda, California

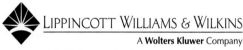
LIPPINCOTT WILLIAMS & WILKINS
A **Wolters Kluwer** Company
Philadelphia · Baltimore · New York · London
Buenos Aires · Hong Kong · Sydney · Tokyo

Editor: Neil Marquardt
Developmental Editor: Kathleen H. Scogna
Marketing Manager: Scott Lavine
Senior Project Editor: Paula C. Williams
Designer: Risa Clow
Compositor: Maryland Composition, Inc.
Printer: DRC

351 West Camden Street
Baltimore, Maryland 21201-2436 USA

530 Walnut Street
Philadelphia, Pennsylvania 19106-3621 USA

Printed in the United States of America

Obstetrics and gynecology / editors, Mark Morgan, Sam Saddighi – 5th ed.
    p.; cm.—(National medical series for independent study)
  Includes index.
  ISBN 0-7817-2679-4
   1. Obstetrics—Outlines, syllabi, etc. 2. Gynecology—Outlines, syllabi, etc.
  3. Obstetrics—Examinations, questions, etc. 4. Gynecology—Examinations, questions, etc.
  I. Title: Half-title: NMS obstetrics and gynecology. II. Morgan, Mark, 1955– III. Siddighi,
  Sam. IV. Series.
   [DNLM: 1. Obstetrics—Examination Questions. 2. Obstetrics—Outlines.
  3. Gynecology—Examination Questions. 4. Gynecology—Outlines. WQ 18.2 O141 2004]
  RG112.O73 2004
  618–dc22

                                                                                2004044189

To purchase additional copies of this book call our customer service department at **(800) 638-3030** or fax orders to **(301) 824-7390.** International customers should call (301) 714-2324.

Visit Lippincott Williams & Wilkins on the Internet: http://www.lww.com. Lippincott Williams & Wilkins customer service representatives are available from 8:30 am to 6:00 pm, EST, Monday through Friday, for telephone access.

04 05 06
1 2 3 4 5 6 7 8 9 10

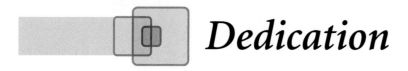

Dedication

In Memory of Michelle Battistini, MD and Dedicated to Sorraya Siddighi.

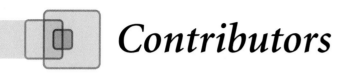

Contributors

Janice Asher, MD
University of Pennsylvania Medical Center
Student Health
Obstetrics and Gynecology
Philadelphia, PA

Christina Bandera, MD
Assistant Professor
Division of Gynecologic Oncology
Brigham and Women's Hospital
Dana Farber Cancer Institute
Harvard Medical School
Boston, MA

Kurt Barnhart, MD
University of Pennsylvania Medical Center
Reproductive Endocrinology and Infertility
Philadelphia, PA

William Beck, MD
University of Pennsylvania Medical Center
Polson, MT

Michelle Berlin, MD, MPH
Oregon Health and Science University
Department of Obstetrics and Gynecology
Portland, OR

Catherine Bradley, MD
University of Pennsylvania Medical Center
Division of Urogynecology
Philadelphia, PA

Samantha Butts, MD
University of Pennsylvania Medical Center
Reproductive Endocrinology & Infertility
Philadelphia, PA

Peter J. Chen, MD
University of Pennsylvania Medical Center
Department of Obstetrics and Gynecology
Philadelphia, PA

Doris Chou, MD
University of Pennsylvania Medical Center
Maternal/Fetal Medicine
Philadelphia, PA

Christina Chu, MD
University of Pennsylvania Medical Center
Division of Gynecologic Oncology
Philadelphia, PA

Scott Edwards, MD
University of Pennsylvania Medical Center
Department of Obstetrics and Gynecology
Philadelphia, PA

Mohammed Elkousy, MD
University of Pennsylvania Medical Center
Maternal/Fetal Medicine Division
Philadelphia, PA

Melissa Esposito, MD
Shady Grove Fertility
Rockville, MD

Clarisa Gracia, MD
University of Pennsylvania Medical Center
Reproductive Endocrinology & Infertility
Philadelphia, PA

Alfredo Gil, MD
University of Pennsylvania Medical Center
Department of Obstetrics and Gynecology
Philadelphia, PA

Ann Honebrink, MD
Pennsylvania Hospital
Philadelphia, PA

Jane Houdeshel, MSN, RN, CRNP
University of Pennsylvania Medical Center
Division of Gynecologic Oncology
Philadelphia, PA

Sami I. Jabara, MD
University of Michigan
Women's Hospital
Ann Arbor, MI

Jack Ludmir, MD
Pennsylvania Hospital
Chairman of Obstetrics and Gynecology
Maternal/Fetal Medicine
Philadelphia, PA

George A. Macones, MD
University of Pennsylvania Medical Center
Maternal/Fetal Medicine
Philadelphia, PA

Dominic Marchiano, MD
University of Pennsylvania Medical Center
Maternal/Fetal Medicine Division
Philadelphia, PA

Sara J. Marder, MD
Washington University School of Medicine
Department of Obstetrics and Gynecology
St. Louis, MO

Emmanuelle Pare, MD
University of Pennsylvania Medical Center
Maternal/Fetal Medicine
Philadelphia, PA

Samuel Parry, MD
University of Pennsylvania Medical Center
Maternal/Fetal Medicine Division
Philadelphia, PA

Samantha Pfeifer, MD
Reproductive Endocrinology and Infertility
University of Pennsylvania Medical Center
Philadelphia, PA

Joanne N. Quinones, MD
University of Pennsylvania Medical Center
Maternal/Fetal Medicine Division
Philadelphia, PA

Sally Y. Segel, MD
Emory University Health System
Department of Obstetrics and Gynecology
Atlanta, GA

Harish Sehdev, MD
Pennsylvania Hospital
Philadelphia, PA

Steven Sondheimer, MD
Reproductive Endocrinology and Infertility
University of Pennsylvania Medical Center
Philadelphia, PA

Ann Steiner, MD
Penn Medicine at Radnor
Radnor, PA

Richard Tureck, MD
Reproductive Endocrinology and Infertility
University of Pennsylvania Medical Center
Philadelphia, PA

Serdar Ural, MD
Maternal/Fetal Medicine
University of Pennsylvania Medical Center
Philadelphia, PA

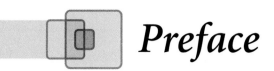

Preface

The fifth edition of NMS Obstetrics and Gynecology has the same primary goal of the previous edition, and indeed, the entire NMS series in general: to provide the most up-to-date and relevant information in an easy-to-understand outline format for both students and residents. Basic scientific information is balanced by clinical relevance, and a wealth of more than 200 USMLE-formatted questions allows readers to test their knowledge prior to their board examinations.

This fifth edition represents a collaborative effort between the many contributors who revised existing chapters or wrote new chapters for this edition, and the two new co-editors, Mark Morgan, MD, and Sam Siddighi, MD, who orchestrated and oversaw the text revision (Dr. Morgan) and completely revamped the USMLE questions and comprehensive examination (Dr. Siddighi) to reflect current Step 2 formats and content areas. The 52 questions in the comprehensive examination have been written at a slightly higher level of difficulty than the USMLE-formatted questions in the chapters. Some of the answers, therefore, require a level of knowledge that goes beyond the information presented in the book. The examination thus provides a rigorous and comprehensive review of content.

Information in all of the chapters has been thoroughly updated, and a new chapter on benign breast disease has been added. In addition, the order of the chapters has been slightly rearranged to make the order of presentation more logical, although the chapters can be used in any order. Two new case studies have been added in this edition, and a third, on hormone replacement therapy, has been rewritten to encompass current research findings. A new feature in this edition is the test question CD-ROM, which places the USMLE questions from the text in an electronic interface that mimics the actual USMLE test environment.

This edition would not have been possible without the assistance of several people. Carmen Lord, editorial assistant to the Division of Gynecologic Oncology at the University of Pennsylvania, was instrumental in organizing, coordinating, and collating the vast amount of information that went into this edition. Martha Cushman, freelance editor, imposed order and clarity on the manuscript and perfected the outline format that is the hallmark of this series.

In addition, Dr. Siddighi wishes to acknowledge the mentors and teachers at Loma Linda University Medical Center for sharing their knowledge and wisdom, and also extends special thanks to Jeff Cao, MD and Glenn Rouse, MD for their contributions to the book.

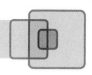

Table of Contents

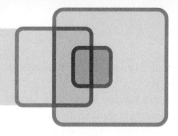

chapter 1

Endocrinology of Pregnancy

SAMUEL PARRY AND DOMINIC MARCHIANO

I   INTRODUCTION

Endocrine changes in pregnancy are largely dependent on the concerted production of protein and steroid hormones by the fetoplacental unit. These endocrine changes support the successful establishment, maintenance, and termination of pregnancy.

A Endocrine changes during pregnancy. The most important endocrine changes involve the production of **protein hormones** (human chorionic gonadotropin [hCG] and **human placental lactogen** [hPL]) and **steroid hormones** (**estrogen** and **progesterone**). Levels of hormones in pregnant women differ from those in nonpregnant women because of the presence of:

1. A **placenta,** which has a diverse secretory repertoire that surpasses that of any other endocrine organ.

2. A **fetus,** whose endocrine structures (e.g., pituitary gland, thyroid, adrenal cortex, pancreas, and gonads) function as early as the eleventh week of pregnancy.
   a. In the **male fetus,** the testes, in response to placental gonadotropin, produce testosterone, which is necessary for normal male development.
   b. In the **female fetus,** although the ovaries are responsive to placental gonadotropins, normal development is not dependent on the production of fetal ovarian steroids. The ovaries in the fetus produce small but progressively greater amounts of estrogen.

3. **Increased levels of circulating estrogens,** which have the following effects:
   a. To increase the maternal hepatic production of binding proteins such as **thyroid-binding globulin (TBG)** and **cortisol-binding globulin (CBG)**
      (1) These proteins bind **thyroxine** and **cortisol** and raise their total levels in the maternal circulation.
      (2) However, the free fraction changes little. Thus, the metabolic processes that are dependent on these hormones usually are unaltered.
   b. To inhibit maternal pituitary gonadotropin synthesis and release, thus making placental gonadotropins primarily responsible for gonadotropic function
   c. To enhance placental production of 11β-hydroxysteroid dehydrogenase (11β-HSD), which inactivates maternal cortisol, thereby isolating the fetal pituitary and adrenal from maternal influences

B Significant characteristics of hormones during pregnancy

1. Chemical nature
   a. **Protein hormones** (e.g., hCG, hPL, prolactin)
   b. **Steroids** (e.g., progesterone, estrogen, fetal adrenal steroids)
2. Source
   a. The **mother** is the exclusive source of certain hormones (such as estrogen and progesterone) early in pregnancy.

    b. By the end of the first trimester, the **fetus** and **placenta** are important sources of sex steroids and protein hormones.

        (1) The **fetus** produces thyroid hormones, pituitary tropic hormones, and gonadal steroids.

        (2) The **placenta** secretes large quantities of estrogen and progesterone along with many releasing and inhibiting hormones, including **gonadotropin-releasing hormone (GnRH)**, **corticotropin-releasing hormone (CRH)**, and **thyrotropin-releasing hormone (TRH)**.

    c. Occasionally, hormones have multiple sources. For example, the mother, the placenta, and the fetus all produce estradiol.

  3. Secretion patterns. Recognizing normal patterns of hormone activity throughout pregnancy can help distinguish abnormal pregnancies and fetal compromise.

  4. Biologic functions. Understanding the function of a particular hormone may illuminate its role in reproductive physiology, particularly in maintaining pregnancy and fetal well-being. For example, it is possible to correct hormone deficiencies that are harmful in pregnancy with the use of exogenous hormones, and the presence of certain hormones may serve as markers for gestational abnormalities. Although deficiencies in estriol or hPL late in gestation have been correlated with fetal growth restriction and fetal demise, obstetricians are advised to use more traditional methods of monitoring to document fetal well-being.

    a. Unusually high levels of hCG suggest a trophoblastic neoplasm, because hCG originates in trophoblastic tissue.

    b. Progesterone deficiency early in pregnancy suggests corpus luteum insufficiency, because progesterone is produced by the corpus luteum in early pregnancy.

II   HUMAN CHORIONIC GONADOTROPIN (hCG)

A **Chemical nature.** hCG is a glycoprotein composed of two subunits, α and β, that are noncovalently linked.

  1. The α-subunit is biochemically similar to pituitary gonadotropins and thyrotropin.

  2. The β-subunit is similar to luteinizing hormone (LH).

B **Source**

  1. hCG is almost exclusively the product of the trophoblastic tissue, specifically the syncytiotrophoblast.

  2. hCG is produced by normal placental tissue as early as 6 to 8 days postconception.

C **Secretion patterns**

  1. Normally, hCG rises rapidly 8 days postconception, doubling every 2 to 3 days and reaching a peak at approximately 9 to 10 weeks gestation. It declines after 10 weeks' gestation to a plateau for the remainder of pregnancy and remains detectable throughout pregnancy.

    a. Significance of abnormally high levels of hCG

        (1) Multiple placentas (multiple gestation)

        (2) Hydatidiform mole by virtue of trophoblastic proliferation

        (3) Choriocarcinoma

    b. Significance of abnormally low levels of hCG

        (1) Ectopic pregnancy

        (2) Miscarriage

  2. Detection of hCG in the serum or urine is the basis of **contemporary pregnancy tests.**

    a. Serum hCG assays are able to detect pregnancy within 8 to 12 days of ovulation.

    b. Urine hCG assays detect hCG within 14 to 18 days of ovulation.

3. After delivery at term, hCG can normally be detected in the maternal serum or urine for up to 4 weeks.

4. After first-trimester miscarriage or elective termination of pregnancy, hCG can be detected in the maternal serum or urine for as long as 10 weeks.

D Biologic functions

1. Signals the ovary to **maintain the corpus luteum** and continue progesterone production

2. Regulates **fetal testicular testosterone production,** which is critical in the development of male external genitalia

3. Possesses some TSH-like properties and can cause hyperthyroidism when present in high levels (as in trophoblastic neoplasms)

4. Clinical uses
   a. **Treatment for anovulation.** Based on its biologic similarities to that of LH, hCG can be used to **induce ovulation.**
   b. **Assessment of viability of pregnancy.** Quantitative serum hCG values may be correlated with transvaginal ultrasound findings. When the serum hCG value exceeds 1000 IU/L, an intrauterine pregnancy should be visible; otherwise, ectopic pregnancy is suspected.
   c. **Multiple marker screen. Maternal serum hCG** in conjunction with α-fetoprotein (**AFP,** the primary serum protein in fetuses before mid-gestation) and unconjugated **estriol,** is used in the prenatal diagnosis of fetal chromosomal abnormalities (see Chapter 4).
      (1) Allows detection of approximately 60% of fetuses with Down syndrome.
      (2) During the second trimester, elevated hCG is the most sensitive serum marker for Down syndrome.
   d. **Observing patients with trophoblastic neoplasia.** hCG determinations are used to follow the course of patients treated for this condition.

III HUMAN PLACENTAL LACTOGEN (hPL)

A Chemical nature. hPL, or **human chorionic somatomammotropin (hCS),** is a nonglycosylated protein hormone.

B Source. hPL is formed by the placenta as early as 3 weeks postconception and is secreted by the syncytiotrophoblast.

C Secretory patterns. hPL can be detected in maternal serum as early as 6 weeks postconception. Like most hormones produced by the syncytiotrophoblast, hPL is secreted primarily into the maternal bloodstream. hPL levels rise in maternal serum until 34 weeks gestation and then plateau.

D Biologic function

1. **Diabetogenic effect of pregnancy.** hPL induces lipolysis and **increases maternal free fatty acids,** ketones, and glycerol, which provide energy for the mother.
   a. In the fed state, free fatty acids **interfere with insulin-directed entry of glucose into cells.**
   b. In the fasting state, ketones can cross the placenta and serve as fuel for the fetus.
   c. However, recent findings suggest that hPL is not responsible for acute changes in maternal lipolysis and glycemic control. Therefore, the integrated role of hPL in modulating maternal metabolism is probably chronic.

2. **Increased insulin levels.** hPL **raises plasma insulin** by upregulating pancreatic islet function.

3. **Clinical use.** Although early studies have shown that low maternal serum levels of hPL are associated with fetal growth restriction and nonreassuring fetal heart rate patterns, subsequent studies have been unable to substantiate the value of hPL monitoring for detecting fetal complications secondary to uteroplacental insufficiency.

IV PROLACTIN

A **Chemical nature.** Prolactin is a protein hormone that circulates in different molecular sizes.

B **Source.** The **three potential sources** of prolactin during pregnancy are the:

1. Anterior lobe of the maternal pituitary gland, which is the primary source of elevated maternal serum prolactin levels

2. Anterior lobe of the fetal pituitary gland

3. Decidual tissue of the uterus, from which prolactin is secreted primarily into the amniotic fluid

C **Secretory patterns**

1. In the nonpregnant state, prolactin levels normally range between 8 and 25 ng/mL.

2. In pregnancy, maternal prolactin levels increase under the influence of estrogen to a maximum of 200 ng/mL in the third trimester.

3. Levels of prolactin in pregnancy should not be interpreted as indicative of pituitary adenoma growth. However, women with prolactin-secreting adenomas who conceive should be monitored by visual field determinations for the possibility of enlargement.

D **Biologic function**

1. **Preparing the mammary glands for lactation**
   a. Stimulates the growth of mammary tissue.
   b. Stimulates production and secretion of milk into the alveoli. Lactation does not occur during pregnancy because estrogen inhibits the action of prolactin on the breast.

2. Decidual prolactin is thought to be important for fluid and electrolyte regulation of the amniotic fluid.

V PROGESTERONE

A **Chemical nature.** Progesterone is a **21-carbon steroid** hormone.

B **Source.** All steroid hormones are derived from cholesterol.

1. **In nonpregnant women, progesterone is produced by all steroid-forming glands,** including the ovaries, testes, and adrenal cortex. It serves as an intermediary for other hormones (e.g., aldosterone, cortisol, estrogen, and testosterone) and as an end-product when it is produced by the corpus luteum.

2. In the **pregnant state, progesterone has a dual source.** It is produced by the **corpus luteum** until the seventh to tenth week of pregnancy; then the **placenta** assumes its production until parturition.
   a. This **shift in production** occurs at approximately the **eighth week of pregnancy,** after which the corpus luteum becomes an insignificant source of progesterone.
   b. This point has **clinical significance,** because progesterone produced by the corpus luteum is essential for pregnancy maintenance until the eighth week. Consequently, progesterone suppositories are generally prescribed to women with suspected corpus luteum deficiency for the first 8 to 10 weeks of gestation.

3. The human placenta operates in close communication with the developing fetus (i.e., **fetal adrenal cortex, fetal liver**) in the biosynthesis and actions of all steroid hormones (Fig. 1-1). In the placenta, cholesterol is metabolized to **pregnenolone,** which is converted to progesterone and not metabolized to other steroids.

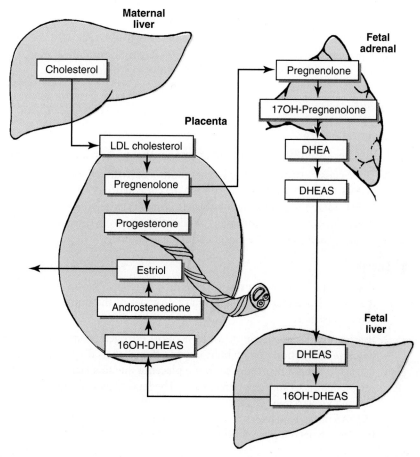

FIGURE 1-1 Schematic representation of estrogen and progesterone synthesis in late pregnancy. DHEA, dehydroepiandrosterone; DHEAS, DHEA sulfate; LDL, low-density lipoprotein.

C **Secretory patterns**

1. Because progesterone originates initially from the corpus luteum, it is present at ovulation. In a nonconception cycle, the peak production of progesterone reaches 25 mg/day, and levels measure approximately 20 to 25 ng/mL in peripheral blood.

2. In the late luteal phase in a conception cycle, progesterone levels increase slowly because of hCG stimulation.

3. As placental progesterone supplements corpus luteal progesterone, levels increase more rapidly.

4. Progesterone concentrations in the blood continue to increase up until the time of parturition, at which time the placenta produces 300 mg/day; most of the progesterone produced enters the maternal circulation.

5. Progesterone is produced in larger quantities in the presence of multiple gestation.

D **Biologic functions.** The primary function of progesterone is to **support pregnancy**.

1. It **prepares the endometrium for implantation of the embryo.**

2. It **relaxes the myometrium.**
   a. Progesterone suppresses the calcium–calmodulin–myosin light chain kinase system in smooth muscle.

  b. These effects of progesterone appear to be receptor-mediated and can be blocked by the progesterone receptor antagonist **mifepristone (RU486)**, which is used as an abortifacient in the first trimester.

  3. It **prevents rejection of the fetus** by the maternal immune system. Specifically, progesterone suppresses lymphocyte production of cytolytic cytokines.

VI ESTROGENS

A Chemical nature

  1. Estrogens are **18-carbon steroid hormones that possess an aromatic ring**.

  2. Three classic estrogens differ by the number of hydroxyl groups they contain:
   a. Estrone, a relatively weak estrogen, has one hydroxyl group.
   b. Estradiol, the most potent estrogen, contains two hydroxyl groups.
   c. Estriol, a very weak estrogen, contains three hydroxyl groups. Estriol is produced in extremely large quantities by the placenta during pregnancy.

B Source

  1. Role of fetal adrenal glands. Because the placenta cannot convert pregnenolone to androgens, the fetal adrenal cortex is the primary provider of the immediate **androgen precursors of placental estrogens**.

  2. Production. Estriol accounts for 80% of the estrogen produced during pregnancy. Its synthesis involves integration of metabolic steps in the mother, the placenta, and the fetus (see Fig. 1-1). Estrogens cannot be produced in the **placenta** due to a lack of the enzyme necessary to convert pregnenolone to androgen precursors. The **fetal adrenal cortex** converts pregnenolone to dehydroepiandrosterone (DHEA) and DHEA sulfate (DHEAS), which is then converted to 16-OH DHEAS in the **fetal liver**. 16-OH DHEAS is then converted to androgen precursors and aromatized to estrogen in the **placenta**.

C Secretory patterns

  1. The estrone:estradiol:estriol ratio produced by the placenta is approximately 14:5:81. Estradiol is largely bound to sex hormone–binding globulin in the maternal serum, whereas **estriol remains unbound**. Therefore, estriol is more rapidly excreted in the urine, and maternal serum levels of estriol and estradiol are similar.

  2. Early in pregnancy, estradiol is the major form of estrogen produced by the maternal ovaries.

  3. Later in pregnancy, estrone and estradiol are produced primarily by the placenta; estriol is produced almost exclusively by the placenta.

  4. Significant amounts of estriol are produced early in the second trimester, and levels continue to rise until parturition, increasing 1000-fold over the nonpregnant levels.

  7. Extremely low levels or no estriol may be associated with:
   a. Fetal demise.
   b. Anencephaly. The **limited ACTH production** results in atrophy of the fetal zone of the adrenal cortex after 20 weeks' gestation.
   c. Maternal ingestion of corticosteroids. However, placental 11β-HSD limits the transfer of cortisol to the fetus.
   d. Placental sulfatase deficiency.

D Biologic activities.
  Because placental estrogen formation is dependent on androgenic precursors produced by the fetal adrenal cortex, the fetus appears to be ultimately responsible for many of the maternal physiologic effects mediated by estrogen.

1. Estrogen **stimulates** receptor-mediated **LDL uptake by the placenta** and placental expression of enzymes that are important in steroidogenesis.
2. Estrogen **increases blood flow to the uterus.**
   a. Effects are mediated in part by prostanoids.
   b. Effects are tonic and do not elicit acute changes in blood flow.
3. Estrogen **regulates end-of-gestation events.**
   a. **Parturition.** Estrogen activates oxytocin secretion and myometrial gap junction formation. Consequently, maternal salivary estriol levels have been used to predict preterm birth. Conversely, **labor and delivery may be delayed in anencephalic fetuses and fetuses with placental sulfatase deficiency.**
   b. **Lactation.** Estrogen stimulates epithelial cell proliferation in human breast tissue. However, milk release is delayed until estrogen levels decrease after delivery.
4. Because estriol is an index of normal function of the fetus and the placenta, **reduced maternal estriol levels may reflect abnormalities in fetal or placental development.**
   a. Conditions that may occur include fetal demise, hypertensive disease during pregnancy, preeclampsia and eclampsia, and intrauterine growth retardation.
   b. When estriol levels are reduced below normal or fail to increase during pregnancy, fetal and placental well-being may be studied by supplemental tests, including ultrasonography, fetal heart rate testing, and biophysical profile.

Study Questions for Chapter 1

Directions: Each of the numbered items or incomplete statements in this section is followed by answers or by completions of the statement. Select the ONE lettered answer or completion that is BEST in each case.

1. A 26-year-old woman, gravida 1, para 0 with history of one ectopic pregnancy, presents to your clinic because she missed her last period. According to her records, 4 years ago her unruptured ectopic was resolved by a linear salpingostomy procedure. You send off a serum β-hCG level, which returns elevated (β-hCG = 900 IU/l). Radiologic images obtained in the emergency department are unremarkable. What is the next best step in the management of this patient?

- [A] Formal transvaginal ultrasound
- [B] Formal transabdominal ultrasound
- [C] Urine hCG
- [D] Repeat serum β-hCG in 2 days
- [E] Repeat linear salpingostomy

2. A 36-year-old woman, gravida 3, para 2 at 8 weeks' gestation presents to your clinic reporting painless vaginal bleeding. Her vital signs are as follows: T = 99.9, BP = 162/94, P = 100, and R = 18. Her uterus is consistent with a 14-week pregnancy. Her serum β-hCG level is 320,000 IU/l. Which of the following endocrine glands is most likely to be affected by β-hCG?

- [A] Adrenal cortex
- [B] Hypothalamus
- [C] Ovary
- [D] Parathyroid
- [E] Thyroid

3. A 29-year-old woman, gravida 3, para 1, with a history of two ectopic pregnancies presents to your office for an annual physical examination. Her last menstrual period was 33 days ago. She tells you that her periods are regular, usually occur every 28 days, and last for 4 days. She has not been on any form of contraception for the last 6 months. You perform a β-hCG level today and ask her to return for a repeat β-hCG level in 3 days. The results are as follows: day 0, β-hCG = 1000 IU/l; and day 3, β-hCG = 1700 IU/l. Which of the following is the most likely diagnosis?

- [A] Ectopic pregnancy
- [B] Therapeutic abortion
- [C] Hydatidiform mole
- [D] Choriocarcinoma
- [E] Multiple gestation

4. A 38-year-old nulligravid woman and her 39-year-old husband have been attempting to get pregnant for the last 3 years. They have tried every type of over-the-counter medicine and herbal remedy to increase their fertility, but nothing has worked. Initial workup demonstrated that her husband has normal sperm parameters and that the cause of infertility may be the wife's inability to ovulate. She has been taking clomiphene citrate to help induce development of ovarian follicles. Injection of which of the following is necessary at midcycle prior to "egg retrieval" for intrauterine insemination (IUI) or in vitro fertilization–embryo transfer (IVF-ET)?

- [A] FSH
- [B] LH
- [C] β-hCG
- [D] TSH
- [E] Estrogen

QUESTIONS 5–15

For each of the following questions, match the hormone with the description that best fits. Answer choices can be used once, more than once, or not at all.

- **A** hCG
- **B** hPL
- **C** Prolactin
- **D** Progesterone
- **E** Estriol

5. Increases myometrial gap junction formation

6. Suppresses maternal lymphocyte activity

7. Necessary for development of male external genitalia

8. Most sensitive marker for abnormal karyotype

9. Elevates ketone levels

10. Produced by the uterus

11. Inhibits lactation during pregnancy

12. Lack of this hormone can cause spontaneous abortion in the first trimester

13. Lack of this hormone is associated with an enzyme deficiency in the placenta

14. Elevated levels of this hormone are associated with twin pregnancy

15. Anencephaly causes lack of production of this hormone

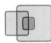

Answers and Explanations

1. The answer is D [II C 1]. Eight days after conception, hCG doubles every 2 to 3 days in a normal pregnancy (not in an ectopic or a destined miscarriage). Performing a formal (i.e., performed and interpreted by a radiologist with expertise in ultrasonography) transvaginal ultrasound at a serum β-hCG level less than 1000 IU/l is not useful because both the fallopian tubes and the uterus appear empty even though a developing embryo may be present. The transvaginal ultrasound is not sensitive enough to detect a gestational sac at hCG levels below 1000 IU/l. The transabdominal ultrasound is even less sensitive. It can detect a gestational sac reliably at hCG levels of less than 6500 IU/l. The qualitative urine hCG is not as sensitive as a quantitative serum β-hCG level. A linear salpingostomy may not be required if, in 2 days (when β-hCG level has doubled), a gestational sac is detected inside the uterus rather than inside the fallopian tube.

2. The correct answer is E [II D 3]. The clinical scenario (i.e., vaginal bleeding, early pregnancy-induced hypertension, enlarged uterus, and exaggerated β-hCG levels) is consistent with a molar pregnancy. Because of morphologic similarities between hCG and TSH (the alpha subunit is homologous to the alpha subunit of TSH), hCG possesses TSH-like properties and can cause hyperthyroidism. The other endocrine glands are not affected by a molar pregnancy.

3. The answer is A [II C 1 b (1)] . This patient's menses occur every 28 days with regularity, and she has not been on any form of hormonal contraception that could disrupt the regularity of her cycles. Therefore, she may be pregnant. Given her history of two ectopic pregnancies, she is at high risk for a third ectopic pregnancy. A serum β-hCG rise of less than double in 3 days is highly suspicious for an abnormal pregnancy (either ectopic or a miscarriage). A transvaginal ultrasound can differentiate between an ectopic pregnancy and a miscarriage. A therapeutic abortion (TAB) is not the same as a miscarriage (i.e., a spontaneous abortion [SAB]). Abnormally high levels of hCG are found in hydatidiform mole, choriocarcinoma, or multiple gestation.

4. The correct answer is C [II D 4 a]. During a normal spontaneous menstrual cycle, the LH surge is responsible for ovulation. During ovulation induction, however, β-hCG is injected at midcycle to induce ovulation because hCG is morphologically analogous to LH and is more readily available. FSH can be used for ovarian follicle stimulation instead of clomiphene (and FSH is a more potent follicle stimulant), but it does not cause ovulation induction. Estrogen is produced by the developing follicles, and thus its levels can be used to follow follicle development. TSH is not involved in these processes.

The answers are: 5-E [VI D 3 a], **6-D** [V D 3], **7-A** [II D 2], **8-A** [II D 4c (2)], **9-B** [III D 1 b], **10-C** [IV B 3], **11-E** [IV D 1 b], **12-D** [V B 2 b], **13-E** [VI C 7 d], **14-A** [II C 1 a (1)], **15-E** [VI C 7 b].

Estrogen activates oxytocin secretion and myometrial gap junction formation. Progesterone suppresses production of maternal lymphocytic cytokines, which contribute to immune rejection of the fetus. HCG regulates fetal testicular testosterone production, which is critical for the development of male external genitalia. Elevated hCG is the most sensitive serum marker for Down syndrome. HPL induces lipolysis, which provides energy for the mother in the form of fatty acids. HPL also provides energy for the fetus by elevating ketone levels. Prolactin is produced not only by the decidual tissue of the uterus, but also by the maternal and fetal pituitary glands. Lactation does not occur during pregnancy because estrogen inhibits the action of prolactin on the breast. Progesterone produced by the corpus luteum is essential for pregnancy maintenance until the eighth week. Progesterone suppositories are prescribed during the first 8 weeks of gestation in women with suspected corpus luteum deficiency. Low levels of estriol are associated with placental sulfatase deficiency. Abnormally high levels of hCG are seen in multiple gestation (twins). Anencephaly contributes to lack of ACTH production; therefore, the fetal adrenal cortex is not stimulated properly to convert pregnenolone to DHEA and DHEAS, which are essential in the production of estriol.

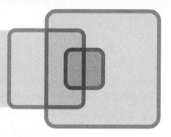

chapter **2**

Fetal Physiology

SARA J. MARDER

<table><tr><td>**I**</td><td>**INTRODUCTION**</td></tr></table>

The normal growth and development of the fetus depends on the successful integration of the functions of the placenta, umbilical cord, amniotic fluid, and fetal organ systems.

<table><tr><td>**II**</td><td>**PLACENTA**</td></tr></table>

A **Structure**

1. Villi
   a. These structures, the functioning units of the placenta, are formed by invading placental tissue (trophoblast) and contain the terminal fetal capillaries of the umbilical arteries.
   b. The villi are surrounded by the intervillous space into which maternal blood from the decidual (uterine) arteries is forced by maternal arterial pressure.
   c. Gases and nutrients pass **from the maternal blood** in the intervillous space, across the plasma membrane of the trophoblast to the basement membrane of the fetal capillary, and then through the single endothelial cell layer of the fetal capillary **to the fetal blood.** The fetal capillaries drain into the fetal veins that join to form the umbilical vein. Maternal blood drains from the intervillous space into the maternal veins.

2. **Placental cotyledons (lobes)** are formed from the branching villi supplied by one terminal arterial branch and its partner venous branch of the fetal umbilical vessels. On average, about 20 cotyledons make up the fetal side of the placenta. The maternal side of the placenta is divided by septa into lobes.

B **Function.** The placenta transfers nutrition and oxygen from the mother to the fetus, removes metabolic waste products from the fetus to be eliminated by the mother, and synthesizes proteins and hormones that support fetal development and important maternal physiologic changes.

1. **Mother-to-fetus transfer of nutrients**
   a. The essential substances for growth and development move from the mother to the fetus in four ways:
      (1) **Active transport:** amino acids, calcium
      (2) **Facilitated transport:** glucose
      (3) **Endocytosis:** cholesterol, insulin, iron, immunoglobulin G (IgG)
      (4) **Sodium pumps and chloride channels:** ions
   b. Solute size and lipid solubility are also important factors that influence transport.

2. **Gas exchange.** This process involves supplying oxygen to the fetus and removing carbon dioxide from the fetus.

3. **Secretion** of proteins and steroid hormones (see Chapter 1)
   a. **Progesterone** is produced by the placenta from maternal cholesterol, is secreted into the maternal circulation, and is important for maintaining pregnancy.

11

    b. Estrogen is converted from circulating fetal androgens (dehydroepiandrosterone sulfate [DHEAS] produced in the fetal adrenal glands. Estrogen plays an important role in maternal physiologic changes in pregnancy, labor, and lactation.

    c. Numerous **proteins, peptides,** and **growth factors** are produced in the placenta. They are important for placental growth, fetal growth and development, and the maternal physiologic changes necessary to ensure adequate nutrition to the fetus.

    4. Immunology. Invading placental cells express a unique antigen, HLA-G, which is not recognized as a "foreign" antigen by the mother. Other unique antigens and local immune suppression contribute to the prevention of rejection of the fetal–placental unit.

    C Metabolism. Glucose is the primary substrate for placental aerobic metabolism.

III UMBILICAL CORD

A Umbilical arteries. Two umbilical arteries originate from the fetal aorta. They supply fetal blood to all portions of the placenta for gas and solute exchange. A single umbilical artery is associated with low birth weight and chromosomal anomalies in about 10 to 15% of infants.

B Umbilical vein. One umbilical vein returns nutrient-rich, oxygen-rich blood to the fetus.

IV AMNIOTIC MEMBRANES AND FLUID

A Membranes

    1. Amnion. The amnion is a single layer of epithelial cells surrounding the fetus and containing the amniotic fluid.

    2. Chorion. The chorion, which lies adjacent to the uterine endometrium, is exterior and fused to the amnion.

B Fluid

    1. Fetal lung fluid appears to be important for the successful development of the bronchial tree, but the amniotic fluid volume derives primarily from the fetal urine.

    2. Early in gestation, the fluid surrounding the embryo is probably transudative. By the second trimester, the fetal lungs and kidneys produce the amniotic fluid. Fluid resorption mainly results from fetal swallowing. Fluid volume increases with increasing gestational age until the middle of the third trimester, after which the volume stays stable and may decrease somewhat at term.

V FETUS

A Metabolism. Fetal metabolism is primarily oxidative. Normal metabolism is necessary to maintain the normal function of existing tissue and to support the acquisition of new tissue.

    1. Requirements

      a. Glucose. The principal sugar in fetal blood is glucose; it is a major nutrient for growth and energy in the fetus. The maternal blood (via the placenta) is the source of fetal glucose, and the fetal glucose level is determined by the maternal level.

      b. Oxygen. Fetal oxygen consumption is approximately 8 mL/kg/min compared to an adult oxygen consumption of about 3/mL/kg/min.

      c. Amino acids. The fetus synthesizes protein from amino acids from maternal blood.

    2. Hormones important for fetal growth. Hormones produced in the fetus, placenta, and mother function together to promote the growth and development of the fetus.

      a. Human placental lactogen (hPL) or **human chorionic somatomammotropin (hCS).** This maternal hormone increases resistance to insulin and blocks the peripheral uptake and use of glucose by maternal tissues, allowing placental transfer of glucose to the fetus.

    b. Insulin. The fetus produces its own insulin.

    c. Insulin-like growth factors I and II, human placental growth hormone, and other growth factors. Growth factors produced in the placenta are responsible for the regulation of cell proliferation and cell differentiation in the fetus.

B **Organ systems**

  1. Cardiovascular

    a. Unique features of the fetal circulation (Fig. 2-1)

      (1) Umbilical vein. The umbilical vein carries oxygenated, nutrient-rich blood from the placenta to the fetus. The umbilical vein gives off branches to the liver and becomes the ductus venosus.

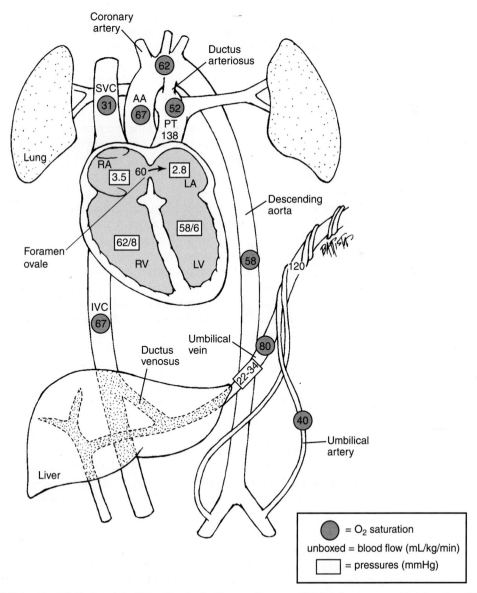

FIGURE 2-1 **Hemodynamics of the fetus (in utero).** AA, ascending aorta; IVC, inferior vena cava; LA, left atrium; LV, left ventricle; PT, pulmonary trunk; RA, right atrium; RV, right ventricle; SVC, superior vena cava.

      (2) Ductus venosus. The ductus venosus brings oxygenated blood from the placenta to the inferior vena cava. Blood from the portal vein flows into the ductus venosus, thereby decreasing the overall oxygen content of the blood entering the inferior vena cava. Thus, blood flowing into the right ventricle is not as well oxygenated as blood coming directly from the placenta.

      (3) Foramen ovale. The foramen ovale is a right-to-left intracardiac (atrial) shunt. Well-oxygenated blood carried by the inferior vena cava from the ductus venosus streams preferentially across the foramen ovale into the left atrium and then to the left ventricle, brain, and upper body. Less-oxygenated blood returning from the systemic circulation also forms a stream in the inferior vena cava that joins blood from the superior vena cava to flow preferentially across the tricuspid valve.

      (4) Ductus arteriosus. Blood from the systemic circulation is delivered preferentially to the right ventricle. From the right ventricle, blood flows into pulmonary artery. The ductus arteriosus connects the left pulmonary artery to the arch of the aorta.

        (a) The high vascular resistance in the fetal lungs is greater than the aortic pressure that diverts blood away from the lungs and into the ductus and the aorta. The umbilical arteries deliver the blood from the aorta to the placenta for gas exchange.

        (b) Prostaglandins, such as prostaglandin E, play a role in maintaining patency of the ductus arteriosus. Prostaglandin inhibitors promote closure of the ductus.

  b. Circulatory adjustments to neonatal life. At birth, the lungs expand and pulmonary vascular resistance decreases. With closure of the ductus arteriosus, pulmonary blood flow increases. Right atrial pressure decreases, and the foramen ovale closes. The ductus arteriosus, ductus venosus, and umbilical vein are no longer patent and become known as the ligamentum arteriosum, ligamentum venosum, and the ligamentum teres, respectively. The intra-abdominal portion of the umbilical arteries becomes the lateral umbilical ligaments.

  c. Heart rate and cardiac output. Cardiac output of the fetal heart is 200 mL/kg/min, which is higher than the cardiac output of the adult (about 70 mL/kg/min). The cardiac output of the right ventricle is greater than that of the left ventricle (60% versus 40%), resulting in a right ventricular dominance. The normal fetal heart rate is 120 to 160 beats per minute.

  d. Regulation of blood flow and pressures. The cardiovascular system is controlled by a complex integration of autonomic and hormonal effects. The stimulation of baroreceptors (by changes in blood flow) and chemoreceptors (by changes in oxygenation) is responsible for the initiation of autonomic reflexes and the secretion of hormones to coordinate the regulation of blood flow, pressure, and heart rate in the fetus.

2. Respiratory

  a. The fetal lungs play no role in gas exchange. Oxygen and carbon dioxide are exchanged between fetal and maternal blood across the placenta. The partial pressure of oxygen in intervillous blood is lower in the fetus compared with the mother, which favorably influences the transfer of oxygen from maternal to fetal blood. Similarly, physiologic maternal respiratory changes result in a lower partial pressure of carbon dioxide in the maternal circulation, which favors the transfer of carbon dioxide from the fetus to the mother.

  b. At about 34 weeks of gestation, the fetal lungs produce **surfactant**, a combination of glycerophospholipids, from the type II pneumocytes. Surfactant is essential for successful respiration because it lowers the surface tension in the alveoli to prevent alveolar collapse.

3. Gastrointestinal/hepatic

  a. Although the fetus swallows amniotic fluid, gastrointestinal absorption is not a fetal source of nutrients. The fetal intestine absorbs water from the swallowed amniotic fluid.

  b. Meconium is composed of intestinal tract secretions and desquamation of intestinal epithelial cells.

  c. The fetal liver is the major source of fetal cholesterol.

d. The majority of unconjugated bilirubin is removed from the fetal circulation by the placenta, where it is transferred to the maternal circulation, conjugated by the maternal liver, and excreted. At term, fetal hepatic conjugation of bilirubin is relatively deficient, and a mild **hyperbilirubinemia** may be seen in the term neonate in the first few days of life.

4. Renal
    a. Fetal urine production begins in the first trimester and is important for maintaining amniotic fluid volume as gestation advances.
    b. Fetal urine is hypotonic.
    c. Most ion exchange occurs in the placenta.

5. Hematologic
    a. Hematopoiesis occurs in the yolk sac in the second week of gestation, in the liver and spleen in the fifth week, and in the bone marrow by the eleventh week.
    b. Hemoglobin
        (1) The hemoglobin concentration is high in the term fetus (16 to 18 g/dL) compared to that in the mother.
        (2) Fetal hemoglobin is composed of two α- and two γ-globin chains. It differs from adult hemoglobin, which is composed of two α- and two β-globin chains.
        (3) Adult hemoglobin is found in the fetus by 12 weeks gestation and increases with length of gestation. However, at term, 70% of the circulating hemoglobin is fetal hemoglobin.
        (4) Fetal hemoglobin has a high affinity for oxygen, resulting in an oxygen dissociation curve that is shifted to the left compared with that in adults (Fig. 2-2). Because of the high affinity of fetal hemoglobin for oxygen, fetal red blood cells efficiently extract oxygen from the maternal blood in the placenta.
    c. Erythropoietin originates in the fetal liver and is highest in utero.

6. Endocrine (see Chapter 1)
    a. Thyroid gland. Adequate thyroid function is important for normal neurologic development. Thyroid function is detectable by the end of the first trimester and thyroxine levels steadily increase from midgestation until term.

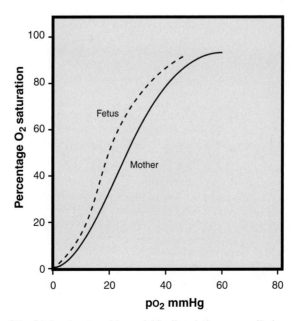

FIGURE 2-2 Comparison of the fetal and maternal hemoglobin dissociation curves. (Redrawn from Gabbe SG. Obstetrics: Normal and Problem Pregnancies, 4th Ed. New York: Churchill Livingstone, 2002:49.)

    b. Adrenal gland. DHEAS is secreted by the fetal zone of the adrenal in response to stimulation by adrenocorticotropic hormone (ACTH) and human chorionic gonadotropin (hCG). The fetal adrenal gland also produces cortisol and catecholamines.

C Immune system

1. Although the fetus produces macrophages and granulocytes, the cellular immunity of the fetus and neonate is not as active or efficient as adult cellular immunity. Similarly, the fetus cannot mount adult-level antibody responses to antigen stimulation.

2. In response to infection, fetal IgM increases. In the absence of infection, fetal levels of IgA and IgM are much lower than adult levels.

3. The majority of immunoglobulin found in the fetus is IgG and is due to transplacental passage from the mother. IgG is the only immunoglobulin isotype that crosses the placenta.

Study Questions for Chapter 2

Directions: Each of the numbered items or incomplete statements in this section is followed by answers or by completions of the statement. Select the ONE lettered answer or completion that is BEST in each case.

1. A 24-year-old woman, gravida 4, para 3, and at 18 weeks' gestation dated by her last menstrual period, receives an ultrasound to confirm her "due date" and to evaluate fetal anatomy. Her first pregnancy was complicated by delivery of an infant with spina bifida. Her other two pregnancies were uncomplicated. After confirmation of her gestational age using biparietal diameter, abdominal circumference, and femur length data, you scan the fetal ductus venosus. Using ultrasound, which structure would you see leading <u>into</u> and <u>out of</u> the ductus venosus, respectively?

- A Pulmonary artery ; aorta
- B inferior vena cava ; portal vein
- C umbilical vein ; portal vein
- D portal vein ; inferior vena cava
- E right atrium ; left atrium

2. A 37-year-old woman, gravida 1, para 1 just delivered at term, a viable male infant weighing 3980 grams with APGARs (American Pediatric Gross Assessment Records) of 9 and 9 at 1 and 5 minutes, respectively. Delivery was via spontaneous vaginal delivery without any complications. After clamping of the umbilical cord, the baby takes his first breath. Which event(s) is/are directly responsible for most efficient oxygenation of blood inside the lungs?

- A Closure of foramen ovale
- B Closure of ductus arteriosus
- C Closure of foramen ovale and ductus arteriosus
- D Closure of umbilical vein and artery
- E Closure of ligamentum arteriosum and ligamentum teres

3. You are listening to a discussion between two medical students about fetal oxygen consumption and fetal cardiac output. The first student claims that the fetal cardiac output is at least two times that of adult cardiac output since the average heart rate in the fetus is 140 beats per minutes (two times an adult heart beat). The second student claims that the fetal oxygen consumption is probably half of adult oxygen consumption because fetal hemoglobin has twice the affinity for oxygen than adult hemoglobin. The cardiac output and oxygen consumption in a fetus is approximately what multiple/fraction of that compared with an adult, respectively?

- A 2 and 2
- B 3 and 3
- C 1/2 and 1/2
- D 1/3 and 1/3
- E 2 and 1/2

4. The most oxygenated blood is found in which part of the fetal circulation?

- A Ductus venosus
- B Portal vein
- C Inferior vena cava
- D Ductus arteriosus
- E Descending aorta

QUESTIONS 5–8

For each substance listed below, select its route of transfer across the placenta. Each answer choice may be used once, more than once, or not at all.

- A Endocytosis
- B Facilitated transport
- C Passive diffusion
- D Active transport
- E Ion pumps

5. Glucose

6. Iron

7. Amino acids

8. Carbon dioxide

QUESTIONS 9–13

For each statement below, match the trimester during which the event occurs. Each answer can be used once, more than once, or not at all.

- A First trimester
- B Early second trimester (weeks 14–21)
- C Late second trimester (weeks 22–28)
- D Third trimester

9. Highest concentration of hemoglobin containing two α and two β chains

10. Amniotic fluid volume derived from transudation

11. Significant amniotic fluid volume contribution from the lung

12. Production of red blood cells by the spleen

13. Thyroxine levels first detectable in serum

Answers and Explanations

1. The answer is D [V B 1 a (2), 1 a (3)]. Oxygenated blood from the umbilical vein and deoxygenated blood from the portal vein flow into the ductus venosus, which connects to the inferior vena cava through the hepatic veins. From there, blood goes to the right atrium via the inferior vena cava. A large percentage of the oxygenated blood is shunted to the left atrium via the foramen ovale. A small percentage of blood from the inferior vena cava joins the deoxygenated blood from the superior vena cava and flows into the right ventricle. The right ventricle pumps blood via the pulmonary artery through the patent ductus arteriosus into the aorta because the lung is a high-resistance system in the fetus.

2. The answer is C [V B 1 b]. When the baby takes his first breath, resistance in the pulmonary vessel circuit is substantially reduced, and thus blood can flow through the pulmonary artery to the lungs (instead of to the aorta through the ductus arteriosus) to become oxygenated. This event also decreases the pressure in the right atrium, allowing closure of the foramen ovale. Both of these events are necessary for the most efficient oxygenation of blood (closure of the foramen ovale allows all of the blood returning to the heart to be oxygenated). Conditions such as atrial septal defect (ASD) do not allow for the most efficient oxygenation of blood returning to the heart because a small percentage of that deoxygenated blood is shunted to the left atrium and into systemic circulation instead of into the lungs to become oxygenated. The ligamentum arteriosum is the closed (non-patent) ductus arteriosus, and the ligamentum teres is the closed (non-patent) umbilical vein.

3. The answer is B [V A 1 b and V B 1 c]. Fetal cardiac output is approximately 200 mL/kg/min, whereas an average adult's cardiac output is 70 mL/kg/min. Fetal oxygen consumption is approximately 8 mL/kg/min, whereas adult oxygen consumption is approximately 3 mL/kg/min.

4. The answer is A [V B 1 a (2)]. The umbilical vein carries the most well-oxygenated blood from the placenta. The ductus venosus carries slightly less oxygen because it mixes with the portal venous blood. The inferior vena cava carries blood from both the ductus venosus and the systemic circulation; it therefore carries less oxygen overall than the ductus venosus. The ductus arteriosus and descending aorta receive blood returning from the systemic circulation and therefore have less oxygen then the other choices.

The answers are 5-B [II B 1 a (2)], **6-A** [II B 1 a (3)], **7-D** [II B 1 a (1)], **8-C** [II B 2]. Glucose is transported across the placenta via facilitated transport. Iron is transported via endocytosis. Amino acids are transported via active transport. Carbon dioxide passively diffuses across the placenta.

The answers are 9-D [V B 5 b (2)], **10-A** [IV B 2], **11-B** [IV B 2], **12-A** [V B 5 a], **13-A** [V B 6 a]. The highest concentration of adult hemoglobin is near term. However, even near term, fetal hemoglobin makes up the majority of circulating hemoglobin (almost 70%). Amniotic fluid is a transudative during early pregnancy. In the second trimester, the lung and the kidneys both contribute to amniotic fluid volume. The contribution of the kidney steadily increases until it is the major contributor of amniotic fluid volume by the end of second trimester and in the third trimester. Hematopiesis occurs in the yolk sac in the second week of gestation, in the liver and spleen in the fifth week, and in the bone marrow by the eleventh week. Thyroid hormones are first detectable in serum near the end of the first trimester.

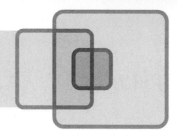

chapter 3

Normal Pregnancy, the Puerperium, and Lactation

PETER J. CHEN

I   DIAGNOSIS OF PREGNANCY

A   Presumptive symptoms

1. **Amenorrhea.** Amenorrhea, or the abrupt cessation of spontaneous, cyclic, and predictable menstruation, is strongly suggestive of pregnancy. Because ovulation can be late in any given cycle, the menses should be **at least 10 days late** before their absence is considered a reliable indication.

2. **Breast changes.** In very early pregnancy, women report tenderness and tingling in the breasts. Breast enlargement and nodularity are evident as early as the second month of pregnancy. The nipples and areolae enlarge and become more deeply pigmented.

3. **Nausea (with or without vomiting).** The so-called **morning sickness of pregnancy** usually begins early in the day and lasts for several hours, although occasionally it persists longer and may occur at other times. Gastrointestinal disturbances begin at 4 to 6 weeks' gestation and usually last no longer than the first trimester. Excessive nausea and vomiting (i.e., **hyperemesis gravidarum**) can result in dehydration, weight loss, electrolyte imbalance, and the need for hospitalization; intravenous hyperalimentation may be indicated in severe cases.

4. **Disturbances in urination.** Early in pregnancy, the enlarging uterus puts pressure on the bladder, causing **frequent urination.** This condition improves as the uterus grows and moves up into the abdomen but returns late in pregnancy when the fetal head settles into the pelvis against the bladder.

5. **Fatigue.** Tiredness is one of the earliest symptoms of pregnancy. Fatigue usually persists into the second trimester; the need for sleep returns to normal by the sixteenth to eighteenth week.

6. **Sensation of fetal movement.** Between the sixteenth and twentieth week after the last menstrual period (LMP), a woman begins to feel movement in the lower abdomen, described as a fluttering or gas bubbles. This is known as **quickening.**

B   Clinical evidence

1. **Enlargement of the abdomen.** By the end of the twelfth week of pregnancy, the uterus can be felt above the symphysis pubis. By the twentieth week, the uterus should be at the level of the umbilicus. Between the twentieth week and the thirty-seventh week, the fundal height in centimeters should correspond, within 2 cm, to the gestational age in weeks (Fig. 3-1).

2. **Uterine and cervical changes.** The uterus enlarges and softens early in pregnancy (at approximately 6 weeks' gestation), and lateral uterine vessel pulsations are palpable on vaginal examination. The softening between the cervix and the uterine fundus causes a sensation of separateness between these two structures (**Hegar sign**). The vaginal mucosa has a bluish color within the first 6 to 8 weeks of pregnancy (**Chadwick sign**).

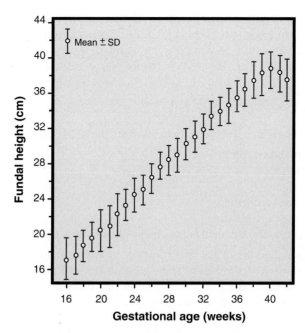

FIGURE 3-1 Fundal height versus gestational age. (Reprinted with permission from Gabbe SG. Obstetrics: Normal and Problem Pregnancies. 3rd Ed. New York: Churchill Livingstone, 1996:181.)

3. **Endocrine tests for pregnancy.** These tests depend on **human chorionic gonadotropin (hCG)** levels in maternal plasma and excretion of hCG in the urine, which are identified by a number of immunoassays and bioassays. The presence of hCG can be demonstrated in maternal plasma or urine by 8 to 9 days after ovulation.

   a. **Urine pregnancy tests** detect the presence of hCG. This depends on the recognition of hCG or its β-subunit by an antibody to the hCG molecule or the β-subunit.

   b. **Serum pregnancy tests** quantify the β-subunit of hCG, thus providing greater sensitivity than the urine tests and allowing serial determinations to observe increases and decreases in the level of hCG.

C **Confirming the diagnosis of pregnancy**

1. **Identification of a heart beat.** The diagnosis of pregnancy is confirmed with the identification of the fetal heartbeat, which ranges from 120 to 160 beats per minute. The fetal heart can be identified by the tenth week with an ultrasound fetal heart monitor and at 17 to 19 weeks by auscultation with a stethoscope.

2. **Ultrasonographic recognition of the fetus**

   a. After 5 weeks of amenorrhea, an early **chorionic (gestational) sac** is visible as a small, fluid-filled structure surrounded by an echogenic rim of tissue on transvaginal ultrasound. The **embryo** is apparent within the gestational sac after 6 weeks of amenorrhea.

   b. **Fetal heart activity** is seen by real-time ultrasonography after 6 weeks of gestation. The normal heart rate may be as low as 90 beats per minute at 6 weeks and increases during the first trimester.

D **Pregnancy dating.**   The **estimated date of delivery (EDD)**, or due date, is based on the assumption that a woman has a 28-day cycle, with ovulation on day 14 or 15. Pregnancy lasts for 280 days (40 weeks) from the LMP. The EDD is therefore 9 calendar months plus 7 days from the start of the LMP; it is customary to estimate the **EDD** by counting back 3 calendar months and adding 7 days to the LMP (**Nägele rule**). Because ovulation does not always occur at midcycle (the postovulatory phase in any cycle lasts for 14 days), the EDD must be adjusted accordingly. For example, ovulation in a woman with a 35-day cycle occurs on approximately day 21; therefore, the EDD in such a woman is later than that predicted by the Nägele rule (see Chapter 6 regarding ultrasound dating).

II PREGNANCY

A **First trimester.** This period extends from the LMP through the first 12 to 13 weeks of pregnancy.

1. **Signs and symptoms**
   a. Nausea
   b. Fatigue
   c. Breast tenderness
   d. Frequent urination
   e. Minimal abdominal enlargement (the uterus is still in the pelvis)

2. Bleeding occurs in the first trimester of approximately 25% of all pregnancies; spontaneous abortion occurs in half of these pregnancies, and the other half continues without problems. Uterine cramping with bleeding in the first trimester is more suggestive of impending abortion than either bleeding or cramping alone.

B **Second trimester.** This period extends from 14 weeks of pregnancy through 27 weeks of pregnancy.

1. **Signs and symptoms**
   a. **General well-being.** The second trimester is often the most comfortable time for a pregnant woman because the symptoms of the first trimester have disappeared, and the discomfort of the last trimester is not yet present.
   b. **Pain.** As the uterus grows, a certain amount of pulling and stretching of pelvic structures occurs. Round ligament pain, which results from the stretching of the round ligaments that are attached to the top of the uterus on each side and the corresponding lateral pelvic wall, is common.
   c. **Contractions.** Palpable uterine contractions (**Braxton Hicks contractions**) that are mild and irregular can begin during the second trimester.

2. **Bleeding.** A low-lying placenta that causes bleeding at this stage usually moves away from the cervix as the uterus grows.

3. **Fetus.** The fetus attains a size of almost 1000 g (more than 2 lb) by the twenty-eighth week.
   a. **Motion.** Quickening (see I A 6) begins between the sixteenth and twentieth week.
   b. **Viability.** Infants born at the end of the second trimester have an 80% to 90% chance of survival. If death occurs, it is usually from respiratory distress due to lung immaturity.

4. **Complications of second-trimester pregnancies** include an incompetent cervix (i.e., painless dilation of the cervix in the second trimester). Resulting conditions include:
   a. **Premature rupture of the membranes** (PROM) can occur without labor or with an incompetent cervix and can result in serious bacterial infections in both the mother and fetus.
   b. **Premature labor** can occur without an incompetent cervix. When dilation or effacement of the cervix occurs, tocolytic agents are necessary to prevent delivery (see Chapter 15).

C **Third trimester.** This period extends from 28 weeks of pregnancy until term, or 40 weeks' gestation.

1. **Symptoms**
   a. **Braxton Hicks contractions** (see II B 1 c) become more apparent in the third trimester.
   b. **Pain in the lower back and legs** is often caused by pressure on muscles and nerves by the uterus and fetal head, which fills the pelvis at this time.

    c. Lightening is the descent of the fetal head to or even through the pelvic inlet due to the development of a well-formed lower uterine segment and a reduction in the volume of amniotic fluid.

  2. Fetus

    a. Weight. The fetus gains weight at a rate of approximately 224 g (0.5 lb) per week for the last 4 weeks and weighs an average of 3300 g (7.0 to 7.5 lb) at term.

    b. Motion

      (1) A decrease in fetal motion usually occurs because of the size of the fetus and lack of room within the uterus. However, some decreased fetal activity may indicate fetal compromise due to uteroplacental insufficiency.

      (2) The fetal mortality rate decreases from 44/1000 to 10/1000 as measured by a fetal movement screening method. (This commonly used method [daily fetal kick count] requires maternal perceptions of at least 10 fetal movements in 2 hours daily in the third trimester.)

  3. Bleeding

    a. Bloody show, a discharge of a combination of blood and mucus caused by thinning and stretching of the cervix, is a sure sign of the approach of labor.

    b. Heavy bleeding suggests a more serious condition such as **placenta previa** (the placenta developing in the lower uterine segment and completely or partially covering the internal os, usually **painless** bleeding) or **abruptio placentae** (premature separation of the normally implanted placenta, usually **painful bleeding**) (see Chapter 9).

  4. Rupture of membranes is either a sudden gush or a slow leak of amniotic fluid that can happen at any time without warning.

    a. Brownish or greenish fluid may represent meconium staining of the fluid, the sign of a **fetal bowel movement** that may or may not represent fetal stress.

    b. At term, **labor** usually begins within 24 hours after rupture of membranes.

    c. At term, **induction of labor** is indicated if there is no labor within 6 to 24 hours of rupture or if there is any evidence of infection (**chorioamnionitis**).

  5. Labor. Contractions that occur at decreasing intervals with increasing intensity cause the progressive dilation and effacement of the cervix.

III   STATUS OF THE FETUS

A   Growth and development

  1. Weight. A normal fetus weighs approximately 1000 g (more than 2 lb) at 26 to 28 weeks, 2500 g (5.5 lb) at 36 weeks, and 3300 g (7.0 to 7.5 lb) at 40 weeks.

  2. Lung maturity. Fetal lung maturity can be assessed by measuring surface-active lipid components of surfactant (e.g., lecithin and phosphatidylglycerol), which are secreted by the type II pneumocytes of fetal lung alveoli. Fetal lung maturity is essential for normal respiration immediately after birth. These measurements are made by laboratory examination of **amniotic fluid.**

    a. Lecithin to sphingomyelin (L/S) ratio. Studies have shown that when the level of lecithin in amniotic fluid increases to at least **twice** that of sphingomyelin (at approximately 35 weeks), the risk of respiratory distress is very low (Fig. 3-2).

    b. Phosphatidylglycerol. The presence of phosphatidylglycerol in the amniotic fluid provides even more definite assurance of lung maturity.

    c. Respiratory distress syndrome (RDS). Infants born before phosphatidylglycerol appears in surfactant, even with an L/S ratio of 2:1, may be at risk for RDS.

    d. Early fetal lung maturation (32 to 35 weeks) is seen with maternal hypertension, PROM, and intrauterine growth retardation, all of which are stressful to the fetus. This stress increases **fetal cortisol secretion,** which in turn accelerates fetal lung maturation.

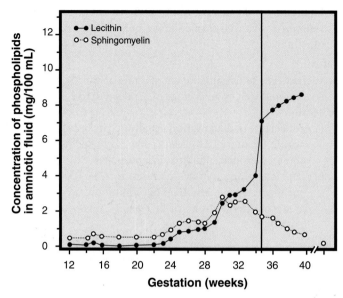

FIGURE 3-2 Changes in mean concentrations of lecithin and sphingomyelin in amniotic fluid during gestation in normal pregnancy. (Reprinted with permission from Cunningham FG, MacDonald PC, Gant NF, et al. Williams Obstetrics. 20th Ed. New York: McGraw-Hill, 1997:970, Figure 42-2.)

   e. **Glucocorticoids.** Administration of glucocorticoids to mothers between the twenty-fourth and thirty-fourth week of pregnancy effects an increase in the rate of maturation of the human fetal lung and is associated with a reduced rate of respiratory distress in their prematurely born infants.

B **Lie of the fetus** is the relation of the long axis of the fetus to the long axis of the mother and is either longitudinal or transverse.

   1. **Longitudinal lie.** In most labors (more than 99%) at term, the fetal head is either up or down in a longitudinal lie.

   2. **Transverse lie.** The fetus is crosswise in the uterus in a transverse lie.

   3. **Oblique lie.** This indicates an unstable situation that becomes either a longitudinal or transverse lie during the course of labor.

C **Fetal presentation** is determined by the portion of the fetus that can be felt through the cervix.

   1. **Cephalic presentations** are classified according to the position of the fetal head in relation to the body of the fetus.
      a. **Vertex.** The head is flexed so that the chin is in contact with the chest, and the occiput of the fetal head presents. A vertex presentation occurs in 95% of all cephalic presentations (Fig. 3-3).
      b. **Face.** The neck is extended sharply so that the occiput and the back of the fetus are touching, and the face is the presenting part (Fig. 3-4).
      c. **Brow.** The fetal head is extended partially but converts into a vertex or face presentation during labor (Fig. 3-5).

   2. **Breech presentations** are classified according to the position of the legs and buttocks, which present first. Breech presentations occur in 3.5% of all pregnancies (Fig. 3-6).
      a. In a **complete breech,** both the legs and the hips are flexed.
      b. In an **incomplete breech,** one hip is not flexed, and one foot or knee lies below the breech (i.e., one foot or knee is lowermost in the birth canal).
      c. In a **frank breech,** the hips are flexed and the legs are extended.

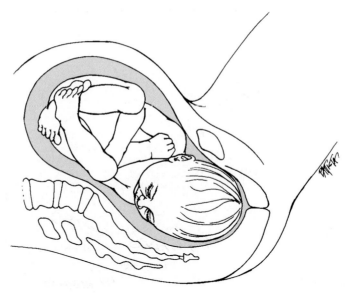

FIGURE 3-3 Vertex presentation. (Redrawn from Cunningham FG, MacDonald PC, Gant NF, et al. Williams Obstetrics. 20th Ed. New York: McGraw-Hill, 1997:320, Figure 12-1 #2.)

IV PUERPERIUM

This period of 4 to 6 weeks starts immediately after delivery and ends when the reproductive tract has returned to its nonpregnant condition. Multiple anatomic and physiologic changes occur during this time, and the potential exists for significant complications, such as infection or hemorrhage.

A Physiology

1. **Involution of the uterus.** The uterus regains its usual nonpregnant size within 5 to 6 weeks, shrinking from 1000 g immediately postpartum to 100 g. This rapid atrophy occurs because of

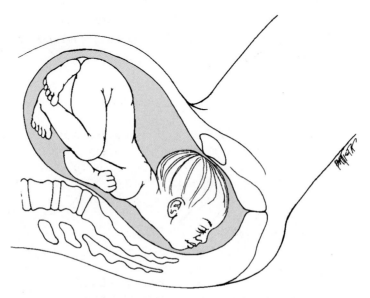

FIGURE 3-4 Face presentation. (Redrawn from Gabbe SG. Obstetrics: Normal and Problem Pregnancies. 3rd Ed. New York: Churchill Livingstone, 1996:473, Figure 16-9.)

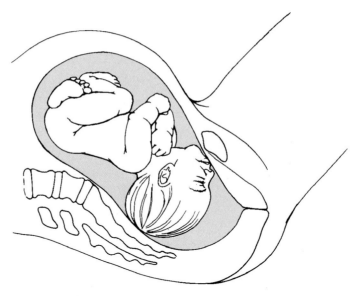

FIGURE 3-5 Brow presentation. (Redrawn from Gabbe SG. Obstetrics: Normal and Problem Pregnancies. 3rd Ed. New York: Churchill Livingstone, 1996:475, Figure 16-10.)

the marked decrease in size of the muscle cells rather than the decrease in their total number. Breastfeeding accelerates involution of the uterus because stimulation of the nipples releases oxytocin from the neurohypophysis; the resulting contractions of the myometrium facilitate the involution of the uterus.

  a. Afterpains. The uterus contracts throughout the period of involution, which produces afterpains, especially in multiparous women and nursing mothers. In primiparous women, the uterus tends to remain contracted tonically, whereas in multiparous women, the uterus contracts vigorously at intervals.

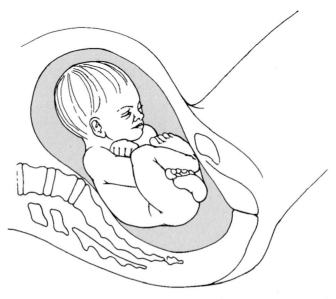

FIGURE 3-6 Breech presentation. (Reprinted with permission from Gabbe SG. Obstetrics: Normal and Problem Pregnancies. 3rd Ed. New York: Churchill Livingstone, 1996:479, Figure 16-14.)

    b. Lochia. This uterine discharge follows delivery and lasts for 3 or 4 weeks. Foul-smelling lochia suggests infection.

        (1) Lochia rubra. This blood-stained fluid lasts for the first few days.

        (2) Lochia serosa. This discharge appears 3 to 4 days after delivery. It is paler than lochia rubra because it is admixed with serum.

        (3) Lochia alba. After the tenth day, because of an admixture with leukocytes, the lochia assumes a white or yellow-white color.

2. Involutional changes of the renal system. The puerperal bladder has an increased capacity and a relative insensitivity to intravesical fluid pressure.

    a. Incomplete emptying, resulting in excessive residual urine, and overdistention may lead to a postpartum urinary tract infection.

    b. Diuresis usually occurs between the second and fifth postpartum day.

    c. Anatomic changes, such as the dilation of the calyces, renal pelvis, and ureters, that are characteristic of pregnancy may persist as long as 8 weeks postpartum. Functionally, the increased renal plasma flow, glomerular filtration rate, and creatinine clearance rate associated with pregnancy return to normal by 6 weeks after delivery.

3. Cardiovascular changes. The changes that occurred during pregnancy (e.g., increases in heart rate, cardiac output, and blood volume) generally return to baseline by approximately 6 weeks postpartum. Peripheral vascular resistance also returns to the prepregnancy level by this time. Most of these parameters return to normal within the first 2 weeks postpartum.

4. Blood. A marked **leukocytosis** occurs during and after labor. The leukocytosis, primarily a granulocytosis, may be as high as 30,000/mm^3.

Pregnancy-induced changes in **blood coagulation factors** persist for variable periods of time after delivery. Elevated plasma fibrinogen levels are maintained at least through the first week of the puerperium.

5. Ovulation and menstruation

    a. Nonlactating women. The first menstrual flow usually returns within 6 to 8 weeks after delivery, with ovulation occurring at 2 to 4 weeks postpartum.

    b. Lactating women. Ovulation is much less frequent in women who breast feed compared with those who do not. The first menstrual flow may occur as early as the second month or as late as the eighteenth month after delivery.

        (1) Amenorrhea during lactation is due to a lack of appropriate ovarian stimulation by pituitary gonadotropins.

        (2) Nevertheless, pregnancy can occur with lactation. Nursing mothers must understand that the contraception afforded by lactation possesses risk of ovulation and pregnancy even in amenorrheic women.

6. Family planning. Methods of contraception should be fully reviewed and implemented (see Chapter 24).

    a. Nonlactating mothers may begin using a contraceptive soon after delivery if they wish to avoid becoming pregnant. **Combination oral contraceptives** may be prescribed, or depot medroxyprogesterone acetate can be injected before discharge.

    b. Lactating mothers may begin using oral contraceptives as soon as their milk supply is established. **Progesterone-only contraceptives** do not appear to have adverse effects on lactation.

        (1) Intrauterine devices (IUDs) do not interfere with breast milk. However, IUDs are generally not inserted until 4 to 6 weeks postpartum.

        (2) Diaphragms or cervical caps cannot be fitted adequately during the immediate postpartum period, and their use should be delayed until after the 4- to 6-week examination.

        (3) Spermicides and barrier methods have no effect on breastfeeding. Lubricated condoms may offset vaginal dryness secondary to breastfeeding.

c. Patients for whom the use of oral contraceptives is contraindicated or who prefer other methods of contraception, such as foam or condoms, should also be offered instructions in their use. Fertility awareness methods, such as the rhythm method, are difficult to practice accurately before the resumption of menses and therefore are not recommended.

B **Complications.** The most common complications include hemorrhage, genital tract infections, urinary tract infections, and mastitis.

1. **Postpartum hemorrhage** is defined as a blood loss in excess of 500 mL during the first 24 hours after delivery.
   a. Causes
      (1) **Trauma to the genital tract** because of:
         (a) Episiotomy
         (b) Lacerations of the cervix, vagina, or perineum
         (c) Rupture of the uterus
      (2) **Failure of compression of blood vessels at the implantation site** of the placenta because of:
         (a) An **atonic uterus** due to general anesthesia; overdistention of the uterus from a large fetus, hydramnios (excess amniotic fluid), or multiple fetuses; prolonged labor; very rapid labor; high parity; or a labor vigorously stimulated with oxytocin. **The most common cause of postpartum hemorrhage is uterine atony.**
         (b) **Retention of placental tissue,** as seen in placenta accreta, a succenturiate placental lobe, or a fragmented placenta
      (3) **Coagulation defects,** either congenital or acquired, as seen in hypofibrinogenemia or thrombocytopenia
   b. Management
      (1) **Vigorous massage** of the uterine fundus
      (2) **Use of uterine contracting agents**
         (a) **Oxytocin** 20 U in 1000 mL of lactated Ringer's solution intravenously
         (b) **Methylergonovine** 0.2 mg intramuscularly or intravenously. Because methylergonovine may cause hypertension, it should be avoided in patients with preeclampsia.
         (c) **Prostaglandin** $F_{2\alpha}$ 0.25 mg intramuscularly up to eight doses at 20-minute intervals
      (3) **Manual exploration** of the uterine cavity for retained placental fragments or uterine rupture
      (4) **Inspection** of the cervix and vagina for lacerations
      (5) **Curettage** of the uterine cavity
      (6) Hypogastric artery **ligation; embolization** of the uterine vessels; and, rarely, **hysterectomy**
2. **Puerperal infection** is defined as any infection of the genitourinary tract during the puerperium accompanied by a temperature of **100.4°F (38°C) or higher** that occurs for at least 2 of the first 10 days postpartum, **exclusive of the first 24 hours.** Prolonged rupture of the membranes accompanied by multiple vaginal examinations during labor is a major predisposing cause of puerperal infection.
   a. Pelvic infections
      (1) **Endometritis (childbed fever),** the most common form of puerperal infection, involves primarily the endometrium and the adjacent myometrium.
      (2) **Parametritis,** infection of the retroperitoneal fibroareolar pelvic connective tissue, may occur by:
         (a) Lymphatic transmission of organisms
         (b) Cervical lacerations that extend into the connective tissue
         (c) Extension of pelvic thrombophlebitis
      (3) **Thrombophlebitis** results from an extension of puerperal infection along pelvic veins.

b. Urinary tract infections are common during the puerperium because of:
  (1) Trauma to the bladder from a normal vaginal delivery
  (2) A **hypotonic bladder** from conduction anesthesia
  (3) Catheterization
c. Management. Precise identification of bacteria specifically responsible for any puerperal infection can be difficult. Historically, genital tract cultures were obtained; however, they are now of little clinical utility because many of the same pathogens were also found in the uterine cavity in clinically healthy puerperal women. Blood and urine cultures may be useful to identify some of these pathogens, especially in women who have undergone cesarean section.
  (1) Antibiotics should be administered according to the sensitivity of the infecting organism to the drug. Broad-spectrum antibiotics, which include anaerobic coverage, are recommended for those pelvic infections in which identification of the offending organism is impossible. **Common organisms include:**
    (a) Aerobic (group B *Streptococcus, Enterococcus,* and *Escherichia coli*)
    (b) Anaerobic (*Peptococcus, Peptostreptococcus, Bacteroides,* and *Clostridium*)
  (2) Heparin should be administered when thrombophlebitis is suspected and a spiking temperature does not respond to intravenous antibiotics.

V LACTATION

A Physiology. Progesterone, estrogen, placental lactogen, prolactin, cortisol, and insulin act together in stimulating the growth and development of the breast's milk-secreting apparatus.

1. Prolactin, which is released from the anterior pituitary gland, **stimulates milk production.**
  a. Initiation of lactation. The delivery of the placenta causes a sharp decrease in the levels of estrogens and progesterone, which, in turn, leads to the release of prolactin and the consequent stimulation of milk production.
  b. Continued prolactin production. A stimulus from the breast (e.g., a suckling infant) curtails the release of prolactin-inhibiting factor from the hypothalamus, thus inducing a transiently increased secretion of prolactin.

2. Oxytocin is responsible for the **let-down reflex** and the subsequent release of breast milk. Stimulation of the nipples during nursing causes oxytocin to be released from the posterior pituitary gland.

B Nursing. Breast milk is ideal for the newborn because it provides a balanced diet. It contains protective maternal antibodies, and the maternal lymphocytes in breast milk may be important to the infant's immunologic processes. Most drugs given to the mother are secreted in low concentrations in the breast milk. Water-soluble drugs are excreted in high concentrations into colostrum, whereas lipid-soluble drugs are excreted in high concentrations into breast milk.

C Mastitis. This parenchymatous inflammation of the mammary glands seldom appears before the end of the first week postpartum and not until the third or fourth week postpartum.

1. Symptoms. Engorgement of the breasts is accompanied by a temperature increase, chills, and a hard, red tender area on the breast.

2. Etiology. The most common offending organism is *Staphylococcus aureus* from the infant's nose and throat, which usually enters the breast through the nipple at the site of a fissure or abrasion during nursing.

3. Therapy

   a. Gram-positive antibiotic coverage (e.g., penicillin and ampicillin) is recommended; erythromycin is recommended for penicillin-resistant organisms.

   b. Heat should be applied to the breast.

   c. Nursing from the affected breast should continue to decrease engorgement.

   d. The abscess should be drained if the mastitis has progressed to suppuration.

4. Prevention. The use of an emollient cream is recommended to help prevent cracking of the nipple.

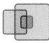

Study Questions for Chapter 3

Directions: Each of the numbered items or incomplete statements in this section is followed by answers or by completions of the statement. Select the ONE lettered answer or completion that is BEST in each case.

1. A 23-year-old primigravida woman just delivered an infant weighing 4,350 g by spontaneous vaginal delivery. After 5 minutes of gentle traction on the umbilical cord, you deliver the placenta, which appears to be intact. You begin massaging the uterine fundus and ask the nurse to run 20 U of oxytocin in 1000 mL of LR solution as fast as possible. After careful inspection of the genital tract, you notice a second-degree laceration and a 2-cm left lateral vaginal wall laceration, which you attempt to repair. Suturing is difficult because of brisk bleeding from above the site of laceration. Physical examination reveals a soft, boggy uterine fundus. Her vitals are as follows: T = 98.9, BP = 164/92, P = 130, R = 18. Which of the following is the next best step in management?

- [A] Oxytocin 10 U direct IV infusion
- [B] Methylergonovine 0.2 mg IM
- [C] Prostaglandin $F_{2\alpha}$ 0.25 mg IM
- [D] Manual exploration
- [E] Curettage

2. Forty hours ago, a 19-year-old primigravida delivered a viable female infant weighing 3,600 g. The baby's APGARs (American Pediatric Gross Assessment Records) were 9 and 9 at 1 and 5 minutes, respectively. The patient is breastfeeding and reports minimal lochia. Review of her labor records reveals that her membranes were ruptured 7 hours before delivery of her infant. Her vital signs before discharge from the hospital are as follows: T = 100.8, P = 105, BP = 110/70, R = 16. Her physical examination is remarkable for slight tenderness in the area of the uterus; nonerythematous, nontender firm breasts; and nontender calves. Which of the following is the best initial step before treatment with antibiotics?

- [A] Urinalysis and culture
- [B] Genital tract culture
- [C] Blood culture
- [D] Incentive spirometry
- [E] Uterine curettage

3. A 27-year-old woman, gravida 2, para 1 presents for her first prenatal visit after testing positive on a home pregnancy test. She reports regular cycles every 35 days. She denies use of birth control pills, Depo-Provera, or other contraceptive in the last 7 months. The first day of her last menstrual period was April 1, 2003 and the last day was April 5, 2003. She says her periods always last 4 to 5 days. What is the best estimate of her due date?

- [A] January 1, 2004
- [B] January 8, 2004
- [C] January 12, 2004
- [D] January 15, 2004
- [E] June 23, 2004

4. A 16-year-old primigravida presents to labor and delivery with reports of abdominal pain. Her pain is constant and located in both the right lower quadrant and the left lower quadrant. There is no radiation and no associated symptoms other than constipation. The patient ate lunch a few hours ago without any problems. Her vital signs are as follows: T = 97.8, BP = 108/74, P = 96, R = 14. Physical examination of the abdomen reveals bilateral tenderness in the lower abdomen. There is no rebound tenderness or guarding, and costovertebral angles are nontender. Her cervix is closed and uneffaced, and fetal vertex is high. Urinalysis reveals +1 protein, 0 leukocytes, 0 nitrites, 0 bacteria, and 0-1 blood. Amylase, lipase, and liver enzymes are within normal range except for elevated alkaline phosphatase. Her complete blood cell count is within normal range except for a white blood cell count of 14,000/mm^3. Which of the following is the best explanation for her abdominal pain?

- A Braxton Hicks
- B Round ligament
- C Urinary tract infection
- D Uterine leiomyoma
- E Liver disease

5. A 20-year-old woman presents to labor and delivery in labor. She has not had any prenatal care. On examination of her cervix, you palpate a bulging membrane but no fetal parts. The cervix is 4 cm dilated. Ultrasound demonstrates that the fetal head is in the fundus, the fetal spine is parallel to mother's spine, and the knees and hips are flexed. Both arms are flexed at the elbows. Which of the following is the best description of fetal lie?

- A Complete breech
- B Incomplete breech
- C Frank breech
- D Vertex
- E Longitudinal

Answers and Explanations

1. The answer is C [IV B 1 b (2) (c)]. Uterine atony is the most common cause of postpartum hemorrhage. Because vigorous massage and dilute oxytocin have not been successful in ceasing her bleeding (i.e., uterus is soft and boggy), the next best step is to add another uterotonic agent. Methylergonovine is contraindicated because this patient is hypertensive despite brisk blood loss. The next best agent is prostaglandin $F_{2\alpha}$. Infusion of undiluted oxytocin 10 U intravenously would cause severe hypotension. Manual exploration would be appropriate if you suspect laceration as cause of bleeding. Here the diagnosis is most likely uterine atony. Curettage is appropriate for delayed postpartum bleeding when you suspect retained products of conception.

2. The answer is A [IV B 2 b and c]. Incomplete emptying results in excessive residual urine, overdistension, and stasis, and intermittent or Foley catheterization during labor. The postpartum bladder is therefore prone to infections. Slight uterine tenderness can be normal in a postpartum uterus, and one should not automatically assume postpartum endomyometritis. Even when endomyometritis is suspected, genital tract cultures have little usefulness because the same organisms can be found in clinically healthy puerperal women. Blood culture is appropriate in the workup of postpartum fevers, but it is not the initial step. Incentive spirometry is used for immediate postoperative patients to promote lung expansion and decrease atelectasis and initial postoperative temperature elevation. Uterine curettage is used to treat postpartum hemorrhage.

3. The answer is D [I D]. The calculated due date of 9 months plus 7 days from the last menstrual period is based on the assumption that a woman has 28-day cycles and that ovulation occurs on day 14 (thus no recent contraception which may change pattern of ovulation). Using Naegele's rule, count back 3 months (April minus 3 months = January) and add 7 days to the first day (not the last day) of the last menstrual period (1 plus 7 = 8). So far, you have January 8. However, this date is based on a 28-day cycle. Because this patient has 35 day cycles and because the luteal phase of the menstrual cycle is always constant (14 days), ovulation occurred on day 21 rather than day 14 (7 days later than you predicted). Therefore, her due date is January 15.

4. The answer is B [II B 1 b]. Round ligament pain is common during the second trimester. It results from stretching of the round ligaments that are attached to the top of the uterus on each side and the corresponding lateral pelvic wall. Braxton Hicks contractions can begin during second trimester but are more common later in pregnancy. Braxton Hicks contractions usually are not described as a "constant" type of pain. Urinary tract infection is unlikely given that her urinalysis was normal. Uterine leiomyoma that degenerates can cause severe pain, but the pain is usually not bilateral. The history or physical examination would be suggestive of that diagnosis. Liver disease is not likely because all of her liver enzymes are normal. An elevated alkaline phosphatase would be expected during normal pregnancy because of placental production of this enzyme.

5. The answer is A [III C 2]. Lie of the fetus is the relation of the long axis of the fetus to the long axis of the mother. The presentation described in this question is a complete breech. Vertex is a subtype of cephalic presentation.

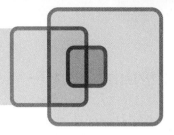

chapter **4**

Antepartum Care

ALFREDO GIL

I   **INTRODUCTION**

Pregnancy is a normal physiologic state. The objective of prenatal care is the delivery of a healthy infant and the maintenance of a healthy mother.

A **Preconception care.**   Optimal prenatal care begins when a woman is considering pregnancy. The following elements should be addressed (Table 4-1 for summary of tests):

1. **Identification of preconceptional risks and assessment of history**—reproductive, family, and medical. The genetic history of the prospective father, as well as the mother, is important.

2. **Nutritional status**

3. **Environmental and occupational exposure** and **social concerns** (e.g., occurrence of **physical abuse**)

4. **Current medications** (prescription and nonprescription)

5. **Substance use**, including alcohol, tobacco, and illicit drugs

6. **Rubella status.** Immunize susceptible patients.

7. **Hepatitis B status.** Offer to immunize patients.

8. **Toxoplasmosis status.** Screen patients with cats for toxoplasmosis.

9. **Varicella status.** Screen patients for varicella.

10. **HIV status.** Offer HIV testing.

11. **Genetic disorders**
    a. Prospective parents should be screened for the following conditions based on racial and ethnic background: sickle hemoglobinopathies, β-thalassemia, α-thalassemia, Tay-Sachs disease, and Canavan disease.
    b. Screening for other genetic disorders should be performed based on family history (e.g., cystic fibrosis, fragile X for family history of nonspecific mental retardation, Duchenne muscular dystrophy).

12. **Use of vitamins.** Start prenatal vitamins and folic acid.

B **Definitions**

1. **Parity.** It is customary to summarize past obstetrical history using a series of digits connected by dashes. The first digit refers to the number of term infants delivered (T), the second to the number of preterm infants (P), the third to the number of abortions (A), and the fourth to the number of children currently alive (L). Abortions can be either therapeutic or spontaneous (i.e., miscarriage). A woman who is para 5-2-1-4 (TPAL) has had 5 term pregnancies, 2 premature deliveries, 1 abortion (or miscarriage), and has 4 living children
    a. A **primipara** is a woman who has completed one pregnancy (single or multiple gestation) to the stage of viability.

TABLE 4-1   Summary of Antepartum and Peripartum Tests

Test	1st Visit	16–20 Weeks	20–24 Weeks	24–28 Weeks	28–32 Weeks	35–37 Weeks
PAP smear	X					
CBC	X				X	
Urine analysis and culture	X					
Type and screen	X			X Rh neg patients		
Rubella	X					
Syphilis	X				X*	
HIV	X					
Hepatitis	X					
Gonorrhea and chlamydia	X				X*	
Hemoglobin electrophoresis**	X					
PPD	X					
Triple marker		X				
Amnioscentesis***		X				
Ultrasound		X				
1 hour glucose tolerance test	X*			X		
Rhogam, if antibody negative					X	
Group B Strep screen						X
Fetal kick count						X

* As indicated or in high risk populations
** Offered to African American patients, must consider in Asians
*** Offered to women over 35 years old at delivery and patients with increased risk of chromosomal defects on triple marker

   b. A **multipara** is a woman who has completed two or more pregnancies to viability. The number of pregnancies that reached viability, not the number of fetuses delivered, determines parity.
   c. A **nulligravida** is a woman who is not now, and never has been, pregnant.
   d. A **gravida** is a woman who is or has been pregnant irrespective of the pregnancy outcome. A **primigravida** is a woman in her first pregnancy. A **multigravida** is a woman on her successive pregnancy.
   2. **Parturient.** This term refers to a woman in labor.
   3. **Puerpera.** This term refers to a woman who has just given birth.

II   REPRODUCTIVE HISTORY (see Chapter 5 regarding medical, family and socioeconomic history)

A Determine estimated due date (EDD).

   1. Calculation of EDD is most accurate when a woman has regular menses. Precise determination of the gestational age is extremely important in the management of the pregnancy.
      a. According to **Nägele's rule,** the EDD is estimated by subtracting 3 months and adding 1 week to the last menstrual period (LMP). This rule assumes a 28-day cycle with ovulation occurring on day 14.
      b. The **pregnancy wheel** is based on 10 lunar months (term pregnancy is 280 days) from the first day of the LMP.
      c. **Birth control pills.** This calculation is unreliable in women using birth control pills for contraception who become pregnant in the first post-pill cycle. Ovulation may have occurred more than 2 weeks after the onset of the LMP.

2. **Ultrasound** can be used to calculate or confirm the EDD.
   a. At **6 to 10 weeks**, the **crown–rump length** is used, and the measured EDD is accurate to ± 3 to 7 days.
      (1) Fetal heart activity can be detected by vaginal probe ultrasound at 5 to 6 weeks from the LMP or when the human chorionic gonadotropin (hCG) reaches a level of 1500 to 2000 mIU/mL.
      (2) With abdominal ultrasound, the fetal heart rate can be detected at hCG levels of 5000 to 6000 mIU/mL.
   b. At **12 to 28 weeks**, the **biparietal diameter** is used, and the measured EDD is accurate to ± 8 to 14 days.
   c. In the **third trimester**, the **biparietal diameter or the femur length** is used, and the measured EDD is accurate to ± 21 days.

B **Review previous pregnancies.**
   1. **Obtain a history of each pregnancy.** Note the following information:
      a. **Weeks of gestation at delivery**
      b. **Weight of infant**
      c. **Anesthesia used**
      d. **Mode of delivery**
         (1) Spontaneous vaginal delivery
         (2) Forceps-assisted vaginal delivery
         (3) Vacuum-assisted vaginal delivery
         (4) Cesarean section, including the indication:
            (a) Low transverse (patient may undergo labor in subsequent pregnancies)
            (b) Classical (these patients have had a vertical incision in the muscular body of the uterus and should not undergo labor in subsequent pregnancies and will need a repeat cesarean section for delivery)
      e. **History of diabetes mellitus.** Note whether the disease was controlled by diet or insulin and if it was present prior to pregnancy.
   2. **Complications of previous pregnancies**
      a. **Premature labor.** The timing of labor onset, interventions performed, and eventual delivery dates should be documented.
      b. **Premature rupture of membranes (PROM).** Time of rupture to time of delivery should be documented. Screening for bacterial vaginosis and other vaginal infections should be performed because treatment of these infections may prevent PROM.
      c. **Preeclampsia.** Document when the onset of disease occurred and whether the woman received magnesium sulfate.

III **PHYSICAL EXAMINATION**

A **General examination.** Height, weight, and blood pressure measurements should be recorded during the first visit. Funduscopic, heart, lung, breast, abdominal, and rectal examination should be performed. The extremities should also be examined.

   1. A **systolic flow murmur** at the left sternal border is normal.

   2. **Edema** is common in pregnancy.
      a. Normal if confined to feet and ankles
      b. Abnormal in face, hand, or abdomen

B **Pelvic examination.** A speculum examination permits visualization of the vagina and cervix.
   1. **Vagina and cervix**
      a. **Chadwick sign** is a blue-red passive hyperemia of the cervix seen in the first trimester.
      b. **Normal vaginal discharge is** a moderate amount of white mucous.

    c. Abnormal vaginal discharge

        (1) Foamy white liquid with a strawberry discoloration of the cervix suggests *Trichomonas.*

        (2) White curdy discharge suggests *Candida.*

        (3) Foul-smelling, gray discharge may indicate **bacterial vaginosis.** It is important to identify patients who may be infected because untreated patients may have a higher incidence of PROM and preterm delivery.

    d. A Papanicolaou smear and cultures for gonorrhea and chlamydial infection should be obtained.

2. Uterus

    a. Uterine size should be estimated and correlated with the expected weeks of gestation.

    b. Hagar sign is a softening of the isthmus of the uterus and gives the impression that the uterus and cervix are separate.

3. Pelvis

    a. The **configuration and capacity of the bony pelvis** are evaluated by clinical pelvimetry (Fig. 4-1).

        (1) True conjugate is a measure from the sacral promontory to the anterior **superior** pubic symphysis, which can be obtained only with radiographs.

        (2) Diagonal conjugate is a measure from the sacral promontory to the anterior **inferior** pubic symphysis, which can be obtained clinically.

        (3) Obstetrical conjugate is a measure from the sacral promontory to the posterior pubic symphysis. This measurement is typically 1.5 to 2 cm less than the diagonal conjugate. The obstetrical conjugate is the shortest anterior posterior diameter through which the fetal head must pass.

    b. Women have **four basic types of pelvises** (Fig. 4-2):

        (1) Gynecoid pelvis. This type is the most common pelvis type (50% of women). The overall shape is round, with divergent ischial spines and a wide pubic arch.

        (2) Android pelvis. This type is found in 33% of white women and 15% of nonwhite women. The overall shape of an android pelvis is heart-like, with prominent ischial spines and a narrow pubic arch.

        (3) Anthropoid pelvis. This type is found in 25% of white women and 50% of nonwhite women. The overall shape is long and oval, with prominent ischial spines and a narrow pubic arch.

        (4) Platypelloid pelvis. This type is found in less than 3% of women. The overall shape is flat and oval, with widely spaced ischial spines.

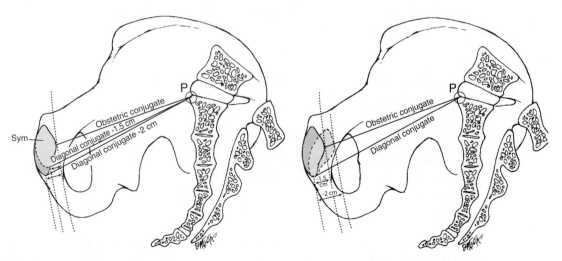

FIGURE 4-1 Variations in length of diagonal conjugate dependent on height and inclination of the symphysis pubis (P, sacral promontory; Sym, pelvic symphysis). (Reprinted with permission from Cunningham FG, MacDonald PC, Gant NF. Williams Obstetrics. 21st Ed. New York: McGraw-Hill, 2001:59, Figure 3-29.)

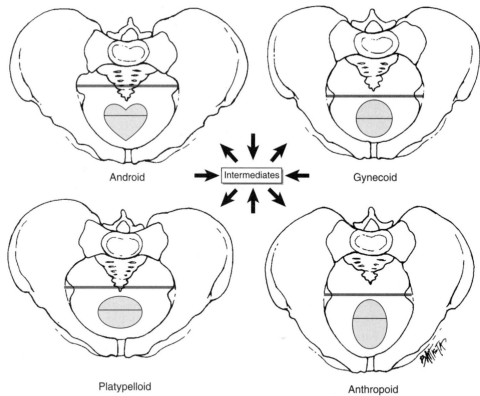

Android   Intermediates   Gynecoid

Platypelloid   Anthropoid

FIGURE 4-2 The four parent pelvic types of the Caldwell-Moloy classification. A line passing through the widest diameter divides the inlet into posterior and anterior segments. (Reprinted with permission from Cunningham FG, MacDonald PC, Gant NF. Williams Obstetrics. 21st Ed. New York: McGraw-Hill, 2001:57, Figure 3-27.)

C **Abdominal examination** allows for ongoing evaluation of the growth and status of fetus.

1. Between 18 and 30 weeks, measurement from the pubic symphysis to the top of the uterus in centimeters correlates well with the weeks of gestation.

2. Fetal heart tones can be identified by Doppler ultrasound at 12 to 14 weeks and by fetoscope at 18 to 20 weeks.

IV **ANTEPARTUM MANAGEMENT**

A **Laboratory tests** (see Chapter 5)

1. **Initial screening** should include the following studies:
   a. Hemoglobin and hematocrit levels
   b. Urinalysis and urine culture
   c. Blood group and Rh type
   d. Antibody screening
   e. Rubella titers. Nonimmune patients should be immunized in the postpartum period.
   f. Serologic test for syphilis and hepatitis B
   g. Cervical culture for gonorrhea and chlamydial infection
   h. Cervical cytologic analysis
   i. Sickle cell test for at-risk women
   j. Skin test for tuberculosis for exposed women or for women from endemic areas
   k. One-hour glucose tolerance test, particularly for women with a history of gestational diabetes or a history of delivery of large infants (more than 4000 g)

2. **Maternal serum α-fetoprotein (MSAFP)** levels are measured between 15 and 20 weeks' gestation. The values are reported as the multiple of the mean (MOM).
    a. **Elevated MSAFP** (2.5 MOM or more) may indicate:
        (1) Open neural tube defects (e.g., anencephaly, spina bifida, or meningomyelocele)
        (2) Ventral wall defects (e.g., omphalocele or gastroschisis)
        (3) Multiple gestation
        (4) Duodenal atresia
        (5) Calculations of MSAFP based on incorrect dates
    b. **Depressed MSAFP** (0.7 MOM or less) is associated with Down syndrome. The mothers of 15 to 20% of infants with Down syndrome have low MSAFP values.
    c. The MSAFP can be either high or low with no obvious reason and with a normal fetus.
    d. Some cases of high MSAFP have been associated with nonspecific placental abnormalities. Patients with unexplained high levels of MSAFP should undergo weekly nonstress tests starting at 32 to 34 weeks.

3. The **triple screen examination** (also called multiple marker screen) is a screening test for Down syndrome (trisomy 21) and Edward syndrome (trisomy 18). Performed between 15 and 20 weeks' gestation in women younger than 35 years of age, it measures MSAFP, hCG, and estriol.
    a. The **mothers of 60% of infants with Down syndrome** have an abnormal triple screen test, with low MSAFP, high hCG, and low estriol.
    b. The mothers of 80% of **Edward syndrome** have abnormal triple screen test, with low MSAFP, low hCG, and low estriol.

4. **Third-trimester routine screening** should include the following studies:
    a. Repeat hemoglobin and hematocrit levels
    b. Diabetes screening with a 50-g glucose tolerance test (28 weeks)
    c. Repeat antibody screen at 28 weeks. If the patient is Rh negative, she should receive prophylactic Rh_o (anti-D) immune globulin (300 μg) to reduce the incidence of Rh isoimmunization in an Rh-negative woman and the father of an Rh-positive fetus.
    d. Group B streptococcus vaginal and perineal swab (35 to 37 weeks)

B **Office visits**

1. Frequency
    a. In an **uncomplicated pregnancy**, a woman should be seen every 4 weeks for the first 28 weeks, every 2 weeks until 36 weeks, and weekly thereafter until delivery.
    b. **High-risk pregnancies** with medical or obstetric problems require close surveillance at intervals determined by the severity of the problem.

2. Monitoring
    a. Mother
        (1) Blood pressure taken at every visit
        (2) Urine dip for protein and glucose
        (3) Weight
        (4) Presence of headache, pain, nausea, vomiting, bleeding, loss of fluid, and dysuria
        (5) Height of the uterine fundus above the pubic symphysis
        (6) Position, consistency, effacement, and dilation of the cervix (starting after 38 weeks)
    b. Fetus
        (1) Fetal heart rate
        (2) Size of fetus
        (3) Fetal activity
        (4) Presenting part (late in pregnancy), as determined by the Leopold maneuvers (palpation)

3. **Special instructions.** Patients are instructed about the following danger signals, which should be reported immediately whenever they occur.
   a. Any vaginal bleeding
   b. Swelling of the face or hands
   c. Severe continuous headaches
   d. Blurring of vision
   e. Abdominal pain
   f. Persistent vomiting
   g. Chills or fever
   h. Dysuria
   i. Loss of fluid from the vagina
   j. Decrease in the frequency of fetal movements. Normal is at least 10 fetal movements in a 2-hour period.

V NUTRITION

A The **recommended weight gain in a normal pregnancy** is **11.5 to 16 kg (25 to 35 lb)**, although these numbers remain controversial.

1. Pregnancy-induced changes account for about 9 to 10 kg (20 to 22 lb) of the weight gain in normal conditions in the following approximate distributions:
   a. Fetus: 3.4 kg (7.5 lb)
   b. Placenta plus membranes: 0.7 kg (1.5 lb)
   c. Amniotic fluid: 0.9 kg (2 lb)
   d. Increase in weight of the uterus: 1.1kg (2.5 lb)
   e. Increase in blood volume: 1.6 kg (3.5 lb)
   f. Breasts: 0.45 kg (1 lb)
   g. Lower extremity fluid: 1.1 kg (2.5 lb)

2. **Failure to gain weight** may be a dangerous sign.

B **Calories.** The pregnant woman requires approximately **300 kcal/day** above her prepregnant needs.

C **Protein.** Inadequate intake of protein may lead to suboptimal growth of the fetus, a decrease in the size of various organs, and perhaps increased prenatal morbidity and mortality. The majority of protein is best obtained from animal sources, such as meat, milk, eggs, cheese, poultry, and fish, because they supply amino acids in optimal combinations. During pregnancy, about **1 kg** of protein is deposited, half to the fetus and placenta and half to the mother.

D **Minerals**

1. Iron
   a. Many women have **inadequate iron stores** because of blood loss during menses. During pregnancy, iron stores are further depleted.
   b. **Supplemental iron** is needed for both the mother and the fetus.
      (1) **Recommended intake** for the mother is 30 to 60 mg of elemental iron per day. Iron is found in liver, red meat, dried beans, green leafy vegetables, whole grain cereal, and dried fruits.
      (2) The fetus maintains normal hemoglobin levels at the mother's expense.

2. Calcium
   a. **Recommended intake** of calcium is 1200 mg daily. Calcium is best obtained from calcium-rich foods in the diet, such as milk, cheese, yogurt, and tofu; supplements may be necessary if dietary sources are insufficient. Calcium may also be obtained from calcium-containing antacid tablets.
   b. **Leg cramps** at night are the classic symptom of calcium deficiency in a pregnant woman.

3. Sodium. A restriction of sodium intake, which was advocated in the past, is no longer advised because of the natriuretic effects of progesterone.

E | Vitamins

1. **Folic acid** is required for the formation of heme, the iron containing protein in hemoglobulin. Deficiency in folic acid may cause megaloblastic anemia.
   a. Approximately **1 mg of folic acid per day** is required during pregnancy. Folic acid is found in many of the same foods that contain iron, such as green, leafy vegetables.
   b. For women with a history of infant or fetal **neural tube defect, 4 mg of folic acid per day** should be consumed daily, starting 1 month before conception.
   c. All fertile women should take 0.4 mg/day of folic acid.

2. **Vitamin B$_{12}$** occurs naturally in foods of animal origin. Supplements may be necessary in vegetarians who may be deficient in this area.

3. **Vitamin C** is readily available in the normal diet. The recommended daily allowance in pregnancy is **70 mg/day.**

VI | LIFESTYLE MODIFICATIONS

A | Exercise.
It is not necessary for a pregnant woman to limit her exercise, provided she does not become excessively tired. Maternal heart rate should be monitored and kept below 148 beats per minute; fetal decelerations have been identified at higher maternal heart rates. Restrictions in exercise may be necessary in situations such as placenta previa, cervical incompetence, pregnancy-induced hypertension, premature labor, and multiple gestation.

B | Travel.
No harmful effects have been ascribed to travel. A pregnant woman should move around every 2 hours to prevent venous stasis and thrombus formation.

C | Bowel habits.
a. **Bowel habits during pregnancy tend to become erratic because of progesterone-induced** gastrointestinal smooth muscle relaxation, leading to increased transit time. Late in the pregnancy, compression on the bowel by the **presenting part** may cause constipation. Women may avoid constipation by liberal fluid intake; exercise; and taking stool softeners, bulking agents, and mild laxatives.
b. Nausea and vomiting are common in the first and second trimester, usually worse in the morning. Nonpharmacologic therapy is advocated initially. This includes small, frequent meals and avoidance of strong odors.

D | Coitus.
Sexual intercourse does no harm at any time in the pregnancy, provided there are no pregnancy complications such as placenta previa, rupture of membranes, preterm labor, or premature cervical dilation. Prostaglandin in ejaculate may cause transient contractions.

E | Smoking.
Women who smoke often have smaller infants (average of 200 g) with increased perinatal morbidity. Mothers should be encouraged to quit smoking completely during pregnancy. The adverse effects are thought to be a function of the following factors:

1. **Carbon monoxide** and its inactivation of fetal and maternal hemoglobin

2. **Vasoconstrictor effect of nicotine,** causing reduced perfusion to the placenta, which may lead to growth restriction

3. **Reduced appetite** and **reduced caloric intake**

F **Alcohol.** The current recommendation is that no alcohol be consumed during pregnancy. The fetal abnormalities associated with drinking are known as fetal alcohol syndrome, which includes craniofacial defects, limb and cardiovascular defects, prenatal and postnatal growth restriction, and mental retardation (see Chapter 8).

G **Caffeine.** Most studies in pregnancy show no increase in teratogenic or reproductive risk.

H **Medications.** Most drugs administered during pregnancy cross the placenta and reach the fetus. Exceptions are large organic ions such as heparin and insulin. The Food and Drug Administration (FDA) created five categories based on risk to the fetus in pregnancy (see Chapter 7). Package inserts that include FDA classification should be consulted when prescribing medication in pregnancy.

1. **Category** A (e.g., levothyroxine, folic acid). Well-controlled studies in pregnant women show no risk to the fetus in any trimester of pregnancy.

2. **Category** B (e.g., ondansetron, penicillins). Well-controlled studies in pregnant women have shown no increased risk of fetal abnormalities despite adverse findings in animals. Drugs are also placed in this category if, in the absence of adequate human studies, animal studies show no fetal risk. The chance of fetal harm is remote but possible.

3. **Category** C (e.g., prochlorperazine, trimethoprim–sulfamethoxazole). Well-controlled human studies are lacking, and animal studies are lacking as well or have shown a risk to the fetus. There is a **chance of fetal harm if the drug is administered in pregnancy.** However, the potential benefits may outweigh the potential risk.

4. **Category** D (e.g., phenytoin, carbamazepine). Studies in humans have demonstrated a risk to the fetus; therefore, the **drug should not be administered during pregnancy.** However, the potential benefits may be acceptable in cases of a life-threatening situation or serious disease for which a safer drug cannot be used or has proven ineffective.

5. **Category** X (e.g., diethylstilbestrol, thalidomide). Studies in animals or human have demonstrated **evidence of fetal abnormalities or risk** that clearly outweigh any possible benefit to the patient.

Study Questions for Chapter 4

Directions: Each of the numbered items or incomplete statements in this section is followed by answers or by completions of the statement. Select the ONE lettered answer or completion that is BEST in each case.

1. A woman presents to your office for prenatal care. She has had two abortions, two second-trimester miscarriages, one ectopic pregnancy, a fetal demise at 37 weeks' gestation, and two live births. Her son, who is now 13 years old, was delivered at 34 weeks' gestation by spontaneous vaginal delivery. Her daughter, who is now 10 years old, was delivered at 38 weeks by cesarean section secondary to fetal distress during labor. What are her "Gs and Ps" by simple notation and by TPAL notation, respectively?

- A $G_8 P_2$ and $G_8 P_{1142}$
- B $G_8 P_3$ and $G_8 P_{2142}$
- C $G_9 P_3$ and $G_9 P_{2142}$
- D $G_8 P_3$ and $G_8 P_{1142}$
- E $G_9 P_3$ and $G9 P_{2152}$

2. A 34-year-old woman, gravida 2, para 1 at 32 weeks' gestation presents to your office for routine prenatal care. She delivered her daughter vaginally at 39 weeks without any complications. Her past medical history is unremarkable, and her current pregnancy has been uncomplicated other than occasional Braxton Hicks and increasing vaginal discharge that is nonpruritic, the same color as her cervical mucous, and has been present during most of her pregnancy. Her BP = 108/73, her temperature is 96.8°, her fundus measures at 33 weeks, she is 5 feet 4 inches tall, her prepregnancy weight was 120 lbs, and she now weighs 135 lbs. She is Rubella non-immune, Hepatitis B surface antigen negative, O + / antibody −, Veneral Disease Research Laboratory nonreactive, and gonorrhea culture/chlamydia negative. What is the next best step in management?

- A Rubella antibody test
- B 50 g glucose tolerance test
- C 300 μg anti-D immune globulin
- D Follow-up in 2 weeks
- E Counseling about appropriate weight gain

3. A 28-year-old woman, gravida 3, para 2 at 5 weeks' gestation presents to you for confirmation of pregnancy and possible prenatal care. Her first pregnancy resulted in vaginal delivery of a viable female infant weighing 3,900 g at term. Her daughter has a bilateral hearing deficit. Her second pregnancy resulted in cesarean section delivery of a viable male infant weighing 2,900 g at 34 weeks because of pregnancy-induced hypertension. Her son was born with mild myelomeningocele. She denies family history of any diseases or problems. She tells you that she is a lacto-ovo vegetarian. What is the most appropriate advice during this prenatal session?

- A Supplement your diet with additional iron
- B Supplement your diet with additional vitamin B_{12}
- C Increase your folic acid intake to ten times your prepregnancy amount
- D Eat plenty of green, leafy vegetables
- E Increase your calcium intake to 1,200 mg per day

4. You discover two medical students in the low-risk obstetric clinic debating over the recommended weight gain in normal pregnancy and the two largest contributions to weight gain during a normal pregnancy. You agree that the recommended weight gain during normal pregnancy is about 30 lbs give or take a few pounds depending on the prepregnancy weight. Aside from the weight of the fetus, what is the largest contributor to weight gain during pregnancy?

- A Blood volume
- B Uterus
- C Placenta
- D Amniotic fluid
- E Breasts

5. A 24-year-old woman, gravida 2, para 1 at 27 weeks' gestation presents to you for routine prenatal care. She reports plenty of fetal movement and denies spotting or regular contractions. She does report increasing vaginal discharge that is white to yellow in color and has a distinct odor. Her temperature today is 98.2° and her BP = 100/60. The fundus measures 28 cm above the symphysis pubis. Her last pregnancy was uncomplicated. She has no known drug allergy. Her past medical history is remarkable for asthma (about two wheezing episodes per week and symptom-free at nights). You perform a sterile speculum examination and you notice homogenous, adherent, white-yellow discharge in the posterior fornix and the cervix but the mucosa does not appear inflamed. The pH of the discharge is 5.5. Wet mount displays 30% clue cells. The potassium hydrochloride (KOH) prep is nondiagnostic but has a strong odor. Which of the following is the best diagnosis and treatment combination, respectively?

- A Normal discharge and follow-up in 4 weeks
- B Trichomonas and metronidazole
- C Bacterial vaginosis and clindamycin
- D Chlamydia and erythromycin
- E Candida and fluconazole

Answers and Explanations

1. The answer is C [I B 1]. Remember that "parity" refers to the number of pregnancies that reached viability (23 or more weeks of gestation) and not the number of pregnancies resulting in a live-born. Additionally, The route of delivery (vaginal versus cesarian section) does not change the parity. In this question's scenario, the woman has been pregnant nine times (her current pregnancy = 1, two abortions = 2, two miscarriages = 2, one ectopic = 1, one fetal demise = 1, and two live-births = 2; 1+2+2+1+1+2 = 9). Only three pregnancies reached viability (fetal demise at 37 weeks, her preterm delivery at 34 weeks, and her term delivery at 38 weeks). For the **TPAL** notation, **T** refers to the number of term infants delivered regardless of outcome (fetal demise at 37 weeks and term delivery at 38 weeks = 2); **P** stands for preterm (preterm delivery at 34 weeks = 1); **A** stands for abortions, either elective or miscarriages (it does not include ectopic pregnancies) (2 abortions + 2 miscarriages = 4); and **L** refers to number of living offspring (son and daughter = 2). With multiple gestation pregnancies, the parity does not increase by the number of babies delivered (e.g., a patient who has been pregnant once and delivered twins at 38 weeks would be noted as G_1P_1 and G_1P_{1002}).

2. The answer is D [IV B 1]. In an uncomplicated pregnancy, as in this case, a woman should be seen every 4 weeks for the first 28 weeks, every 2 weeks until 36 weeks, and weekly thereafter until delivery. Although this patient is Rubella non-immune, no action needs to be taken until after she delivers. You can assume that by 32 weeks of gestation, she should have already had a 50 g glucose tolerance test because the recommended time to perform the screening is between 24 and 28 weeks of gestation. This patient does not need anti-D immune globulin because she is Rh +. For her height and prepregnancy weight, it is appropriate to have gained 15 lbs up to this point in pregnancy.

3. The answer is C [V E 1 b]. The most appropriate advice during this session is to remind the patient to increase her folic acid intake to 4 mg per day because she has a history of delivering a child with neural tube defect. Although it is appropriate to counsel every pregnant patient to supplement with iron, to increase their intake of green leafy vegetables, and to try to consume 1200 mg of calcium per day, these are not the most important to convey in this first prenatal counseling session (you can counsel her about these during the next visit, along with reinforcing folic acid supplementation). Strict vegans (not lacto-ova vegetarians) are at risk for vitamin B_{12} deficiency.

4. The answer is A [V A 1]. The top four contributors to weight gain during pregnancy are as follows: #1, fetus (7.5 lbs); #2, blood volume (3.5 lbs); #3 uterus and lower extremity edema (2.5 lbs); and #4, amniotic fluid (2 lbs). The placenta contributes only about 1.5 lbs, and the breasts contribute only 1 lb.

5. The answer is C [III B 1 c]. A foul-smelling discharge that is grayish in color (sometimes), whose pH is less than 4.5, with more than 15% clue cells on wet mount field, and a positive whiff test (KOH on discharge has fishy odor) is most likely bacterial vaginosis. This condition can be treated with either metronidazole (first choice) or clindamycin. There is no way of diagnosing chlamydia without a culture or test such as ligase chain reaction or an enzyme immunoassay. All the other answers listed (normal vagina, candida, and trichomonas) have a vaginal pH of 4.5 or less.

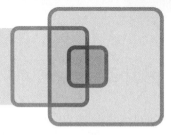

chapter **5**

Identification of the High-Risk Pregnant Patient

JACK LUDMIR

I INTRODUCTION

For the majority of women, pregnancy and childbirth are a normal physiologic process that results in the delivery of a healthy infant; however, certain circumstances may place a mother or infant at risk for morbidity. A pregnancy is defined as **high risk** when the likelihood of an adverse outcome is greater than in the general pregnant population. A program of routine prenatal care may optimize pregnancy outcome by achieving the following goals:

A Providing **advice, reassurance, education,** and **support** for the woman and her family

B Managing the **minor ailments** of pregnancy

C Providing a **screening** program to confirm that a woman continues to be at low risk

D **Preventing, detecting,** and **managing** factors that adversely affect the health of mother and infant

II MATERNAL AND PERINATAL MORTALITY

A Definitions

1. **Maternal death** occurs either during pregnancy or within 42 days of the termination of pregnancy.

2. **Maternal mortality ratio** is the number of maternal deaths per 100,000 live births. Maternal mortality in the United States has decreased substantially in the past few decades—from 582/100,000 live births in 1935 to 8.4/100,000 live births in 1997. The maternal mortality rate for African Americans has also declined, but it remains **three times higher** than Caucasian women. Major causes of maternal death in nonabortive pregnancies (excluding ectopic pregnancies) are, in descending order, **pulmonary embolism**, hypertensive disorders of pregnancy, obstetric hemorrhage, and sepsis.

3. **Perinatal mortality** is the combination of fetal deaths (after 20 weeks or weighing more than 500 g) and neonatal deaths (up to 28 days after birth)/1000 live births. The perinatal mortality rate has fallen drastically in the last 25 years, from about 29/1000 in 1970 to 13/1000 in 1995. Women without prenatal care have higher rates of perinatal mortality.

III PRECONCEPTION CARE

A Preconception care involves identifying those conditions that could affect a future pregnancy but may be ameliorated by early intervention, such as hypertension, diabetes mellitus, or other metabolic and inherited disorders.

B Women (and their partners) who are contemplating pregnancy should be evaluated for conditions that may affect a future pregnancy. Reproductive, family, genetic, and medical histories should be reviewed (see Chapter 4).

IV INITIAL PRENATAL VISIT

A General history

1. **Socioeconomic status. Low socioeconomic status** increases the risk of perinatal morbidity and mortality.

2. **Age** is an identifiable risk factor.
   a. **Maternal age younger than 20 years of age** increases the risk of the following conditions:
      (1) Premature births
      (2) Late prenatal care
      (3) Low birth weight
      (4) Uterine dysfunction
      (5) Fetal deaths
      (6) Neonatal deaths
   b. **Maternal age older than 35 years of age** increases the risk of the following conditions:
      (1) **First-trimester miscarriage.** The miscarriage rate for women older than 40 years is three times higher than for women younger than 30 years.
      (2) **Genetically abnormal conceptuses.** The risk for fetal chromosomal anomalies increases in direct proportion to maternal age. (This increase may also explain, in part, the increase in first-trimester miscarriages.) **Trisomy 21** represents 90% of the chromosomal abnormalities, but the incidence of other autosomal trisomies (i.e., 13 and 18) and sex chromosomal anomalies also increase with advancing age.
      (3) **Medical complications**
          (a) **Hypertension**
          (b) **Diabetes**
          (c) **Preeclampsia.** The incidence of preeclampsia increases with age; it is 6% at 25 years of age, 9% at 35 years of age, and 15% at 40 years of age.
      (4) **Multiple gestation.** The incidence of multiple gestation increases with age. The rate of dizygotic twins is 3/1000 live births in women younger than 21 years of age, and it increases to 14/1000 live births in women 35 to 40 years of age.
      (5) **Higher rate of cesarean section.** Part of the increase may be attributed to a greater incidence of placenta previa, abnormal presentations, multiple gestations, and medical complications.
      (6) **Fetal morbidity and mortality.** Women older than 40 years of age have higher rates of stillbirth and low birth weight compared with younger women.

3. **Substance Abuse** (see Chapter 8)
   a. **Tobacco.** A dose-response relationship exists between heavy cigarette smoking and increased fetal morbidity and mortality.
   b. **Drugs.** The maternal and fetal consequences of drug addiction in pregnancy depend on the drug ingested. Many (e.g., cocaine, opioids, or marijuana) are associated with low birth weight, and drugs such as cocaine and opioids are associated with neonatal withdrawal. Cocaine is also associated with premature labor and abruptio placentae.
   c. **Alcohol.** Not only does alcohol abuse undermine maternal health, but a pattern of abnormalities known as the **fetal alcohol syndrome** manifests in varying degrees of severity in the fetus. Regular screening for alcohol abuse should be carried out using tools such as the T-ACE questionnaire (Table 5-1).

Table 5-1   Alcohol Abuse Screening: The T-ACE Questionnaire
T: **T**olerance; How many drinks does it take to make you feel "high?" Or how many drinks can you hold? (A positive response is two or more drinks.)
A Have people **a**nnoyed you by criticizing your drinking?
C Have you ever felt you ought to **c**ut down on your drinking?
E Have you ever had a drink first thing in the morning to steady your nerves or to get rid of a hangover (*eye-opener*)?
Scoring: The tolerance question carries substantially more weight (2 points) than the three other questions (1 point each).
These questions were found to be significant identifiers of risk drinking in pregnancy (i.e., alcohol intake potentially sufficient to damage the embryo/fetus).
From Sokol RJ, Martier SS, Ager JW.. The T-ACE questions: practical prenatal detection of risk-drinking. *Am J Obstet Gynecol* 1989;160:863.

     d. Caffeine. Caffeine-containing beverages, including coffee, are frequently consumed by pregnant women. There is no increased risk of congenital anomalies; however, a recent study suggested higher rates of spontaneous abortion with caffeine intake.

  4. Environmental risks

     a. Noxious chemicals may cause unpleasant symptoms in the mother (i.e., headache, nausea, and lightheadedness). There is no evidence of increased rate for birth defects.

     b. Radiation and radioactive compounds have been associated with spontaneous abortion, birth defects, and childhood leukemia.

  5. Domestic violence. Victims of domestic violence are more likely to be abused while pregnant. Such assaults may lead to placental abruption, fetal fractures, rupture of the uterus, spleen or liver, and preterm labor. It estimated that 8% of obstetric patients are physically assaulted while pregnant. Questions on personal safety and violence should be addressed during the prenatal period (Fig. 5-1).

B **Obstetric history.**   Previous obstetric and reproductive history is essential to care in subsequent pregnancy.

  1. Parity

     a. Nullipara. Nulliparous women are at high risk for development of specific problems, including pregnancy-induced hypertension and possible complications caused by relative lack of knowledge of the pregnancy state.

     b. Multipara. Grand multiparous women (five or more pregnancies resulting in viable fetuses) appear to be at increased risk for placenta previa, postpartum hemorrhage secondary to uterine atony, and increased incidence of dizygotic twins (which may occur because grand multiparas are usually of advanced age).

  2. Ectopic pregnancy. A woman with a history of ectopic pregnancy has an increased risk of another ectopic pregnancy. It is imperative that she be evaluated by 6 weeks' gestation by pelvic examination or vaginal ultrasound so that the site of pregnancy can be confirmed immediately.

  3. Preterm delivery. The incidence of preterm delivery, which correlates well with past reproductive performance (Table 5-2), increases with each subsequent preterm delivery. The recurrence rate for preterm labor is 25 to 40%. Recently, a short cervical length (less than 2.5 cm), as determined by ultrasound at 24 weeks, has been associated with increased risk of preterm birth.

Abuse Assessment Screen (Circle YES or NO for each question)		
1. Have you ever been emotionally or physically abused by your partner or someone important to you?	YES	NO
2. Within the last year, have you been hit , slapped, kicked, or otherwise physically hurt by someone?	YES	NO

If YES, by whom? (circle all that apply)

      Husband   Ex-husband   Boyfriend   Stranger   Other   Multiple

Total number of times _____

3. Since you've been pregnant, have you been hit, slapped, kicked, or otherwise physically hurt by someone?   YES   NO

If YES, by whom? (circle all that apply)

      Husband   Ex-husband   Boyfriend   Stranger   Other   Multiple

Score each incident according to the following scale:

1 = Threats of abuse, including the use of a weapon

2 = Slapping, pushing; no injuries and/or lasting pain

3 = Punching, kicking, bruises, cuts, and/or continuing pain

4 = Beaten up, severe contusions, burns, broken bones

5 = Head, internal, and/or permanent injury

6 = Use of weapon, wound from weapon

(If any of the descriptions for the higher number apply, use the higher number)

4. Within the last year, has anyone forced you to have sexual activities?   YES   NO

If YES, by whom? (circle all that apply)

      Husband   Ex-husband   Boyfriend   Stranger   Other   Multiple

Total number of times _____

5. Are you afraid of your partner or anyone you listed above?   YES   NO

FIGURE 5-1 Determination of frequency and severity of physical abuse during pregnancy. (From McFarlane J, Parker B, Solken K, et al. Assessing for abuse during pregnancy. *JAMA* 1992;267(23):3176–3178. Copyright 1992, American Medical Association.)

4. **Second-trimester pregnancy loss.** Such loss could be the result of an abnormality in the fetus (chromosomal or infectious) or manifestation of a recurrent condition in the mother, such as cervical incompetence. This condition is characterized by premature delivery associated with painless cervical dilation. Ultrasound evaluation of the cervix during gestation is an objective way to identify patient at risk for this condition. These patients may benefit from therapeutic interventions, such as cervical cerclage.

5. **Large infant (more than 4000 g).** Large size may indicate previously undetected or uncontrolled glucose intolerance and may be associated with subsequent intrapartum complications, such as:
   a. Difficult vaginal delivery caused by shoulder dystocia
   b. Cesarean section for arrest of dilation or descent
   c. Postpartum complications for the neonate, such as hypoglycemia (see Chapter 17 regarding gestational diabetes)

    6. Perinatal death (stillborn or neonatal). A pregnancy that follows a perinatal death should be observed closely to avoid a similar outcome. Perinatal death may indicate an underlying problem that may or may not have been detected previously, such as:

      a. Glucose intolerance

      b. Collagen vascular disease

      c. Congenital anomalies

      d. Chromosomal abnormality

      e. Preterm labor

      f. Hemolytic disease

      g. Abnormal labor

      h. Antiphospholipid syndrome (APS)

      i. Thrombophilia

    7. Cesarean section

      a. A woman who has had a **previous cesarean section** should be encouraged to attempt a vaginal delivery with a subsequent pregnancy, provided there are no medical or surgical contraindications, such as:

        (1) Classical uterine incision. A trial of labor is contraindicated in patients with a previous incision into the body of the uterus (classical) because of the high risk of uterine rupture (6 to 8%).

Table 5-2 System for Determining Risk of Spontaneous Preterm Delivery

Points Assigned	Socioeconomic Factors	Previous Medical History	Daily Habits	Aspects of Current Pregnancy
1	Two children at home Low socioeconomic status	Abortion × 1 Less than 1 year since birth	Works outside home	Unusual fatigue
2	Maternal age > 20 years or > 40 years Single parent	Abortion × 2	Smokes > 10 cigarettes per day	Gain of < 10 lb by 32 weeks
3	Very low socioeconomic status Height < 150 cm	Abortion × 3	Engages in heavy or stressful work Takes long, tiring trip	Breech at 32 weeks Weight loss of 5 lb Head engaged at 32 weeks Febrile illness
4	Maternal age < 18 years	Pyelonephritis		Bleeding after 12 weeks Effacement Dilation Uterine irritability
5		Uterine anomaly Second-trimester abortion Exposure to diethylstilbestrol Cone biopsy		Placenta previa Hydramnios
10		Preterm delivery Repeated second-trimester abortions		Twins Abdominal surgery

Modified from Creasy RK, Gummer BA, Liggins GC. System for predicting spontaneous preterm birth. *Obstet Gynecol* 55:692, 1980.

(2) An **active herpes infection** at term

(3) **Myomectomy** with penetration into the endometrium

b. **Labor in a successive pregnancy** is usually safe in patients with one prior transverse scar should be offered a trial of labor. The chance of uterine rupture is less than 1%. Currently, not enough data is available to establish the safety of a trial of labor in women with two or more transverse uterine scars.

8. **Pregnancy-induced hypertension (preeclampsia and eclampsia)**

a. There appears to be a familial tendency (higher rate for women with affected sisters, mothers, and grandmothers).

b. Women with a history of severe preeclampsia early in pregnancy may have an increased risk for development of preeclampsia in subsequent pregnancies.

C **Medical history**

1. **Chronic hypertension** (higher than 140/90 mmHg). Patients with chronic hypertension are at risk of the following conditions:

a. Superimposed preeclampsia

b. Abruptio placentae

c. Perinatal loss

d. Maternal mortality

e. Myocardial infarction

f. Uteroplacental insufficiency

g. Cerebrovascular accident

2. **Cardiac disease.** Cardiac disorders have both maternal and fetal implications.

a. **Heart disease may develop or worsen in pregnant women.** Because of the hemodynamic changes associated with pregnancy, some cardiac lesions are particularly dangerous, such as Eisenmenger syndrome, primary pulmonary hypertension, Marfan syndrome, and hemodynamically significant mitral or aortic stenosis.

b. **Fetal growth and development** depend on an adequate supply of well-oxygenated blood. If this supply is limited, as it appears to be with certain cardiac lesions, then the fetus is at risk of abnormal development and even death.

c. **Offspring of parents with cardiac disease** have an increased risk of developing cardiac disease in their lifetimes. This is sometimes identified in utero with fetal echocardiography after 20 weeks.

3. **Pulmonary disease.** Maternal respiratory function and gas exchange are affected by the associated biochemical and mechanical alterations that occur in a normal pregnancy. The effect of pregnancy on pulmonary disease is often unpredictable. Diseases such as asthma should be managed as they would be normally. When pulmonary disease affects maternal well-being or compromises the supply of well-oxygenated blood to the fetus, there is need for concern.

4. **Renal disease**

a. In a normal pregnancy, the renal system undergoes certain potentially stressful physiologic, anatomic, and functional changes; therefore, **continuous assessment is necessary** in patients with preexisting or developing renal disease.

b. With proper medical supervision and control of blood pressure, most women with underlying renal disease can have an **uneventful pregnancy** without adverse effects on either the primary disease or the ultimate prognosis, **provided that the woman's creatinine level is below 1.5 mg/100 mL.**

5. **Diabetes.** The cornerstone of management for women with diabetes is rigid metabolic control to make patients as consistently euglycemic as possible. Ideally, these efforts should begin before conception and continue throughout the pregnancy. The following fetal problems may complicate the pregnancy of a diabetic:

a. **Congenital anomalies** (two to three times higher than in individuals without diabetes)

b. Fetal mortality

c. Neonatal morbidity, including:
  (1) Respiratory distress syndrome
  (2) Macrosomia
  (3) Hypoglycemia
  (4) Hyperbilirubinemia
  (5) Hypocalcemia

6. Thyroid disease. Untreated hypothyroidism or hyperthyroidism may profoundly alter pregnancy outcome. The fetal thyroid is autonomous and is unaffected by maternal thyroid hormone; however, treatment of thyroid disease during pregnancy can be complicated because the fetal thyroid responds to the same pharmacologic agents as does the maternal thyroid.

7. Thromboembolic disease. Pregnancy is associated with increased production of clotting factors by the liver; this places patients at risk for thromboembolic disease. Patients with prior history of thromboembolism or thrombophilia may benefit from anticoagulation during gestation and puerperium.

8. Systemic lupus erythematosus. This condition increases the risk of placental abruption, growth restriction, and superimposed preeclampsia.

9. Genetic disorders
  a. Genetic disorders in the mother, such as phenylketonuria, increase the risk of fetal malformation. Proper maternal diet during conception and pregnancy reduces the risk.
  b. Historical factors may help identify the at-risk pregnancy.
    (1) Consanguinity. Marriage between close relatives results in a large pool of identical genes, thereby increasing the possibility of sharing similar mutant genes, resulting in an:
      (a) Increased risk of miscarriage
      (b) Increased risk of rare recessive genetic disease in offspring
    (2) Ethnicity. Specific ethnic groups are more prone to specific diseases.
      (a) Tay-Sachs disease (Ashkenazi Jews, French Canadians)
      (b) Canavan disease (Ashkenazi Jews)
      (c) Thalassemias (Mediterranean, Southeast Asian, Indian, or African people)
      (d) Sickle cell anemia (African, Mediterranean, Caribbean, Latin American, or Indian people)
      (e) Cystic fibrosis (Caucasians)

10. Infectious diseases. In addition to rubella and syphilis, for which pregnant women are routinely screened, the following infections during pregnancy place the mother and infant at high risk for potential morbidity and mortality. The **TORCH** syndrome refers to an infection developing in a fetus or newborn caused by Toxoplasmosis, Rubella, or Herpes Simplex.
  a. Cytomegalovirus results in **increased risk of congenital anomalies** with primary infection during gestation and risk of a small-for-gestational-age infant.
  b. Herpes simplex virus may result in **increased risk of neonatal infection** if active viral lesions are present at birth and the infant is born vaginally.
  c. Toxoplasmosis leads to **increased risk of congenital anomalies** in the fetus if infection occurs early in pregnancy.
  d. Parvovirus infection may cause severe anemia in the fetus, resulting in **hydrops** and **death.**
  e. Varicella zoster virus infection is associated with a **small risk of** fetal sequelae, such as cutaneous scars and limb hypoplasia, if infection occurs early in the pregnancy. The risk of neonatal infection is greater if infection is present within 5 days of delivery.
  f. Hepatitis B virus (HBV) is associated with **no increased risk of congenital anomalies** but is associated with risk of vertical transmission and neonatal infection (see VI K).
  g. HIV [see VI L]

11. **Autoimmune disorders,** including **APS,** an autoimmune syndrome caused by the lupus anti-coagulant and the anticardiolipin antibody. APS may be expressed as one or more of the following:
    a. Recurrent fetal loss, such as miscarriage or stillbirth
    b. Placental infarction
    c. Preeclampsia early in gestation
    d. Arterial or venous thrombosis, including neurologic disease
    e. Autoimmune thrombocytopenia

D **Medications.** Various medications have adverse effects on the fetus, and it is imperative that the risks and benefits to the mother and fetus be evaluated and discussed with the patient before starting, continuing, or stopping the use of medications. When counseling patients about such risks and benefits, a baseline malformation rate of 2 to 3% in the general population should always be used (see Chapter 8).

V PHYSICAL EXAMINATION

Obstetric patients should undergo a thorough physical examination to assess their general health.

A **General examination.** Maternal size, which may reflect socioeconomic and nutritional status, has become an important predictive index.
1. A pregnant woman who is **short** or **underweight** is at increased risk for:
   a. Perinatal morbidity and mortality
   b. Delivering a low-birth-weight infant
   c. Preterm delivery
2. **Obesity** presents a medical hazard to the pregnant woman and her fetus. Complications that are more likely to develop in an obese woman include:
   a. Hypertension
   b. Diabetes
   c. Aspiration of gastric contents during the administration of anesthesia
   d. Wound complications
   e. Thromboembolism

B **Pelvic examination**
1. The **perineum, vulva, vagina, cervix,** and **adnexa** should be examined and any abnormalities noted that may affect future management (e.g., adnexal masses, cervical lesions, or DES cervical stigmata). A Papanicolaou (Pap) smear should be obtained.
2. **Clinical pelvimetry** should be performed to assess adequacy of the maternal pelvis to facilitate vaginal delivery (see Chapter 4).

C **Evaluation of the uterus.** The size of the uterus is evaluated continuously throughout the pregnancy. The estimated date of delivery should be established at the first prenatal visit so that subsequent discrepancies can be evaluated properly. A strong correlation exists between fundal height in centimeters measured from the symphysis pubis and gestational age in weeks beyond 20 weeks. Reproductive tract abnormalities that may be problematic include:
1. **Leiomyomata (fibroids).** The location and size of the myomas are important in determining possible future sequelae. In general, the pregnancy has an increased risk of being complicated by:
   a. Abortion
   b. Premature labor
   c. Dysfunctional labor
   d. Postpartum hemorrhage
   e. Obstruction of labor by cervical or lower uterine segment myomas

     f. Unstable fetal lie or compound presentation

     g. Pain caused by degeneration

  2. Incompetent cervix. Characterized by premature cervical dilatation in the second trimester, with minimal labor contractions. This is most often identified on physical examination, although ultrasound may aid in the diagnosis.

  3. Uterine anomalies of the bicornuate or septate type may increase the patient's risk of spontaneous miscarriage.

VI   LABORATORY STUDIES

Routine laboratory studies (see Chapter 4) may identify a high-risk pregnancy.

A **Blood type, including antibody screen**

  1. Rh sensitization may have profound consequences for the fetus and the management of the pregnancy. If maternal sensitization of an Rh-negative woman to red blood cell antigens has occurred (e.g., prior transfusions), the resultant antibodies can be transferred to the fetus and cause hemolytic disease in the Rh-positive fetus.

  2. The **antibody screen** is also essential for Rh-positive women because other blood group antigens (e.g., Kell, Kidd, or Duffy) can produce severe hemolytic disease in the fetus.

B **Syphilis test (Venereal Disease Research Laboratory [VDRL]).** Syphilis involves several different stages, and the evaluation of each stage is important in assessing fetal risk. Pregnancy complicated by preexisting or newly acquired syphilis may result in:

  1. An uninfected live infant

  2. A late abortion (after the fourth month of pregnancy)

  3. A stillbirth

  4. A congenitally infected infant

C **Gonorrhea culture.** Screening may be either universal or selective, depending on the prevalence of the disease in the patient population. Gonorrhea during pregnancy may be associated with:

  1. Intrauterine infection, with premature rupture of membranes and preterm delivery

  2. Histologic evidence of chorioamnionitis

  3. Neonatal eye infection (ophthalmia neonatorum)

  4. Clinical diagnosis of sepsis in the neonate

  5. Associated maternal arthritis, rash, or peripartum fever

D **Chlamydia testing.** Screening is recommended for all high-risk or symptomatic patients. Infection during pregnancy may result in:

  1. Ophthalmia neonatorum

  2. Neonatal pneumonia

  3. Postpartum endometritis

E **Rubella titer**

  1. The **clinical course** of rubella is no more severe or complicated in the pregnant woman than in the nonpregnant woman of comparable age. However, active maternal infection does carry risk for the fetus, including:

     a. First-trimester abortion

     b. Fetal infection, resulting in severe congenital anomalies

  2. Maternal infection in the first trimester carries with it the greatest risk to the fetus.

3. Immunization. If a patient is diagnosed as having a rubella titer of less than 1:8, she should be immunized postpartum.

  a. The rubella vaccine is not given during pregnancy because it is a live attenuated vaccine.

  b. There have been no reported cases of congenital rubella from inadvertent administration of the vaccine to pregnant women.

[F] **Complete blood count** with red blood cell indices and platelet count

1. Anemia. If present, anemia should be evaluated further and treated. **Microcytosis** without anemia may represent a thalassemia and should also be investigated.

2. Leukocytosis. A mild leukocytosis is normal in pregnancy; however, a grossly abnormal value needs to be evaluated.

[G] **Urinalysis and culture**

1. Asymptomatic bacteriuria is prevalent in 3 to 5% of pregnant women. Early detection, treatment, and close follow-up must be instituted.

2. Acute systemic pyelonephritis. Asymptomatic bacteriuria predisposes the pregnant woman to the development of acute systemic pyelonephritis, which has serious complications for the mother and fetus and has been associated with premature labor and delivery. Systemic pyelonephritis develops in approximately 20 to 40% of pregnant women with untreated **asymptomatic bacteriuria.**

[H] **Pap smear.**   Baseline cervical cytology should be established. If abnormalities are noted, institute proper evaluation.

[I] **Gestational diabetes screen.**   Screening for this condition should be performed at 24 to 28 weeks' gestation using a 1-hour, 50-g glucose test (see Chapter 17).

[J] **Screening for neural tube defects and trisomies**

1. Using **maternal serum α-fetoprotein (MSAFP), human chorionic gonadotropin (hCG),** and **estriol,** many patients at risk for either trisomy 21 or trisomy 18 may be identified (see Chapter 4, triple screen).

  a. Trisomy 21 is associated with low MSAFP and estriol and high hCG; 60 to 70% of patients may be identified.

  b. Trisomy 18 is associated with low levels of all three markers.

2. Elevated MSAFP is seen in 80 to 90% of pregnancies in which a fetal **neural tube defect** is present (e.g., anencephaly and spina bifida). Other disorders that elevate MSAFP are:

  a. Incorrect dates (i.e., pregnancy further along than anticipated)

  b. Multiple gestation

  c. Fetal demise

  d. Abruptio placentae

  e. Other fetal congenital defects (e.g., omphalocele, gastroschisis, and congenital nephrosis)

3. An unexplained elevated MSAFP may be associated with third-trimester complications.

[K] **HBV testing.**   Screening for HBV should be performed to identify fetuses at risk.

1. Identification of pregnant women who are positive for HBV surface antigen (HBsAg) is essential because vertical transmission of HBV is an important cause of acute and chronic hepatitis.

  a. First-trimester screening programs should be instituted to identify seropositive women (0.01 to 5% of pregnant patients are seropositive). The neonates of women who test positive can then be treated with passive and active immunoprophylaxis.

  b. Groups at high risk for HBV seropositivity include intravenous drug users, HIV-positive women, and Southeast Asian women.

2. **Universal immunization** of **all** neonates, even those of HBsAg-negative mothers, has been recommended by the American Academy of Pediatrics. Immunizations should be given at birth, 1 month of age, and 6 months of age.

L **HIV testing.** HIV testing and counseling of all pregnant women are now recommended by the Centers for Disease Control and Prevention.

1. The rate of **mother-to-infant transmission** has been estimated to be 20 to 30%, regardless of maternal symptoms. Infants born to mothers with HIV infection may become infected via contaminated breast milk in utero; during delivery; and after birth.

2. **Zidovudine (AZT)** given to HIV-positive women during pregnancy has been shown to reduce perinatal transmission to 8.3%.

3. **Elective cesarean section** may further reduce the rate of vertical transmission, particularly in patients with higher viral loads.

M **Sickle-cell screen.** This screen is indicated in all patients of African descent. It should also be considered for those of Indo-Pakistani, Caribbean, Mediterranean, Southeast-Asian, or Latin-American descent.

VII **RISK ASSESSMENT AND MANAGEMENT OF RISK IN PREGNANCY**

Risk is determined based on the patient's history, physical examination, and results of laboratory studies on first prenatal visit or subsequent visits.

Table 5-3   Schematic Risk Factor Management: Past Obstetric History

Risk Factor	Maternal/Fetal Risk	Management
Previous ectopic pregnancy	Recurrence, maternal anxiety	Early ultrasound to confirm intrauterine pregnancy
Previous stillbirth or early neonatal death	Risk depends on cause (not all are recurrent)	Try to establish cause; early review and specific management
Infant weight		
≤2 SD	IUGR	Comprehensive fetal ultrasound Ultrasound for weight
≥2 SD	Gestational diabetes Another large fetus	Random glucose at 28 and 32 weeks Vigilance in labor
Congenital anomaly	Possible recurrence	Obtain details/diagnosis, possible prenatal diagnosis
Blood antibodies	Hemolytic disease	Specific protocol
Preeclampsia	Recurrence	Assess renal function Obtain comprehensive fetal ultrasound Carefully check blood pressure
Preterm delivery	Recurrence	Specific plan depending on cause
Uterine scar	Uterine rupture, cesarean section	Review of mode of delivery at 36 weeks
Short labor	Recurrence and neonatal problems (e.g., trauma, asphyxia, hypothermia)	Specific management plan at 36 weeks
Postpartum hemorrhage	Recurrence	Specific plan at 36 weeks

IUGR, intrauterine growth retardation; SD, standard deviation above the mean for gestation.
Modified from James D. Organization of prenatal care and identification of risk. In *High Risk Pregnancy Management Options*. Edited by James DK, Steer PJ, Weiner CP, Genik B. Philadelphia, WB Saunders, 1994.

Table 5-4 Schematic Risk Factor Management: Factors Arising in Pregnancy

Risk Factor	Maternal/Fetal Risk	Management
Vaginal bleeding		
<20 weeks	Miscarriage	Acute referral to hospital; no long-term additional action
>19 weeks	Placenta previa, abruptio placentae	Acute referral to hospital; long-term fetal surveillance
Blood pressure >140/90 mmHg		
>160/100 mmHg or proteinuria	Preeclampsia	Hospital admission and care using predetermined protocol
<160/100 mmHg or proteinuria	Preeclampsia	Day care using predetermined protocol
Multiple pregnancy	Anemia, hypertension, IUGR, preterm delivery, congenital abnormalities	Iron/folate supplements, vigilance for increased blood pressure and preterm uterine activity, comprehensive fetal assessment, more frequent visits
Small for gestational age	IUGR	Fetal assessment using predetermined protocol
Large for gestational age	Large infant and complications, gestational, diabetes, hydramnios, multiple pregnancy	Fetal assessment using predetermined protocol, random glucose
Polyhydramnios	Large infant and complications, abnormal fetus, diabetes	Fetal assessment using predetermined protocol, random glucose
Malpresentation after 35 weeks	Delivery problems	Look for causes, make plan for labor
Reduced fetal movement	Poor maternal perception, fetal disease	Immediate nonstress test and fetal assessment
Preterm rupture of membranes	Preterm labor, amnionitis	Hospital admission and manage with specific protocol
Urinary infection	Pyelonephritis, preterm labor	Treat (5 days), monthly mid-stream urine

IUGR, intrauterine growth retardation.
Modified from James D, Smoleniec J. Identification and management of the at-risk obstetric patient. *Hosp Update* 1992;18:885–890.

A Once an at-risk patient has been identified, a management plan is implemented to prevent adverse outcome; this plan may be empiric or schematic.

1. **Empiric plan.** The obstetrician decides on the specific management plan on a patient-by-patient basis.

2. **Schematic.** The obstetrician implements a specific, predetermined management scheme every time a risk factor is identified. Tables 5-3 and 5-4 present examples of schematic risk factor management protocols based on past obstetric history and complications arising in pregnancy.

B To date, no studies compare empiric versus schematic risk factor management in regards to outcome, although a schematic approach is arguably more scientific.

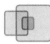

Study Questions for Chapter 5

Directions: Each of the numbered items or incomplete statements in this section is followed by answers or by completions of the statement. Select the ONE lettered answer or completion that is BEST in each case.

1. A 39-year-old woman, gravida 3, para 3 is contemplating pregnancy. She delivered three healthy boys by vaginal delivery at ages 17, 23, and 27 years. Her first pregnancy was complicated by low birth weight. Her second pregnancy was unremarkable. She incurred a third-degree laceration after extension of a midline episiotomy upon delivery of her third boy. Her past medical history is unremarkable other than 3 to 4 asthma exacerbations every month. What is she at highest risk for in her subsequent pregnancy?

- [A] Asthma exacerbation
- [B] Fourth-degree laceration
- [C] Low-birth-weight infant
- [D] Twins
- [E] Uterine dysfunction

2. A 34-year-old primiparous woman is seeing you because she is considering a second pregnancy. She tells you she is afraid to get pregnant given the outcome of her first pregnancy. At 24 years of age, she delivered a term infant with Down syndrome. She wants to file a wrongful birth action because she believes her previous physician did not give her proper genetic counseling or screening for Down syndrome given that a screening test is easy to do and widely available. Had a triple marker screen been performed, which of the following results would have been helpful?

- [A] low MS-AFP, low estriol, low hCG
- [B] low MS-AFP, high estriol, low hCG
- [C] low MS-AFP, low estriol, high hCG
- [D] high MS-AFP, high estriol, low hCG
- [E] high MS-AFP, low estriol, low hCG

3. A 28-year-old woman, gravida 6, para 1 presents to your office because she tested positive on her home pregnancy test. Her last menstrual period occurred 40 days ago. She normally has regular, 28-day cycles and her periods last 3 to 4 days. She delivered a preterm infant with her very first pregnancy at the age of 17 years. Her subsequent pregnancies have been complicated by three miscarriages and an ectopic pregnancy. She denies any medical problems but admits contracting chlamydia during her late teens (which she sought treatment for). Which of the following is the most important initial step in management of this patient?

- [A] Quantitative serum beta hCG
- [B] Triple screen (MS-AFP, estriol, hCG)
- [C] Anticardiolipin antibodies
- [D] Chlamydia antibody levels
- [E] Transvaginal ultrasound

4. A 33-year-old woman, gravida 3, para 2 at 32 weeks' gestation presents to you for her routine prenatal care. She delivered her first baby by cesarean section due to nonreassuring fetal heart rate pattern on the fetal monitor. Her second baby was delivered by cesarean section also because she did not want a trial of labor. Both infants weighed less than 4,000 g and are doing fine now. You obtain operative records of her cesarean sections, which show a Pfannenstiel skin incision and low classical type of incision of the uterus. Currently, she is interested in vaginal delivery. What is the best advice you can give her?

- [A] Vaginal delivery is not recommended because the risk of uterine rupture approaches 8%
- [B] Vaginal delivery is recommended because the risk of uterine rupture is less than 1%

[C] Vaginal delivery is not contraindicated with a history of two previous cesarean sections
[D] Vaginal delivery is a possibility, but risk of rupture is between 0.5% and 4%
[E] Vaginal delivery is a possibility, but risk of uterine rupture is 8%

5. A 41-year-old woman, gravida 8, para 4 at 18 weeks' gestation presents to you for her first prenatal visit. She has a history of three therapeutic abortions as a teenager. She has four healthy children—the first two delivered at 32 weeks' gestation, and her third and fourth children delivered at 37 weeks' gestation. Her past medical history is significant for two episodes of pyelonephritis with her first two pregnancies, as well as a partial bicornuate uterus. What in her history places her at greatest risk for preterm delivery with this pregnancy?

[A] Age
[B] Delivery history
[C] Therapeutic abortions
[D] Pyelonephritis
[E] Uterine anomaly

6. A 25-year-old woman, gravida 2, para 1 at 8 weeks' gestation presents to the high- risk clinic for prenatal care. Her first pregnancy was complicated by delivery of a premature infant with respiratory problems. Her past medical history is remarkable for severe asthma (more than 20 exacerbations per week) for which she uses albuterol and steroid inhalers. She has type II diabetes mellitus that was treated with oral hypoglycemic agents before pregnancy. She also tells you she acquired hepatitis C a few years ago when she used to inject intravenous heroine. She is 5′ 5″ tall and weighs 90 lbs. Her blood pressure is 180/98, and her urine dipstick is negative. Which of the following predisposes her to delivery of an infant with congenital anomalies?

[A] Weight
[B] Liver disease
[C] Diabetes mellitus
[D] Hypertension
[E] Intravenous drug history

Answers and Explanations

1. The answer is D [IV A 2 b (4)]. Maternal age greater than 35 years is at risk for multiple gestation, especially dizygotic. The effect of pregnancy on lung diseases is unpredictable; therefore, you cannot assume that her mild asthma will worsen. A third-degree laceration does not necessarily lead to a fourth-degree laceration in a subsequent pregnancy. Laceration degrees depend on obstetrical factors, such as size of the baby and length of a midline episiotomy. Teenage pregnancies are at risk for delivery of low-birth- weight infants and uterine dysfunction.

2. The answer is C [VI J 1 a]. Trisomy 21 is associated with low MS-AFP, low estriol, and high hCG. It is a screening test that can identify up to 70% of pregnancies with Down syndrome. Triple-marker screens with high MS-AFP are associated with neural tube defects. Triple marker with low levels of all three markers is associated with trisomy 18.

3. The answer is E [IV B 2]. The most important initial step in a patient with a history of an ectopic pregnancy and possible pelvic inflammatory disease history (history of chlamydial infection) who may be pregnant is to perform a transvaginal ultrasound to rule out another ectopic pregnancy and to rule in an intrauterine pregnancy. A quantitative serum β-hCG can be helpful. However, given that patient has had a positive home pregnancy test, an in-office, ultrasensitive urine hCG is sufficient to confirm pregnancy. The triple screen is not useful when performed before 16 weeks' gestation. Anticardiolipin antibodies may be helpful in the future along with other parameters if the patient is interested in delineating the cause of her recurrent spontaneous abortions. Chlamydia antibody levels are not necessary because you already know that the patient has had a chlamydial infection in the past.

4. The answer is A [IV B 7 a (1) and 7 b]. A classical uterine incision (vertical uterine incision through the muscular portion of the uterus) is a contraindication to a trial of labor and vaginal delivery with a subsequent pregnancy. Women with one previous cesarean section are candidates for a vaginal delivery with a subsequent pregnancy, especially if the reason for having the initial cesarean section is non-repetitive (i.e., breech). Currently, not enough data is available to establish the safety of trial of labor with two or more previous transverse uterine scars.

5. The answer is B [IV B 3]. A history of two previous preterm deliveries is the strongest risk factor for spontaneous preterm delivery with a subsequent pregnancy. Premature birth is a risk factor with teenage pregnancies, not advanced maternal age pregnancies. Therapeutic abortions, pyelonephritis, and uterine anomalies are all significant risk factors for spontaneous preterm delivery.

6. The answer is C [IV C 5 a]. Pre-gestational diabetes may increase the risk of birth defects by a factor of three. Anomalies of the heart and central nervous system are the most common problems. The patient with diabetes should be counseled extensively with the aim of achieving good sugar control prior to conception in an attempt to reduce the number of birth defects. Being below ideal body weight does not increase the risk of congenital anomalies. A previous history of intravenous drug use is not significant enough to contribute to congenital anomalies during a current pregnancy. Asthma, hypertension, and liver disease do not increase baseline malformation rate.

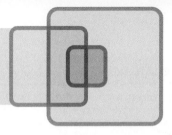

chapter **6**

Prenatal Diagnosis and Obstetric Ultrasound

EMMANUELLE PARE AND SERDAR H. URAL

I INTRODUCTION

The baseline incidence of congenital malformations in the general population is 2 to 3%. Prenatal diagnosis is indicated when the risks of having an affected child exceed this value or when a risk factor for a specific congenital anomaly has been identified.

A **Currently available procedures for prenatal diagnosis.** **Noninvasive** procedures include ultrasound and fetal echocardiography. **Invasive** procedures include preimplantation diagnosis, chorionic villus sampling, amniocentesis, and percutaneous umbilical blood sampling (PUBS).

B **Genetic counseling.** It is important to assess the risk of a woman giving birth to a child with a genetic or congenital birth defect and to interpret this risk. Genetic counseling helps parents make decisions on contraception, sterilization, adoption, artificial insemination, carrier detection, and referrals to agencies concerned with handicapped children, prenatal diagnosis, and pregnancy termination.

II INDICATIONS FOR PRENATAL DIAGNOSIS

A **Chromosomal abnormalities**
1. **Advanced maternal age** (i.e., at least 35 years of age at time of delivery) (Table 6-1)
2. **Previously affected child**
3. **Chromosomal translocation or inversion in either parent**
4. **Abnormal ultrasound findings**
   a. **Congenital malformations** involving a major organ system
   b. **Markers for aneuploidy,** which can be seen in normal fetuses on ultrasound but are observed with an increased frequency in fetuses with chromosomal abnormalities
      (1) Increased nuchal thickness, even isolated, indicates invasive prenatal diagnosis.
      (2) Pyelectasis, echogenic bowel, short femur, or short humerus warrant a detailed ultrasound examination to search for anomalies and other markers but may not require invasive prenatal diagnosis if they are isolated findings.

B **Congenital malformations**
1. **Congenital heart defects** are the most common congenital malformation and occur in 8/1000 live births.
   a. Inheritance is multifactorial.
   b. Risk factors include familial history of congenital heart defects, pregestational maternal diabetes, maternal rubella infection during the first trimester, and exposure to teratogens such as alcohol and some antiseizure medications (e.g., phenytoin).

TABLE 6-1 Relationship of Maternal Age to Occurrence of Trisomy 21	
Maternal Age (Years)	**Occurrence Per Live Births**
15–19	1/1250
20–24	1/1400
25–29	1/1100
30	1/900
35	1/350
40	1/100
45+	1/25

2. **Neural tube defects (NTDs)** are one of the most common congenital malformations and occur in 1 to 2/1000 live births.
   a. Inheritance is multifactorial.
   b. Risks factors include familial history of NTDs, pregestational maternal diabetes, maternal seizure disorder, and maternal intake of some antiseizure medications (e.g., carbamazepine).
   c. The incidence of NTDs may be reduced by maternal folic acid supplementation at least 3 months before conception and during the first 3 months of pregnancy.
      (1) A 0.4-mg dose reduces the incidence of NTDs in the general population by 50%.
      (2) A 4-mg dose reduces the risk of NTD recurrence by 70% in women with a previous affected child.

C Mendelian abnormalities
   1. **Inborn errors of metabolism**
      a. Mucopolysaccharidoses
      b. Mucolipidoses
      c. Lipidoses
      d. Amino acid disorders
      e. Miscellaneous biochemical disorders
   2. **Abnormalities in DNA structure**
      a. Congenital adrenal hyperplasia
      b. Gaucher disease
      c. Ehlers-Danlos types IV, VI, and VII
      d. Niemann-Pick disease
      e. Osteogenesis imperfecta congenita
      f. Xeroderma pigmentosum

D Abnormal maternal serum α-fetoprotein (MSAFP) or multiple markers screen

E Fragile X syndrome.   This condition is the most common cause of inherited mental retardation.
   1. Inheritance is X-linked recessive.
   2. Women who have a child with or a familial history of mental retardation or developmental delay should be tested to see if they carry the mutation, and if so, they should be offered prenatal diagnosis.

III   COMMONLY SCREENED GENETIC DISORDERS

In the United States, universal screening for NTDs and aneuploidy with the triple screen (which includes MSAFP) should be offered during the second trimester to every pregnant woman younger than 35 years of age. After age 35, women have the option of invasive prenatal diagnosis with amniocentesis or chorionic villus sampling. The most common selectively screened genetic disorders are Tay-Sachs disease, sickle cell anemia, and the thalassemias.

A **Tay-Sachs disease.** Congenital absence of the enzyme hexosaminidase A results in an overaccumulation of sphingolipids.

1. Inheritance is autosomal recessive.
2. The carrier rate is 1 in 31 in Ashkenazi Jews and 1 in 277 in non-Ashkenazi Jews. Prenatal diagnosis should be offered if both parents are carriers.

B **Hemoglobinopathies.** Approximately 2 to 2.5 million individuals in the United States have inherited hemoglobin abnormalities.

1. **Normal hemoglobin** is composed of three types of hemoglobin:
   a. Hemoglobin A has two α- and two β-chains and makes up 95% of adult hemoglobin.
   b. Hemoglobin A_2 has two α- and two δ-chains and makes up 2 to 3.5% of adult hemoglobin.
   c. Hemoglobin F has two α- and two γ-chains and makes up the remainder of adult hemoglobin.
2. **Sickle cell screening.** All prospective parents of African descent should undergo sickle cell screening. If the results are positive, hemoglobin electrophoresis is warranted.
   a. Inheritance of **sickle cell disease** is **autosomal recessive.** Prenatal diagnosis should be offered if both parents have **sickle cell trait** (are carriers).
   b. The frequency of sickle cell trait in the adult African-American population is approximately 1 in 12.
   c. **Sickle hemoglobin (HbS)** results from a substitution from glutamic acid to valine at the sixth position in the β-globin chain. In the oxygenated state, HbS functions normally. In the deoxygenated state, hydrophobic bonds are formed, which causes red blood cell distortion, or sickling. This leads to vaso-occlusion, tissue infarction, and anemia.
3. **Thalassemias.** For all individuals at risk, screening should begin with the mean corpuscular volume (MCV). If the MCV is 80 fL or less, patients should undergo hemoglobin electrophoresis (see Chapter 17).
   a. α-thalassemia
   (1) Groups at risk are of Asian, Mediterranean, or African descent.
   (2) Production of the α-globin chains is decreased.
   b. β-thalassemia
   (1) Groups at risk are of Mediterranean, southeast Asian, or African descent.
   (2) Production of the β-globin chains is decreased.

C **Cystic fibrosis.** This disease is the most common inherited disorder in Caucasians.

1. The carrier rate is 1 in 25 in North American Caucasians.
2. Screening is indicated when family history is positive for cystic fibrosis (CF). The most common mutation in the CF gene is ΔF508, which accounts for approximately 70% of mutations found in North American Caucasians. There are more than 800 known mutations in the CF gene, but most laboratories screen for 28–31 mutations, which account for 90 to 95% of mutations in these individuals.
3. Inheritance is autosomal recessive. Prenatal diagnosis should be offered if both parents are carriers.

IV TECHNIQUES OF PRENATAL DIAGNOSIS

A **Maternal markers.** Maternal **serum** may be evaluated for **NTDs, Down syndrome,** and **trisomy 18.**

1. The **MSAFP screen** may be performed at 15 to 22 weeks' gestation.
   a. An **elevated value** is indicative of an increased risk of **NTDs and other disorders** (Table 6-2).
   b. A **low value** indicates an increased risk of **Down syndrome.**

TABLE 6-2   Conditions Characterized by Elevated α-Fetoprotein
Multiple gestation
Bladder extrophy
Congenital nephrosis
Fetal bowel obstruction
Underestimated gestational age
Abdominal wall defects (omphalocele and gastroschisis)
Fetal death
Cystic hygroma
Aneuploidy
Sacrococcygeal teratoma

2. The **multiple markers screen** is offered at the same time as the MSAFP screen. The most widely used multiple markers screen is the **triple screen,** which includes **MSAFP, human chorionic gonadotropin (hCG),** and **estriol.** All three values are adjusted for gestational age and are used in conjunction with maternal age to calculate the risk of Down syndrome and trisomy 18. Amniocentesis is offered when the risk of these chromosomal anomalies is higher than the risk of the procedure itself.

    a. The risk of Down syndrome is increased when MSAFP is decreased, hCG is increased, and estriol is decreased.

    b. The risk of trisomy 18 is increased when the three markers are all lower than normal.

B **Ultrasound.**   This technique, the most commonly used method of pregnancy assessment, is a valuable tool in the prenatal diagnosis of congenital anomalies. Ultrasound uses low-energy, high-frequency sound waves. Transabdominal ultrasounds performed for prenatal diagnosis operate at frequencies between 3.5 and 5 MHz.

1. Safety

    a. Epidemiologic studies in pregnant women have failed to reveal any association of ultrasound with congenital anomalies or adverse pregnancy outcome.

    b. Most instruments used for diagnosis produce energies far lower than the supposedly safe level of ultrasound exposure to tissues.

2. Indications for ultrasound during pregnancy

    a. Evaluation of gestational age

    b. Assessment of fetal viability

    c. Evaluation of multiple gestations

    d. Screening for fetal anomalies, especially in the presence of an abnormal MSAFP or triple screen

    e. Evaluation and follow-up of fetal growth and size

    f. Vaginal bleeding of undetermined etiology

    g. Suspected oligohydramnios or polyhydramnios

    h. Assessment of fetal well-being

    i. Determination of fetal presentation

    j. Guidance during amniocentesis, chorionic villus sampling, or PUBS

    k. Evaluation for ectopic or molar pregnancy

    l. Pelvic mass

3. Ultrasound examinations provide **different information depending on gestational age. Fetal anatomy** is best evaluated during the **second trimester,** and most routine ultrasounds are performed at this time. Although some first-trimester ultrasound examinations are ordered routinely (e.g., for accurate determination of gestational age), most are performed for specific indications, such evaluating a possible ectopic pregnancy. Likewise, third-trimester ultrasound examinations may be routine (e.g., to estimate fetal weight and to detect growth abnormalities); however, most are performed for specific indications, such as evaluating the location of the placenta in the case of third-trimester bleeding.

4. **First-trimester ultrasound** may be performed transvaginally or transabdominally and should:
   a. Document location of the gestational sac. An intrauterine sac is visible transvaginally as early as 5 weeks' gestation.
   b. Document fetal number.
   c. Confirm fetal viability. Fetal **cardiac activity** can be detected transvaginally as early as **6 weeks' gestation.**
   d. Evaluate gestational age. Measurement of the fetal crown–rump length between 6 and 10 weeks' gestation can estimate fetal age within 5 days (Fig. 6-1).
   e. Evaluate the uterus and adnexal structures.

5. **Second-trimester ultrasound** is usually performed transabdominally. It is routinely performed between 16 and 20 weeks' gestation to evaluate fetal anatomy, gestational age, placental location, and amniotic fluid volume.
   a. The **fetal anatomic survey** should include, but not be limited to:
      (1) Intracranial anatomy with visualization of the lateral ventricles, thalamus, and cerebellum
      (2) Face views
      (3) Longitudinal and coronal views of the spine

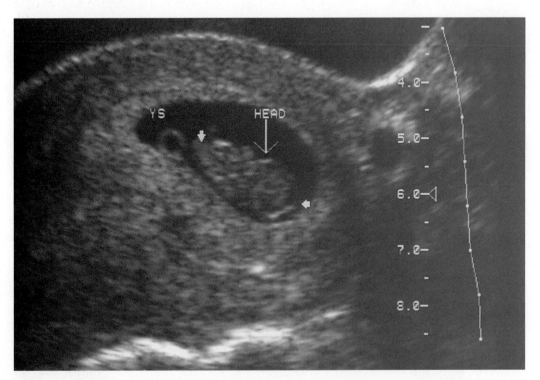

FIGURE 6-1 Ultrasound of the fetal crown–rump length. The fetus is surrounded by amniotic fluid (*dark shadow*). *Thick arrows* = ends of crown–rump length; YS, yolk sac.

      (4) Thorax, diaphragm, and four-chamber view of the heart

      (5) Visualization of the stomach

      (6) Visualization of the kidneys and bladder

      (7) Umbilical cord insertion on an intact abdominal wall and determination of the number of vessels of the umbilical cord (normally two small arteries and one large vein)

      (8) Upper and lower extremities

  b. Fetal biometry includes:

      (1) The **biparietal diameter** (BPD), which is measured at the level of the thalamus and the cavum septum pellucidum. The BPD is the most accurate measurement of gestational age between 12 and 18 weeks' gestation. The correlation of the BPD with gestational age decreases as the pregnancy advances because the biologic variability of fetal head size increases dramatically (Fig. 6-2).

      (2) The **head circumference** is measured at the same level as the biparietal diameter.

      (3) The **abdominal circumference** is measured at the level of the umbilical vein entering the liver.

      (4) The **femur length** is measured.

      (5) Fetal weight may be estimated by composite measurement of the BPD, head circumference, femur length, and abdominal circumference.

  c. Placental location should be assessed. Previa, marginal, or low-lying placenta diagnosed in the second trimester should be reevaluated in the third trimester; many of these conditions resolve.

  d. Amniotic fluid volume can be assessed by semiquantitative methods.

      (1) Measurement of the **deepest single pocket of amniotic fluid**

        (a) If the pocket is less than 2 cm vertically, **oligohydramnios** is present.

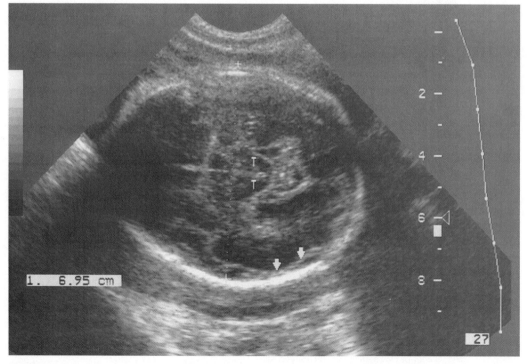

FIGURE 6-2 Ultrasound of a biparietal diameter (6.95 cm) measured between the calipers. T, thalamus (which always points posteriorly); *thick arrows* = edge of sylvian fissure.

TABLE 6-3   Fetal Malformations Associated with Polyhydramnios

Central nervous system
Anencephaly
Hydrocephaly
Encephalocele
Gastrointestinal system
Gastroschisis
Omphalocele
Esophageal atresia
Duodenal atresia
Diaphragmatic hernia
Respiratory system
Cystic adenomatoid malformation of the lung
Chylothorax
Musculoskeletal system
Myotonic dystrophy
Skeletal dysplasia

  (b) If the pocket is 2 to 8 cm vertically, the amniotic fluid volume is adequate.
  (c) If the pocket is more than 8 cm vertically, **polyhydramnios** is present. Polyhydramnios is associated with a higher incidence of congenital abnormalities (Table 6-3).
  (2) The **amniotic fluid index** is calculated by adding the measurements of the vertical depths of amniotic fluid in the four quadrants of the uterus. Normal values range from 6 to 24 cm.
6. **Third-trimester ultrasound** is approached transabdominally.
  a. **Fetal weight** is estimated as previously described (see IV A 5 b [5]). The margin of error is approximately 15% and may be even higher in term fetuses.
    (1) If the estimated fetal weight is below the 10th percentile for gestational age, the fetus is **small-for-gestational age.** Intrauterine growth restriction is suspected.
    (2) If the estimated fetal weight is greater than the 90th percentile for gestational age, the fetus is large-for-gestational age. Macrosomia is suspected.
  (2) **Amniotic fluid volume** is assessed as previously described (see IV A 5 d).
  (3) **Fetal well-being** is assessed using the BPD.
    (a) The **biophysical profile** evaluates **five** components: amniotic fluid volume, fetal tone, fetal movement, fetal breathing, and nonstress test.
    (b) A score of 2 (normal) or 0 (abnormal) is assigned to each component. A total score of 8 to 10 is normal. An abnormal score of less than 8 is managed according to gestational age and clinical situation.

C **Fetal echocardiography.**   This detailed ultrasound examination of the heart is useful in the detection, diagnosis, and follow-up of congenital heart defects and fetal arrhythmias. It is usually performed between 20 and 22 weeks' gestation. Indications include:
1. Risk factors for congenital heart defects (family history of congenital heart defects, maternal diabetes, or exposure to cardiac teratogens)
2. Suspected congenital heart defects on ultrasound examination
3. Suspected fetal arrhythmia on ultrasound examination or heard on Doptone
4. Other congenital anomalies detected on ultrasound examination
5. Nonimmune hydrops fetalis

D **Amniocentesis.** This transabdominal, fine-needle aspiration of amniotic fluid usually involves the removal of 10 to 30 mL of fluid. Amniotic fluid contains fetal cells, which can be cultured and evaluated for chromosomal abnormalities and used for molecular testing. Specific markers can also be measured in the amniotic fluid.

1. Amniocentesis should be performed under **ultrasound guidance.**

2. **Genetic amniocentesis** is usually performed between **15 and 18 weeks'** gestation, at which time ample fluid is present. Diagnostic tests may be performed, and elective termination, if desired by the patient, is still possible.
   a. The **risk of fetal loss** is **0.25% to 0.5%.**
   b. Amniotic fluid can be assessed for MSAFP and acetylcholinesterase levels in the evaluation of NTDs.
   c. Chromosomal abnormalities such as Down syndrome (trisomy 21), trisomy 18, trisomy 13, triploidy, Turner syndrome (45,XO), and Klinefelter syndrome (47,XXY) can be identified.
      (1) Karyotype is obtained from cultured cells, and chromosomes are counted and analyzed for structural alterations.
      (2) Fluorescence in situ hybridization can be used for more rapid identification of additional or missing chromosomes.
   d. DNA of the fetus may be retrieved, and the presence of specific diseases may be detected.
      (1) If the precise molecular basis of the disease is known (e.g., mutation from adenine to guanine in the codon for the sixth amino acid in the gene coding for β-globin), then specific probes may be used.
      (2) If the precise molecular basis of the disease is not known, prenatal diagnosis is still possible in a given family using restriction fragment length polymorphisms. This method can be used for Huntington chorea; adult-onset polycystic kidneys; adrenal 21-hydroxylase deficiency; and some forms of Duchenne muscular dystrophy, hemophilia A or B, and β-thalassemia.

3. **Amniocentesis can also be performed later in pregnancy** for other indications.
   a. The **risk of preterm delivery** from a third-trimester amniocentesis is **1 to 2%.**
   b. The degree of fetal anemia may be evaluated indirectly using spectrophotometry to measure the level of bilirubin in the amniotic fluid, which reflects fetal hemolysis. This method is used in the management of alloimmunization. (see Chapter 17).
   c. Evaluation of fetal lung maturity is performed using the lecithin-to-sphingomyelin ratio and presence of phosphatidyl glycerol.
   d. Diagnosis of in utero infections is warranted if maternal infection has been documented or fetal infection is suspected based on ultrasound examination.

4. Rh-negative women who are not sensitized must receive Rho(D) immune globulin after the procedure.

E **Chorionic villus sampling.** This procedure is usually performed at **10 to 12 weeks'** gestation. Fetal cells can be obtained using either a transabdominal or a transcervical approach. The major benefit of this procedure is earlier prenatal diagnosis.

1. The **risk of fetal loss** is **1%.**

2. The accuracy is comparable to that of amniocentesis.

3. Chromosomal analysis and fetal DNA analysis are possible; however, amniotic fluid levels of markers such as MSAFP cannot be measured with this method.

4. **Limb reduction defects** have been associated with this procedure.

5. Rh-negative women must receive Rho(D) immune globulin after the procedure.

F **Other techniques**

1. **PUBS** or cordocentesis is used to sample fetal blood for karyotype, DNA-based analysis, hemoglobin electrophoresis and diagnosis of fetal infection, anemia, or thrombocytopenia.

    a. PUBS must be performed under ultrasound guidance.

    b. The reported **risk of fetal loss** is **1 to 3%** but varies greatly depending on indication.

    c. Rh-negative women must receive Rho(D) immune globulin after the procedure.

2. **Preimplantation diagnosis** requires the use of in vitro fertilization techniques and is performed on one or two embryo cells at a very early stage.

3. **Fetal skin sampling** may be performed to obtain fetal cells.

Study Questions for Chapter 6

Directions: Each of the numbered items or incomplete statements in this section is followed by answers or by completions of the statement. Select the ONE lettered answer or completion that is BEST in each case.

QUESTIONS 1–2

1. A 32-year-old woman, gravida 1, para 1 presents to you for genetic counseling. Her firstborn had sickle cell disease. She has since remarried and requests prenatal testing. She has no known medical problems. The next best step in management during the appropriate gestational age is

    A Maternal serum α-fetoprotein
    B Second-trimester ultrasound
    C Maternal hemoglobin electrophoresis
    D Paternal hemoglobin electrophoresis
    E Amniocentesis

2. A 23-year-old woman, gravida 1, para 0 at 16 weeks' gestation presents to you because a second-degree relative has Huntington's chorea. She insists on prenatal diagnosis before the fetus reaches viability. The best step in management is

    A Maternal serum α-fetoprotein
    B Amniocentesis
    C Chorionic villus sampling
    D Percutaneous umbilical blood sampling
    E Transabdominal ultrasound

Directions: Choose the laboratory results that have the greatest sensitivity and specificity for detection of the listed condition.

QUESTIONS 3–4

    A Maternal serum–AFP ↓, E3 ↓, hCG ↑
    B Maternal serum–AFP ↑, E3 ↑, hCG ↓
    C Maternal serum–AFP ↓, E3 ↓, hCG ↓
    D Amniotic fluid–AFP ↑, acetylcholinesterase ↑
    E Amniotic fluid–AFP normal, acetylcholinesterase ↑

3. Trisomy 21 (Down syndrome)

4. Meningomyelocele

Directions: Match the statement below with the approximate number above. Each answer may be used once, more than once, or not at all.

QUESTIONS 5–8

A Less than 1
B 1
C 5
D 10
E 20

5. Incidence of congenital heart defect in general population

6. Best gestational age to perform chorionic villus sampling

7. Best gestational age to perform echocardiograph of fetal heart

8. Risk of fetal loss with chorionic villus sampling

Answers and Explanations

1. The answer is D [III B 2]. This woman must be a heterozygous carrier of sickle cell disease since she is asymptomatic and has an affected child (hence, maternal serum electrophoresis is unnecessary). Her previous husband must also be a carrier. Her new husband should undergo hemoglobin electrophoresis to evaluate his carrier status. MSAFP and second-trimester ultrasound cannot detect sickle cell disease. Amniocentesis is too invasive at his point and may not be needed if the new father is not a carrier of sickle cell.

2. The answer is B [IV D 2 d 2]. At 16 weeks of gestation, the best test to perform is an amniocentesis and not a chorionic villus sampling (which is usually performed between 10 and 12 weeks of gestation). A genetic amniocentesis and then restriction fragment polymorphisms can diagnose Huntington's chorea. Percutaneous umbilical blood sampling has a high fetal loss rate (approximately 3%) and thus is not preferable to amniocentesis for this diagnosis. There is no way to diagnose Huntington's chorea by maternal serum alpha-fetoprotein (MS-AFP) or transabdominal ultrasound.

3. A [IV A] **4. D** [IV D 2 b]. The risk of Down syndrome is increased when the α-fetoprotein and estriol levels are lower than normal and the hCG is higher than normal. Amniotic fluid acetylcholinesterase and α-fetoprotein levels are more sensitive and specific than MS-AFP in predicting neural tube defects (meningomyelocele is an example of a NTD).

5. A [II B 1] **6. D** [IV E] **7. E** [IV C] **8. B** [IV E 1]. The incidence of congenital heart defect (which is the most common congenital malformation) is 8 in 1000 or 0.8. The best gestational age to perform chorionic villus sampling is 10 to 12 weeks. The best time to do a fetal echocardiograph is between 20 and 22 weeks. The risk of fetal loss with chorionic villus sampling is 1% (which is slightly higher than with amniocentesis).

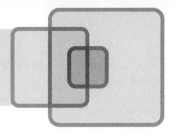

chapter 7

Teratology

DORIS CHOU AND GEORGE A. MACONES

I   INTRODUCTION

Teratology is the **study of abnormal fetal development.** Major birth defects occur in approximately 3% of all deliveries. A teratogenic agent, which can be identified in less than 50% of the cases, is any chemical (drug), infection, physical condition, or deficiency that, on fetal exposure, can alter fetal morphology or subsequent function. Teratogenicity appears to be related to genetic predisposition (both maternal and embryonic), the developmental stage of the fetus at the time of exposure, and the route and length of administration of the teratogen. Because any woman in her reproductive years may be pregnant, all women should be warned of any teratogenic potential associated with a drug. In cases of known teratogens, women and their physicians have a responsibility to effectively prevent pregnancy.

A **Genetic susceptibility.**   Species differences in response to teratogens have been demonstrated. Human newborns exposed to the tranquilizer thalidomide in utero demonstrated major malformation of the arms (phocomelia), whereas laboratory animals (rats) showed no effect at similar doses. Animal studies, although helpful, do not always reliably predict the response in humans.

B **Developmental stage at time of exposure**   (Fig. 7-1). Susceptibility of the conceptus to teratogenic agents depends on the developmental stage at the time of exposure.

1. **Resistant period.** From day 0 to day 11 of gestation (postovulation), the fetus exhibits the "all or none" phenomenon with regard to major anomalies; that is, it will either be killed by the insult or survive unaffected. This is the period of predifferentiation when the aggregate of totipotential cells can recover from an injury and continue to multiply.

2. **Maximum susceptibility (embryonic period).** From days 11 to 57 of gestation, the fetus is undergoing organ differentiation and, at this time, is most susceptible to the adverse effects of teratogens. The particular malformation depends on the time of exposure. After a certain time in organogenesis, it is thought that abnormal embryogenesis can no longer occur. For example, because the neural tube closes between days 22 and 28 postconception (5 weeks after the last menstrual period), a teratogen must be active before or during this period to initiate development of a neural tube defect (e.g., spina bifida or anencephaly).

3. **Lowered susceptibility (fetal period).** After 57 days (8 weeks) of gestation, the organs have formed and are increasing in size. A teratogen at this stage may cause a reduction in cell size and number, which is manifested by:
   a. Growth retardation
   b. Reduction of organ size
   c. Functional derangements of organ systems

C **Administration of teratogen.**   The route and length of administration of a teratogen alter the type and severity of the malformation produced. Abnormal developments increase in frequency and degree as the dosage increases. Agents may be less teratogenic if systemic blood levels are reduced by the route of administration (e.g., poor gastrointestinal antibiotic absorption may account for lower blood levels in pregnancy).

D **Definition.** Teratogenicity of an agent or factor is defined by the following criteria:

1. **Presence of the agent during the critical period of development when the anomaly is likely to appear.** Malformations are caused by intrinsic problems within the developing tissues at a specific time in organogenesis.

2. **Production of the anomaly in experimental animals when the agent is administered during a stage of organogenesis similar to that of humans.** Teratogenicity may not become apparent for several years; for example, in utero exposure to diethylstilbestrol is known to cause genital tract abnormalities, such as adenosis and carcinoma, but these abnormalities may not become apparent until the reproductive years.

3. **Ability of the agent to act on the embryo or fetus either directly or indirectly through the placenta.** For example, heparin is not teratogenic because, unlike warfarin, it cannot cross the placenta because of its large molecular weight.

E **Structural defects.** These defects have been categorized into three groups (Fig. 7-2).

1. **Malformations** are morphologic defects of an organ or other part of the body resulting from an abnormality in the process of development in the first trimester. This leads to incomplete or aberrant morphogenesis (e.g., ventricular septal defect).

2. **Deformations** are abnormal forms, shapes, or positions of a body part caused by constraint within the uterus, usually occurring in the second or third trimester. An example is club feet from oligohydramnios.

3. **Disruptions** are defects from interference with a normally developing organ system, usually occurring later in gestation (i.e., in the second or third trimester, after organogenesis). An example is amniotic band syndrome.

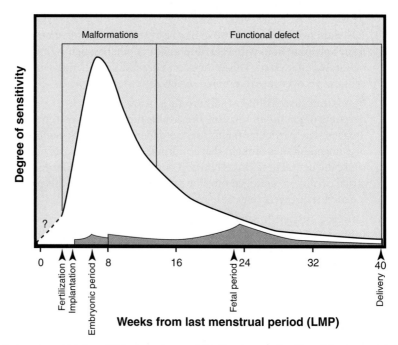

FIGURE 7-1 Embryonic and fetal sensitivity to environmental influences as a function of developmental state. (Reprinted with permission from Creasy RK, Resnik R. Maternal–Fetal Medicine: Principles and Practice. Philadelphia: WB Saunders, 1984:95.)

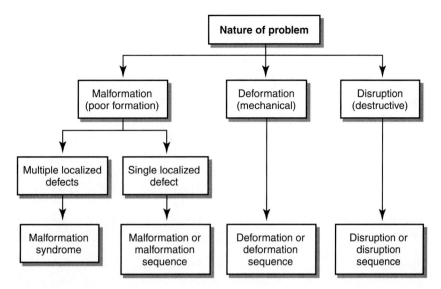

FIGURE 7-2 Categories of structural defects. (Adapted from Graham JM, Jr. Smith's Recognizable Patterns of Human Deformation. Philadelphia: WB Saunders, 1988:4.)

II TERATOGENIC AGENTS

A Ionizing radiation

1. **Acute high dose (more than 250 rad).** The dose of radiation and the gestational age during exposure are predictive of the adverse neonatal effects: microcephaly, mental retardation, and growth retardation. For example, the in utero victims of the atomic explosions in Hiroshima and Nagasaki have suffered from both birth defects and leukemia. However, follow-up studies have shown that most children with these adverse effects were those exposed before 15 weeks' gestation, during the period of organogenesis, whereas most of the children exposed during the third trimester had growth retardation but normal intelligence.

   a. **Time of exposure.** Fetal effects depend on the gestational age (postovulation) at the time of exposure.

      (1) At 2 to 4 weeks, either the fetus is normal or a spontaneous abortion occurs.

      (2) At 4 to 12 weeks, microcephaly, mental retardation, cataracts, growth retardation, or microphthalmia may occur.

      (3) At 12 to 16 weeks, mental retardation or growth retardation occurs.

      (4) After 20 weeks, the effects are the same as with postnatal exposure and include hair loss, skin lesions, and bone marrow suppression.

   b. **Dose effect**

      (1) After exposure to less than 5 rad, and probably less than 10 rad, an adverse fetal outcome is unlikely to result.

      (2) After exposure to 10 to 25 rad, there some adverse fetal effects may result.

      (3) After exposure to more than 25 rad, classic fetal effects, including growth retardation, structural malformations, and fetal resorption, may be detected. At this level of exposure, elective abortion should be offered as an option.

2. **Chronic low dose**

   a. In **diagnostic radiation,** the dose to the conceptus should be calculated by the hospital's radiation biologist (Table 7-1). Such a dose rarely adds up to significant exposure, even if several radiographic studies are performed.

TABLE 7-1   Doses to the Uterus and Embryo for Common Radiologic Procedures

Study	View	Dose/View (mrad)	Films/Study	Dose/Study (mrad)
Skull	AP, PA	<0.01		
	Lat	<0.01	4.1	<0.05
Chest	AP, PA	0.01–0.05	1.5	0.02–0.07
	Lat	0.01–0.03		
Mammogram	CC	0.1–0.5	4.0	
	Lat	3–5		7–20
Lumbar spine	AP (7″ × 17″)	30–58	2.9	51–126
	14″ × 17″			
	Lat	33–65		
		11–32		
Lumbosacral	AP	92–187	3.4	168–359
spine	PA	40–97		
	Lat	12–33		
Abdomen	AP	80–163	1.7	122–245
	PA	23–55		
	Lat	29–82		
Intravenous pyelogram	AP	130–264	5.5	686–1398
	PA	43–104		
	Lat	13–37		
Retrograde pyelogram	AP	109–220	1.0	
Hip	AP	72–140	2.0	103–213
	Lat	18–51		

   b. **Associated risk of teratogenicity**
      (1) The mutagenic effects of radiation, if present, have proved to be very small. The estimated risk of leukemia for children exposed in utero to radiation during maternal radiographic pelvimetry increases from 1 in 3000 among unexposed children to 1 in 2000.
      (2) The results of several studies provide no conclusive evidence linking preconception low-dose radiation exposure with an increased risk of delivering an infant with a chromosomal abnormality.
   3. **Radioactive iodine.** Radiation exposure from radioisotopes administered internally for organ visualization is roughly equal to that of radiographic procedures; however, after the tenth week of gestation, fetal thyroid development can be retarded in addition to any adverse effects of radiation.

B **Drugs and medications.**   In the United States, surveys show that 45 to 95% of pregnant women ingest either over-the-counter or prescription drugs other than iron and vitamins during their pregnancy. Many are taken before a woman realizes that she is pregnant or are taken without the advice of a physician. The prohibition of all medications during pregnancy is impossible and is likely to be more harmful to the patient. However, the issue of whether a medication is harmful to the fetus is raised in most pregnancies. Physicians caring for women of childbearing age should be aware of potential teratogenicity of medications and should be able to address questions arising from the accidental or intentional ingestion of drugs during pregnancy.
   1. Approximately 3 to 5% of newborns have **congenital malformations** caused by a host of environmental and genetic factors, most of which are unable to be identified. Drugs and medications account for less than 1% of these malformations.

2. **Access to the fetoplacental unit** is critical in the causation of developmental anomalies. Factors affecting access of the drug or medication to the fetus include:
   a. Maternal absorption
   b. Drug metabolism
   c. Protein binding and storage
   d. Molecular size (molecules with a molecular weight of more than 1000 dalton do not cross the placenta easily)
   e. Electrical charge
   f. Lipid solubility

3. **Animal research** can help identify teratogenic potential, but results may be misleading because of species variation.
   a. The most striking example is **thalidomide,** in which exposure in the animals tested (mice and rats) failed to produce limb defects but caused severe limb reduction defects in humans, monkeys, and rabbits. Although the thalidomide-associated embryopathy led to the belief that human teratogenicity could not be predicted by animal studies, it is erroneous.
   b. **Every drug found to be teratogenic in humans has subsequently been shown to cause similar defects in animals,** although species variation exists. It is worth noting that drugs that cause teratogenesis in animals often do so at much higher doses than used clinically in humans, where similar outcome are not seen. Of the 1600 drugs that have been tested in animals, about one half cause congenital anomalies; however, there are only 30 documented human teratogens.

4. **Human research.** Case reports once suggested that drugs such as warfarin, diethylstilbestrol, and isotretinoin were teratogenic. Other studies have led to the "mislabeling" of safe drugs (e.g., Bendectin). Pharmaceutical companies also play a role in the identification of teratogens by participating in postmarketing surveillance studies. To learn more about the teratogenic effects of certain drugs, women can call centers that monitor exposure to prescription and over-the-counter medications.
   a. **Formal epidemiologic studies** are designed to assess whether mothers who took a drug during pregnancy have larger numbers of malformed children than those who did not (cohort studies) or whether mothers of children with a specific malformation took the drug more often than mothers of children without the malformation (case-control studies). Long-term studies are also important; it is becoming increasingly clear that adverse affects of drugs on neurodevelopmental behavior may be more serious than structural defects.
   b. Difficulties occur with the study of teratogens. Because most malformations occur rarely, large sample sizes of exposed individuals are necessary. Maternal illnesses that require the use of medications may be a confounding factor in the study of the teratogenicity of any drug used to treat that disorder. Recall bias also confounds the study of drugs and their potential teratogenic affects, because women whose children have abnormalities are much more likely to recall an exposure (especially in case-control studies).

5. **Risk factors for adverse fetal effects** have been assigned to all drugs based on the teratogenic risk that the drug poses to the fetus. The Food and Drug Administration has proposed the following classification scheme, which is generally accepted by manufacturers and authors (see Chapter 4).

6. **Known teratogenic drugs.** The list of proven teratogens is surprisingly short. Certain commonly used agents should be avoided even while a patient is trying to conceive. These include the vitamin A isomer isotretinoin or doses of vitamin A higher than 8000 IU daily; alcohol; excess caffeine; and some of the sex steroids. The live virus vaccines, such as rubella, should never be prescribed if a patient is possibly pregnant or planning to conceive within 3 months. However, if the aforementioned drugs are inadvertently given, the outcome is still usually favorable.

7. A **dose threshold** is a theoretic dose for each teratogen below which no adverse effects have been noted.

8. **"Recreational" drugs** (see Chapter 8). Because most recreational drugs are taken with other agents, such as alcohol or tranquilizers, the precise effect is difficult to ascertain. Listed below are commonly used drugs and their potential effects.

   a. **Alcohol.** Consumption of alcohol in pregnancy is the most common known teratogenic cause of mental retardation. Both abortion and stillbirth are increased in heavy drinkers. **Fetal alcohol syndrome,** which manifests as mental retardation, growth retardation, abnormal facies, ocular and joint anomalies, and cardiac defects, has been associated with the ingestion of 1 oz or more of absolute alcohol per day.

      (1) The **threshold dose** of alcohol (the point at which congenital anomalies are induced) is unknown; therefore, alcohol consumption in pregnancy can never be regarded as "safe."

      (2) **Early exposure.** The critical period for facial dysmorphology has been found to be around the time of conception.

      (3) **Late exposure.** Exposure late in gestation or in small quantities may result in isolated effects, such as learning or behavioral disorders.

      (4) **Heavy alcohol consumption** (more than 3 oz of absolute alcohol or six drinks daily) is associated with some or all of the features of fetal alcohol syndrome, including:

         (a) **Prenatal or postnatal growth retardation.** Growth retardation is usually prenatal in onset, but postnatal catch-up generally does not occur. It is manifested by decreased birth weight, length, and head circumference.

         (b) **Central nervous system (CNS) involvement** includes small brain size and brain malformations. Functional deficits, such as moderate mental retardation, delayed motor development, poor coordination, tremulousness, hyperactivity, and poor attention spans, have been noted.

         (c) **Characteristic facial dysmorphology** includes a shortened palpebral fissure (observed in more than 90% of affected children); a short, upturned nose; a hypoplastic maxilla; and a thinned upper lip. One study linked craniofacial abnormalities with prenatal alcohol exposure in a dose-response manner.

      (5) **Risk of fetal alcohol syndrome.** A large number of children whose mothers drank moderately or heavily during pregnancy may exhibit features of prenatal alcohol exposure, such as developmental delay, but not the full-blown syndrome.

         (a) Approximately 30% of children born to chronic alcoholic women have fetal alcohol syndrome.

         (b) The risk of major or minor congenital anomalies in infants of mothers who ingest excessive amounts of alcohol but do not meet the criteria for chronic alcoholism is around 32%.

         (c) Intrauterine fetal growth retardation is increased 2.7 times in pregnant women who drink excessively.

   b. **Marijuana.** There is no evidence that smoking marijuana is teratogenic, although the adverse effects of smoking in pregnancy should not be overlooked (see Chapter 8).

   c. **Heroin** has not been shown to cause birth defects, but the drugs that are often taken with heroin are associated with congenital anomalies. The principal adverse fetal effect in heroin addicts is severe neonatal withdrawal, causing death in 3 to 5% of neonates. Methadone is used to replace heroin, and, although it is not teratogenic, it is associated with severe neonatal withdrawal.

   d. **Phencyclidine (PCP),** or "angel dust," is a hallucinogenic agent associated with facial abnormalities in a small percentage of exposed infants.

   e. **Cocaine** is rapidly becoming the most abused drug in pregnancy, second only to alcohol. One study showed an increased risk of congenital malformations, stillbirths, and low-birth-weight infants in cocaine users. A clear causal relationship exists between cocaine use and abruptio placentae because of the drug's vasoconstrictive properties (see Chapter 9).

9. **Cancer chemotherapy.** Although there is a high incidence of fetal loss, including spontaneous abortion and stillbirth, the incidence of congenital malformations is surprisingly low.
   a. When cancer chemotherapy is administered during the first trimester of pregnancy, there are varied and unpredictable effects, ranging from severe deformity to no abnormality.
   b. After the period of organogenesis, there is no teratogenic risk from chemotherapy in pregnancy.

C **Hyperthermia.** Studies suggest that sustained maternal hyperthermia (body temperature of more than 102°F [38.9°C] for more than 24 hours between 4 and 14 weeks' gestation), rather than spiking fevers, is teratogenic. Malformations noted in infants of mothers who were febrile from infectious agents or who frequented saunas in the first trimester include the following:

1. Growth restriction

2. CNS defects, such as mental deficiency, microcephaly, hypotonia, and anencephaly, and increased risk of neural tube defects

3. Facial anomalies, including midfacial hypoplasia, cleft lip and palate, microphthalmia, micrognathia, and external ear anomalies

4. Minor limb anomalies, such as syndactyly

D **Maternal medical disorders.** Women with medical disorders should be counseled about the teratogenic risks both from the condition being treated and from the treatment. In some cases, the untreated medical disorder poses greater risks to the fetus than the teratogenic potential of the specific drug therapy.

1. **Diabetes mellitus.** Infants of insulin-dependent diabetic mothers have up to a 22% incidence of cardiac, renal, gastrointestinal, CNS, and skeletal malformations. Most of the malformations occur between the third and sixth week postconception and are increased if there is hyperglycemia during that stage of gestation.
   a. The level of risk may be estimated by obtaining glycosylated hemoglobin (hemoglobin A_{Ic}) in the first trimester. Levels greater than 8% (depending on the laboratory) have been associated with a significantly increased risk. Strict glucose control preconceptually has been shown to decrease the frequency of malformations.
   b. Two particular **malformations** are found in infants of diabetic mothers:
      (1) **Caudal regression syndrome** with hypoplasia of the caudal spine and lower extremities.
      (2) **Congenital heart disease,** most commonly ventricular septal defects.
   c. Because neural tube defects occur more frequently in infants of diabetic mothers, maternal serum α-fetoprotein (MSAFP) screening should be performed at 16 weeks' gestation. An extensive anatomic survey by ultrasound at 18 to 22 weeks' gestation should identify most of the major anomalies (i.e., cardiac and spinal defects) in an affected fetus.

2. **Hypothyroidism.** This endocrine disorder has been associated with a twofold increase in stillbirths and congenital anomalies. Cretinism is the result of maternal, fetal, and neonatal thyroid hormone deficiency in iodine-poor areas. Severe cretinism is characterized by mental retardation, deaf mutism, spasticity, strabismus, and abnormal sexual maturation. Congenital hypothyroidism occurs in severely iodine deficient areas. Maternal subclinical hypothyroidism has recently been observed to possibly decrease several points of IQ scores in their offspring.

3. **Phenylketonuria (PKU).** This genetic disorder is characterized by a deficiency of phenylalanine hydroxylase, a liver enzyme that catalyzes the conversion of phenylalanine to tyrosine. The resulting high levels of phenylalanine in maternal serum result in high levels in the fetus. A special diet low in phenylalanine beginning before conception can prevent the adverse effects (mental retardation) of this disorder. Children born to mothers with PKU who have neglected their special diets are at risk for the following conditions:
   a. Mental retardation (92% incidence)
   b. Microcephaly (73% incidence)

    c. Congenital heart disease (12% incidence)

    d. Low birth weight (40% incidence)

4. Virilizing tumors (arrhenoblastoma). This condition can have masculinizing effects on the mother and produce pseudohermaphroditic changes in the female fetus, including fusion of the labia and clitorimegaly.

5. Epilepsy. This condition is a classic example of the contribution of a disease process and its treatment to an increase in birth defects. Management of epilepsy is complicated by the fear that anticonvulsants may cause fetal abnormalities.

    a. In general, infants born to epileptic mothers have a **6 to 7% incidence of major and minor congenital abnormalities.**

    b. The **most commonly observed malformations** in infants of mothers who take anticonvulsants are **cleft lip, cleft palate, and congenital heart disease.** Some studies have suggested that increased seizure frequency leads to higher incidence of malformations. Other research has indicated that malformations may also be inherent to the seizure disorder itself; mothers who take phenytoin for indications other than epilepsy did not have a higher incidence of malformations.

6. Psychotropic drug use in pregnancy. Most psychotropic medications readily cross the placenta. Although no psychotropic drug has yet been specifically approved for use in pregnancy, continued use of the agent may prevent maternal relapse of psychiatric disease. Studies of patients taking antipsychotic medications show that the rate of malformation in exposed patients is similar to that in unexposed patients; however, the rate is still approximately two times that in the general population. This suggests that some other factor may be responsible for the higher incidence of malformations.

    a. Lithium has been associated with 10 to 20 times the normal rate of Ebstein anomaly after first-trimester exposure.

    b. Benzodiazepines are associated with a very small (less than 1%) risk of associated cleft anomalies.

    E **Infections.** Exposure to viral infections during gestation has been recognized as a significant cause of birth defects. Most infants, if infected during the first trimester, suffer from a syndrome of congenital malformations and are small for gestational age.

1. Rubella virus (German measles). When rubella infections occur in the first month of pregnancy, there is a 50% chance of anomalous development. This chance decreases to 22% in the second month and to 6 to 10% in the third to fourth month. The timing of infection is important. If infection occurs during week 6, cataracts may form. Deafness occurs when infection takes place between weeks 7 and 8. If a mother is infected at the time of delivery, the newborn may contract pneumonitis or encephalitis. **Congenital rubella syndrome** includes the following symptoms:

    a. Neuropathologic changes

        (1) Microcephaly

        (2) Mental and motor retardation

        (3) Meningoencephalitis

    b. Cardiovascular lesions

        (1) Persistent patent ductus arteriosus

        (2) Pulmonary artery stenosis

        (3) Atrioventricular septal defects

    c. Ocular defects

        (1) Cataracts

        (2) Microphthalmia

        (3) Retinal changes

        (4) Blindness

    d. Inner ear problems, resulting in sensorineural deafness

    e. Symmetric **intrauterine growth retardation**

2. **Cytomegalovirus (CMV).** This ubiquitous virus infects 1 to 2% of all infants in utero. Between 1 in 5000 to 20,000 infants suffer severe problems that are recognizable at birth.

    a. The risk of severe complications is much greater for infants of mothers who had a primary infection in pregnancy compared with those who had a recurrent infection.

        (1) Seronegative mothers infected with primary CMV transmit the infection to the fetus in 30 to 40% of cases. Of those infected, 2 to 4% are severely symptomatic at birth.

        (2) Seropositive mothers who have a recurrent infection transmit the infection to the fetus in only 1% of cases, and 99% of these infants appear normal at birth. Later in life, these affected infants may suffer from delayed speech development and learning difficulties due to sensorineural hearing loss. A small group has chorioretinitis.

    b. A specific relation between time of exposure and subsequent deficit has not been demonstrated, although the most damage seems to occur early in pregnancy. Gestational age at the time of exposure does not appear to influence the rate of fetal infection. The neonatal effects of fetal CMV infection include the following:

        (1) Microcephaly and hydrocephaly

        (2) Chorioretinitis

        (3) Hepatosplenomegaly

        (4) Cerebral calcification

        (5) Mental retardation

        (6) Heart block

        (7) Petechiae

3. **Herpes simplex virus type 2 (HSV-2).** Although mucocutaneous herpetic infection is common, less than 1 in 7500 infants suffer from perinatal transmission of HSV-2. Fetal transmission occurs by hematogenous spread during a maternal viremia or by direct contact during passage through an infected birth canal; however, congenital infection, which causes fetal malformations, is rare. It is thought that fetal infection during the first trimester results in miscarriage. In a few cases, a syndrome was described that resembled other infants with viral infections during the first trimester, including the following fetal anomalies:

    a. Growth retardation

    b. Microcephaly

    c. Chorioretinitis

    d. Cerebral calcification

    e. Microphthalmia encephalitis

4. **Toxoplasmosis.** This disease, which is caused by a protozoan, *Toxoplasma gondii*, may be transmitted from mother to fetus antepartum. Although infection is most common outside the United States (e.g., in Sweden), the incidence of congenital infection in the United States ranges from 1 to 6 cases per 1000 live births. Approximately 30% of infected women transmit the disease to their unborn children. The disease can be contracted by changing infected cat litter or eating poorly cooked meat. In a population of 550 French women who acquired toxoplasmosis during pregnancy, 61% of the neonates had evidence of congenital infection; of these neonates, 6% died, 5% had severe clinical illness, 9% had mild disease, and 41% had subclinical disease.

    a. Fetal infection early in pregnancy increases the severity of infection.

        (1) The pregnancy may result in a spontaneous abortion, perinatal death, severe congenital anomalies, abnormal growth, and residual handicaps.

        (2) In severe disease, the characteristic triad of anomalies includes chorioretinitis; hydrocephaly or microcephaly; and cerebral calcification, resulting in psychomotor retardation.

    b. Transmission to the fetus is more likely later in pregnancy, although the neonatal handicap is much more benign and, in fact, is often subclinical.

5. **Syphilis** (*Treponema pallidum*). The incidence of syphilis in pregnant women is increasing. The rise in congenital syphilis has paralleled the increase in primary and secondary syphilis in adults. Several hundred cases of congenital syphilis are diagnosed each year; half of these infants are born to women with no prenatal care. *T. pallidum* appears to be able to cross the placenta at any time during pregnancy. Because the fetus has an immature immune system, it is rarely infected before 16 to 18 weeks' gestation. Before this time, antibiotic therapy is highly successful.

   a. The incidence of congenital infection is inversely proportional to the duration of maternal infection and to the degree of spirochetemia.

      (1) Recent or secondary infection in the mother confers the greatest risk of fetal infection. All infants born to women with primary and secondary infection are infected, but 50% are asymptomatic.

      (2) Only 40% of infants born to women with early latent disease are infected, and the incidence drops to 5 to 15% for late latent infection.

   b. In utero infection may result in:

      (1) Preterm delivery or miscarriage

      (2) Stillbirth

      (3) Neonatal death in up to 50% of affected infants

      (4) Congenital infection (asymptomatic or symptomatic), which, when symptomatic, can manifest as:

         (a) Hepatosplenomegaly

         (b) Joint swelling

         (c) Skin rash

         (d) Anemia

         (e) Jaundice

         (f) Snuffles

         (g) Metaphyseal dystrophy

         (h) Periostitis

         (i) Cerebrospinal fluid changes

   c. **Adequate antibiotic therapy** for the pregnant woman is generally thought to provide adequate therapy for the unborn child. However, several case reports have described congenitally infected infants born to mothers treated with benzathine penicillin G. The risk of treatment failure appears to be greater for women who are treated for secondary syphilis or who are in the last trimester of pregnancy.

6. **Varicella zoster virus (VZV).** This condition, which can take the form of **chickenpox** and, later, **herpes zoster,** is an uncommon virus, occurring in 1 to 7 of 10,000 pregnancies. The infection is much more severe in adults than in children, and pregnancy does not seem to alter this risk. Transplacental transmission of VZV is now well documented and occurs in about 24% of cases after maternal varicella in the last month of pregnancy and in 0% of cases of maternal zoster (see II E 6 c). The frequency of fetal infection in the first trimester is less than 5%.

   a. Inconclusive reports have described an increased risk of leukemia in infants born with gestational varicella. One case also describes chromosome breaks in the leukocytes of a child whose mother had varicella in pregnancy.

   b. Multiple cases of congenital malformations may occur in the offspring of women who have chickenpox during the first 20 weeks of pregnancy. These include abnormalities of several organ systems.

      (1) **Cutaneous**

         (a) Cicatricial skin scarring with denuded skin and limb hypoplasia

         (b) Vesicular rash (hemorrhagic rash) if infection occurs in the last 3 weeks of pregnancy

      (2) **Musculoskeletal**

         (a) Limb hypoplasia (unilateral) involving the arm, mandible, or hemithorax

         (b) Rudimentary digits

         (c) Club foot

    (3) **Neurologic**
      (a) Microcephaly
      (b) Cortical and cerebellar atrophy
      (c) Seizures
      (d) Psychomotor retardation
      (e) Focal brain calcifications
      (f) Autonomic dysfunction, such as loss of bowel and bladder control, dysphagia, and Horner syndrome
      (g) Ocular abnormalities, such as microphthalmia, optic atrophy, cataracts, and chorioretinitis
    (4) **Other**
      (a) Symmetric intrauterine growth retardation
      (b) Fever, vesicular rash, pneumonia, and widespread necrotic lesions of the viscera, leading to death if infection occurs in the last 3 weeks of pregnancy
  c. No good evidence proves that **herpes zoster** causes congenital anomalies. A few case reports have described microcephaly, microphthalmia, cataracts, and talipes equinovarus in infants born to mothers suffering from zoster during pregnancy; however, these cases may represent chance occurrences.

7. Mumps. Mumps infection is not strictly teratogenic; however, after maternal exposure, neonates have been born with endocardial fibroelastosis, ear and eye malformations, or urogenital abnormalities.

8. Enteroviruses (Coxsackie B). Serious or fatal illness (40%) in the fetus results from maternal exposure to Coxsackie B virus. Surviving infants may exhibit cardiac malformations; hepatitis, pneumonitis, or pancreatitis; or adrenal necrosis.

Study Questions for Chapter 7

Directions: *Each of the numbered items or incomplete statements in this section is followed by answers or by completions of the statement. Select the ONE lettered answer or completion that is BEST in each case.*

1. A 23-year-old woman who was seen in the emergency department yesterday for a superficial gunshot wound to the wrist tested positive on a routine serum β-hCG screen. Her cycles have always been regular and occur every 28 days and 4 days in duration. She believes she is on day 23 of her current cycle. She denies past medical history. She does not smoke or consume any alcohol. She does take mega doses of vitamins, which include 20,000 IU of vitamin A daily. Which of the following is the most likely outcome of this pregnancy?

 [A] Facial abnormalities
 [B] Myelomeningocele
 [C] Cataracts
 [D] Fetal demise
 [E] Ventricular septal defect

2. A 28-year-old woman, gravida 2, para 1 at 11 weeks of gestation who just moved from another state is seeing you for her first prenatal visit. She has an idiopathic respiratory disease that predisposes her to recurrent lung infections. She tells you that she can't even count how many radiographs she has received in the last 2 months. You contact her previous hospital's radiation biologist who calculates her radiation exposure at approximately 260 mrad. Which of the following is the likely possible outcome of this pregnancy?

 [A] No adverse outcome
 [B] Growth retardation
 [C] Spontaneous abortion
 [D] Bone marrow suppression
 [E] Mental retardation

3. A 28-year-old woman just tested positive on a home pregnancy test even though she and her husband use condoms regularly. Her last menstrual period was 36 days ago. Her periods usually occur every 30 days. Her past medical history is unremarkable and she denies use of tobacco, alcohol, or drugs. Her only concern is that 3 weeks ago she received a Rubella vaccine and was told by her doctor to not become pregnant for the next 3 months after administration of the vaccine. Which of the following is the best advice?

 [A] You should schedule an elective termination as soon as possible
 [B] You have the option of having a therapeutic abortion within the first trimester
 [C] Rubella vaccine is not harmful to your fetus
 [D] Pregnancy outcome is usually favorable even after exposure to this vaccine
 [E] Live viral vaccines are associated with a fourfold increased risk of malformation

4. A 19-year-old woman, gravida 1, para 0 presents to you at 7 weeks of gestation by her last menstrual period for prenatal care. Her history and physical examination are completely unremarkable. You educate her about nutrition and exercise during pregnancy and perform an in-office transvaginal ultrasound to confirm her gestational age. You then order routine prenatal labs. While chatting with her, you discover that she has a stressful job and likes to use the hot tub at least several times a day in excess of 4 hours. What is the best advice to give to this patient?

 [A] You should not use hot tubs during pregnancy
 [B] Hot tub use in pregnancy is associated with fetal growth restriction
 [C] Minimize hot tub use in the first trimester because it may cause malformations

[D] Hot tub use during pregnancy is acceptable as long as it is in short intervals
[E] Hot tub use is acceptable as long as water temperature is below 102.5°F

QUESTIONS 5–9

Match the statement below with the teratogenic agent above that best describes it. Each answer may be used once, more than once, or not at all.
[A] Rubella
[B] Cytomegalovirus
[C] Herpes simplex
[D] Herpes zoster
[E] Mumps

5. Persistent patent ductus arteriosus

6. Endocardial fibroelastosis

7. Triad of heart, eye, and ear defects or malformations

8. Skin scarring and shortened limbs

9. Infection during labor may cause newborn pneumonia

QUESTIONS 10–15

Match each description below with the number above that most closely pertains to it. Each answer may be used once, more than once, or not at all.
[A] 3
[B] 6
[C] 10
[D] 30
[E] 50

10. Exposure to ___ rad may have some adverse fetal effects

11. After week ___, exposure to radioactive iodine may affect fetal thyroid development

12. Baseline risk of major congenital anomaly is _____

13. Intrauterine fetal growth retardation is increased ≈ ___ times in excessive drinkers

14. Infants born to epileptic mothers have ___% incidence of congenital abnormalities

15. Rate of congenital anomalies in pregnant women taking antipsychotic medications is _____

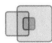

Answers and Explanations

1. The correct answer is D [I B 1 and II B 6]. A positive β-hCG is indicative of pregnancy. If she became pregnant near the time of ovulation, the pregnancy does not exceed 11 days, and therefore exposure to the teratogen occurred within the resistant period. The possible outcomes are either fetal death or continuation of pregnancy. Because continuation of pregnancy is not an option, fetal demise is the next best answer. All the other answer choices are congenital malformations that can occur after exposure to a teratogen during the embryonic period.

2. The correct answer is A [II A 1 b (1)]. Exposure to 260 mrad (260×10^{-3} rads) at 11 weeks of gestation is unlikely to result in any problems—exposure to radiation of 5 rad or less has not been associated with adverse fetal outcomes. Large dose radiation (more than 250 rads) during weeks 4 through 12 may cause mental retardation or cataracts. Spontaneous abortion may occur if fetus is exposed to more than 250 rad during weeks 2 through 4. Growth retardation may occur if fetus is exposed to large dose of radiation during weeks 12 through 16. Bone marrow suppression is seen when the fetus is exposed to large dose radiation after 20 weeks of gestation or postnatally.

3. The correct answer is D [II B 6]. Even if known teratogenic agents, such as live viral vaccines (rubella), excess caffeine, alcohol, isotretinoin, and excess vitamin A are inadvertently taken during pregnancy, the outcome is still usually favorable. Simple exposure to a live viral vaccine is not an indication for therapeutic abortion. The rubella vaccine can be harmful to the fetus. The risk for congenital malformations is different between various live viral vaccines (rubella, mumps, measles, etc.).

4. The correct answer is C [II C]. Sustained maternal hyperthermia (over 102° F) for more than 24 hours during the first trimester is associated with growth restriction and CNS defects, such as microcephaly, anencephaly, and mental deficiency. As her physician, you should not prohibit use of saunas if is important to her for stress relief. Simply telling the patient that "hot tub use is associated with fetal growth restriction" is not the best advice even though it is a true statement. Answer choices D and E are not the best answers. Simply revealing the parameters (over 102°F, more than 24 hours, short intervals rather than sustained hyperthermia) of studies that have shown an association between sustained maternal hyperthermia and pregnancy outcomes is not the best advice.

The answers are 5-A [II E 1 b (1)], **6-E** [II E 7], **7-A** [II E 1 b, 1 c, 1 d], **8-D** [II E 6 b 1, b 2], and **9-A** [II E 1].

Congenital rubella infection can cause a triad of ocular defects (cataracts, blindness), inner ear problems (sensorineural deafness), and cardiovascular lesions, such as persistent patent ductus arteriosus, pulmonary artery stenosis, and atrioventricular septal defects. Maternal infection with rubella at the time of delivery can result in newborn pneumonia and encephalitis. Although rare, after maternal exposure to mumps, neonates have been born with endocardial fibroelastosis, ear and eye malformations, or urogenital abnormalities. Infection with chickenpox during first 20 weeks of gestation may result in congenital malformations, such as cicatricial skin scarring and limb hypoplasia.

The answers are 10-C [II A 1 b (2)], **11-C** [II A 3], **12-A** [I], **13-A** [II B 8 a 5 (c)], **14-B** [II D 4 a], **15-B** [II D 5].

Exposure to less then 5 rad (and probably less than 10 rad) is unlikely to cause an adverse outcome. However, exposure to 10 to 25 rads may have some adverse fetal effects. After the 10th week of gestation, fetal thyroid development can be retarded in addition to any adverse effects of radiation. Major birth defects occur in approximately 3% of all deliveries. Intrauterine growth retardation is increased 2.7 times in pregnant women who drink excessively. Infants born to epileptic mothers have 6% incidence of congenital malformations. The rate of congenital anomalies in pregnant women taking antipsychotic medications is two times that in general population (which is 3%).

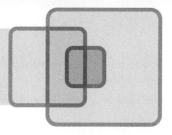

chapter **8**

Substance Abuse in Pregnancy

SERDAR H. URAL AND EMMANUELLE PARE

I · INTRODUCTION

Substance abuse during pregnancy is currently a significant problem in modern obstetrics. It is common to abuse more than one substance at a time.

A **Frequency of occurrence.** Use of illicit substances in the general population has become so prevalent that the obstetrician and neonatologist are faced daily with the effects of these drugs on their patients. The true prevalence of drug use in pregnancy is difficult to determine. In the United States, prevalence based on urine toxicology is a minimum of 10%. This number is probably much higher because the urine test is valid for recently used drugs only, and its sensitivity is low.

B **Substances most likely to be abused.** **Alcohol and cocaine** have become the leading abused substances, with alcohol being the most common potentially teratogenic substance in pregnancy. Although other substances are abused in pregnancy, these two substances are examples of how a significant social problem can affect obstetric practice.

C **Problems related to substance abuse.** Women who abuse substances while pregnant tend to have other related problems, including sexually transmitted diseases, poor nutrition, and poor prenatal care.

II · DEFINITION

Substance abuse is divided into three stages: use, abuse, and dependence.

A **Use** involves taking low, infrequent doses of illicit substances for experimentation or social reasons. Damaging consequences are rare or minor.

B **Abuse** is the persistent or repeated use of a psychoactive substance for more than 1 month, despite the persistence or recurrence of adverse social, occupational, psychological, or physical effects.

C **Dependence** is present if **three or more of the following criteria** are met continuously for 1 month or repeatedly in a given year:

1. Abandonment of social, occupational, or recreational activities
2. Continued substance use despite knowledge of social, psychological, or physical problems exacerbated by drug use
3. Substance is taken to relieve or avoid withdrawal symptoms
4. Withdrawal symptoms
5. Persistent desire or one or more unsuccessful attempts to control substance use
6. Substance taken in larger amounts or over a longer period than intended

7. Frequent intoxication or withdrawal symptoms occur when the individual is expected to fulfill obligations at work, school, or home

8. Significant time spent obtaining or taking the substance or recovering from the effects of its use

III SIGNS AND SYMPTOMS OF SUBSTANCE ABUSE

A Disorientation, euphoria, sedation, and agitation

B Hallucinations, hypertension, tachycardia, inflamed nasal mucosa, track marks, and pupil abnormalities

C Unusual infections, such as cellulitis and hepatitis

IV PSYCHOACTIVE SUBSTANCES

A Opiates

1. **Examples** include heroin, morphine, methadone, and codeine.
2. **Effects** include euphoria, relaxation, mood elevation, drowsiness, and respiratory depression.

B Depressants

1. **Examples** include barbiturates, methaqualone, and diazepam.
2. **Effects** include euphoria, relaxation, mood elevation, drowsiness, mood volatility, respiratory depression, and impaired coordination.

C Stimulants

1. **Examples** include cocaine and amphetamine.
2. **Effects** include euphoria, alertness, sense of well-being, suppression of fatigue and hunger, increased sexual arousal, increased pulse and blood pressure, tremor, insomnia, paranoia, psychosis, cardiac arrest, abruptio placentae, and fetal growth retardation.

D Hallucinogens

1. **Examples** include lysergic acid diethylamide (LSD), mescaline, and psilocybin.
2. **Effects** include altered perception, detachment, increased blood pressure, tremor, impaired judgment, and panic.

E Phencyclidine (PCP) and related compounds

1. One **example** is ketamine hydrochloride. Street names include angel dust and crystal.
2. **Effects** include detachment, mental numbness, distorted perception, anxiety, and impaired coordination.

F Cannabinoids

1. **Examples** include marijuana and hashish.
2. **Effects** include euphoria, relaxation, altered perception, sexual arousal, increased appetite, disorientation, impaired judgment, incoordination, and paranoia.

V ALCOHOL USE IN PREGNANCY

A Alcohol use is the leading cause of teratogenesis by drugs or environmental agents (see Chapter 7). Ethanol crosses the placenta and the fetal blood-brain barrier freely. It is thought to cause toxicity both directly and indirectly by its metabolites.

B Women who drink during pregnancy are often older and have higher rates of other illicit drug use, less education, and lower social status.

1. **Fetal alcohol syndrome** is a congenital syndrome involving a triad of growth retardation, facial abnormalities, and central nervous system (CNS) dysfunction. The **most common abnormalities** are:
   a. Prenatal and postnatal growth deficiency
   b. Mental retardation
   c. Behavioral disturbances
   d. Atypical facial appearance: short palpebral fissure, epicanthal folds, flat midface, and hypoplastic philtrum
   e. Congenital heart defects

2. In the United States, the incidence is 1 in 500 to 1 in 1000 deliveries.

C **Threshold of alcohol abuse.** There is **no safe level of alcohol use in pregnancy.** Patients should be advised that even though occasional drinking may not be harmful, it is safest not to consume any alcohol during pregnancy. The daily consumption of 1 to 2 ounces of absolute alcohol (moderate-to-heavy drinking) may result in infants who show characteristics of fetal alcohol syndrome. Use of smaller amounts of alcohol has also been related to fetal alcohol syndrome. Alcohol is excreted in breast milk. There is evidence that drinking alcohol during breastfeeding may have a detrimental effect on the baby's motor development.

VI COCAINE USE IN PREGNANCY

The rise in the use of cocaine among the general population has spawned a rise in use among pregnant women, thus making the maternal and fetal complications associated with cocaine use more common. In addition, the increase in rates of crack cocaine for sex has increased the number of cocaine-complicated pregnancies.

A **Use in general population.** Cocaine use has increased among the general population because of the availability of inexpensive "**crack**" cocaine, a highly purified form of cocaine that is named for the cracking or popping sound made when the crystals are heated in a test tube. Cocaine can be smoked as crack, taken intranasally, or injected intravenously.

B **Pharmacologic effects**

1. Cocaine produces **complex cardiovascular effects** that depend on an intact sympathetic nervous system and direct stimulation of the myocardium and vasculature.

2. Cocaine **blocks dopamine and norepinephrine reuptake at the postsynaptic junction,** thereby increasing CNS irritability.

3. This leads to **maternal and fetal vasoconstriction and tachycardia,** as well as **stimulation of uterine contractions.**

C **Maternal complications**

1. Neurologic
   a. Seizures
   b. Rupture of intracranial aneurysm
   c. Postpartum intracerebral hemorrhage
   d. Cerebral infarction

2. Cardiovascular
   a. Myocardial infarction
   b. Hypertension
   c. Arrhythmias

      d. Rupture of the ascending aorta

      e. Sudden death

  3. Infectious

      a. Intravenous use predisposes the patient to bacterial endocarditis, hepatitis, and HIV exposure.

      b. Sexually transmitted diseases, such as gonorrhea, chlamydia, human papillomavirus, and syphilis, are common, frequently because of the exchange of sex for drugs or sex for money to buy drugs.

  4. Obstetric

      a. Possible increase in spontaneous abortions

      b. Increased incidence of preterm labor and delivery

      c. Intrauterine growth restriction

      d. Abruptio placentae

      e. Increased risk of intrauterine fetal demise

      f. Increased risk of fetal distress

      g. Congenital anomalies

        (1) Fetal microcephaly

        (2) Nonduodenal intestinal atresia–infarction

        (3) Limb reduction defects

        (4) Genitourinary tract anomalies

        (5) Cerebral infarctions in utero

      h. Neonatal and infant behavioral disturbances (e.g., sudden infant death syndrome)

      i. Increased incidence of premature rupture of membranes (PROM)

      j. Meconium-stained amniotic fluid

D **Management**

  1. Detection

      a. Consider drug abuse in the differential diagnosis.

      b. Educate patients about drug use and its effects on the mother and developing infant.

      c. Ask patients directly about types of psychoactive substances used.

      d. Examine patients for **inflammation of nasal alae and intravenous injection sites,** especially in patients who do not keep prenatal appointments or who show signs of anemia, fetal growth retardation, or preterm labor.

      e. Consider **urine toxicology screening.** Although this can be used as a method of monitoring and instructing pregnant women about drug use, some states require that these results be reported to government authorities.

        (1) A **patient-physician alliance** can be best forged through directly confronting a patient about the suspected drug abuse. At that time, the physician can impress on the patient the need to treat the problem in the interest of both herself and the developing infant.

        (2) Urine screening can then be obtained through reasoned persuasion rather than deception.

  2. Treatment

      a. Refer the patient to a chemical dependency treatment center. Ideally, treatment center options should include individual and group counseling, intensive day treatment, and residential treatment. Optimally, residential treatment should include obstetric facilities.

      b. Use the assistance of social services to coordinate a management plan, because a patient's hostile home and social environment (e.g., pervasive poverty, easy access to drugs, or positive opinion of drug culture) can lead to conditions that compound complications caused by cocaine use (e.g., lack of prenatal care and poor nutrition). Dealing effectively with the patient's environment may determine the success or failure of any medical intervention.

      c. Prevent premature labor and intrauterine growth retardation using education, nutrition counseling, ultrasound, and fetal testing. Choose magnesium sulfate rather than β-mimetics to treat preterm labor, because magnesium sulfate does not have stimulating effects on the heart muscle.

d. With **symptoms of abdominal pain,** differentiate between abruptio placentae appendicitis and bowel ischemia. Laboratory evaluation and fetal monitoring clarify the diagnosis and point to the best treatment option (see Chapter 9). Drug screening is essential.

e. With **cocaine overdose,** control seizures, hyperthermia, and hypertension by reducing CNS irritability and sympathetic nervous system overactivity. In addition, evaluate the patient's cardiovascular system.

  (1) Obtain a urine toxicology screen, a complete blood count, and coagulation studies, and measure cardiac and liver enzymes, electrolytes, and arterial blood gas.

  (2) Administer oxygen and consider intubation for intractable seizures.

  (3) Monitor urine output, vital signs, and fetal heart rate.

  (4) Use ice baths or cooling blankets to treat hyperthermia.

  (5) Treat seizures with magnesium sulfate or diazepam.

  (6) Maintain normotension and normal heart rate.

f. **Consider hospitalization for detoxification,** treatment of psychological disorders, and coordination of further therapy.

g. Once **abstinence** has been achieved, perform periodic urine screens to monitor continued abstinence.

VII OTHER SUBSTANCES ABUSED IN PREGNANCY

A Marijuana

1. Marijuana is the most commonly used illicit substance among pregnant women.

2. There is no evidence that marijuana is associated with congenital anomalies in humans.

3. Maternal smoking level may correlate with increased perinatal mortality, preterm delivery, PROM, and infants of lower birth weight. This correlation may be because marijuana is commonly abused along with other substances.

B Heroin

1. Heroin causes no increase in congenital anomalies.

2. Intrauterine growth retardation, stillbirth, prematurity, and perinatal death are increased.

3. Neonatal withdrawal, behavioral disturbances, and mild developmental delay have been reported.

4. The poor nutritional status of many heroin addicts may be as important as the heroin use.

C Methadone

1. Methadone causes no increase in congenital anomalies.

2. Methadone use is associated with low-birth-weight infants.

D Tobacco (nicotine)

1. 25% of reproductive-age women are smokers.

2. Concurrent use with other substances is a likely possibility.

3. Spontaneous abortion, abruptio placentae, PROM, preterm delivery, and lower-birth-weight infants are increased.

4. No increase in congenital anomalies has been seen.

VIII SUBSTANCE ABUSE AND PRENATAL CARE

A Prenatal care may **reduce the adverse effects of substance abuse** for the mother and fetus.

B A **multidisciplinary approach,** including social workers, is essential; substance abusers probably have nonmedical problems that tend to complicate pregnancy.

C Treatment for substance abuse should be offered.

D Intensive counseling on the risks associated with substance abuse is essential.

E Laboratory studies, ultrasound examinations, and frequent visits may be necessary; frequency should be determined on a case-by-case basis.

F Counseling on breastfeeding and exposure of the infant to substances used by the mother is important.

Study Questions for Chapter 8

Directions: Each of the numbered items or incomplete statements in this section is followed by answers or by completions of the statement. Select the ONE lettered answer or completion that is BEST in each case.

1. An 18-year-old student enjoys drinking once or twice a week with her college friends. Lately, she has been drinking more than 10 mixed alcoholic beverages each time she goes out. Although she gets a severe "hangover" after each night of drinking, she still enjoys drinking alcohol and doesn't believe it causes any harm to her body. She is an average student at school and is able to keep a part-time job without any difficulty. She has many friends and is well liked. She claims that everybody around her drinks as much as she does. She doesn't have a thirst for alcohol throughout the day, but admits that a month ago she only had to drink four drinks to get the same "buzz" she gets now with six drinks. Her pattern of alcohol consumption is best described as

- [A] Use
- [B] Abuse
- [C] Tolerance
- [D] Dependence
- [E] Withdrawal

2. A 30-year-old woman, gravida 2, para 1 at 8 weeks of gestation likes to drink one glass of red wine at night with dinner and doesn't believe it will harm her developing fetus. She drank the same amount throughout her last pregnancy and she delivered a normal healthy neonate weighing 8 pounds 4 ounces. Her past medical history is unremarkable other than an appendectomy. When performing her ultrasound at 18 weeks of gestation, the ultrasonographer should pay close attention to the anatomy of the baby's

- [A] Bones
- [B] Brain
- [C] Heart
- [D] Kidneys
- [E] Vertebrae

3. A 20-year-old woman, gravida 4, para 3 presents to you at 22 weeks of gestation for routine prenatal care. She has missed her last two appointments. All of her previous pregnancies were complicated by preterm labor and delivery of small infants with significant respiratory distress. She has a history of a small inferiolateral myocardial infarct from the previous year. In the office she appears anxious. Her vital signs are as follows: T = 99.0, BP = 170/96, P = 135, R = 18. The rest of her physical examination is unremarkable other than what she describes as "stretch marks" on her ante-cubital fossa. Which of the following obstetrical complications is most likely to occur during this pregnancy?

- [A] Cerebral infarction
- [B] Chorioamnionitis
- [C] Placenta previa
- [D] Placental abruption
- [E] Seizures

4. A 25-year-old woman, gravida 1, para 0 at 13 weeks of gestation presents to you for routine prenatal care. She says her baby moves frequently and keeps her up part of the night. She also reports increasing vaginal discharge that is odorless and otherwise asymptomatic. Upon measuring the fundal height you smell alcohol on her breath. She fails the finger to nose test. The rest of the physical examination is unremarkable. She has no medical history and denies smoking, alcohol, or drug use. What is the initial best step?

|A| Alcohol and drug screen
|B| Prescribe metronidazole and follow-up in 4 weeks
|C| Refer her to a social worker
|D| Confront her about your findings
|E| See her back in 4 weeks

5. A 35-year-old woman, gravida 3, para 2 at 20 weeks of gestation is seeing you for a routine prenatal visit. Today she has no complaints. Her previous pregnancies have been unremarkable. She has chronic hypertension and a history of a cholecystectomy. She has no known drug allergies. She is a successful attorney who admits to smoking marijuana several times a week for relaxation and says she has read several papers that show no increased risk of congenital anomalies. Her vitals are as follows: T = 97.9, BP = 108/68, P = 100, R = 16. Doppler shows fetal heart rate at 156 bpm. What is the best course of action during this prenatal visit?

|A| Educate her about the possibility of delivering a small infant
|B| Refuse to see her if she does not stop using marijuana
|C| Refer her to a social worker for possible substance abuse
|D| Acknowledge that she is correct about no increased risk of congenital anomalies
|E| See her back at 24 weeks of gestation

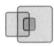

Answers and Explanations

1. The answer is B [II B] . This teenager is abusing alcohol because she consumes alcoholic beverages despite recurrent adverse physical effects (i.e., hangover). Alcohol "use" would imply low, infrequent quantities of consumption. Although she is beginning to build up tolerance (needing six drinks instead of four to get the same effect), "tolerance" is not the best term to describe her entire pattern of alcohol consumption and its effect on her lifestyle. She doesn't meet most of the criteria for alcohol dependence. She does not have problems at work or school, she does not have withdrawal symptoms, nor does she spend excessive time obtaining or drinking alcohol. Alcohol withdrawal can be serious. It involves autonomic hyperactivity, tremor, agitation, insomnia, and even seizures. The student doesn't have these symptoms.

2. The answer is C [V B 1 e] . There is no safe level of alcohol use in pregnancy. Although the chances of congenital anomalies are small with small amounts of alcohol use during pregnancy, there is still a slight possibility of an anomaly. Heavy alcohol use during early first trimester has been associated with congenital heart defects (especially ventricular septal defect). The anatomy of bone in the developing fetus is not changed; however, its growth velocity is affected by alcohol. Although fetal alcohol syndrome causes mental retardation, brain anatomy is infrequently changed to the point of detection on a routine 18-week ultrasound. Alcohol is rarely associated with kidney and spine anomalies.

3. The answer is D [VI C 4 d] . High blood pressure, anxiety, needle-track marks, and history of repetitive preterm deliveries and myocardial infarct in a young, healthy woman are suspicious for drug use. Cocaine use is associated with much higher rates of placental abruption than in the general pregnant population. Cerebral infarction and seizures can occur in both the mother and the developing infant because of cocaine use. Neither is, however, an "obstetric" complication; seizures and infarction are both maternal and fetal/neonatal complications. No association exists between cocaine use and placenta previa or chorioamnionitis.

4. The answer is D [VI D 1 e (1)]. A patient-physician alliance can be best forged through directly confronting a patient about the suspected drug abuse. Alcohol and drug screen can be obtained after confronting the patient rather than through deception. This patient's discharge is normal during pregnancy and most likely doesn't require antibiotic treatment. Referring her to a social worker is premature if you have not confronted her about the possibility of alcohol abuse. A multi-disciplinary approach is important for long-term treatment and maintenance of abstinence, but is not the initial best step. Seeing her back in 4 weeks without addressing the issue of alcohol use during pregnancy would be inappropriate.

5. The answer is A [VI D 1 b and VII A 3]. Educating patients about drug use and its effects and establishing a strong patient-physician relationship is key to successfully managing substance abuse during pregnancy. This educated patient would benefit from knowing that her newborn may be of lower birth weight because of her use of marijuana during pregnancy. Refusing to see a patient without at least a 30-day notice and referral to another physician sets grounds for a lawsuit. A social worker consult may be helpful later but not at this initial visit. Acknowledging that she is correct about her facts without addressing the consequence on low birth weight with marijuana use is not the best of course of action. It is not proper to see her back in 4 weeks without addressing the issue of illicit substance use.

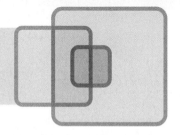

chapter 9

Antepartum Bleeding
ALFREDO GIL

I INTRODUCTION

Antepartum bleeding complicates 4% of all pregnancies, and hemorrhage remains a leading cause of maternal death. Early in pregnancy, bleeding is associated with spontaneous abortion, ectopic pregnancy, and molar pregnancy (see Chapters 18 and 31). In the third trimester, bleeding is most often associated with placental abnormalities.

II PLACENTA PREVIA

A **Definition.** In placenta previa, the placenta is implanted in the lower segment of the uterus and covers the internal cervical os (Fig. 9-1). There are three types of placenta previa:

1. **Total or complete placenta previa.** The placenta completely covers the internal os. Complete previa presents the greatest maternal risk and is associated with the largest amount of blood loss.

2. **Partial previa.** The placenta partially covers the internal os.

3. **Marginal previa.** The placenta extends to the margin of the internal cervical os. Marginal previa is generally not associated with large amounts of vaginal bleeding.

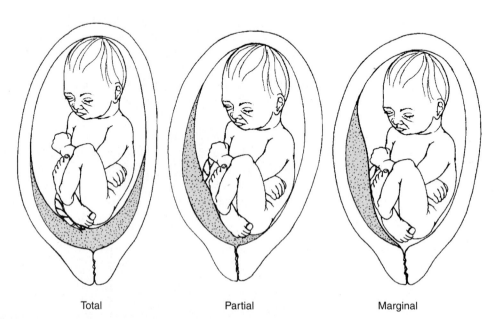

Total   Partial   Marginal

FIGURE 9-1   Variations of placenta previa. (From Niebyl JR, Simpson JL, Gabbe SG. Obstetrics: Normal and Problem Pregnancies. 4th Ed. London: Churchill Livingstone, 2001.)

TABLE 9-1 Ultrasonic Identification of Placenta Previa and Subsequent Clinical Outcome	
Gestational Age at Sonography (wk)	**Previa or Hemorrhage at Delivery (%)**
<20	2.3
20–25	3.2
25–30	5.2
30–35	24

Reprinted with permission from Cunningham F, Gant N, Gilstrap L, et al. Williams Obstetrics. 21st Ed. New York: McGraw-Hill, 2001:634.

B **Incidence.**   Placenta previa occurs in approximately **1 in 200 live births** (0.5%). When detected before 30 weeks' gestation on ultrasound, placenta previa rarely persists until delivery (Table 9-1).

C **Etiology.**   Little is known about the cause of placenta previa. Although previous history of placenta previa is rare, several risk factors have been identified.

1. **Previous cesarean section.** The incidence of placenta previa increases with an increasing number of cesarean sections; it is 1.9% after two prior cesarean sections and 4.1% after three or more cesarean sections. This change represents a three- to fivefold increase compared with the general obstetric population.

2. **Multiparity.** Approximately 80% of cases of placenta previa occur in multiparous patients.

3. **Advanced maternal age.** Women older than 35 years of age, regardless of parity, are more likely to have a placenta previa than women younger than 25 years of age.
    a. 1 in 300 in women: 20 to 29 years of age
    b. 1 in 100 in women: More than 35 years of age 1 in 50 in women: More than 40 years of age

4. **Increased placental surface** may occur in the following conditions:
    a. **Multiple gestations** caused by increased placental mass
    b. **Erythroblastosis fetalis** (Rh isoimmunization), which may be accompanied by a large hydropic placenta

5. **Smoking.** The relative risk of placenta previa **increases twofold** in pregnant women who smoke more than 20 cigarettes a day.

D **Clinical presentation.**   **Painless vaginal bleeding** in the third trimester in a previously normal pregnancy is the most characteristic sign. Bleeding may occur in the following circumstances:

1. During rest or activity (70% of bleeding occurs during rest)

2. After trauma, coitus, or pelvic examination

3. During labor, when the lower uterine segment begins to efface and dilate. The tearing of the placental attachments at or near the internal cervical os causes the bleeding.

E **Diagnosis.**   Placenta previa should be suspected in all patients who present with vaginal bleeding after 24 weeks. Women suspected of having a placenta previa should undergo an **ultrasound** to determine the position of the placenta. Digital and pelvic examination is deferred until the diagnosis of placenta previa is excluded by ultrasound.

1. **Ultrasound. Transabdominal ultrasound is up to 95% accurate** in diagnosing placenta previa. **Transvaginal ultrasound** may also be performed when the diagnosis is still in question.

2. **Examination.** Definitive diagnosis of placenta previa can be made by clinical palpation of placenta tissue though the cervical os. This clinical technique is called the **double set-up** examination, and it may precipitate a hemorrhage. Therefore, it is performed only when:
    a. Delivery is contemplated at the time of the examination.

   b. The examination is performed in the operating room with the patient prepped for surgery, an anesthesiologist present, the surgeon scrubbed, and blood cross-matched and available.

   c. The pregnancy is at or near term.

F **Management.** Treatment depends on gestational age, amount of vaginal bleeding, maternal hemodynamic status, and fetal condition.

  1. Expectant management. This approach is justifiable if the fetus is preterm (less than 37 weeks) and can benefit from further intrauterine development. Expectant management should proceed as follows:

   a. Hospitalization until bleeding subsides. The patient may be discharged after the bleeding lessens and a physician judges that the fetus is healthy.

   b. Careful speculum examination to rule out any vaginal or cervical lesions

   c. Twice-daily fetal monitoring strips

   d. Steroids for fetal lung maturity if gestational age is less than 34 weeks

   e. Tocolysis (see Chapter 15) may be safely undertaken in patients with placenta previa before 34 weeks. The agent of choice is magnesium sulfate because it is associated with fewer hemodynamic alterations.

  2. Delivery. Decisions concerning delivery are made based on the gestational age of the fetus and the amount of vaginal bleeding. Indications for **cesarean section** include:

   a. Elective

    (1) When the gestational age is **37 weeks**

    (2) When **fetal lung maturity** is demonstrated by amniocentesis

   b. Emergent

    (1) When the amount of bleeding presents a threat to the mother regardless of gestational age or fetal size

    (2) When fetal nonreassuring testing is observed on the fetal monitoring strip

G **Maternal and fetal complications.** Maternal and fetal morbidity may be from placenta previa and may be significant.

  1. Maternal morbidity

   a. Maternal shock can result from acute blood loss

   b. Severe postpartum hemorrhage (PPH) can occur after the delivery because the placental implantation is in the lower uterine segment, which has decreased muscle content. Thus, muscle contraction may be less effective in controlling the bleeding. PPH may lead to the following conditions:

    (1) Renal damage (acute tubular necrosis), which may result from prolonged hypotension

    (2) Pituitary necrosis (Sheehan syndrome) and resulting panhypopituitarism

   c. Placenta accreta (growth of placenta into the myometrium), or any of its variations, due to the absence of decidua basalis. Placenta accreta should always be considered in the presence of placenta previa.

    (1) The incidence of placenta accreta (with placenta previa) is 4%. The incidence of placenta accreta increases to 16 to 25% after a previous cesarean section.

    (2) The presence of a placenta accreta may necessitate a cesarean hysterectomy to control the blood loss. There are three types of placenta accreta (Fig. 9-2):

     (a) Placenta accreta. The placenta is attached directly to the myometrium.

     (b) Placenta increta. The placenta invades the myometrium.

     (c) Placenta percreta. The placenta penetrates completely through the myometrium.

  2. Fetal morbidity. Preterm delivery may be necessary secondary to maternal bleeding, and the infant may experience the complications of prematurity (see Chapter 15).

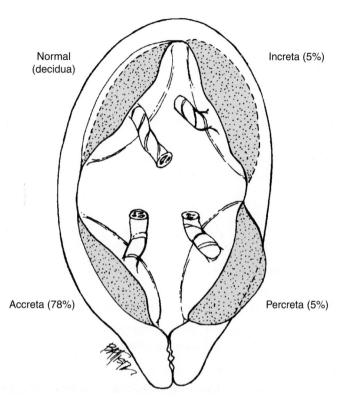

FIGURE 9-2 Uteroplacental relationships found in abnormal placentation. (From Niebyl JR, Simpson JL, Gabbe SG. Obstetrics: Normal and Problem Pregnancies. 4th Ed. London: Churchill Livingstone, 2001.)

III ABRUPTIO PLACENTAE (PLACENTAL ABRUPTION)

A Definition. Abruptio placentae is **premature separation of a normally implanted placenta** after 20 weeks' gestation.

1. **Pathophysiology.** Initiated by bleeding into the decidua basalis, the bleeding splits the decidua, and the hematoma that forms causes further splitting.
   a. The process may be **self limited,** with no further complication to the pregnancy.
   b. If the initial point of separation is in the center of the placenta, the blood follows the path of least resistance. This may result in extravasations of blood into the myometrium, causing a bluish discoloration of the uterus (**Couvelaire uterus**).

B Incidence

1. The reported incidence of abruptio placentae is about **1 in 75 to 1 in 200 births.**
2. Abruptio placentae severe enough to kill the fetus occurs in **1 in 400 births.**

C Etiology. The primary cause of abruptio placentae is uncertain; several associated conditions have been identified.

1. **Maternal hypertension,** either chronic or pregnancy induced, has been implicated and is most often identified as a risk factor.
2. **Cocaine** use is associated with both an increase in maternal hypertension and vasoconstriction of the placental vasculature. Recent increases in cocaine use have led to an increase in the number of cases of abruptio placentae.

3. **Preterm premature rupture of membranes (PROM)** has been associated with cases of abruptio placentae. The incidence of abruptio placentae is 5% in pregnancies between 20 and 36 weeks complicated by PROM.

4. **Maternal trauma** accounts for a small number of cases of abruptio placentae. Clinical evidence of abruption is not always immediately apparent. A period of prolonged monitoring is required to exclude developing abruptio placentae.

5. Either **sudden decompression** of the uterus by rupture of membranes in a patient with polyhydramnios, or delivery of a first twin, can lead to a shearing effect on the placenta as the uterus contracts, thus causing abruptio placentae.

6. **Cigarette smoking** is associated with decidual necrosis on pathologic examination and an increased risk of abruptio placentae.

7. **Uterine fibroids** may contribute to abruptio placentae when the placenta is implanted directly over the fibroid.

8. **History of abruptio placentae** predisposes patients to subsequent abruptions; the risk is increased 10-fold (0.4 to 4%).

D **Clinical presentation.** The clinical signs of abruptio placentae vary with the type and degree of placental separation.

1. With **peripheral detachment,** the bleeding is usually less severe.

2. With **central detachment,** the bleeding may be concealed and the patient may present in hypovolemic shock or disseminated intravascular coagulation (DIC).

E **Diagnosis.** The basis of diagnosis consists of history, clinical examination, and a high index of suspicion. The triad of external bleeding through the cervical os, uterine or back pain, and fetal distress is common.

1. **Fetal heart rate monitoring** may reveal loss of variability or may have late decelerations. The uterine tone may be increased without periods of relaxation.

2. **Premature contractions** that are unresponsive to tocolytics may suggest either abruptio placentae or intra-amniotic infection.

3. **Ultrasound** is most useful in making the diagnosis of placenta previa as the cause of third-trimester bleeding. However, a normal ultrasound does not rule out the possibility of abruptio placentae.

4. **Laboratory tests** are nonspecific but may reveal thrombocytopenia, hypofibrinemia, and an increase in fibrin split products. These abnormalities usually occur relatively late in the course of a placental abruption.

F **Management.** Treatment depends on the condition of the mother and on the gestational age of the fetus.

1. **Maternal hospitalization** with continuous fetal monitoring should be considered.
   a. **Delivery may be delayed** if the fetal heart rate tracing is reassuring and the maternal condition remains stable.
   b. **Immediate delivery is necessary** in the following conditions:
      (1) The fetal heart rate tracing is nonreassuring and the gestational age is greater than 24 weeks.
      (2) The maternal condition deteriorates regardless of gestational age.
   c. **Vaginal delivery is desirable** if the maternal and fetal condition permits.

2. **Tocolytic drugs** (see Chapter 15) may be used if the pregnancy is less than 37 weeks and the status of the mother and fetus is reassuring.
   a. **Magnesium sulfate** is the tocolytic of choice because of its efficacy and side-effect profile.

    b. β-mimetic tocolytics should be avoided in cases of suspected abruptio placentae because they may mask maternal hypovolemia by causing tachycardia.

    c. Prostaglandin inhibitors should be used with caution because they are associated with a theoretic risk of platelet dysfunction.

  3. Complications

    a. Hemorrhagic shock may occur either from external bleeding or from concealed clots. Treatment includes:

      (1) Aggressive intravenous fluid replacement

      (2) Replacement of blood loss and coagulation factors

      (3) Prompt delivery after maternal stabilization

    b. Consumptive coagulopathy (DIC) may occur in 30% of cases of severe abruptio placentae that lead to fetal demise.

    c. Renal failure, in the form of acute tubular necrosis, may result from intrarenal vasospasm or from massive hemorrhage and ensuing hypotension.

    d. Couvelaire uterus results from extravasation of blood into the myometrium. The hematoma seldom interferes with uterine contractions, and the uterus responds well to uterotonic agents. A Couvelaire uterus is not an indication for hysterectomy.

    e. Fetal maternal hemorrhage or the presence of fetal red blood cells in the maternal circulation is more commonly seen with traumatic instances of abruptio placentae. Rh-negative patients should receive RhoGAM (anti-D immune globulin).

IV   OTHER CAUSES OF THIRD-TRIMESTER BLEEDING

A   Obstetric causes

  1. Bloody show is a normal part of labor, bleeding is usually minimal, and the blood is mixed with mucus.

  2. Rupture of a vasa previa is a rare but very serious cause of vaginal bleeding. The bleeding is fetal in origin.

    a. The **cause** of ruptured vasa previa is rupture of a placental vessel with a velamentous cord insertion.

    b. Diagnosis is made using the **Apt test,** which involves:

      (1) Collecting blood from vagina

      (2) Adding a small amount of tap water

      (3) Centrifuging the sample

      (4) Adding the pink supernatant to 1 mL of a sodium hydroxide solution

      (5) "Reading" the treated sample in 2 minutes

        (a) Pink color: present of fetal hemoglobin

        (b) Yellow-brown color: presence of adult hemoglobin

  3. A ruptured uterus must be considered if a patient has a history of previous uterine surgery or fetal parts are palpable abdominally.

B   Nonobstetric causes

  1. Vaginal lacerations from trauma

  2. Vaginal infections, such as bacterial vaginosis or trichomonas

  3. Cervical pathology, such as gonorrhea, chlamydia, cervical polyps, or cervical cancer

Study Questions for Chapter 9

Directions: Each of the numbered items or incomplete statements in this section is followed by answers or by completions of the statement. Select the ONE lettered answer or completion that is BEST in each case.

1. A 25-year-old woman, gravida 2, para 1 at 36 and 4/7th weeks of gestation with twin gestation is in the operating room for a double set-up examination. Labor has been unremarkable thus far. She is fully dilated, 100% effaced, vertex of twin A is at +1 station, membranes have been ruptured for 20 minutes, and the fluid was clear after amniotomy. Twin B is also cephalic presentation. The fetal heart rate baseline for both twins is between 140 bpm and 150 bpm with good variability and reactivity. After delivery of twin A and artificial rupture of the second membrane, a large gush of clear fluid is followed by painless vaginal bleeding. Fetal heart rate patterns have not changed. What is the most likely cause of the bleeding?

- [A] Trauma
- [B] Cervical polyp
- [C] Placenta previa
- [D] Placental abruption
- [E] Uterine rupture

2. A 27-year-old woman, gravida 1, para 0 just delivered a viable female infant weighing 4100 g with APGARs of 9 and 9 at 1 and 5 minutes, respectively. After delivery of the complete placenta previa by cesarean section, intravenous dilute oxytocin is infused and the uterus and the abdominal layers are closed. In the recovery room, the patient continues to have brisk vaginal bleeding. Her vitals are as follows: T = 97.2, BP = 110/74, P = 102, R = 16. Her uterine fundus is firm. What is the most likely reason for her bleeding?

- [A] Cervical laceration
- [B] Lack of response to oxytocin
- [C] Retained placental fragments
- [D] Coagulopathy
- [E] Lower uterine segment bleeding

3. A 20-year-old woman, gravida 3, para 2 at 36 weeks of gestation arrives to labor and delivery reporting continuous vaginal bleeding and back pain. She denies sexual intercourse within the last 48 hours. She also denies trauma to the abdomen. You perform a pelvic ultrasound and note the fetus in cephalic presentation, amniotic fluid index of 10, and an anterior-fundal placenta. The fetal monitoring strip displays coupled contractions and up to six contractions in a 10-minute period. The fetal heart rate baseline is 130 with decreased variability. Her vitals are as follows: T = 96.8, BP = 100/60, P = 105, R = 16. Examination of the abdomen reveals tenderness over the uterus. What is the next step in management?

- [A] Magnesium sulfate
- [B] Cesarean section
- [C] Oxytocin
- [D] Fibrinogen level
- [E] Fibrin split products

4. A 34-year-old woman, gravida 2, para 1, at 34 and 2/7th weeks of gestation presents to labor and delivery reporting painless vaginal bleeding. You immediately perform a transvaginal ultrasound and note placenta completely overlying the internal os, a fetus in cephalic presentation, and an amniotic fluid index of 14. The cervical length appears 2.5 cm with funneling of the internal os. Her blood pressure is 110/78 and her pulse is 106. She has slow, continuous bleeding from her vagina. Fetal monitoring reveals one uterine contraction every 30 minutes, and the fetal heart rate is reactive. What is the next best step in management?

    A Magnesium sulfate
    B Hospitalization
    C Vaginal delivery
    D Cesarean section
    E Dexamethasone

5. A 28-year-old woman, gravida 3, para 1 at 37 weeks of gestation presents to labor and delivery for a scheduled repeat cesarean section with possible cesarean hysterectomy. She has a history of two previous low transverse cesarean sections. The first was because of fetal distress during labor, and the second was an elective repeat cesarean section. Her current pregnancy has been complicated with complete placenta previa with occasional spotting and recent hospitalization. Delivery by low transverse cesarean section is complicated by hemorrhage and hypotension. The patient receives 20 units of pRBCs. Which of the following organs is most likely to malfunction?

    A Adrenal cortex
    B Hypothalamus
    C Kidney
    D Liver
    E Heart

Answers and Explanations

1. The answer is D [III C 5]. Sudden decompression of the uterus by rupture of membranes or delivery of a first twin can lead to a shearing effect on the placenta as the uterus contracts, thus causing abruption placentae. Although there is a "double set-up" and "painless" vaginal bleeding, it is not automatically a placenta previa. Double set-up is also used in situations other than placenta previa. The only reliable diagnosis of placenta previa is via transvaginal ultrasound visualization of the placenta in the lower uterine segment covering the internal os. Uterine rupture usually occurs in patients with a previous history of a classical (vertical incision of uterus) cesarean section.

2. The answer is E [II G 1 b]. One of the complications of complete placenta previa is severe postpartum hemorrhage. Bleeding can occur after delivery because the placental implantation was in the lower uterine segment, which has decreased muscle content. Thus, muscle contraction may be less effective in controlling the bleeding. There is no mention of cervical laceration, which is unlikely because the fetus was delivered via a cesarean section rather than via vaginal delivery. Lack of response to oxytocin is less likely because physical examination reveals a firm uterine fundus. Retained placental fragments are unlikely after cesarean section because the uterus is exteriorized and manually curetted. Coagulopathy may occur with placental abruption or after severe blood loss. Decreasing fibrinogen levels, increasing PT and PTT, and increased fibrin split products would hint at this diagnosis.

3. The answer is D [III E 4, F 1 a]. The clinical scenario is describing placental abruption (painful bleeding, uterine contraction coupling, uterine tenderness, etc.). The most important blood test after clinical diagnosis of placental abruption is a coagulation profile to predict disseminated intravascular coagulation (DIC), especially by obtaining fibrinogen levels, which are the most sensitive of all coagulation parameters. Because the mother's vital signs are stable, the fetus is equivocal (lack of deep variable decelerations or repetitive late decelerations of fetal monitoring strip), and labor is preterm, you have time to perform a fibrinogen level. Although this patient is preterm (less than 37 weeks of gestation), she may need to be delivered if placental abruption causes fetal distress, if the mother's vital signs become unstable, or if decreasing fibrinogen levels indicate impending DIC. Both cesarean section and oxytocin induction of labor would be appropriate once the decision has been made to deliver the infant. Therefore, delivery would be the second step in management. Fibrin split products are useful for diagnosis of DIC but are not as sensitive as fibrinogen levels.

4. The answer is B [II F 1 a]. Expectant management is justifiable if the fetus is preterm (less than 37 weeks) and can benefit from further intrauterine development. Hospitalization is appropriate until the bleeding subsides. The patient may be discharged after the bleeding lessens and the physician judges that the fetus is healthy. Tocolysis (magnesium sulfate) is not necessary because the patient is not having significant, regular uterine contractions and the cervix is closed. Vaginal delivery or cesarean section is not necessary at this point because the pregnancy is preterm, the mother's vital signs are stable, and the fetus is stable (reactive on fetal monitoring strip). Steroids (dexamethasone or betamethasone) for advancement of fetal lung maturity are useful only between 24 to 34 weeks of gestation in a pregnancy with intact membranes.

5. The answer is C [II G 1 b 1]. After severe hemorrhage (e.g., 20 u pRBC and severe hypotension during surgery), renal damage in the form of acute tubular necrosis is most likely to occur. This patient is also at risk for Sheehan syndrome, which is pituitary necrosis (not hypothalamus). Injury to the liver, heart, and adrenal glands can occur but are less likely.

chapter 10

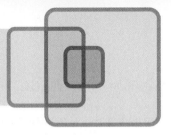

Labor and Delivery

PETER J. CHEN

I THEORIES OF THE CAUSES OF LABOR

The exact mechanism by which labor is initiated spontaneously, at either term or preterm, is not known. Many theories have been proposed.

A **Oxytocin stimulation.**   Oxytocin is known to cause uterine contractions when administered late in pregnancy; therefore, endogenously produced oxytocin may play a role in the spontaneous onset of labor.

1. Levels of oxytocin in maternal blood in early labor are higher than before the onset of labor, but there is no evidence of a sudden surge.

2. Oxytocin influence must therefore rely on the presence of oxytocin receptors.
   a. Receptors are found in the nonpregnant uterus.
   b. There is a sixfold increase in receptors at 13 to 17 weeks' gestation and an 80-fold increase at term.
   c. In preterm labor, receptor levels are two to three times higher than would be expected at the same gestational age in the absence of labor.

B **Fetal cortisol levels.**   Fetal cortisol levels and the proper functioning of the fetal adrenal gland may influence the spontaneous onset of labor.

1. In sheep, infusion of either cortisol or adrenocorticotropic hormone into a fetus with an intact adrenal gland causes premature labor. Hypophysectomy, adrenalectomy, or transection of the hypophyseal portal vessels in a sheep fetus results in prolonged gestation.

2. In humans, an anencephalic fetus has a prolonged gestation caused by faulty brain-pituitary-adrenal function.

C **Progesterone withdrawal.**   Although, in rabbits, the withdrawal of progesterone is followed by the prompt evacuation of the contents of the pregnant uterus, there is no decrease in the human maternal blood levels of progesterone at term. However, the progesterone level at the placental site may decrease before the onset of labor and assist in the synthesis of prostaglandin.

D **Prostaglandin release.**   Prostaglandins, particularly $PGF_{2\alpha}$ and PGE_2, have long been believed to be involved in the spontaneous onset of labor. Recent evidence suggests that this may not be true. Although prostaglandin levels are increased in amniotic fluid during labor, there seems to be **no parturition-related increase prior** to the onset of labor. The normal processes of labor appear to result in **inflammation,** which results in increased prostaglandin synthesis. Prostaglandins produced in myometrial tissue may contribute to the effectiveness of myometrial contractions during labor.

II DEFINITION AND CHARACTERISTICS OF LABOR

A **Definition.**   Labor is characterized by contractions that occur at with increasing frequency and intensity, causing dilation of the cervix.

B **Myometrial physiology**

1. **Contraction of uterine smooth muscle** is caused by the interaction of the proteins **actin** and **myosin.**
   a. The interaction of actin and myosin is regulated by the enzymatic phosphorylation of myosin light chains.
   b. The phosphorylation of myosin light chains is catalyzed by the enzyme myosin light-chain kinase, which is activated by calcium ion (Ca^{2+}).

2. **Gap junctions** are important cell-to-cell contacts that facilitate communication between cells via electrical or metabolic coupling.
   a. Myometrial gap junctions, which are virtually absent during pregnancy, increase in size and number before and during labor.
   b. Gap junctions facilitate synchronization of the contraction of individual cells, which permits the simultaneous recruitment of large numbers of contractile units during excitation.
   c. Progesterone appears to prevent and estrogen appears to promote gap junction formation.
   d. Prostaglandins are believed to be important stimulators of gap-junction formation. If prostaglandins are inhibited, gap-junction formation is inhibited as well.
   e. Oxytocin does not stimulate gap junction formation.

3. **Substances that interfere with the physiology of the myometrium** can inhibit contractions.
   a. **Tocolysis** or pharmacologic inhibition of uterine activity occurs with the following agents:
      (1) **Antiprostaglandin agents,** such as indomethacin and acetylsalicylic acid, inhibit the synthesis of prostaglandin, which, in turn, decreases uterine contractions and inhibits gap-junction formation. If the drugs are discontinued by 34 weeks' gestation, premature closure of the fetal ductus arteriosus does not occur.
      (2) **Calcium channel blockers** (e.g., nifedipine and magnesium sulfate) inhibit calcium influx.
      (3) β-mimetic agonists stimulate cyclic adenosine monophosphate (cAMP) generation. An increase in intracellular cAMP stimulates calcium uptake in various cellular organelles, including the sarcoplasmic reticulum, thereby lowering intracellular free calcium.
   b. **Potential complications associated with tocolytic agents** (Table 10-1)
   c. **Contraindications to tocolytic agents in preterm labor** (Table 10-2)

TABLE 10-1 Potential Complications of Tocolytic Agents

β-Adrenergic agents	Cardiac arrest[a]
Hyperglycemia	Maternal tetany[a]
Hypokalemia	Profound muscular paralysis[a]
Hypotension	Profound hypotension[a]
Pulmonary edema	
Cardiac insufficiency	**Indomethacin**
Arrhythmias	Hepatitis[b]
Myocardial ischemia	Renal failure[b]
Maternal death	Gastrointestinal bleeding[b]
Magnesium sulfate	**Nifedipine**
Pulmonary edema	Transient hypotension
Respiratory depression[a]	

[a] Effect is rare; seen with toxic levels.
[b] Effect is rare; associated with chronic use.
From the American College of Obstetricians and Gynecologists. ACOG Technical Bulletin, No. 206, June 1995:6.

TABLE 10-2   Contraindications to Tocolytic Agents in Preterm Labor*ᵃ*

General Contraindications
Acute fetal distress (except intrauterine resuscitation)
Chorioamnionitis
Eclampsia or severe preeclampsia
Fetal demise (singleton)
Fetal maturity
Maternal hemodynamic instability

Contraindications to Specific Tocolytic Agents
  β-Mimetic agents
  Maternal cardiac rhythm disturbance or other cardiac disease
  Poorly controlled diabetes, thyrotoxicosis, or hypertension
Magnesium sulfate
  Hypocalcemia
  Myasthenia gravis
  Renal failure
Indomethacin
  Asthma
  Coronary artery disease
  Gastrointestinal bleeding (active or past history)
  Oligohydramnios
  Renal failure
  Suspected fetal cardiac or renal anomaly
Nifedipine
  Maternal liver disease

ᵃ Relative and absolute contraindications to tocolysis based on clinical circumstances should take into account the risks
  of continuing the pregnancy versus those of delivery.
From the American College of Obstetricians and Gynecologists. ACOG Technical Bulletin, No. 206, June 1995:5.

C **Stages of labor**

1. **First stage.** The first stage of labor entails effacement and dilation. It begins when uterine contractions become sufficiently frequent, intense, and long to initiate obvious effacement and dilation of the cervix. The first stage of labor is further divided into a relatively flat latent phase and a rapidly progressive active phase (Fig. 10-1).

2. **Second stage.** The second stage of labor involves the expulsion of the fetus. It begins with the complete dilation of the cervix and ends when the infant is delivered.

3. **Third stage.** The third stage of labor involves the separation and expulsion of the placenta. It begins with the delivery of the infant and ends with the delivery of the placenta.

D **True labor and false labor** are compared in Table 10-3.

E **Characteristics of uterine contractions**

1. **Effective uterine contractions** last for 30 to 90 seconds, create 20 to 50 mmHg of pressure, and occur every 2 to 4 minutes.

2. The **pain of contractions** is thought to be caused by one or more of the following:
   a. Hypoxia of the contracted myometrium
   b. Compression of nerve ganglia in the cervix and lower uterus by the tightly interlocking muscle bundles

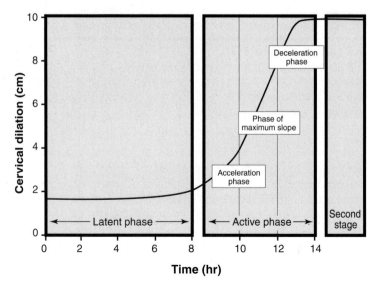

FIGURE 10-1 Composite of the average dilation curve for nulliparous labor. The first stage is divided into a relatively flat latent phase and a rapidly progressive active phase. In the active phase, three identifiable component parts include an acceleration phase, a linear phase of maximum slope, and a deceleration phase. (From Pritchard JA, MacDonald PC, Gant NF. Williams Obstetrics. 21st Ed. New York: McGraw-Hill, 2001:428, Figure 18-4.)

    c. Stretching of the cervix during dilation

    d. Stretching of the peritoneum overlying the uterus

  3. During labor, **contractions cause the uterus to differentiate** into two parts.

    a. The **upper segment of the uterus** becomes thicker as labor progresses and contracts down with a force that expels the fetus with each contraction.

    b. The **lower segment of the uterus** passively thins out with the contractions of the upper segment, promoting effacement of the cervix.

F Changes of the cervix before or during labor

  1. Effacement of the cervix is the shortening of the cervical canal from a structure of approximately 2 cm in length to one in which the canal is replaced by a more circular orifice with almost paper-thin edges. Effacement occurs as the muscle fibers near the internal os are pulled upward into the lower uterine segment.

  2. Dilation of the cervix involves the gradual widening of the cervical os. For the head of the average fetus at term to be able to pass through the cervix, the canal must dilate to a diameter of approximately 10 cm. When a diameter is reached that is sufficient for the fetal head to pass through, the cervix is said to be **completely or fully dilated.**

TABLE 10-3　True Versus False Labor

	True Labor	False Labor
Contractions	Regular intervals 2–4 minutes apart; intensity gradually increases and can last for 1 minute	Irregular intervals; no pattern; intensity remains steady
Discomfort	Back and abdomen	Lower abdomen
Dilation	Progressive	No change in cervix
Effect of sedation	Contractions are not affected	Contractions are relieved or stopped

III NORMAL LABOR IN THE OCCIPUT PRESENTATION

A **Occiput (vertex) presentations** occur in approximately 95% of all labors (Fig. 10-2). The occiput may present in the transverse, anterior, or posterior position. **Position** refers to the relation of an arbitrarily chosen portion of the fetus (**in this case, the occiput of the fetal head**) to the right or left side of the maternal birth canal. Positions of the occiput presentation include the following:

1. **Occiput transverse.** On vaginal examination, the sagittal suture (in the midline front to back) of the fetal head occupies the transverse diameter of the pelvis more or less midway between the sacrum and the symphysis.
   a. In the **left occiput transverse positions,** the smaller posterior fontanelle is to the left in the maternal pelvis, and the larger anterior fontanelle is directed toward the opposite side.
   b. In the **right occiput transverse positions,** the reverse is true.
2. **Occiput anterior.** The head enters the pelvis with the occiput rotated either 45° anteriorly from the transverse position, right occiput anterior or left occiput anterior.

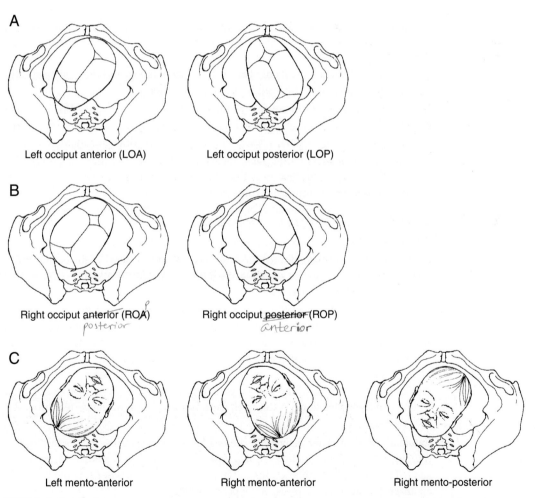

FIGURE 10-2 Occiput and face presentations in labor. **A.** Left positions in occiput presentations, with the fetal head viewed at a cross-section of the pelvis from below. **B.** Right positions in occiput presentations. **C.** Left and right positions in face presentations. (From Pritchard JA, MacDonald PC, Gant NF. Williams Obstetrics. 21st Ed. New York: McGraw-Hill, 2001:294–296.)

3. **Occiput posterior.** The incidence of posterior positions is approximately 10%. The right occiput posterior position is more common than the left occiput posterior position. The posterior positions are often associated with a narrow forepelvis.

   a. In the **right occiput posterior position,** the sagittal suture occupies the right oblique diameter. The small posterior fontanelle is directed posteriorly to the right of the midline, whereas the large anterior fontanelle is directed anteriorly to the left of the midline.

   b. In the **left occiput posterior position,** the reverse is true.

B The mechanism of labor and delivery involves **seven cardinal movements** (Fig. 10-3). A process of positional adaptation of the fetal head to the various segments of the pelvis is required to complete childbirth. These positional changes occur sequentially in the following order:

1. **Engagement.** The biparietal diameter of the fetal head, the greatest transverse diameter of the head in occiput presentations, passes through the pelvic inlet.

   a. **When engagement occurs,** the lowest point of the presenting part is, by definition, at the level of the ischial spines, which is designated as **0 station.** Levels 1, 2, and 3 cm above the spines are designated as **−1, −2, and −3 stations,** respectively; levels 1, 2, and 3 cm below the spines are designated as **+1, +2, and +3 stations,** respectively. At +3, the presenting part is on the perineum.

   b. **Engagement may take place during the last few weeks of pregnancy, or it may not occur until labor begins.** It is more likely to happen before the onset of labor in a primigravida than in a multigravida.

   b. **When the fetal head is not engaged at the onset of labor,** and the fetal head is **freely movable** above the pelvic inlet, the head is said to be **floating.**

2. **Descent.** The first requirement for the birth of an infant is descent. When the fetal head is engaged at the onset of labor in a primigravida, descent may not occur until the start of the second stage. In a multiparous woman, descent usually begins with engagement.

3. **Flexion.** When the descending head meets resistance from either the cervix, the walls of the pelvis, or the pelvic floor, flexion of the fetal head normally occurs.

   a. The chin is brought into close contact with the fetal thorax.

   b. This movement causes a smaller diameter of fetal head to be presented to the pelvis than would occur if the head were not flexed.

4. **Internal rotation.** This movement is always associated with descent of the presenting part and usually is not accomplished until the head has reached the level of the ischial spines (0 station). The movement involves the gradual turning of the occiput from its original position anteriorly toward the symphysis pubis.

5. **Extension of the fetal head.** This extension is essential during the birth process. When the sharply flexed fetal head meets the vulva, the occiput is brought in direct contact with the inferior margin of the symphysis.

   a. Because the vulvar outlet is directed upward and forward, extension must occur for the head to pass through.

   b. The expulsive forces of the uterine contractions and the woman's pushing, along with resistance of the pelvic floor, result in the anterior extension of the vertex in the direction of the vulvar opening.

6. **External rotation.** After delivery of the head, restitution occurs. In this movement, the occiput returns to the oblique position from which it started and then to the transverse position, left or right. This movement corresponds to the rotation of the fetal body, bringing the shoulders into an anteroposterior diameter with the pelvic outlet.

7. **Expulsion.** After external rotation, the anterior shoulder appears under the symphysis and is delivered. The perineum soon becomes distended by the posterior shoulder. After delivery of the shoulders, the rest of the infant's body is extruded quickly.

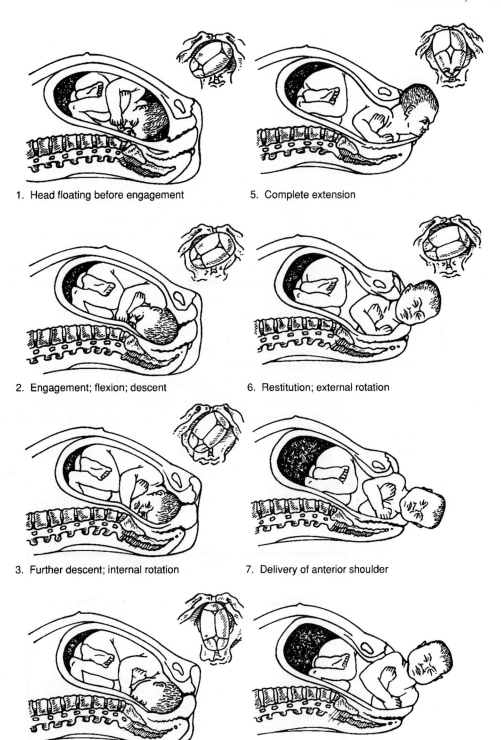

1. Head floating before engagement
2. Engagement; flexion; descent
3. Further descent; internal rotation
4. Complete rotation; beginning extension
5. Complete extension
6. Restitution; external rotation
7. Delivery of anterior shoulder
8. Delivery of posterior shoulder

FIGURE 10-3 Principal movements in labor and delivery, left occiput anterior position. (From Cunningham FG, MacDonald PC, Gant NF. Williams Obstetrics. 21st Ed. New York: McGraw-Hill, 2001:302, Figure 12-13.)

IV   CONDUCT OF LABOR

A **Detection of ruptured membranes.**   Ruptured membranes are signified at any time during pregnancy by either a sudden gush or a steady trickle of clear fluid from the vagina. In a term pregnancy, labor usually follows within 24 hours of membrane rupture. The risk of intrauterine infection (chorioamnionitis) increases if the patient has ruptured membranes for longer than 24 hours, with or without labor.

1. **Nitrazine test.** Nitrazine paper changes color, depending on the pH of the fluid being tested. Amniotic fluid, which is alkaline, turns Nitrazine paper deep blue.

2. **Ferning.** Amniotic fluid, like many body fluids, has a high sodium content, which causes a ferning pattern when the fluid is air-dried on a slide. Other vaginal secretions do not have such a ferning pattern. A positive fern test confirms ruptured membranes because the Nitrazine paper can turn blue with alkaline cervical mucus or blood in the absence of ruptured membranes.

B **First stage of labor.**   On average, the first stage of labor lasts for approximately 12 hours in the primigravida and approximately 7 hours in the multigravida, although there is great patient-to-patient variability. A graph of cervical dilation and descent versus time produces a characteristic sigmoid pattern in normal labor (Fig. 10-4).

1. **Fetal monitoring.** The fetal heart tones should be monitored immediately after a uterine contraction because a sudden drop to less than 120 beats per minute (bpm) or an increase to above 180 bpm may indicate fetal distress.

2. **Amniotomy.** Artificial rupture of the membranes reveals the color of the amniotic fluid (whether it is stained by **meconium,** a sticky, dark-green substance found in the intestine of the full-term fetus) and often shortens the length of labor if a woman is already contracting regularly.

3. **Latent phase of labor.** During the latent phase, the uterine contractions typically are infrequent; somewhat uncomfortable; and, in some cases, irregular. However, they generate sufficient force to cause slow dilation and some effacement of the cervix. A prolonged latent phase is more than 20 hours in the primigravida and more than 14 hours in the multigravida.

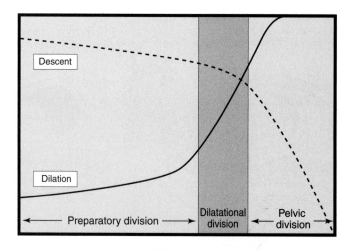

Time

FIGURE 10-4   Graph of cervical dilation and descent versus time. (From Cunningham FG, MacDonald PC, Gant NF. Williams Obstetrics. 21st Ed. New York: McGraw-Hill, 2001:428, Figure 18-2.)

TABLE 10-4 Abnormal Labor Patterns, Diagnostic Criteria, and Methods of Treatment

Labor Pattern	Diagnostic Criterion		Preferred Treatment	Exceptional Treatment
	Nulliparas	**Multiparas**		
Prolongation disorder (prolonged latent phase)	>20 hr	>14 hr	Therapeutic rest	Oxytocin or cesarean delivery for urgent problems
Protraction disorders				
Protracted active phase dilatation	<1.2 cm/hr	<1.5 cm/hr		
Protracted descent	<1.0 cm/hr	<2 cm/hr	Expectant management and support	With CPD: cesarean delivery
Arrest disorders				
Prolonged deceleration phase	>3 hr	>1 hr	Without CPD: oxytocin	Rest if exhausted
Secondary arrest of dilatation	>2 hr	>2 hr		
Arrest of descent	>1 hr	>1 hr	With CPD: cesarean delivery	Cesarean delivery
Failure of descent	No descent in deceleration phase of second stage of labor	Cesarean delivery	Cesarean delivery	

CPD, cephalopelvic disproportion.
From Cunningham FG, MacDonald PC, Gant NF. Williams Obstetrics. 21st Ed. New York: McGraw-Hill, 2001:431, Table 18-4.

4. **Active phase of labor.** The active phase, or clinically apparent labor, follows the latent phase and is characterized by progressive cervical dilation. A prolonged active phase is seen in the primigravida who dilates less than 1.2 cm per hour and in the multigravida who dilates less than 1.5 cm per hour.

5. **Dysfunctional labor patterns.** Uterine dysfunction in any phase of cervical dilation is characterized by lack of progress because one of the cardinal features of normal labor is its progression. Abnormal labor patterns, diagnostic criteria, and methods of treatment are summarized in Table 10-4.

C **Second stage of labor.**   On the average, the second stage lasts for approximately 50 minutes in the primigravida and approximately 20 minutes in the multigravida. However, second stages that last 2 hours, especially in the primigravida, are common. The second stage is characterized by intense pushing on the part of the patient.

1. **Spontaneous vaginal delivery**
   a. **Delivery of the head.** With each contraction, the vulvar opening is dilated by the head. The encirclement of the largest diameter of the fetal head by the vulvar ring is known as **crowning.** The head is then delivered slowly with the base of the occiput rotating around the lower margin of the symphysis pubis.
   b. **Delivery of the shoulders.** In most cases, the shoulders appear at the vulva just after external rotation and are delivered spontaneously. If the shoulders are not delivered spontaneously, gentle traction is used to engage and deliver the anterior and then the posterior shoulders. Excessive traction with extension of the infant's neck can result in temporary or permanent injury to the brachial plexus, known as Erb palsy.

TABLE 10-5   Types of Episiotomy

Type	Advantages	Disadvantages
Median	Ease of repair Faulty healing is rare Dyspareunia is rare Good anatomic result Small blood loss	Extension through anal sphincter and into rectum is relatively common
Mediolateral	More space at vaginal outlet for breech or shoulder dystocia Rare extension through anal sphincter	Faulty healing is common Difficulty of repair Occasional dyspareunia Occasional faulty anatomic result Greater blood loss than with median episiotomy

2. **Episiotomy** is the most common operation in obstetrics (Table 10-5). It involves an incision in the perineum that is either in the midline (**median episiotomy**) or begun in the midline but directed laterally away from the rectum (**mediolateral episiotomy**). The episiotomy substitutes a straight, clean surgical incision for the ragged laceration that may otherwise result. An episiotomy is easier to repair and heals better than a tear, shortens the second stage of labor, and spares the infant's head from prolonged pounding against the perineum.

D **Third stage of labor.**   The placenta usually is delivered within 5 minutes of the delivery of the infant.

1. **Signs of placental separation**
   a. The uterus becomes globular and firm.
   b. There often is a sudden gush of blood.
   c. The uterus rises in the abdomen because the placenta, having separated, passes down into the lower uterine segment and vagina, where its bulk pushes the uterus upward.
   d. The umbilical cord protrudes farther out of the vagina, indicating that the placenta has descended.

2. **Uterine hemostasis.** The mechanism by which hemostasis is achieved at the placental site is **vasoconstriction,** produced by a well-contracted myometrium. Intravenous or intramuscular **oxytocin** (10 U intramuscularly or 20 U in a 1000-mL intravenous bottle), **ergonovine** (0.2 mg intramuscularly or intravenously), or **prostaglandin** $F_{2\alpha}$ (0.25 mg intramuscularly and repeated if necessary at 15- to 90-minute intervals up to a maximum of eight doses) helps the uterus contract and decreases blood loss. These medications are administered after the placenta has been delivered.

E **Lacerations of the birth canal.**   There are four types of vaginal or perineal lacerations, all of which are less likely to occur with an appropriate episiotomy.

1. **First-degree lacerations** involve the fourchette, perineal skin, and vaginal mucosa, but not the fascia and muscle.

2. **Second-degree lacerations** involve the skin, mucosa, fascia, and muscles of the perineal body, but not the anal sphincter.

3. **Third-degree lacerations** extend through the skin, mucosa, perineal body, and involve the anal sphincter.

4. **Fourth-degree lacerations** are extensions of the third-degree tear through the rectal mucosa to expose the lumen of the rectum.

Study Questions for Chapter 10

Directions: *Each of the numbered items or incomplete statements in this section is followed by answers or by completions of the statement. Select the ONE lettered answer or completion that is BEST in each case.*

1. A 26-year-old woman, gravida 2, para 1 at 39 weeks of gestation is admitted to the hospital in labor. Her cervix is dilated 5 cm and is 100% effaced, and fetal vertex is at +1 station. You perform amniotomy and obtain 3+ meconium. You place a fetal scalp monitor and an intrauterine pressure catheter and you start amnioinfusion with normal saline. Fetal monitoring strip reveals five contractions in 10 minutes, and each contraction produces 50 mmHg of pressure. Three hours later, her cervix is 5 cm dilated and 100% effaced, and fetal vertex is at +1 station. What is the next best step in management?

- [A] Augmentation with oxytocin
- [B] Cesarean section
- [C] Vacuum delivery
- [D] Magnesium sulfate
- [E] Methergine

2. A 22-year-woman, gravida 1, para 0 at 40 weeks of gestation presents to labor and delivery reporting regular contractions for the last 2 hours. She denies loss of fluid from the vagina and reports fetal movement. Her cervix is dilated 2.5 cm and 50% effaced, and fetal vertex is at 0 station. The fetal monitoring strip shows regular uterine contractions every 2 to 3 minutes that are uncomfortable but not painful. The fetal heart rate baseline is 154 bpm without decelerations and is reactive. What is the next step in management?

- [A] Cesarean section
- [B] Oxytocin
- [C] Fundal massage
- [D] Walk for 1 to 2 hours
- [E] Meperidine

3. A 29-year-old woman, gravida 2, para 1 at 32 weeks of gestation presents to labor and delivery reporting flank pain, fever, chills, and cramping. She is having contractions every 3 to 4 minutes, and the fetal heart rate baseline is 180. You check her cervix and discover a dilation of 3.5 cm, 100% effacement, and you see that the fetal head is floating. Three injections of terbutaline are administered every 15 minutes while you continue your evaluation. From the physical examination and from results of the urinalysis, you conclude that she has pyelonephritis and admit her to the hospital for intravenous antibiotics, magnesium sulfate, and steroids. Several hours later, you are paged because she is having trouble breathing. Her vitals are follows: T = 102.1, BP = 110/78, P = 105, R = 28, and oxygen saturation is 96% on room air. Physical examination reveals that heart is regular rate and rhythm and without murmurs. You hear bilateral rales over the lung bases. Her abdomen is soft, gravid, and non-tender. She still has costovertebral angle tenderness. There is 2+ pedal edema. Which of the following is the most likely diagnosis?

- [A] Complication of pyelonephritis
- [B] Congestive heart failure
- [C] Pulmonary embolus
- [D] Pulmonary edema
- [E] Respiratory muscle paralysis

4. A 24-year-old woman, gravida 1, para 0 at 39 weeks of gestation is crowning. The fetal head is not emerging from the vagina after two pushes. You palpate a thick hymenal ring of tissue at the introitus.

Fetal monitoring strip shows bradycardia after the third push, so you decide to cut a 3-cm episiotomy that extends through the hymenal ring and vagina and ends laterally in the perineum. What is the advantage of this type of episiotomy?

- [A] Clean surgical incision
- [B] Avoids fourth-degree laceration
- [C] Less dyspareunia
- [D] Commonly used when distance between posterior introitus and anus is large
- [E] Easier to repair

5. A professor of obstetrics is explaining the seven cardinal movements of labor: first—the greatest transverse diameter of the fetal head passes through the pelvic inlet; second—fetal head descends; third—the fetal chin is brought into close contact with the fetal thorax; fourth—turning of the occiput toward 12 o'clock position; fifth—the uterine contractions extend fetal vertex anteriorly. What is the next step?

- [A] Delivery of the head
- [B] Rotation of occiput to transverse position
- [C] Rotation of occiput to posterior position
- [D] Delivery of anterior shoulder
- [E] Expulsion

Answers and Explanations

1. The answer is B [IV B 4 and Table 10-4]. This is a clinical scenario where the patient has had arrest of dilation (i.e., there has been no change in dilation in the last 2 hours in this multiparous patient). Augmentation with oxytocin is not necessary because she has adequate contraction frequency (every 2 to 3 minutes) and intensity (50 mmHg) in a 10-minute period. This patient is not a candidate for vacuum delivery. To perform a low vacuum delivery, the cervix must be fully dilated, the station must be +2 or greater, the rotation of fetal head is unnecessary, and a valid indication for use of vacuum must be present (i.e., fetal distress, prolonged second stage of labor, or maternal disease process [e.g., heart condition or brain aneurysm], which benefit from reduction in pushing during the second stage of labor). There is no need to use a tocolytic to slow down labor. You want to achieve the opposite. Methergine is used for postpartum hemorrhage.

2. The answer is D [II D and Table 10-3]. This patient is in stage 1, latent phase of labor. It is difficult to predict when a person will make the transition from latent phase to active phase of labor. At this point, you cannot tell if this patient is in true labor or if this is pseudo-labor. By having the patient walk for 1 to 2 hours and then return to check her cervix, you are able to diagnose labor if the cervical dilation changes. For example, if she returns in 2 hours and her cervix is dilated to 4 cm, then you can diagnose labor because her regular uterine contractions have produced cervical change. There is no need to augment her contractions with oxytocin in this stage of labor. She is not a candidate for cesarean section because there are no fetal or maternal indications. A fundal massage is a maneuver useful immediately after delivery of the placenta to help contract the uterus. Meperidine would be useful if the patient had prolongation of the latent phase of labor; that is, if she was having regular, painful uterine contractions for more than 20 hours (in nulliparas = "para 0") and did not have change in her cervix.

3. The answer is D [Table 10-1]. This patient has many risk factors for noncardiogenic pulmonary edema. She has pyelonephritis and has been given terbutaline and subsequently magnesium sulfate (both of these have pulmonary edema as a complication). She has bilateral lung rales because of exudation of fluid from the capillaries into the alveoli of the lung bases. There is no reason to think she has a heart problem (she is young, there is no mention of family history, heart examination is normal, and pedal edema is found in normal pregnancy). Pulmonary embolism is always a possibility and must be ruled out because she is pregnant and has tachypnea, but it is lower down in the differential diagnosis. Pyelonephritis can lead to sepsis and adult respiratory distress syndrome (ARDS), but again this is lower down in the differential because there is no mention of blood culture results, her blood pressure is stable, oxygen saturation is high, and there is no mention of her level of distress. Respiratory muscle paralysis occurs at very high levels of magnesium sulfate (there is no mention of her serum magnesium level).

4. The answer is B [IV C 2; Table 10-5]. A mediolateral episiotomy is cut if there is not enough space in the introitus for emergence of fetal head and if there is a short distance between the posterior introitus and anus (because a median episiotomy as high risk of extending into the anal sphincter and even rectal mucosa). A median episiotomy is easier to repair, has less blood loss, causes less dyspareunia, heals better, and has better anatomic results. Clean surgical incision is obtained with both median and mediolateral episiotomy.

5. The answer is B [III B 6]. The sixth cardinal movement begins with delivery of the fetal head by extension and ends with rotation of the occiput from anterior position to oblique and then to transverse position. Expulsion and delivery of anterior shoulder is the seventh cardinal movement.

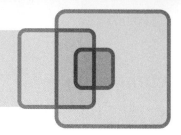

chapter **11**

Intrapartum Fetal Monitoring

JOANNE N. QUINONES AND SARA J. MARDER

I   INTRODUCTION

A The fetal heart rate (FHR) is under the control of the autonomic nervous system (ANS). An intact ANS reflects **normal fetal oxygenation** and results in a **normal FHR pattern.**

B Intrapartum FHR monitoring is used to **assess fetal well-being** during labor. It closely **quantifies and interprets the FHR** to obtain reassurance that fetal oxygenation is normal.

1. A reassuring FHR pattern is usually associated with **adequate oxygenation** of the fetus and a newborn that is vigorous at birth. When the FHR pattern is **reassuring:**
   a. A clinician can safely allow labor to proceed.
   b. There is a **low risk of perinatal asphyxia,** which refers to **damaging acidemia, hypoxia, and metabolic acidosis** associated with **neonatal neurologic sequelae** and other organ dysfunction.
2. A nonreassuring FHR pattern is a sign of potential **hypoxia.** When the FHR pattern is **nonreassuring:**
   a. A clinician must obtain other reassurance of fetal well-being.
   b. It may be necessary to expedite delivery.

II   PATHOPHYSIOLOGY OF FETAL HYPOXIA

A Normal fetal oxygenation

1. Uterine blood flow, intervillous blood flow, and **transplacental gaseous exchange are reduced** during normal labor, temporarily resulting in relative fetal hypoxemia.
2. Transient, sometimes repetitive, episodes of **hypoxemia and hypoxia,** even at the level of the central nervous system (CNS), are **common during normal labor** and are **usually well tolerated** by the fetus.
3. **Greater fetal oxygen-carrying capacity** allows adequate delivery of oxygen to the fetal tissues despite the low fetal arterial partial pressure of oxygen (PO_2) for the following reasons:
   a. Higher fetal cardiac output
   b. Higher systemic blood flow rate (compared with adults)
   c. Greater affinity of fetal hemoglobin for oxygen

B Fetal hypoxia

1. When uterine or umbilical blood flow is impaired, fetal tissue perfusion is decreased and **oxygen transfer is diminished.**
2. Carbon dioxide accumulates in the fetal circulation, causing a **decline in pH, resulting in acidemia.**
3. Prolonged periods of decreased uterine or placental perfusion lead to **metabolic acidosis** as the fetus becomes dependent on anaerobic glycolysis to meet its energy requirements.

    4. As pyruvic and lactic acids accumulate, there is a further drop in fetal pH, eventually resulting in **asphyxia** if unresolved.

III   TYPES OF FETAL HEART RATE MONITORING

A **Continuous monitoring.**   The FHR pattern can be continuously evaluated in two ways.

    1. An **external ultrasound device** placed on the maternal abdomen emits and receives the reflected **ultrasound signal from the movement of the fetal heart valves.** The reflected sound waves return to the transducer, permitting an assessment of the FHR activity.

    2. A **fetal scalp electrode** measures **consecutive R-R wave intervals** of the fetal QRS complex, directly measuring the FHR. The signal is transmitted to a monitor, where it is amplified, counted, and recorded.

B **Intermittent FHR auscultation.**   This method is **equivalent to continuous monitoring** in assessing fetal condition when performed at specific intervals with a 1:1 nurse-patient ratio. However, continuous monitoring is more commonly used in the United States because it is convenient and less expensive.

    1. During the **active phase of labor,** auscultation is recorded **at least every 15 minutes** after a contraction.

    2. During the **second stage of labor,** auscultation is recorded **every 5 minutes.**

IV   INTERPRETATION OF FETAL HEART RATE PATTERNS

When describing the FHR tracing in labor, the clinician evaluates the **baseline FHR, variability, contraction frequency,** and **periodic changes.**

A **Baseline FHR.**   The FHR is the heart rate that occurs between contractions, regardless of accelerations or decelerations.

    1. Normal
      a. **Normal baseline FHR is 120 to 160 beats per minute (bpm).**
      b. The baseline FHR decreases gradually from 16 weeks' gestation to term as the parasympathetic system develops.

    2. Tachycardia
      a. **Baseline tachycardia is an FHR greater than 160 bpm** for periods of 10 minutes or more.
      b. Recurrent tachycardia can be associated with the following conditions:
        (1) Hypoxia
        (2) Maternal fever
        (3) Chorioamnionitis
        (4) Prematurity
        (5) Drugs (e.g., ritodrine, atropine)
        (6) Fetal stimulation
        (7) Fetal arrhythmias
        (8) Maternal anxiety
        (9) Maternal thyrotoxicosis

    3. Bradycardia
      a. **Baseline bradycardia is an FHR of less than 120 bpm** for periods of 10 minutes or more.
      b. Recurrent bradycardia can be associated with the following conditions:
        (1) Hypoxia
        (2) Drugs (e.g., mepivacaine, β-blockers)
        (3) Autonomic mediated reflex (e.g., to pressure on fetal head)

    (4) Arrhythmias

    (5) Hypothermia

B **FHR variability**

1. **Baseline variability** is defined as deflections from the baseline FHR resulting from the continuous interaction between fetal sympathetic and parasympathetic nervous systems. **Normal variability** is one of the best indicators of **intact integration** between the fetal CNS and the heart.

2. Causes of **loss of variability**

    a. Hypoxia

    b. Fetal sleep state (sleep cycles of 30 minutes or less)

    c. CNS depressants (e.g., atropine, scopolamine, tranquilizers, narcotics, barbiturates, anesthetics)

    d. Prematurity

    e. Baseline tachycardia

    f. Fetal cardiac abnormalities or arrhythmias

    g. Fetal CNS abnormalities

3. Characterization of variability

    a. Absent: undetectable amplitude

    b. Minimal (Fig. 11-1): Detectable amplitude but less than 5 bpm

    c. Moderate (Fig. 11-2): Amplitude of 6 to 25 bpm

    d. Marked: Amplitude of more than 25 bpm

C **Contractions.**   Assessment occurs in two ways.

1. **Tocodynamometer**

    a. A pressure-sensitive tocodynamometer is placed around the maternal abdomen.

    b. The tocodynamometer measures **only the frequency of contractions,** not their intensity or strength.

2. **Intrauterine pressure catheter (IUPC).** This method allows internal monitoring of contractions.

    a. After the catheter is introduced into the uterine cavity, it is attached to a strain gauge, which measures the pressure generated by the uterine contractions.

    b. IUPC measures **both the frequency and strength of contractions.**

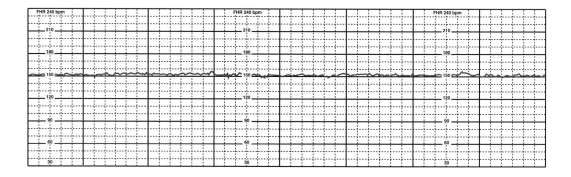

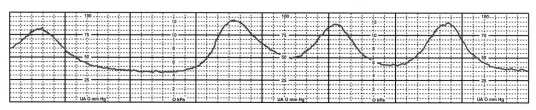

FIGURE 11-1 Minimal variability.

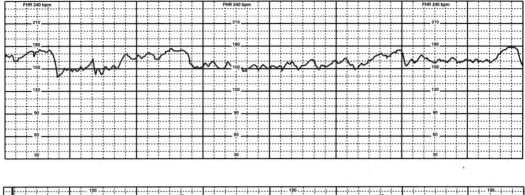

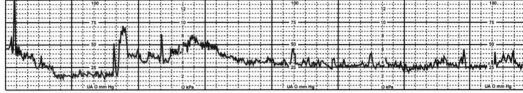

FIGURE 11-2   Moderate variability.

D FHR accelerations (Fig. 11-3) are defined as abrupt increases in baseline FHR (onset to peak FHR in less than 30 seconds).

1. **Before 32 weeks' gestation,** accelerations are defined as having a peak **of at least 10 bpm** above baseline, **lasting for 10 seconds or more.**

2. **After 32 weeks' gestation,** accelerations are defined as having a peak **of at least 15 bpm** above baseline, **lasting between 15 seconds and 2 minutes.**

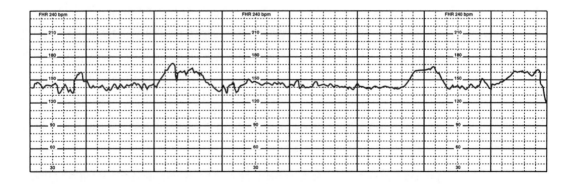

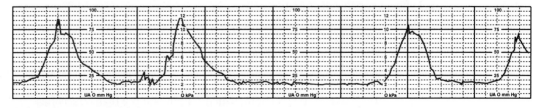

FIGURE 11-3   Accelerations are defined as abrupt increases in baseline fetal heart rate, which peak in less than 30 seconds.

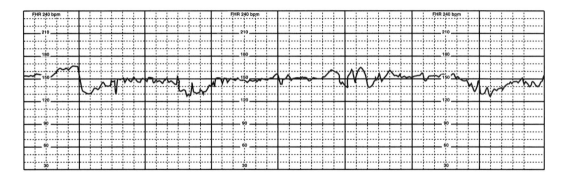

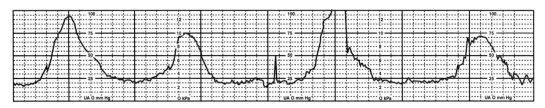

FIGURE 11-4 Early decelerations reach their lowest point at the peak of the contraction.

E **FHR decelerations.** The **three patterns of periodic decelerations** are based on the waveform configuration and the **timing of the deceleration in relation to the uterine contraction.**

1. **Early decelerations** (Fig. 11-4)
   a. **Definition.** Early decelerations begin with the onset of uterine contractions, **reach their lowest point (never less than 100 bpm) at the peak of the contraction,** and return to baseline as the contraction ends.
   b. **Mechanism.** Early decelerations are thought to be caused by local changes in cerebral blood flow, which result in stimulation of the **vagal centers,** with acetylcholine release at the sinoatrial node.
   c. **Associated conditions.** Early decelerations can occur when the **fetal head is compressed** as it moves down the birth canal. The decelerations are considered physiologic and are **not associated** with fetal acidemia.

2. **Variable decelerations**
   a. **Definition.** Variable decelerations are **abrupt decreases in FHR** with a rapid return to baseline (onset of deceleration to nadir less than 30 seconds) that may **occur before, during, or after** the onset of uterine contractions.
   b. **Mechanism.** Variable decelerations involve **reflex-mediated changes** in the FHR controlled by the vagus nerve.
   c. **Associated conditions.** Variable decelerations are generally caused by **umbilical cord compression** between fetal parts or between fetal parts and the uterine wall. They can also be seen in patients with **oligohydramnios.**
   d. **Types of variable decelerations**
      (1) **Mild** (Fig. 11-5)
         (a) Duration of less than 30 seconds
         (b) Minimal clinical significance
      (2) **Moderate** (Fig. 11-6)
         (a) Two types
            (i) Nadir of 70 to 80 bpm, with duration of more than 60 seconds
            (ii) Nadir of less than 70 bpm, with duration of 30 to 60 seconds

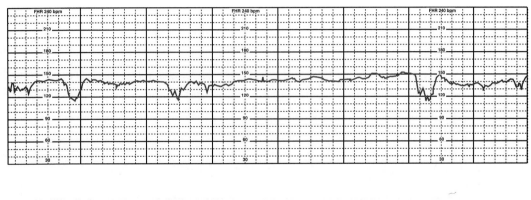

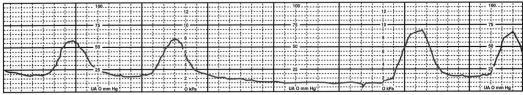

FIGURE 11-5 Mild variable decelerations last less than 30 seconds.

   (b) Persistent moderate variable decelerations can lead to a reduction in fetal oxygenation, resulting in hypoxemia and acidemia.

  (3) Severe (Fig. 11-6)

   (a) Nadir of less than 70 bpm, with duration of more than 60 seconds

   (b) Prolonged or severe variable decelerations may lead to a significant reduction in respiratory gas exchange with subsequent fetal hypoxemia and acidemia.

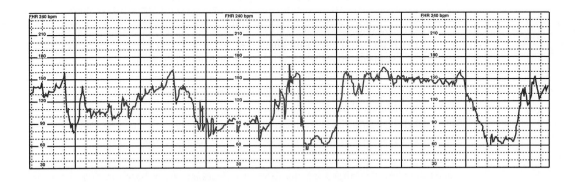

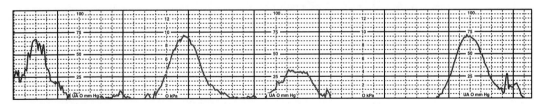

FIGURE 11-6 Moderate and severe variable decelerations.

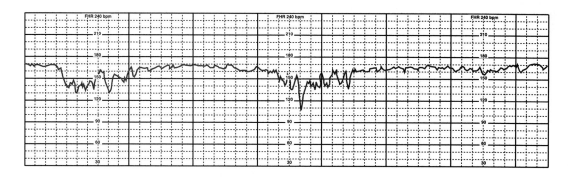

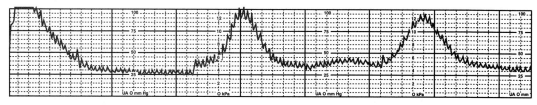

FIGURE 11-7 Late decelerations. The nadir of each deceleration occurs after the peak of the contraction.

3. **Late decelerations** (Fig. 11-7)
   a. **Definition.** Late decelerations are gradual decreases and returns to baseline FHR associated with uterine contractions (onset to nadir is 30 seconds or more). The **nadir occurs after the peak of the contraction.**
   b. **Mechanism and associated conditions**
      (1) Late decelerations associated with **normal variability** represent reflex responses mediated via the vagus nerve. They may be seen with **mild transient hypoxia.**
      (2) Late decelerations associated with **decreased variability** can result from direct myocardial depression and can be seen with **prolonged hypoxia and acidemia.**
      (3) **Uteroplacental insufficiency,** which results from decreased uterine perfusion or decreased placental function, can lead to repetitive late decelerations and minimal variability. Conditions that may lead to uteroplacental insufficiency include:
         (a) Postdates pregnancy
         (b) Maternal diabetes mellitus
         (c) Maternal hypertension (chronic or pregnancy-induced)
         (d) Abruptio placentae
         (e) Maternal anemia
         (f) Maternal sepsis
         (g) Hypertonia (excessive uterine tone)
         (h) Hyperstimulation (excessive uterine contractions)
4. **Prolonged decelerations**
   a. **Definition.** Prolonged decelerations are decreases from baseline of 15 bpm or more, which last 2 to 10 minutes.
   b. **Mechanism.** Prolonged decelerations can result from the following factors:
      (1) **Vagus nerve discharge** (e.g., head compression during rapid descent)
      (2) **Fetal hypoxia** caused by mechanisms such as:
         (a) Uterine hyperactivity
         (b) Sympathetic blockade from regional anesthesia
         (c) Supine hypotension
         (d) Unrelieved cord compression
         (e) Maternal respiratory arrest

V   FETAL HEART RATE TRACINGS: ASSESSMENT AND MANAGEMENT IN LABOR

A **Reassuring FHR patterns.** When FHR tracings are reassuring, practitioners allow labor to continue. FHR accelerations contribute to the reassurance of fetal well-being.

B **Nonreassuring FHR patterns**
1. Characteristics
   a. Repetitive decelerations
   b. Abnormal baseline FHR
   c. Absence of accelerations
   d. Loss of variability
   e. Repetitive late decelerations; repetitive, moderate-to-severe variable decelerations; and absent variability or baseline tachycardia
2. **Further evaluation** is necessary.
   a. Evaluate for the **potential causes** of the nonreassuring FHR pattern.
   b. Obtain information and reassurance about the fetal well-being.
   c. Perform intrauterine resuscitation to improve placental perfusion and oxygen transfer to the fetus.

C **Management of women with nonreassuring FHR patterns**
1. Change in maternal position
   a. In the **supine position**, the uterus obstructs blood flow through the aorta and the inferior vena cava, potentially leading to decreased placental perfusion.
   b. Placement in a lateral recumbent position during labor causes the uterus to fall away from the great vessels, which should improve fetal oxygenation.
2. **Oxygenation. Maternal hyperoxia** may increase the maternal-fetal oxygen gradient, potentially improving the FHR pattern. Oxygen should be given by mask.
3. Reversal of anesthetic effects
   a. **Sympathetic blockade** from epidural anesthesia may result in decreased venous return and cardiac output, maternal hypotension, and decreased uteroplacental perfusion.
   b. Administration of intravenous fluids or ephedrine to the mother may improve uterine blood flow and, therefore, the FHR tracing.
4. Regulation of uterine activity
   a. **Hyperstimulation or excessive uterine activity** from prostaglandin or oxytocin stimulation may lead to incomplete uterine relaxation and possibly decreased fetal oxygenation.
   b. Intravenous hydration, **discontinuation of the uterotonic agent,** or uterine relaxation with terbutaline (β-sympathomimetic) may improve the FHR pattern.
5. **Correction of cord compression.** Variable decelerations, which are caused by **umbilical cord compression,** may be corrected with the following maneuvers:
   a. Change in maternal position, which may relieve the compression
   b. Placement of an **amnioinfusion**, which is an intrauterine catheter through which saline is infused into the uterine cavity. Theoretically, an amnioinfusion "pads" the cord, protecting it from compression.

D **Further assessment of fetal well-being.** After optimization of the maternal position, maternal vital signs, and labor pattern, further evaluation of fetal well-being should take place.
1. **Vibroacoustic stimuli (VAS).** An artificial larynx is placed on the maternal skin over the fetal head, and the fetus is stimulated by noise for 1 second.
   a. The presence of fetal accelerations in response to VAS is considered reassuring.
   b. The fetus is restimulated if no accelerations occur within 10 seconds. The VAS test may be repeated up to four times.

    2. Scalp stimulation test. The examiner rubs the fetal scalp during a digital examination.

      a. An acceleration is usually seen in the FHR tracing of the uncompromised, nonacidotic fetus. The presence of an **acceleration** is associated with an intact ANS and a fetal scalp **blood pH greater than 7.20.**

      b. If an acceleration is not obtained after scalp stimulation, fetal scalp blood can be sampled to measure the fetal pH.

    3. Fetal scalp blood sampling. The fetal scalp is visualized through the dilated cervix, and blood is collected in heparinized capillary tubes after making a tiny stab on the scalp with a small blade. The capillary tubes are sent to the laboratory for pH measurement. The normal fetal capillary pH is 7.25 to 7.35 in the first stage of labor.

      a. A **fetal scalp pH greater than or equal to 7.20** is reassurance that **the fetus is not acidotic.** Labor can proceed for 20 to 30 minutes.

        (1) If a nonreassuring FHR pattern persists after 20 to 30 minutes and scalp stimulation is ineffective, the fetal scalp pH may be repeated to obtain reassurance on fetal well-being.

        (2) In the case of a nonreassuring FHR pattern, the decision to intervene depends on the clinician's assessment of the likelihood of hypoxia and the estimated time to spontaneous delivery.

      b. A **pH of less than 7.20** may represent significant **acidosis.** Delivery is thus indicated by operative (vacuum or forceps-assisted) vaginal delivery, if possible, or cesarean delivery. The clinician must decide on the **most expeditious** way to deliver the patient based on the clinical circumstances.

VI   **NEW DEVELOPMENTS IN INTRAPARTUM MONITORING: FETAL OXYGEN SATURATION MONITORING**

  A **Normal fetal oxygen saturation ranges between 35 and 75%,** with an average level of 55 to 60%. If the fetal oxygen saturation remains **above 30% during labor,** there appears to be **no risk of fetal metabolic acidosis.**

  B The U.S. Food and Drug Administration recently approved the first device for monitoring fetal oxygen saturation.

    1. The sensor is slid through the cervix and lodges against the fetal cheek. It is held in place by the pressure created by the fetal cheek and the pelvic sidewall.

    2. This method is used at some centers but has not yet been broadly instituted. Further research to evaluate its use and impact on current obstetric management is ongoing.

Study Questions for Chapter 11

Directions: Each of the numbered items or incomplete statements in this section is followed by answers or by completions of the statement. Select the ONE lettered answer or completion that is BEST in each case.

1. A 25-year-old woman, gravida 1, para 0 at 39 weeks of gestation has been laboring for a few hours. Her cervix is dilated to 6 cm, 80% effaced, and fetal vertex is at 0 station. Membranes have been ruptured for 20 hours and her labor is being augmented with oxytocin. The intrauterine pressure catheter detects contractions every 1 to 2 minutes at 80 mmHg of pressure and lasting 2 minutes. Fetal heart rate baseline by scalp electrode is 90 bpm for the last 2 minutes (FHR baseline 30 minutes ago was 140 bpm). What is the best next step in management?

- A Penicillin
- B Cesarean section
- C Left lateral position
- D Discontinue oxytocin
- E Amnioinfusion

2. A 22-year-old woman, gravida 2, para 1 at 41 weeks of gestation is in labor. Her cervix is dilated to 5 cm, it is 100% effaced, and fetal vertex is at 0 station with a "bulging bag of water" ahead of fetal vertex. You decide to perform artificial rupture of membranes and obtain large quantities of clear fluid. One hour later, her cervix is dilated to 7 cm. She has 4 to 5 contractions every 10 minutes, and fetal heart rate baseline is 150 bpm with repetitive sharp deceleration to 90 bpm during contractions. What is the best next step in management?

- A Placement of intrauterine pressure catheter (IUPC)
- B Amnioinfusion
- C Terbutaline
- D Change position
- E Oxygen by mask

3. A 27-year-old woman, gravida 1, para 0 at 40 and 3/7th weeks of gestation is in the middle of the first stage of labor. Her cervix is dilated to 4.5 cm and a decision has been made to place an epidural. Prior to placement of the epidural, she receives a 500 cc bolus of LR to prehydrate her, and augmentation with oxytocin is begun. Her vitals are as follows: T = 99.1, BP = 110/74, P = 102, R = 18. The fetal heart rate baseline is 142 bpm with three accelerations every 20 minutes. She is contracting every 3 minutes. After placement of the epidural, fetal heart rate baseline drops to 130 bpm, and no accelerations are seen within a 10-minute period. The fetal heart rate also shows a gradual decline in the middle of each contraction to about 115 bpm and then returns to baseline of 130 bpm. She has contractions every 2 to 3 minutes now. Her vitals at this point are as follows: T = 99.2, BP = 78/56, P = 115, R = 18. What is the best next step in management?

- A Tylenol
- B Penicillin
- C Intravenous hydration
- D Ephedrine
- E Discontinue oxytocin

4. A 22-year-old woman, gravida 2, para 1, at 41 weeks of gestation is laboring. Her cervix is dilated to 8 cm, it is effaced 100%, and fetal vertex is at +1 station. Membranes have been ruptured for more than 24 hours, and labor is being augmented with oxytocin. An amnioinfusion is running because of 3-4 + meconium. Fetal heart rate by scalp electrode has a baseline of 138 bpm with reduced short-term variability and occasional mild variable decelerations. You are suddenly called to evaluate a non-reassuring fetal heart rate. The tocodynamometer shows six contractions in a 10- minute period with a pressure of 70 mmHg, and fetal heart rate is now 70 bpm for more than 3 minutes. She is placed in the left lateral position, oxytocin infusion is stopped, she is given oxygen by mask, and her intravenous fluid rate is increased. Fetal heart rate is now 98 bpm. What is the best next step in management?

- A Cesarean section
- B Vacuum deliver
- C Ephedrine
- D Knee-chest position
- E Terbutaline

5. A 19-year-old woman, gravida 1, para 0 at 38 weeks of gestation is in active labor. Her cervix is dilated to 5 cm and fetal vertex is at +1 station. The tocodynamometer displays contractions every 2 to 3 minutes, lasting 1 minute, and producing 50 mmHg of pressure inside the uterus. The fetal heart rate by scalp electrode has a baseline of 140 bpm with random sharp decelerations to 70 bpm that return to baseline in 60 to 80 seconds. When this type of deceleration occurs, what is the best description of the initial acid-base status of the fetus?

- A Respiratory acidosis
- B Metabolic acidosis
- C Uteroplacental insufficiency
- D Asphyxia
- E Increased P_{CO2}

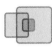 *Answers and Explanations*

1. The answer is D [V C 4 a and b]. This clinical scenario is describing hyperstimulation of the uterus caused by excessive stimulation by oxytocin, which has caused a nonreassuring fetal heart rate (in this case, bradycardia). No level of oxytocin is predictive of hyperstimulation because there are variations in response to oxytocin between individuals and different gestational ages. Remember that normal labor contractions last about 1 minute, produce up to 50 mmHg, and occur every 2 to 3 minutes. When the uterus is hyperstimulated, blood vessels are compressed for an extended period (greater than the fetal reserve), the blood flow to the fetus is reduced, and the fetus becomes hypoxic. None of the other answer choices address the problem of hyperstimulation, which has caused the nonreassuring fetal heart rate pattern.

2. The answer is B [V C 5 b]. After artificial rupture of membranes, a large quantity of fluid flows out of the uterus. The previously cushioned fetus is now vulnerable to every contraction. A lack of fluid cushion and a strong contraction may compress the umbilical cord against the uterus or against a fetal part, thus causing repetitive variable decelerations. Placement of amnioinfusion (which is an intrauterine catheter through which fluid is infused into the uterine cavity) can help. Although amnioinfusion occurs through an IUPC, the latter is not the best next step in managing the problem of repetitive variable decelerations. Although positional changes and oxygen may help, they do not address the root of the problem. Terbutaline is not useful in this circumstance.

3. The answer is D [V C 4 b]. One of the complications with placement of an epidural blockade is hypotension (before the epidural BP = 110/74 and after the epidural BP = 78/56). An epidural blocks sympathetic discharge to vessel walls, and vasoconstriction is inhibited. This causes blood to pool in dependent areas of the body, thus decreasing venous return to the heart. Cardiac output decreases and subsequently results in decreased uteroplacental circulation. To avoid hypotension, anesthesiologists hydrate patients before placement of the epidural and then give ephedrine to keep the BP near its baseline. Although the patient has a low-grade temperature (99.2°), the fever is not the cause of the nonreassuring fetal heart rate; therefore, neither Tylenol nor penicillin are the best choices. Hyperstimulation is not the problem so there is no need to discontinue the oxytocin. This patient has already been prehydrated, so additional hydration would not be as efficacious as giving ephedrine.

4. The answer is E [V C 4 b]. This clinical scenario is describing hyperstimulation. Normal labor contractions have the following property: frequency—every 2 to 3 minutes; duration—45 seconds to a minute; intensity—up to 50 mmHg. In this case, oxytocin has already been stopped, but the nonreassuring fetal heart rate pattern has not resolved because oxytocin is still in the circulation. Thus, before taking the patient for a cesarean section, terbutaline should be tried to reverse the hyperstimulation by tocolysis. This patient is not a candidate for vacuum delivery (she is not even fully dilated yet). Ephedrine is not useful in this case. Knee-chest position is sometimes more useful than left lateral position when there is a nonreassuring fetal heart rate pattern, especially a severe variable deceleration.

5. The answer is A [II B]. This clinical scenario is that of a severe variable deceleration. As the umbilical cord is compressed, decreased perfusion of fetal tissue occurs. This causes the partial pressure of carbon dioxide to increase and the partial pressure of oxygen to decrease. The increased P_{CO_2} decreases the pH, resulting in acidemia. The initial event is therefore respiratory acidosis. When there is prolonged decrease in perfusion, the fetus becomes dependent on anaerobic (not requiring oxygen) glycolysis to meet its energy return and thus produces pyruvic acid and lactic acid. This causes a further drop in the pH, resulting in metabolic acidosis. Eventually, if the acidosis is unresolved, asphyxia occurs. Uteroplacental insufficiency is a term that describes late decelerations. It does not describe the "acid-base" status of the fetus. Although increased PCO_2 (one of the initial occurrences) contributes to respiratory acidosis, it is not the best description of the fetal acid-base status.

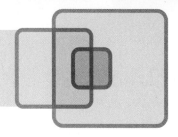

chapter **12**

Operative Obstetrics

DORIS CHOU AND SERDAR URAL

I **CESAREAN BIRTH**

Cesarean section is delivery of a viable fetus through an abdominal incision (laparotomy) and uterine incision (hysterotomy). Cesarean section is the most important surgical procedure in obstetrics. It can be traced to 700 BC in Rome, when the procedure was first used to remove infants from women who died late in pregnancy. The first cesarean section was performed on a living patient in 1610. The maternal mortality rate was high up to the end of the nineteenth century, most often because of hemorrhage and infection. However, advances in surgical and anesthetic techniques, safe blood transfusions, and the discovery of effective antibiotics have led to a dramatic decline in the mortality rate.

A **Incidence.** The incidence of cesarean sections in the United States has continued to increase over the past 30 years. Cesarean section is now the most common operative procedure performed in many hospitals throughout the country.

1. In the United States, **approximately 21% of infants were delivered by cesarean birth in 1997,** compared to 5% in 1960 and 15% in 1970. Several factors contribute to the dramatic increase in cesarean births during this period.
   a. As procedure-related morbidity and mortality rates decreased with advances in anesthetic and operative techniques, the rate of **primary cesarean sections** increased.
      (1) The **widespread use of electronic fetal monitoring** has led to an increased rate of cesarean section for fetal distress.
      (2) The **growing trend of delaying childbirth** in the United States has affected women in labor in two ways. First, a higher proportion of nulliparous women give birth. Second, nulliparity is associated with complications that increase rates of cesarean section, such as dystocia and preeclampsia. The average maternal age has increased in the past 20 years; rates of cesarean section increase with advancing age.
      (3) **Dystocia** or abnormal progress of labor is used more freely as an indication for cesarean section, with a corresponding decline in the rate of forceps deliveries.
      (4) Vaginal **breech** deliveries are not recommended in singleton gestations.
      (5) **Multiple gestation,** an indication for cesarean section, **occurs more frequently.**
   b. As the number of primary cesarean sections increased, previous cesarean section as an indication for a **repeat cesarean section** increased. **Thirty-three** percent of cesarean sections performed in the United States are repeat cesarean sections.
2. **Perinatal mortality.** There is little documentation for an association between the increase in rates of cesarean delivery and a decline in perinatal mortality and morbidity. Although increasing rates of cesarean delivery rates initially led to decreased perinatal mortality, the perinatal mortality rate is not higher in European countries with lower cesarean birth rates. The major causes of perinatal morbidity and mortality continue to be low birth weight and congenital anomalies. In **preterm fetuses weighing greater than 750 g and with malpresentation,** however, cesarean section is believed to **improve** perinatal outcome.

B **Indications.** Compared with vaginal delivery, a properly performed cesarean section carries no increased risk for the fetus; however, the risk of **maternal morbidity and mortality is higher.** Cesarean birth is preferred when the benefits for the mother, fetus, or both outweigh the risk of the procedure for the mother.

1. **Contraindications to labor**
   a. Placenta previa
   b. Vasa previa
   c. Previous classic cesarean section
   d. Previous myomectomy with entrance into the uterine cavity
   e. Previous uterine reconstruction
   f. Malpresentations of the fetus
   g. Active genital herpes infection
   h. Previous cesarean section and patient declines trial of labor

2. **Dystocia and failed induction of labor**
   a. Cephalopelvic disproportion, failure to descend, or arrest of descent or dilation
   b. Failure to progress in normal-size infant, usually because of fetal malposition or posture
   c. Failed forceps or vacuum extractor delivery
   d. Certain fetal malformations that may obstruct labor (i.e., large hydrocephalus, sacrococcygeal tumor)

3. **Emergent conditions that warrant immediate delivery**
   a. Abruptio placentae with antepartum or intrapartum hemorrhage
   b. Umbilical cord prolapse
   c. Nonreassuring antepartum or intrapartum fetal testing
   d. Intrapartum fetal acidemia, with intrapartum scalp pH of less than 7.20
   e. Uterine rupture
   f. Impending maternal death

C **Types of cesarean operations.** Cesarean operations are classified according to the **orientation** (**transverse or vertical**) and the **site of placement** (**lower segment or upper segment**) of the uterine incision.

1. **Low transverse (Kerr).** The low transverse uterine incision is the **preferred** incision and the one **most frequently used** today.
   a. The incision is made in the **noncontractile portion of the uterus,** minimizing chances of rupture or separation in subsequent pregnancies.
   b. The incision requires creation of a bladder flap and lies behind the peritoneal bladder reflection, allowing reperitonealization.
   c. **Uterine closure is accomplished more easily** because of the thin muscle wall of the lower segment, and the **potential for blood loss is lowest** with this type of incision.
   e. This incision may involve potential extension into the uterine vessels laterally and into the cervix and vagina inferiorly.

2. **Low vertical (Sellheim or Krönig).** The vertical incision begins in the noncontractile lower segment but usually extends into the contractile upper segment.
   a. This incision is used **when a transverse incision is not feasible.**
      (1) The lower uterine segment may not be developed if labor has not occurred; the transverse incision may not provide enough room for delivery of the infant.
      (2) Malpresentations of the term or premature infant may necessitate a vertical incision to allow more room for delivery of the infant.
      (3) This incision is sometimes used when an anterior placenta previa is noted to facilitate delivery without cutting through the body of the placenta.

b. This incision also requires creation of a bladder flap and allows reperitonealization.

c. The **risk of uterine rupture** in subsequent pregnancies **is increased** when the upper segment of the uterus is entered.

d. Uterine closure is more difficult, and **blood loss is greater** if the upper segment is involved.

3. **Classic incision (Sanger).** The classic incision is a longitudinal incision in the anterior fundus.

a. This incision is **currently used infrequently** because of the significant **risk of uterine rupture in subsequent pregnancies**, which can occur before labor begins, and higher complication rate.

b. **Indications for this incision** include invasive carcinoma of the cervix, presence of lesions in the lower segment of the uterus (myomas) that prohibit adequate uterine closure, and transverse lie with the back down (most cases). It is the **simplest and quickest incision** to perform.

c. This incision does not require bladder dissection, and reperitonealization is not performed; the potential for intraperitoneal adhesion formation is greater.

d. **Uterine closure is more difficult** because of the thick muscular upper segment, and the **potential for blood loss is greater.**

D Procedure

1. **Patient preparation**
   a. The patient should be **well hydrated.**
   b. The **preoperative hematocrit** should be known, and **blood should be readily available** as indicated.
   c. The **bladder should be empty.** Placement of a Foley catheter is typical.
   d. **Prophylactic antibiotics** are usually given after clamping the umbilical cord.
   e. **Antacids** are also given to reduce the acidity of the stomach contents in the event that the patient aspirates material into the lungs.
   f. **Informed consent** should always be obtained.

2. **Anesthesia.** Most often, anesthesia is regional (spinal or epidural), but it can be inhalational (general) as dictated by the individual situation. General anesthesia may result in depression of the infant immediately after delivery, the degree of which increases with the length of time from incision to delivery. For this reason, the patient is prepared before the induction of general anesthesia (i.e., Foley catheter placement, skin "prep," and draping).

3. **Surgical techniques**
   a. **Abdominal incision**
      (1) The abdominal incision may be **midline, paramedian,** or **Pfannenstiel.**
         (a) **Midline.** The infraumbilical vertical midline incision is less bloody and allows more rapid entry into the abdominal cavity.
         (b) **Paramedian.** A vertical incision lateral to the umbilicus. It is rarely used.
         (c) **Pfannenstiel.** This low transverse incision near the symphysis pubis provides the most desired cosmetic effect and is **used most often.** However, it requires more time to perform.
      (2) The incision is made with the patient on the operating table in a **left lateral tilt** to prevent maternal hypotension and uteroplacental insufficiency, which may result from compression of the inferior vena cava by the uterus when the patient is supine.
      (3) The **approach to the uterus** in reference to the peritoneal cavity can be made in one of two ways:
         (a) The **transperitoneal approach** is **used almost exclusively** today. The parietal peritoneum is opened to expose the abdominal contents and uterus.
         (b) The **extraperitoneal approach** is mentioned for historical purposes; it has been virtually abandoned since the advent of effective antibiotics. This approach was devised for cases of amnionitis to avoid seeding the abdominal cavity in attempts to decrease the risk of peritonitis.

b. Uterine incision. The pregnant uterus is palpated and inspected for rotation. The type of uterine incision is selected depending on development of the lower uterine segment, presentation of the infant, and placental location.

(1) A **bladder flap** is created to approach the lower uterine segment. The reflection of bladder peritoneum is incised and dissected free from the anterior uterine wall, exposing the myometrium. This step is not necessary with a classical incision.

(2) **Incision of the myometrium** is made as indicated.

c. Delivery of the infant

(1) The **infant** is delivered with the hand, forceps, vacuum extraction, or breech extraction.

(2) The **placenta** is delivered spontaneously or can be removed manually.

d. Wound closure

(1) The **uterus is often exteriorized** to massage the fundus, inspect the adnexa, and facilitate visualization of the wound for repair.

(2) The **uterine cavity is cleaned.** Oxytocics are administered as indicated to facilitate contraction of the myometrium and hemostasis.

(3) A **transverse uterine incision** is closed in one or two layers. A **vertical incision** usually is closed in three layers because of the myometrial thickness of the upper segment.

(4) The **peritoneum of the bladder reflection** can be either reattached with fine absorbable sutures or, typically, left open.

(5) The **abdominal incision** is closed in the usual manner.

E Complications. Common postoperative complications include the following conditions:

1. Endomyometritis. Postoperative infection is the most common complication after cesarean section.

a. The average **incidence of endomyometritis** is 34 to 40%, with a range of 5 to 85%.

b. Risk factors include lower socioeconomic status, prolonged labor, prolonged duration of ruptured membranes, and the **number of vaginal examinations.**

c. Infection is **polymicrobial** and includes the following organisms: aerobic streptococci, anaerobic gram-positive cocci, and aerobic and anaerobic gram-negative bacilli.

d. Use of **prophylactic antibiotics** at the time of the procedure **decreases incidence.** With the use of modern, broad-spectrum antibiotics, the incidence of serious complications, including sepsis, pelvic abscess, and septic thrombophlebitis, is less than 2%.

2. Urinary tract infection

a. Urinary tract infections are the **second most common infectious complication** following cesarean delivery after endomyometritis. Incidence varies from 2 to 16%.

b. Practices that decrease risk include preparing the patient properly and minimizing duration of catheter.

3. Wound infection

a. The **incidence** of postcesarean wound infection rates ranges from 2.5 to 16%.

b. Risk factors include prolonged labor, ruptured membranes, amnionitis, meconium staining, morbid obesity, anemia, and diabetes mellitus.

c. Common isolates include *Staphylococcus aureus, Escherichia coli, Proteus mirabilis, Bacteroides* sp., and group B streptococci.

4. Thromboembolic disorders

a. The **incidence** is 0.24% of deliveries, and deep vein thromboses are three to five times more common after cesarean delivery.

b. Diagnosis and treatment are the same as for nonpregnant women. Prompt diagnosis and treatment decrease the risk of complicating pulmonary embolus to 4.5% and that of death to 0.7%.

5. Cesarean hysterectomy

a. Hysterectomy after cesarean delivery is an **emergency procedure** that occurs in less than 1% of cesarean sections.

  b. Indications include uterine atony (43%), placenta accreta (30%), uterine rupture (13%), extension of a low transverse incision (10%), leiomyoma preventing uterine closure, and cervical cancer.

 6. Uterine rupture in future pregnancies

  a. The **risk of rupture** of previous cesarean scar **varies with the location of the incision.**

   (1) Low transverse scar (one): less than 1%

   (2) Low vertical scar: 0.5 to 6.5%

   (3) Classic scar: as high as 10%

  b. Separation of the uterine scar can be categorized as **dehiscence or rupture.**

   (1) A **dehiscence** is a frequently asymptomatic separation and is found incidentally at the time of repeat cesarean or on palpation after a vaginal birth.

   (2) Uterine rupture is a catastrophic event with sudden separation of the uterine scar and expulsion of the uterine contents into the abdominal cavity. Fetal distress is usually the first sign of rupture, followed by severe abdominal pain and bleeding.

F **Vaginal birth after cesarean section.** Previous cesarean section is no longer a contraindication to subsequent labor and a vaginal birth. All women who are candidates should be counseled adequately and encouraged to attempt a vaginal birth.

 1. Considerations. The risks of a vaginal birth after cesarean section, when performed in the proper setting, are less than the risks of a repeat cesarean section.

  a. There is a 60 to 80% rate of successful vaginal delivery after previous cesarean section.

   (1) A previous vaginal delivery is the best prognostic indicator for success.

   (2) Women with "nonrecurring" indications (e.g., breech presentation, fetal distress, or hemorrhage) have higher success rates than women with "recurring" indications (e.g., previous cephalopelvic disproportion or failure to progress). However, as many as 50% of women with previous cesarean section for cephalopelvic disproportion have a successful vaginal birth.

  b. One third of all cesarean births are repeat cesareans, and an effective strategy to decrease the current cesarean section rate is to encourage vaginal births after cesarean section, when safely indicated.

 2. Prerequisites

  a. No maternal or fetal contraindications to labor

  b. Previous low transverse cesarean section, with documentation of the uterine scar

  c. Informed consent regarding risks and benefits of repeat cesarean and vaginal birth

  d. Personnel able to perform emergency delivery and appropriate facility

 3. Contraindications. The risk of vaginal birth after cesarean section in multiple gestations and breech presentations has not been determined.

  a. Previous classic uterine incision

  b. Maternal or fetal contraindications to labor

  c. Trial of labor declined by mother

  d. Previous low vertical scar, unless absence of upper segment extension is well documented

  e. History of more than two prior cesarean sections

II EPISIOTOMY (see Table 10-5)

A **Definition.** An episiotomy is an incision of the perineum made to enlarge the vaginal outlet to facilitate delivery.

 1. It is made at the end of the second stage of labor just before delivery, when indicated.

 2. It increases the area of the outlet for the fetal head during delivery, particularly in assisted deliveries with forceps or the vacuum extractor.

B **Function**

1. An episiotomy is used to prevent major perineal lacerations.

2. Prophylactic episiotomy has been advocated to prevent pelvic relaxation, although this has never been proven.

C **Types**

1. **Median or medial episiotomy.** This incision should be one-half the length of the distended perineum and is cut vertically in the midline of the perineal body.
   a. **Advantages:** less blood loss, easier to repair, more comfortable during healing
   b. **Disadvantage:** possible occurrence of inadvertent cutting or extension into the anal sphincter and rectum. It is important to recognize and repair this complication during repair of the episiotomy so that rectovaginal fistula does not result.

2. **Mediolateral episiotomy.** This incision of the perineum, at a 45° angle to the hymenal ring, extends laterally to the anus onto the inner thigh, allowing more room than a median incision.
   a. **Advantage:** more room with less risk of injury to the rectum and sphincter
   b. **Disadvantages:** more difficult to repair, more blood loss, more discomfort during healing

III   OPERATIVE VAGINAL DELIVERY: FORCEPS AND VACUUM-EXTRACTOR OPERATIONS

A **Definition.** An operative vaginal delivery is defined as the application of direct traction on the fetal head with forceps or a vacuum.

B **Incidence.** The incidence of operative vaginal delivery is approximately 10 to 15%.

C **Indications.** An operative vaginal delivery is performed to shorten the second stage of labor with certain maternal or fetal indications.

1. **Nonreassuring fetal status** based on heart rate pattern, auscultation, lack of response to scalp stimulation, or scalp pH

2. **Prolonged second stage of labor** secondary to malposition, deflexion, or asynclitism (lateral deflection) of the fetal head. A prolonged second stage is defined as follows:
   a. **Nulliparous patient:** More than 3 hours with a regional anesthetic or more than 2 hours without regional anesthesia
   b. **Multiparous patient:** More than 2 hours with a regional anesthetic or more than 1 hour without regional anesthesia

3. Certain **maternal illnesses** (such as heart disease or pulmonary compromise), which make avoidance of voluntary maternal expulsive efforts desirable

4. **Poor voluntary expulsion efforts** because of exhaustion, analgesia, or neuromuscular disease

D **Prerequisites for instrumental delivery.** The successful results of an instrumental delivery depend largely on the skill and judgment of the obstetrician.

1. The cervix must be fully dilated.

2. The membranes must be ruptured.

3. The position and station must be known, and the head must be engaged (0 station; see Chapter 10).

4. The maternal pelvis must be judged adequate in size for delivery.

5. The bladder should be empty.

6. A skilled operator must be present.

7. Adequate anesthesia is needed before forceps or vacuum application.

E **Contraindications**

1. Nonvertex presentation, except for **Piper forceps in the breech delivery**

2. **Nonengagement** of the presenting part

3. Head that cannot be advanced with ordinary traction when using forceps or the vacuum extractor

4. Prematurity, fetal bleeding disorder, or certain maternal infections (i.e., HIV)

F **Classification of forceps deliveries.** Forceps deliveries are classified according to station and rotation.

1. **Outlet forceps.** To be categorized as an outlet forceps delivery, the following criteria must be satisfied:
   a. Scalp is visible at the introitus without separating the labia.
   b. Fetal skull has reached the pelvic floor.
   c. Sagittal suture is in the anteroposterior diameter or right or left occiput anterior or posterior position.
   d. Fetal head is at or on the perineum.
   e. Rotation does not exceed 45°.

2. **Low forceps.** In low forceps delivery, the leading point of the fetal skull has descended to at least +2 station but has not reached the pelvic floor.

3. **Midforceps.** The station is above +2 but the presenting part is engaged.

G **Types of forceps.** The forceps are two matched blades that articulate and lock. The design of the blades provides standard cephalic and pelvic curves; that is, they conform to the shape of the fetal head and to the vaginal canal, respectively. Each matching part of the forceps has three parts: the blade, the shank, and the handle.

1. **Classic.** These forceps are used primarily for traction when there is to be little or no rotation.
   a. Simpson
   b. Elliot
   c. Tucker-McLean

2. **Specialized.** These forceps are designed for rotation or special indications.
   a. Kielland (for rotation)
   b. Barton (for rotation)
   c. Piper (for the aftercoming head in breech deliveries)

H **Vacuum extractors.** There are two types of vacuum extractors, based on the type of cup used for application to the fetal head. Each type has three parts: a cup, a rubber hose, and a vacuum pump.

1. **Malmström vacuum extractor.** This device consists of a metal cup (40 to 60 mm in diameter) that is applied to the fetal scalp. The pump is then used to create a vacuum, not exceeding 0.7 to 0.8 kg/cm². Traction is then applied to bring the infant's head through the introitus.

2. **Plastic cup extractor.** This device, which is **more widely used in the United States**, consists of a flexible Silastic cup that is applied to the fetal scalp more easily and with less trauma than the Malmström extractor. The vacuum pressures attained are about the same, but they can be reached more quickly and with less trauma to the fetal scalp.

I **Complications**

1. **Maternal complications** are usually of minor clinical consequence (incidence, 1.4 to 22%) and include lacerations of the cervix, vagina, and perineum; episiotomy extensions; and associated hemorrhage. More serious complications (incidence, 0.1 to 0.3%) include bladder lacerations, pelvic floor injury, pelvic hematoma, and coccygeal fracture.

2. **Neonatal injury**
   a. **Scalp abrasions or lacerations** are the most common injury associated with vacuum extraction.
   b. **Soft tissue injury** is the most common injury associated with **forceps delivery.**

    c. Cephalohematoma (separation of the fetal scalp from underlying structures) occurs in 0.5 to 2.5% of live births, with an incidence of 14 to 16% in vacuum deliveries and 2% in forceps deliveries.

    d. Subgaleal hemorrhages occur in 26 in 1000 to 45 in 1000 of vacuum deliveries.

    e. Intracranial hemorrhage is a rare complication, occurring in 0.75% of instrumental deliveries.

IV   CERVICAL CERCLAGE

A **Definition:** A suture placed in the cervix to treat **cervical incompetence.**

1. Cervical incompetence is **characterized** by gradual, progressive, painless dilation of the cervix, usually leading to spontaneous pregnancy loss early in the **second trimester.** A minority (15 to 20%) of second-trimester losses are associated with cervical incompetence.

2. Cervical incompetence may be **acquired or congenital.**
   a. **Acquired causes** are primarily result from obstetric or gynecologic trauma to the cervix (e.g., rapid delivery, use of forceps, trauma, surgical dilation, conization, or breech extraction).
   b. **Congenital causes** include anomalies caused by diethylstilbestrol (DES) exposure in utero and other reproductive tract

3. Cervical incompetence is **diagnosed** by a characteristic history of second-trimester spontaneous losses associated with **painless cervical dilation.** The role of ultrasound as a diagnostic modality is being explored.

B **Techniques.** Cervical cerclage involves placing an encircling suture around the **cervical os** using a heavy, nonabsorbable suture or Mersilene tape. The suturing prevents protrusion of the amniotic sac and consequent rupture by correcting the abnormal dilation of the cervix. **Three techniques** for cervical cerclage are used today.

1. **Shirodkar technique.** In the more complicated of the two procedures using a vaginal approach, the suture is almost completely buried beneath the vaginal mucosa at the level of the internal os. It can be left in place for subsequent pregnancies if a cesarean section is performed. This procedure requires dissection of the bladder and is associated with an increased blood loss.

2. **McDonald technique.** This procedure is a simple purse-string suture of the cervix and is simpler, incurring less trauma to the cervix and less blood loss than the Shirodkar procedure.

3. **Abdominal placement.** This uncommon, permanent procedure is used in women with a short or amputated cervix or in those in whom a vaginal procedure has failed. Cesarean birth is necessary for delivery.

C **Timing.** Cerclage is **usually performed** between the **twelfth and sixteenth** weeks of gestation but can be performed as late as the twenty-fourth week. The suture is **removed at the thirty-eighth week** or earlier if labor begins. **Fetal viability and the absence of anomalies** should be documented **before** performing the procedure.

D **Effectiveness.** The **success rate of cerclage** has been stated to be as high as 80 to 90%. However, there have been no randomized trials to define the efficacy and benefit of cerclage; this benefit is probably overstated. Except in women with a strong history consistent with cervical incompetence, the benefit of cerclage has not been proven.

E **Complications**

1. Cervical lacerations occur in 1 to 13% of deliveries after a McDonald cerclage.

2. Cervical dystocia with failure to dilate, requiring a cesarean birth, occurs in 2 to 5% of cases.

3. Displacement of the suture occurs in 3 to 12% of cases. A second cerclage is then attempted, which has a lower success rate.

4. Premature rupture of the membranes complicates cerclage 1 to 9% of cases.

5. Chorioamnionitis complicates 1 to 7% of cases.

6. Early, elective cerclages have a low rate (1%) of infection; cerclage placement with dilation of the cervix has a much higher risk (30%) of infection.

V ▪ ABORTION

The termination of pregnancy before viability, usually designated as 20 weeks' gestation (i.e., before the fetus is capable of surviving outside the uterus) is known as abortion.

A **Spontaneous abortion** is expulsion of the products of conception without medical or mechanical intervention.

1. Incidence. Spontaneous loss occurs in 15% of clinically recognized pregnancies; the risk increases directly with maternal age, advancing paternal age, minority race, increasing gravidity, and history of previous spontaneous losses.

2. Etiology. Chromosomal abnormalities are the most common reason for first-trimester losses, occurring at a 60% frequency. Most chromosomal abnormalities are sporadic defects; in a small percentage of cases, one of the parents carries a balanced translocation. Autosomal trisomies are the most common anomaly, followed by 45,X monosomy (the most common single anomaly seen in abortuses), triploidy, tetraploidy, translocations, and mosaicism.

3. Classification. Spontaneous abortions are classified into five types.
   a. Threatened abortion. This term is traditionally used when bleeding occurs in the first half of gestation without cervical dilation or passage of tissue. Twenty-five percent of pregnant women experience spotting or bleeding early in gestation; 50% of these proceed to lose the pregnancy. An ultrasound is obtained to document viability after 6 weeks' gestation.
   b. Inevitable abortion. This type of pregnancy loss is diagnosed when bleeding or rupture of the membranes occurs with cramping and dilation of the cervix. Suction curettage is performed to evacuate the uterus.
   c. Incomplete abortion. This type of pregnancy loss occurs when there has been partial but incomplete expulsion of the products of conception from the uterine cavity. Therapy is evacuation of remaining tissue by suction curettage.
   d. Missed abortion. Death of the fetus or embryo may occur without the onset of labor or the passage of tissue for a prolonged period. Suction curettage is used to evacuate the first-trimester uterus. Dilation and evacuation (D&E) or prostaglandin induction of labor are methods used to evacuate the early second-trimester uterus.
   e. Recurrent spontaneous abortion. In the past, this condition has been called **habitual abortion** and is defined as three or more spontaneous, consecutive first-trimester losses. This affects 2% of couples. In women with previous liveborn infants who have had a loss, the risk of a subsequent abortion is 25 to 30% regardless of whether she has had one or more losses. In women with no previous liveborn infants, the recurrence risk is 40 to 45%. Evaluation is indicated after three losses (and sometimes after two losses depending on the age of those involved).

4. Workup for spontaneous abortion
   a. Detailed history and physical examination
   b. Chromosomal evaluation of the couple
   c. Endometrial biopsy to exclude luteal phase defect
   d. Thyroid function test and screening for diabetes mellitus
   e. Cervical cultures for *Ureaplasma urealyticum*
   f. Hysterosalpingogram or hysteroscopy to evaluate uterine cavity
   g. Screening test for lupus anticoagulant and anticardiolipin antibody

B **Induced (elective) abortion.** Abortion became legal in 1973 and can be induced up to approximately 24 weeks' gestation, depending on state laws. Legal abortion is one of the most frequently performed surgical procedures in the United States. Therapeutic abortions are terminations of pregnancy that are performed when maternal risk is associated with continuation of the pregnancy or fetal abnormalities are associated with genetic, chromosomal, or structural defects.

1. **Techniques of pregnancy termination.** Techniques used effectively to empty the uterus of the products of conception fall under the categories of surgical evacuation or induction of labor. The preferred procedure depends on gestational age and, in some cases, operator training.

   a. **Surgical evacuation**

      (1) **Suction curettage.** This method of dilation of the cervix and vacuum aspiration of the uterine contents is used for termination of pregnancy at 12 weeks' or less gestational age. Suction curettage is the most common method of pregnancy termination in this country.

         (a) **Hygroscopic dilators** such as laminaria (stems of a brown seaweed that absorb water) can be used when necessary to facilitate gentle dilation of the cervix.

         (b) **Prophylactic antibiotics** administered just before or after the procedure significantly reduce the risk of infection associated with induced abortion.

      (2) **Dilation and extraction (D&E).** This technique is the preferred method of termination at 13 or more weeks of gestation.

         (a) As the length of gestation increases, wider cervical dilation is necessary to accomplish the procedure successfully. Preoperative cervical laminaria may be used.

         (b) **Vacuum aspiration** of uterine contents is usually an adequate method of evacuation between 13 and 16 weeks. After 16 weeks, uterine evacuation is accomplished with forceps extraction. Successful completion of this procedure depends largely on operator skill. Evaluation for major fetal parts is an important component of this procedure.

         (c) **Prophylactic antibiotics** may be given.

      (3) **Other mechanical methods** (now **obsolete**). These methods include sharp curettage, hysterotomy, and hysterectomy (used only when there is another indication for this procedure).

   b. **Induction of labor.** Medical means of inducing abortion include extrauterine and intrauterine administration of abortifacients, such as prostaglandins, urea, hypertonic saline, and oxytocin. These methods are used for second-trimester terminations; frequency of use increases with increasing gestational age.

      (1) **Prostaglandins** are most commonly administered as vaginal tablets of prostaglandin E_2; 90% of abortions are accomplished within 24 hours. Common side effects include fever, nausea and vomiting, diarrhea, and uterine hyperstimulation.

      (2) **Hypertonic solutions of saline** or **urea** are injected directly into the amniotic cavity. This procedure requires amniocentesis and care to avoid intravascular injection.

      (3) Complication rates are lowest when the uterus is successfully evacuated within 13 to 24 hours. Laminaria to facilitate cervical dilation is useful to shorten the length of induction.

   c. **Progesterone antagonists.** These effective agents for pregnancy termination, used in Europe and other countries and previously unavailable in the United States, are now approved by the U. S. Food and Drug Administration.

      (1) **Mifepristone (RU486; Mifeprex),** taken orally, is highly effective in pregnancies with up to 49 days of amenorrhea. Its effectiveness can be increased with the addition of prostaglandin E.

      (2) **Side effects** are minimal, and complication rates, including hemorrhage and retained tissue, are low.

2. **Anesthesia.** Sedation with a local paracervical block is usually used for induced abortion. General anesthesia can be used but is accompanied by a higher incidence of hemorrhage, cervical injury, and perforation because general anesthetics render the uterine musculature more relaxed and, thus, easier to penetrate.

3. **Complications.** The incidence of complications is largely determined by the method of termination and gestational age; incidence varies directly with increasing gestational age.

   a. **Immediate complications.** These complications develop during the procedure or within 3 hours after completion.

      (1) **Hemorrhage.** The incidence of hemorrhage is most accurately determined by the rate of transfusion. Rates vary with method of termination and are reported to be within 0.06 to 1.72%. The lowest rates are seen with suction curettage, and the highest with saline instillation.

      (2) **Cervical injury.** The rates of cervical injury associated with suction curettage are within the range of 0.01 to 1.6%. Factors that decrease the risk of this complication include the use of local anesthetics instead of general anesthesia; use of laminaria; and an experienced operator.

      (3) **Uterine perforation.** The incidence of this potentially serious complication of suction curettage abortions is approximately 0.2%.

         (a) **Risks.** Factors that increase the risk of uterine perforation include multiparity, advanced gestational age, and operator inexperience. The use of laminaria to facilitate cervical dilation decreases the risk.

         (b) **Complications.** Serious consequences of uterine perforation include hemorrhage and damage to intra-abdominal organs. Because of the location of the uterine vessels, lateral perforations may be associated with hemorrhage.

         (c) **Treatment.** Many cases of uterine perforation require only observation. Surgical exploration is indicated when there is evidence of hemorrhage, when injury to abdominal organs is suspected, or when perforation occurs with a suction curette.

      (4) **Acute hematometra.** This complication occurs in 0.1 to 1% of suction curettage procedures and is evidenced by decreased vaginal bleeding and an enlarged, tender uterus. Treatment is repeat curettage and administration of an oxytocic agent.

   b. **Delayed complications**

      (1) **Postabortal infection.** This condition is often associated with retained tissue. The incidence of infection varies with the method of termination.

         (a) **Risks.** Factors that increase the risk of infection include the presence of cervical gonococcal or chlamydial infection, advanced gestational age, uterine instillation methods of termination, and the use of local anesthesia instead of general anesthesia. Infection complicates less than 1% of suction curettage procedures, 1.5% of D&E terminations, and 5.3 to 6.2% of induction terminations.

         (b) **Treatment.** Uterine infection is usually polymicrobial, similar to other gynecologic infections, and is treated with broad-spectrum antibiotics and prompt evacuation of retained tissue. The use of prophylactic antibiotics significantly decreases the risk of infectious complications associated with induced abortions.

      (2) **Retained tissue.** This condition complicates less than 1% of suction curettage abortions.

         (a) **Associated conditions.** Retained tissue may be associated with infection, hemorrhage, or both.

         (b) **Treatment.** Therapy requires repeat curettage and antibiotic administration if infection is present.

      (3) **Rh sensitization.** The risk of sensitization increases with advanced gestational age. The Rh status of every pregnant woman should be known, and Rh immune globulin (Rh$_O$GAM) should be administered to an Rh-negative woman whenever maternal fetal hemorrhage is a possibility.

(a) The estimated risk of sensitization associated with suction curettage is 2.6% if Rh$_O$GAM is not administered appropriately.

(b) The recommended dose for Rh immune globulin prophylaxis is 50 μg up to 12 weeks' gestation, and 300 μg thereafter.

(4) **Future adverse pregnancy outcomes.** The incidences of infertility, spontaneous abortion, and ectopic pregnancy **do not** increase after uncomplicated suction curettage procedures.

4. **Maternal mortality.** The case mortality rate for induced abortion is less than 0.05 per 100,000 procedures. The risk varies with gestational age and method of termination.

   a. The leading cause of death associated with induced abortion is anesthetic complications, followed (in frequency) by hemorrhage, embolism, and infection.

   b. The risk of death is lowest for suction curettage procedures and highest for instillation procedures. Risk increases with advancing gestational age.

Study Questions for Chapter 12

Directions: Each of the numbered items or incomplete statements in this section is followed by answers or by completions of the statement. Select the ONE lettered answer or completion that is BEST in each case.

1. A 26-year-old woman, gravida 2, para 1 at 20 weeks of gestation sees you in the office for prenatal care. Her fundus measures 24 weeks and you are unable to hear fetal heart tone by Doppler. You perform an ultrasound and confirm lack of fetal heart activity and lack of fetal movement or breathing. Her last pregnancy was complicated by severe preeclampsia at 34 weeks that forced her to deliver a preterm baby. She has no medical problems other than mild asthma. Upon further inquiry she tells you she had one episode of spotting 4 weeks ago but did not have cramping nor did she pass any clots or tissue from the vagina. Which of the following is the most descriptive diagnosis?

- [A] Threatened abortion
- [B] Fetal demise
- [C] Incomplete abortion
- [D] Spontaneous abortion
- [E] Missed abortion

2. Chromosomal abnormalities account for the majority of first trimester spontaneous abortions. If one was to analyze the chromosomal composition of the products of conception that are extruded in a spontaneous abortion, which of the following would be the most common finding?

- [A] Balanced translocation
- [B] 45,X monosomy
- [C] Triploidy
- [D] Trisomy
- [E] Mosaicism

3. A 30-year-old woman, gravida 4, para 3 at 12 weeks of gestation is seeing you for prenatal care. Her first pregnancy ended with a successful vaginal delivery, at term, of a healthy boy. Her second pregnancy was uncomplicated and resulted in a cesarean section with low transverse incision of uterus for breech presentation after failed external version. Her last pregnancy resulted in the successful "natural" birth of her daughter. What is the best advice you can give this patient regarding vaginal birth after cesarean section (VBAC)?

- [A] You are not a candidate for VBAC
- [B] You are an excellent candidate for VBAC
- [C] You are an average candidate for VBAC
- [D] You should consider a cesarean section given your risk of uterine rupture
- [E] Your risk of uterine rupture is 1 in 80

4. You are an attending obstetrician in charge of a busy hospital. You are monitoring the progress of a woman (gravida 2, para 0) who has been in labor for the past 24 hours; her membranes have been ruptured for 17 hours. Her cervix is 9 cm dilated and 100% effaced, and fetal vertex has reached pelvic floor and is in left occiput anterior position. She has an epidural. The fetal heart rate tracing is reassuring, and an intrauterine pressure catheter shows contractions every 2 to 3 minutes, 50 seconds in duration, and producing 45 mmHg of pressure. Four hours ago, the patient's cervix was dilated 9 cm, was 100% effaced, and fetal station was the same. What is the best next step in management?

- [A] Outlet vacuum delivery
- [B] Low forceps delivery
- [C] Low transverse cesarean section

[D] Oxytocin augmentation
[E] Penicillin

QUESTIONS 5–11

Match the description below with the best range of numbers above. Each answer choice may be used once, more than once or not at all.

[A] 0–10%
[B] 15–25%
[C] 35–45%
[D] 60–70%
[E] 71–80%

5. Risk of sensitization in Rh-negative woman after D&E if RhoGAM not given

6. Risk of uterine perforation after D&E

7. After three spontaneous abortions (SAB), risk of SAB if no history of liveborn

8. Annual percent of births by cesarean section in the United States

9. Risk of endomyometritis after cesarean section

10. Uterine atony as the indication for a cesarean hysterectomy

11. Success rate for VBAC after one previous low transverse cesarean section for fetal distress and two previous successful VBACs

Answers and Explanations

1. The answer is E [V A 3 d]. The best term to describe this clinical scenario is "missed" abortion. Death of the fetus or embryo (less than 23 weeks and before viability) occurred without onset of labor or passage of tissue and was unrecognized for 4 weeks. Fetal demise is a "missed abortion" that occurs after fetal viability, or 23 weeks or more of gestation. A threatened abortion is an event that is occurring in the present. The fetus is alive inside the uterus but is threatening to abort by causing spotting from the vagina. An incomplete abortion describes an abortion in progress. This means the patient recently had bleeding and cramping, and there was partial or incomplete expulsion of the products of conception. The cervical os is open. A spontaneous abortion is too broad a term. Most of the answer choices are subtypes of "spontaneous abortion."

2. The answer is D [V A 2]. The most common chromosomal abnormality found in spontaneous abortions is autosomal trisomies (for example trisomy 16 or trisomy 21). The most common single anomaly seen in abortuses is 45,X monosomy or Turner's. Don't confuse triploidy (an extra set of 23 chromosomes in humans) with trisomy (one extra chromosome).

3. The answer is B [I F 2]. This patient is an excellent candidate for VBAC for two reasons. She has had one prior successful VBAC with her third pregnancy and she had a cesarean section with her second pregnancy for a "nonrecurring" reason (breech). One should not dissuade a woman wanting a VBAC if the prerequisites are met (1. No maternal or fetal contraindication; 2. Two or less previous low transverse cesarean section(s); 3. Informed consent regarding risks and benefits; and 4. Personnel able to perform emergency delivery). The risk of uterine rupture after one previous low transverse type of cesarean section is less than 1% (i.e., less than 1/100).

4. The answer is C [I B 2 a]. This clinical scenario describes labor dystocia. The patient is gravida 2 but is nulliparous because she has never had a vaginal delivery. She has had arrest of dilation and descent. She does not meet one of the prerequisites for instrumental delivery (vacuum or forceps), which is a fully dilated cervix. Oxytocin is not necessary because she is having adequate labor contractions as measured by the IUPC. Penicillin would be appropriate if she had ruptured her membranes more than 18 hours and she did not have group b streptococcus vaginal-rectal cultures.

5. A [B 3 b3 a], **6. A** [B 3 a 3], **7. C** [V A 3 e], **8. B** [I A 1], **9. C** [I E 1 a], **10. C** [I E 5 b], **11. E** [I F 1 a]. The estimated risk of sensitization (i.e., formation of antibodies against the Rh antigen on red blood cells) associated with curettage is 2.6% if RhoGAM is not administered. The incidence of uterine perforation after a suction curettage is 0.2%. After three spontaneous abortions, a woman with a previous liveborn infant has a 25 to 35% risk of SAB versus 40 to 45% with no history of any liveborn. Approximately 21% of infants were delivered by cesarean birth in 1997. Postoperative infection is the most common complication after cesarean section, especially endomyometritis (incidence 34 to 40%). The most common indication for cesarean hysterectomy is postpartum hemorrhage caused by uterine atony (incidence 43%). There is a 60 to 80% rate of successful vaginal delivery after previous cesarean section, especially if there is a nonrecurring indication (fetal distress) and previous successful VBAC.

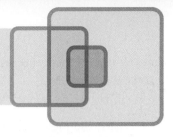

chapter 13

Obstetric Anesthesia

SCOTT EDWARDS

I   INTRODUCTION

[A] In the United States, anesthesia services are commonly used during labor and delivery. In hospitals that perform more than 1500 deliveries per year, the epidural usage rate is nearly 50%.

[B] Obstetric anesthesia includes several techniques. **Analgesia** is the relief of pain without the loss of consciousness. **Local and regional anesthesia** blocks the nerves or nerve roots carrying pain signals from localized areas of the body. **General anesthesia** results in loss of consciousness.

[C] Although obstetric anesthesia allows women to be more comfortable during childbirth and makes surgical procedures possible, it poses unique hazards. Anesthetic complications are a significant cause of maternal morbidity and mortality, and approximately 4% of maternal deaths are attributable to anesthetic complications. The presence of the fetus and changes in maternal physiology must be considered when considering anesthesia in women during childbirth.

II   PHYSIOLOGIC CHANGES IN PREGNANCY

The many physiologic changes that occur during pregnancy may affect how anesthesia is implemented.

[A] **Habitus.**   Increased maternal weight, increased breast size, and airway soft tissue edema make intubation more difficult in gravid women. Airway difficulties are exacerbated in women with additional edema from preeclampsia.

[B] **Cardiovascular changes**
1. By the end of the second trimester, cardiac output increases by 50%, a result of increased heart rate and ejection fraction.
2. The enlarging uterus causes compression of the inferior vena cava, which can decrease venous return.
3. This obstruction of the inferior vena cava also causes diversion of blood through the vertebral venous plexus and paraspinal veins. The engorged veins are more susceptible to injury or inadvertent cannulation during epidural or spinal placement.

[C] **Pulmonary changes**
1. Oxygen consumption increases by 30 to 40% during pregnancy because of the increased metabolic needs of the mother, placenta, and fetus.
2. The functional residual capacity decreases by 20% because the expanding uterus elevates the diaphragm.

3. Minute ventilation increases by 45%, primarily because tidal volume increases. This increase is stimulated by increasing progesterone levels.

   a. The increased ventilation causes the $PaCO_2$ to decrease to 30 mmHg from the nonpregnant baseline value of 40 mmHg.

   b. Metabolic compensation occurs, and the serum bicarbonate concentration decreases to 20 mEq/L.

D **Gastrointestinal changes.** Decreased gastric motility and decreased tone of the lower esophageal sphincter increase the risk of aspiration in pregnant women.

III NEUROPATHWAYS OF OBSTETRIC PAIN

A **Central nervous system**

1. Three membranous layers surround the brain and spinal cord.

   a. The **pia** is a thin vascular membrane investing the brain and spinal cord.

   b. The **arachnoid** is a thin membrane closely attached to the dura and enveloping the cerebrospinal fluid (CSF) and the spinal cord.

   c. The **dura** is a strong, fibroelastic membrane extending from the cranial dura matter through the foramen magnum to about S2. At this point, the filum terminale continues and blends with the periosteum of the coccyx.

2. The **spinal cord ends near the L1 level,** beyond which the spinal nerves continue as the cauda equina and exit through the spinal foramina. Below L1, spinal needles may be introduced into the subarachnoid space with decreased risk of damaging the spinal cord.

3. The epidural space is limited by the dura anteriorly, the ligamentum flavum dorsally, and the vertebral pedicles and foramina laterally. Included in the epidural space are the spinal nerve roots, fat, and lymphatic and blood vessels. The veins within the epidural space are engorged during pregnancy, increasing the chance of inadvertent puncture and decreasing the space available for an anesthetic solution placed within the epidural space.

B **Peripheral nervous system**

1. Pain produced by **uterine contractions** travels through visceral afferent nerve fibers, which travel with the sympathetic nerve fibers and enter the spinal cord at **T10 through L1.**

2. Distention of the **lower vagina and perineum** during the second stage of labor produces pain that is carried via the pudendal nerve to enter the spinal cord at the **S2, S3, and S4** levels.

3. Pain signals are carried through small, unmyelinated A-delta and C fibers to the dorsal horn of the spinal cord. These fibers are more susceptible to nonlipophilic local anesthetics than the heavily myelinated motor neuron fibers.

4. Opiate receptors in the dorsal horn modulate the pain response. Intrathecal and epidural narcotics exert much of their effect at these receptors.

IV AGENTS USED TO PROVIDE ANALGESIA AND SEDATION DURING LABOR

Uterine contractions and cervical dilation cause pain during labor. Medication for pain relief is often indicated to allow the mother to rest between contractions and to experience only moderate discomfort at the peak of a uterine contraction. Opiates help alleviate this pain and are the predominant class of medication used for analgesia during labor.

A **Maternal risks.** Opiates may cause excessive maternal sedation, nausea, vomiting, hypotension, itching, respiratory depression, and impaired protective airway reflexes.

B **Fetal and neonatal risks.** Narcotics given near the time of delivery put newborns at risk for respiratory depression and impaired breastfeeding. Opiates can cause decreased variability on the fetal heart rate tracing, and therefore the variability as index of fetal well-being may be lost. All opiates have similar effects on the fetus and neonate when given in equivalent doses.

C **Specific medications**

1. **Meperidine.** This drug is probably the most widely used narcotic for analgesia during labor.
    a. The usual dose is 50 to 100 mg intramuscularly every 3 to 4 hours or 25 to 50 mg intravenously every 2 to 3 hours. Pain relief occurs within 30 minutes of intramuscular injection and within 5 minutes of intravenous administration.
    b. The greatest risk of neonatal respiratory depression occurs when delivery occurs 2 to 3 hours after meperidine administration.
    c. To minimize nausea, 25 mg of intramuscular promethazine (a phenothiazine) is often given in combination with meperidine.
2. **Fentanyl.** This synthetic opiate is about 100 times as potent as morphine.
    a. The usual dose is 50 to 100 μg intravenously every hour as needed.
    b. Because fentanyl has a rapid onset of action and a short duration of action (20 to 30 minutes), it is often used in patient-controlled analgesia systems.
3. **Morphine.** This powerful opiate is most often used in early labor for analgesia. In doses of 10 to 15 mg intramuscularly, it is a particularly valuable analgesic for patients with a prolonged latent phase and frequent painful contractions.
4. **Nalbuphine and butorphanol.** These synthetic opiate agonist–antagonist medications can be given either intravenously or intramuscularly.
    a. The usual dose of nalbuphine is 10 mg.
    b. The usual dose of butorphanol 1 to 2 mg.
    c. The risk of maternal respiratory depression is less than with meperidine. However, there is no evidence that neonatal respiratory depression is less likely with these agents.
5. **Narcotic antagonists.** When narcotic agents are given close to delivery, newborns may have significant respiratory depression at birth. **Naloxone,** a narcotic antagonist, is capable of reversing this respiratory depression by displacing narcotics from specific receptors in the central nervous system (CNS). The usual dosage for neonates is 0.1 mg/kg intravenously.

V **REGIONAL AND LOCAL ANESTHESIA**

A **Spinal anesthesia.** Spinal anesthesia with local anesthetics is useful when maternal participation is no longer needed, such as in assisted vaginal delivery, cesarean delivery, or extraction of retained placenta. It has a rapid onset and is easier to administer than an epidural block.

1. **Technique**
    a. A narrow-gauge needle is used to place the anesthetic solution directly into the CSF in the spinal canal.
    b. An assisted vaginal delivery requires a spinal block up to the T10 dermatome. A cesarean delivery requires a sensory block up to the T4 dermatome.
    c. Pregnant patients need smaller amounts of anesthetic agents than nonpregnant patients because of the engorgement of the vertebral venous plexus, which reduces the size of the subarachnoid space. Thus, a normal dose of an anesthetic agent could produce a dangerously high level in a pregnant patient.
2. **Complications**
    a. **Hypotension.** The most common complication of spinal anesthesia, hypotension results from the vasodilation caused by the sympathetic blockade. It is compounded by compression of the vena cava by the uterus. Treatment involves:
        (1) Placement in the left lateral decubitus position
        (2) Hydration with intravenous fluids
        (3) Intravenous ephedrine (10 to 15 mg)

    b. High spinal block with respiratory paralysis. This complication may result from excessive spread of a spinal dose of anesthetic or the inadvertent placement of an epidural catheter in the subarachnoid space. Management involves endotracheal intubation and ventilation until the anesthetic has worn off.

    c. Spinal headache. This complication is caused by leakage of CSF from the site of a dural puncture. When the patient stands, there is less CSF to support the cranial structures, and traction on the pia produces the characteristic pain. The pain is worse when sitting or standing and is relieved by lying down.

      (1) Treatment involves hydration, caffeine, analgesics, or abdominal binders.

      (2) If conservative measures fail, a blood patch may be performed. A blood patch uses 15 to 20 mL of the patient's blood introduced into the epidural space to seal the dural puncture and restore pressure within the CSF by increasing the volume within the epidural space.

B **Epidural anesthesia.** Local anesthesia introduced into the epidural space may be used for pain relief during labor and vaginal or cesarean delivery.

  1. Technique

    a. A needle or small catheter is placed into the epidural space to anesthetize the nerve roots exiting the spinal canal at that level. Anesthetic agents can be given as an intermittent bolus or continuously.

    b. The level and intensity of the block can be manipulated to respond to changing needs during labor. Opiates added to the solution allow for the use of a lower concentration of local anesthetic. Newer anesthetic agents, such as ropivacaine and bupivacaine (Marcaine), block sensory fibers more than motor neuron fibers. Therefore, patients can be comfortable and still push effectively.

    c. A combined spinal-epidural technique uses a spinal injection of opiate with or without a dilute local anesthetic during the placement of the epidural catheter. This technique gives prompt pain relief and is particularly useful in early labor because patients can usually remain ambulatory. The epidural catheter can then be used as labor progresses and the initial intrathecal dose wears off.

  2. Complications

    a. Inadvertent spinal anesthesia. This complication may occur with puncture of the dura and injection of the spinal anesthetic. Because the volume of anesthetic used for epidural anesthesia is much greater than for spinal anesthesia (20 to 25 mL versus 1 mL), an intraspinal injection can produce total spinal blockade. To avoid this, a "test dose" is given before giving the entire epidural dose. This test dose contains sufficient local anesthetic to produce a spinal block, if injected intraspinally, and 15 to 20 μg of epinephrine, which produces a transient tachycardia if administered intravascularly.

    b. Intravenous injection of the local anesthetic. This complication can result in **CNS toxicity** with slurred speech, tinnitus, and convulsions. High doses of local anesthetics can cause cardiac arrest.

    c. Hypotension. This condition can result from the sympathetic block as described earlier for the spinal anesthetics (see V A 2 a). However, because an epidural anesthetic can be administered gradually, hypotension can usually be avoided. This method is particularly useful in patients with preeclampsia, who may have volume contraction and are particularly susceptible to spinal-induced hypotension.

    d. Spinal headache. This complication can occur if the dura is inadvertently punctured during placement of an epidural. Treatment involves conservative measures or application of a blood patch (see V A 2 c).

C **Pudendal nerve block.** This technique provides perineal anesthesia by anesthetizing the pudendal nerve. It works well for vaginal delivery and episiotomy repair, but it is not likely to provide adequate anesthesia for a forceps delivery.

1. **Technique.** Administration involves injection of 10 mL of local anesthetic (lidocaine 1% or chloroprocaine 2%) through the sacrospinous ligament near the insertion into the ischial spine. The pudendal nerve is blocked as it passes under the sacrospinous ligament.

2. **Complications.** The pudendal artery travels with the nerve, and care must be taken to avoid intravascular injection of local anesthetic. Rarely, pelvic hematoma, vaginal laceration, or fetal injury can occur.

D Paracervical block. This anesthetic technique is seldom used because of associated complications.

1. **Technique.** The injection of 5 to 10 mL of local anesthetic into the lateral fornices of the vagina blocks the visceral afferent pain fibers. Pain relief lasts 1 to 2 hours.

2. **Complications.** Fetal bradycardia is seen 10 to 25% of the time. This may result from uterine artery vasospasm, uterine hyperstimulation, or the high concentration of the local anesthetic on the CNS or heart of the fetus.

VI GENERAL ANESTHESIA

Because the placenta is not a barrier to general anesthesia, all anesthetic agents that depress the CNS of the mother cross the placenta and depress the CNS of the fetus. General anesthesia is used in obstetric emergencies if the fetus must be delivered quickly; if uterine relaxation is necessary, such as with an entrapped head or uterine inversion; or if medical conditions in the mother, such as coagulation disorders or back problems, prohibit the use of epidural or spinal anesthesia.

A Types

1. **Nitrous oxide.** This is not commonly used in the United States to provide pain relief during labor. However, this method continues to be used in developing countries.
   a. Nitrous oxide does not prolong labor or interfere with uterine contractions.
   b. Modest analgesia can be obtained with a concentration of 50% nitrous oxide and 50% oxygen, with the patient breathing the mixture intermittently while pushing during the second stage of labor.

2. **Volatile anesthetics.** Agents such as **halothane, desflurane,** and **isoflurane** produce significant uterine relaxation. They should be restricted to situations that require a relaxed uterus, such as manipulation of a breech infant during delivery or repositioning of the acutely inverted uterus. Prompt discontinuation of the anesthetic is necessary to prevent hemorrhage from an atonic uterus.

B Aspiration during general anesthesia. Pneumonitis from inhalation of gastric contents is the most common cause of anesthetic death in obstetrics.

1. **Prophylaxis**
   a. The **patient should fast** for as long as possible before the induction of general anesthesia.
   b. After labor has begun, only **clear liquids** should be permitted.
   c. Before the induction of anesthesia, **gastric acidity should be neutralized with antacids,** such as sodium bicitrate.
   d. With **intubation,** cricoid pressure is administered to compress the esophagus just as the patient is being induced with sodium pentothal.

2. **Pathology.** When the pH of aspirated gastric fluid is below 2.5, a severe **chemical pneumonitis** develops.
   a. **Aspiration of particles without acidic fluid** leads to:
      (1) Patchy atelectasis
      (2) Bronchopneumonia

    b. Aspiration of acidic fluid leads to:
        (1) Tachypnea
        (2) Bronchospasm
        (3) Rhonchi
        (4) Rales
        (5) Atelectasis
        (6) Cyanosis
        (7) Hypotension

    c. Exudate into the lung interstitium and alveoli causes:
        (1) Decreased pulmonary compliance
        (2) Shunting of blood
        (3) Severe hypoxemia

3. Treatment

    a. Suction. As much inhaled material as possible must be removed immediately from the mouth, pharynx, and trachea.

    b. Bronchoscopy. This procedure is indicated if large particulate matter is causing airway obstruction.

    c. Oxygen and ventilation. Endotracheal intubation with intermittent positive pressure may be necessary to maintain the arterial P_{O_2} at 60 mmHg. Frequent suction is necessary to remove secretions and edema fluid.

    d. Antibiotics. Infection after aspiration is most frequently caused by **anaerobes.** Therefore, antibiotic coverage with clindamycin or metronidazole is indicated.

Study Questions for Chapter 13

Directions: *For each scenario described below, choose the best type of obstetric anesthesia. Each answer may be used once, more than once, or not at all.*

QUESTIONS 1–4
- [A] Intravenous opiates
- [B] Local anesthetic
- [C] Paracervical block
- [D] Pudendal block
- [E] Epidural
- [F] Spinal
- [G] General

1. A 23-year-old woman, gravida 1, para 0 at 39 weeks of gestation presents in active labor. You check her cervix and realize that her baby is breech presentation. Suddenly her amniotic membranes rupture and the umbilical cord prolapses into the vagina.

2. A 27-year-old woman, gravida 3, para 2 at 40 weeks of gestation presents to labor and delivery. Her cervix is 4 cm dilated and 100% effaced, and fetal vertex is at 0 station. She is uncomfortable and would like pain relief.

3. You just delivered a male neonate weighing 4700 g by vaginal delivery, and you did not have time to cut an episiotomy. After delivery of the placenta, you notice a midline laceration extending from midway inside the vagina, through the anal sphincter and into the rectal mucosa. While deciding how to repair the laceration, you notice the mother bonding with and breastfeeding her infant.

4. A 27-year-old woman, gravida 1, para 0 at 38 weeks of gestation presents to labor and delivery for a scheduled cesarean section because she is HIV positive. She is very sensitive to pain and would like to be comfortable throughout the entire procedure.

Directions: *For each of the normal physiologic phenomenon described below, indicate if and how it changes during pregnancy. Each answer may be used once, more than once, or not at all.*

QUESTIONS 5–12
- [A] ↑
- [B] ↓
- [C] No change
- [D] Need more information
- [E] Unknown

5. Functional residual capacity (FRC)

6. Position of diaphragm within thorax

7. Gastrointestinal motility

8. Subarachnoid space

9. Distance between ligamentum flavum and dura

10. Airway tone

11. Systemic vascular resistance (SVR)

12. Intravascular volume in preeclampsia

Directions: Each of the numbered items or incomplete statements in this section is followed by answers or by completions of the statement. Select the ONE lettered answer or completion that is BEST in each case.

QUESTIONS 13–14

13. A 20-year-old woman, gravida 1, para 0 at 39 3/7 weeks of gestation is sedated before induction of general anesthesia because of an obstetric emergency. Soon it is realized that she has aspirated acidic contents of her stomach. The best step(s) in management is/are _____.

  A Sodium bicarbonate + suction
  B Cricoid pressure + sodium bicarbonate
  C Suction + bronchoscopy + intubation
  D Suction + intubation + clindamycin
  E Bronchoscopy + intubation + ampicillin

14. A patient with epidural anesthesia has adequate pain relief during the first stage of labor but with pushing has significant pain at the perineum. The epidural is less effective in the second stage of labor because _____.

  A Patient has developed tolerance to narcotics given through epidural catheter
  B Valsalva during pushing has displaced the anesthetic from the epidural space
  C Nerves supplying the uterus and perineum arise from different levels of spinal cord
  D Nerve fibers are more sensitive during second stage than during early labor
  E Initial anesthetic is worn off and must be repeated

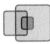

Answers and Explanations

1. G [VI] 2. E [V B] 3. D [V C] 4. F [V A]. General anesthesia is used in obstetric emergencies if the fetus must be delivered quickly (e.g., cord prolapse). Epidural anesthesia may be used for pain relief during vaginal or scheduled cesarean delivery. Pudendal works well for vaginal delivery or episiotomy repair. It is especially useful in this situation because the mother and infant are bonding and placement of an epidural or spinal would interfere with this process. Additionally, local anesthetic injection may not provide adequate analgesia for a fourth degree laceration repair. Spinal anesthesia can be used in vaginal delivery, scheduled cesarean section, and extraction of retained placenta. Spinal anesthesia provides better pain relief than epidural and may be preferred for this patient.

5. B [II C 1] 6. A [II C 1] 7. B [II D] 8. B [V A 1] 9. D [III A 3 and V B] 10. B [II A] 11. B [II C 3] 12. B [V B 2 c]. The FRC decreases by 20% during pregnancy because the expanding uterus elevates the diaphragm. During pregnancy there is decreased gastrointestinal motility and lower resting tone of the lower esophageal sphincter partly because of the smooth muscle relaxing effects of progesterone. Because of the engorgement of the vertebral venous plexus, the size of subarachnoid space decreases during pregnancy. The distance between the ligamentum flavum and the dura depends on the body habitus of the individual and can vary from person to person. Airway edema during pregnancy leads to decreased airway tone during pregnancy. Systemic vascular resistance is reduced during pregnancy because of smooth muscle relaxing effects of progesterone. Intravascular volume is contracted during preeclampsia; therefore, patients are particularly susceptible to spinal-induced hypotension.

13. The answer is D [VI B 3]. Treatment of aspiration during general anesthesia involves 1) *suctioning* as much inhaled material as possible; 2) *bronchoscopy*, if there is a possibility of large particulate matter inhalation; 3) *intubation* and positive pressure ventilation with oxygen to maintain PO_2 over 60 mmHg; and 4) *antibiotics* that cover anaerobes (clindamycin or metronidazole).

14. The answer is C [III B]. Pain signals from uterine contractions travel through nerves that enter the spinal cord at T10 to L1. Pain signals from distension of the lower vagina and perineal body travel through the pudendal nerve, which enters the spinal cord at a different place (S2–S4). Patients do not develop tolerance to local anesthetic or narcotics given during labor. Pushing does not cause the medication to be expelled from the epidural space. Pain signals are carried through the unmyelinated A-delta and C fibers regardless of where they enter the spinal cord. An epidural catheter allows repeated or continuous dosing of local anesthetic.

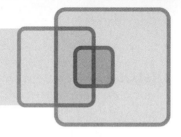
Postterm Pregnancy

MOHAMMED ELKOUSY AND SARA MARDER

I INTRODUCTION

Term gestation is defined as a pregnancy between 37 and 42 completed weeks (260 to 294 days) after the first day of the **last menstrual period (LMP)**. Postterm pregnancy begins when 42 completed (menstrual) weeks have elapsed. The first day of the LMP occurs approximately 2 weeks before conception in a 28-day cycle.

II DETERMINING GESTATIONAL AGE

A **Naegele's rule** uses the first day of the last menstrual period (LMP) to calculate the **estimated date of confinement (EDC)**. Assuming a 28-day cycle, subtract 3 months and add 7 days to the first day of the LMP to determine the delivery date.

B **Quickening** is the maternal perception of fetal movement and begins around 16 to 20 weeks of gestation.

C Uterine size increases with gestational age. The uterus is a pelvic organ until 12 weeks, and the **fundus** can be palpated at the level of the iliac crests. The uterine fundus is palpable at the umbilicus around 20 weeks. Between 20 and 36 weeks, the measurement of the uterus in centimeters from the symphysis pubis to the fundus approximates the gestational age within 2 weeks.

D An electronic doppler ultrasound may detect fetal heart tones as early as 10 to 11 weeks' gestation.

E Ultrasound examination in the first trimester provides the most accurate dating. Measurement of the **crown rump length (CRL)** is accurate to within 5 to 7 days of the actual gestational age. Second- and third-trimester ultrasound uses several parameters for determining gestational age. Those parameters include the **biparietal diameter (BPD)**, the **femur length (FL)**, and the **abdominal circumference (AC)**. In the second trimester, the BPD is the most accurate but only to within 14 days of the actual gestational age. Measurements in the third trimester may have an error up to ±21 days of the actual gestational age.

III ETIOLOGY OF POSTTERM PREGNANCY

Parturition is a complex process that involves events within the fetal brain, adrenals, placenta, amnion, and chorion; it induces changes in the maternal tissues, including the decidua, myometrium, and cervix. The theorized mechanism of parturition begins with a stimulus in the fetal brain, resulting in **activation of the fetal hypothalamic pituitary axis**. **Adrenocorticotropic hormone (ACTH)** production results in stimulation of the **fetal adrenal**. The fetal adrenal increases production of **dehydroepiandrosterone sulfate (DHAS) and cortisol**. The presence of **placental sulfatase** in the placenta is required so that the placenta can convert the DHAS to **estradiol**. Estrogen is thought to be important in increasing myometrial activity, and cortisol is thought to be important in stimulating **prostaglandin** output in the placental tissues. Prostaglandins are important for myometrial contractility. Several disorders may result in delayed parturition and postterm pregnancy. These disorders are all similar in that they are associated with low estrogen production.

A **Anencephaly** is an absence of the fetal cranium with gross abnormalities associated with the fetal brain. The absence and abnormalities of these structures prevent the normal initiation of parturition and result in prolonged gestation.

B **Congenital primary fetal adrenal hypoplasia** has been associated with prolonged gestation. The fetal adrenal is important in the production of cortisol and androgens which help parturition to occur.

C **Placental sulfatase** is required to convert fetal DHAS to estrogen. Deficiency of placental sulfatase leads to decreased estrogen levels and a subsequent delay in parturition. This is an X-linked disorder that affects male fetuses, occurring in 1 in 2500 newborns.

IV CLINICAL SIGNIFICANCE OF POSTTERM PREGNANCY

Postterm pregnancy occurs in approximately 10% of all pregnancies. **Postterm pregnancies have been reported to have a higher incidence of meconium and meconium aspiration, oxytocin induction, shoulder dystocia, macrosomia, oligohydramnios, fetal heart rate abnormalities, and cesarean section.** After 42 completed weeks, an increase in the **perinatal mortality rate** has been observed.

V MANAGEMENT OF THE POSTTERM PREGNANCY

Antenatal **testing** and **induction of labor** are the two most widely used strategies for management of postterm pregnancies. Antenatal testing is used to decrease the risk of adverse perinatal outcome (stillbirth).

A **Antenatal testing** is generally started twice weekly between 41 and 42 weeks' gestation. It can include the **nonstress test (NST)**, the **(CST)**, or the **biophysical profile (BPP)** (see Chapter 6).

   1. The **nonstress test (NST)** is a noninvasive test of fetal activity that correlates with fetal well-being. Fetal heart rate (FHR) accelerations are observed during fetal movement. An external monitor is used to record the FHR, and the mother participates by indicating fetal movements.

     a. A **reactive test** requires **two fetal heart rate accelerations** of at least 15 beats' amplitude of 15 seconds' duration in a 20-minute period.

     b. In one study, 99% of oxytocin challenge tests were negative for signs of fetal distress when performed after a reactive NST.

     c. The most common cause for a nonreactive NST is a period of fetal inactivity or sleep. Studies have shown that the longest interval of fetal inactivity in the healthy fetus is 40 minutes.

     d. If the test is nonreactive after 40 minutes, a contraction stress test (CST) is performed.

     e. Approximately 25% of fetuses that have a nonreactive NST have a positive CST.

   2. The contraction stress test is a test of FHR that indirectly measures placental function in response to uterine contractions. An intravenous infusion of oxytocin is used to stimulate uterine contractions. The nipple stimulation test is an endogenous means of releasing oxytocin in response to manual stimulation of the patient's nipples. It is a noninvasive CST. A CST is performed when the NST is nonreactive.

     a. Criteria for a negative CST consist of three uterine contractions of moderate intensity lasting 40 to 60 seconds over a 10-minute period with no late decelerations in the FHR tracing. A positive CST has late decelerations associated with more than 50% of the uterine contractions. A CST with inconsistent late decelerations is considered suspect.

     b. More often, a favorable outcome follows a negative CST, but as many as 25% of fetuses may experience intrapartum fetal distress after a negative CST.

     c. CSTs have a **25% false-positive rate.**

     d. Studies have shown the incidence of perinatal death within 1 week of a negative CST to be less than 1 in 1000. Most of these deaths are caused by cord accidents or abruptions.

TABLE 14-1 Management Based on Biophysical Profile Score

Score	Interpretation	Management
10	Normal	Repeat testing
8	Normal	Repeat testing
6	Suspect chronic asphyxia	If ≥36 weeks, deliver Repeat testing in 4–6 hours
6	Suspect chronic asphyxia	If ≥32 weeks, deliver Repeat testing in 4–6 hours
0–2	Strongly suspect chronic asphyxia	Extend testing to 120 minutes; if score ≤4, deliver at any gestational age

    e. A positive CST has been associated with an increased incidence of intrauterine death, late decelerations in labor, low 5-minute Apgar scores, intrauterine growth retardation, and meconium-stained amniotic fluid. The overall perinatal death rate after a positive CST is between 7 and 15%.

    f. A suspect CST should be repeated in 24 hours.

  3. Biophysical profile (see Chapter 6) is a composite of tests designed to identify a compromised fetus during the antepartum period (Table 14-1).

    a. Components of the profile

      (1) NST

      (2) Fetal breathing

      (3) Fetal tone

      (4) Fetal motion

      (5) Quantity of amniotic fluid

    b. Scoring of the profile. Each test is given either 2 or 0 points, for a maximum of 10 points. An important feature in the postterm profile is the amniotic fluid profile component. Oligohydramnios is an ominous sign that signifies placental insufficiency.

B Induction of labor. Induction of labor may be performed at 41 weeks if the cervix is favorable. If the cervix is unfavorable, then expectant management with antepartum fetal surveillance should be continued. Generally, at 42 weeks' gestation, if the cervix remains unfavorable, prostaglandins are administered to "ripen" the cervix for induction. A cervix is determined to be favorable by its Bishop's score (Table 14-2). Induction is usually successful with a score of 9 or greater.

C Intrapartum management includes continuous electronic fetal heart rate monitoring. Amnioinfusion may be used if thick meconium is present.

TABLE 14-2 Bishop Scoring System Used for Assessment of Inducibility

	Dilatation	Effacement (%)	Station*	Cervical Consistency	Cervical Position
1	Closed	0–30	−3	Firm	Posterior
2	1–2	40–50	−2	Medium	Midposition
3	3–4	60–70	−1.0	Soft	Anterior
4	≥5	≥80	+1, +2	-	-

Reprinted with permission from Cunningham FG, MacDonald PC, Gant NF. Williams Obstetrics. 21st Ed. New York: McGraw-Hill, 2001:471, Table 20-1.

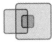

Study Questions for Chapter 14

Directions: *Each of the numbered items or incomplete statements in this section is followed by answers or by completions of the statement. Select the ONE lettered answer or completion that is BEST in each case.*

1. A 33-year-old woman, gravida 2, para 1 who is in the third trimester presents to you for her first prenatal care. She is not sure of her due date because she has been given three different dates by three different doctors. She tells you that her periods are irregular and occur every 21 to 35 days. She has not taken any form of birth control for the past 2 years. The first day of her last menstrual period was July 19, 2002. You obtain a record of an ultrasound performed in the emergency room on September 5, 2002 that showed her to be at 8 0/7 weeks of gestation. You also obtained a record from her last doctor who performed an ultrasound on December 22, 2002, which showed her to be at 24 3/7 weeks of gestation. Which of the following is the best estimate of her due date? (You can use a pregnancy wheel.)

A. April 7, 2003
B. April 8, 2003
C. April 19, 2003
D. April 24, 2003
E. April 26, 2003

2. A 22-year-old woman, gravida 1, para 0 at 15 weeks of gestation by her last menstrual period presents to you for an ultrasound examination to confirm her due date. Which of the following measurements on the fetus is the best at predicting her actual due date?

A. Crown rump length (CRL)
B. Biparietal Diameter (BPD)
C. Abdominal circumference (AC)
D. Femur length (FL)
E. Head circumference (HC)

3. A 25-year-old woman, gravida 3, para 0 at 42 weeks of gestation presents to your clinic for prenatal care. She has accurate dating and has been receiving twice weekly NSTs for the last week. Underdevelopment of which structure in the fetus may contribute to prolongation of this woman's gestation?

A. Cerebral cortex
B. Thalamus
C. Thymus
D. Adrenal cortex
E. Ovary

4. A 21-year-old woman, gravida 4, para 2, SAB 1 at 41 5/7 weeks of gestation presents to labor and delivery for labor check. Her cervix is dilated to 6 cm and is 75% effaced, and fetal vertex is at +1 station. The resident performs an amniotomy and inserts an intrauterine pressure catheter (IUPC). Artificial rupture of membranes (AROM) was performed in this advanced gestational age patient to decrease the incidence of what complication?

A. Meconium aspiration
B. Shoulder dystocia
C. Oligohydramnios
D. Fetal heart tracing abnormalities
E. Macrosomia

5. A 34-year-old woman, gravida 3, para 1, TAB 1 at 42 1/7 weeks of gestation by a week-6 ultrasound presents to your clinic. Her NST is reactive and amniotic fluid volume (AFV) is 8.5. Her cervix is 0.5 cm dilated, 20% effaced, mid-position, and firm, and the fetal vertex is at −4 station. Which of the following is the best next step in management?

[A] Oxytocin
[B] Prostaglandin analogue
[C] Twice weekly NST
[D] Repeat modified BPP (NST and AFV)
[E] Artificial rupture of membranes

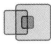

Answers and Explanations

1. The answer is C [II]. Because this patient has irregular periods, estimation of her due date by her last menstrual period is inaccurate. Therefore, Nägele's rule cannot be used to determine her EDC because it assumes a regular 28-day cycle (April 26 is incorrect). Thus, the best estimate of her actual due date is provided by the first trimester ultrasound. Using the pregnancy wheel, if you match September 5 with 8 weeks, then you will see that 40 weeks (due date) corresponds to April 16, 2003 ± 1 day (given inherent error between different pregnancy wheels). Because this is a first trimester ultrasound, there can be a maximum of ± 7 days error. Therefore, the due date must fall between April 8 and April 24 (April 16 ± 8 days). April 19th is the best estimate of the actual due date.

2. The answer is B [II E]. In the second trimester (over 13 weeks), BPD is the most accurate at determining actual gestational age. Crown rump length is the most accurate in the first trimester. None of the other measurements are as useful at estimating gestational age except for the head circumference.

3. The answer is D [III B]. Fetal adrenal hypoplasia has been associated with prolongation of gestation. Anencephaly, not lack of cerebral cortex or thalamus, has been associated with prolongation of gestation. Anencephaly results in lack of hypothalamic-pituitary axis, which is theorized to be responsible for the inception of parturition. The ovary is probably not involved in the initiation of labor. However, estrogen produced by placental conversion of DHAS is thought to increase myometrial activity.

4. The answer is A [IV]. Advanced gestational age and postterm pregnancies are associated with all of the things mentioned in the answer choices. However, AROM as soon as feasible in an advanced gestational age pregnancy allows two things: 1) Assess presence or absence of meconium and how thick (1–4); and 2) Insert IUPC so that you can infuse normal saline (amnioinfusion) if meconium is discovered upon AROM.

5. The answer is B [IV B]. At 42 weeks of gestation, if the cervix remains unfavorable as in this case (her Bishop score is 1 + 1 + 1 + 1 + 2 = 6), prostaglandins will be administered to "ripen" the cervix for induction. Use of oxytocin for induction of an unfavorable cervix results in prolonged labor and increases the possibility of cesarean section. It is not a good idea to AROM if the fetal vertex is very high (−4 station). You should never send a postterm patient (more than 42 weeks) home to follow up with twice weekly NSTs because the perinatal mortality rate is very high. There is no reason to repeat the modified BPP because this one is reassuring.

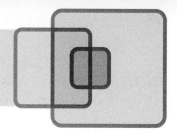

chapter **15**

Preterm Labor

SALLY Y. SEGEL AND GEORGE A. MACONES

I   PRETERM BIRTH

A **Definition.**   Preterm infants are born **before 37 weeks' gestation** (less than 259 days from the date of the last menstrual period). Preterm birth is a major contributor to developmental delay, visual and hearing impairment, chronic lung disease, and cerebral palsy. More than 50% of these condition result from preterm births before 34 weeks' gestation.

B **Epidemiology.**   During the past 15 years, the incidence of premature delivery in the United States has remained stable at approximately 10%. Recently, rates have increased slightly, largely caused by the increase in multifetal gestations. Complications from prematurity account for more than 70% of neonatal and infant deaths in infants without anomalies.

1. **"Spontaneous" preterm birth.** Seventy-five percent of preterm births occur spontaneously after preterm labor and preterm premature rupture of membranes (PPROM).

2. **"Indicated" preterm birth.** Twenty to thirty percent of all preterm births occur because of a medical or obstetric disorder that places the mother or fetus at significant risk for serious morbidity or mortality.

3. Neonatal morbidity and mortality increase as the gestational age at delivery decreases.

II   RISK FACTORS FOR PREMATURE DELIVERY

A **Sociodemographic factors**

1. **Low socioeconomic status.** Low income, low level of education, and poor nutrition are associated with preterm delivery.

2. **Ethnicity.** African Americans have a higher preterm delivery rate than other ethnic groups in the United States.

3. **Age.** Maternal age of 18 years or less or of 40 years or more increases the risk of preterm delivery.

4. **Previous premature birth.** The risk in the subsequent pregnancy after one premature birth is 17 to 37%.

5. **Strenuous work and great personal stress** (variable association)

6. **Tobacco smoking**

7. **Cocaine use**

8. **Complicated obstetric history.** Women with one or more spontaneous second-trimester abortions have an increased risk of premature birth.

B **Maternal medical and obstetric conditions**

1. Uterine conditions
   a. **Müllerian malformations.** Women with unicornuate or bicornuate uteri are at increased risk of preterm delivery.

    b. Cervical incompetence. This painless cervical dilation in the second trimester is associated with eventual pregnancy loss. It can be caused by trauma during an obstetric or gynecologic procedure, diethylstilbestrol exposure in utero, or unknown etiology.

    c. Uterine overdistention

      (1) Polyhydramnios (amniotic fluid index of more than 25 cm)

      (2) Multiple gestation. Twin intrauterine pregnancies have a preterm labor rate of approximately 40%. Triplet intrauterine pregnancies have a 20% risk of delivery prior to 24 weeks' gestation and a 10% delivery rate from 24 to 28 weeks' gestation.

2. Obstetric conditions

  a. Preeclampsia-eclampsia

  b. Placenta abruptio

  c. Placenta previa

  d. Fetal growth restriction

3. Other maternal conditions. These disorders include chronic hypertension, diabetes mellitus type 1, renal disease, osteogenesis imperfecta, and collagen vascular disease.

C | **Infection.** A correlation exists between individual infectious causes of preterm birth and low socioeconomic status. Significant maternal infections that may cause preterm labor and delivery include:

1. Pyelonephritis

2. Pneumonia

3. Asymptomatic bacteriuria

4. Bacterial vaginosis

5. Intra-amniotic infection

6. Sexually transmitted diseases (STDs) (ill-defined relationship with preterm labor)

III **EVALUATION OF PATIENTS IN PRETERM LABOR**

A | **History.** Symptoms of preterm labor include:

1. Uterine cramping or contractions

2. Rhythmic low back pain

3. Pelvic pressure

4. Increased vaginal discharge

5. Vaginal bleeding (bloody show), which may result from cervical dilation

B | **Physical examination**

1. A sterile **speculum examination** is a significant part of the physical examination. The evaluation of fetal membrane status and presence of cervicovaginal infection is determined at this time. If vaginal bleeding is present, an ultrasound must be performed to rule out placenta previa before a digital examination is performed.

  a. Endocervical samples are obtained for gonorrhea and chlamydia testing.

  b. Group B *Streptococcus* cultures are obtained.

  c. Premature rupture of membranes (PROM) is ruled out by doing fern and Nitrazine tests (V D 2).

2. If there is no evidence of PROM, a baseline **digital cervical examination** is performed, and follow-up examinations are warranted with continued uterine contractions.

3. A **urine specimen** is sent for culture.

4. **Fetal heart rate** and **uterine activity monitoring** are used to assess fetal well-being and patterns of uterine contraction. Uterine contractions without cervical change do not constitute preterm labor and may represent uterine irritability.

   a. Intravenous normal saline infusion is started during the initial evaluation.

   b. Parenteral fluids can treat dehydration, which is a cause of uterine irritability.

C **Diagnosis**

1. Regular uterine contractions associated with progressive cervical change (i.e., cervical dilation of 2 cm or more or cervical effacement of 80% or more) must be present.

2. The goal is early identification of pregnant women who develop preterm labor and are at risk for delivery. In women who present with the symptoms of preterm labor, the currently used techniques have only an average positive predictive value. These techniques are mainly used for their high negative predictive values. They are also used to reduce the overdiagnosis of preterm labor.

   a. **Cervical length.** This value can be measured accurately by a transvaginal ultrasound in a woman with an empty bladder. A cervical length of less than 3 cm has a positive predictive value (30 to 50%).

   b. **Fetal fibronectin.** This extracellular matrix glycoprotein found in fetal membranes plays an active role in intercellular adhesion. Fibronectin found in the cervicovaginal fluid in the late second and early third trimesters has been associated with preterm birth. The positive predictive value of the fibronectin assay is approximately 30%.

IV   MANAGEMENT OF PRETERM LABOR

A **Tocolysis.**   Treatment with tocolytic medications may not reduce the rate of preterm birth, but it may delay delivery for 48 hours and reduce the associated complications. The time gained allows for transfer to a tertiary center or corticosteroid administration.

1. **Magnesium sulfate.** This agent is currently the most commonly used tocolytic agent in the United States. Randomized controlled clinical trials suggest that it delays delivery by at least 48 hours.

   a. The **mechanism of action** is unclear. In theory, magnesium acts by competitive inhibition of calcium at the motor end plate or the cell membrane, thereby decreasing calcium influx into the cell. It is cleared from the maternal circulation by the kidneys.

   b. **Administration** involves infusing 2 to 4 g per hour to elevate serum levels to above the normal range. The loading dose is 4 to 6 g given over 30 minutes. Once contractions cease, the infusion is reduced to the lowest possible dose to maintain uterine quiescence.

   c. **Precautions**

      (1) Intravenous fluid is limited to 125 mL per hour, and fluid status is observed closely. An indwelling Foley catheter can be used to monitor urine output accurately.

      (2) Deep tendon reflexes and vital signs should be checked hourly.

      (3) A pulmonary examination should be performed every 2 to 4 hours.

      (4) If signs of magnesium toxicity occur, the infusion should be discontinued and calcium gluconate administered as needed.

   d. **Complications**

      (1) Nausea and vomiting

      (2) Flushing and headache

      (3) Muscle weakness

      (4) Pulmonary edema

      (5) Cardiopulmonary arrest

   e. **Contraindications** to magnesium therapy include renal failure, myasthenia gravis, and hypocalcemia.

2. **β-Mimetics**

    a. These agents stimulate β receptors, leading to smooth muscle relaxation and decreased uterine contractions.

    b. Ritodrine is the only agent approved by the Food and Drug Administration for the treatment of preterm labor. Because of its significant maternal side effects, it is not available in the United States.

    c. Terbutaline is the other β-mimetic tocolytic agent, which may be given subcutaneously, parenterally, or orally.

        (1) Administration is by three routes. The **subcutaneous dose** is 0.25 mg every 20 minutes three times and then every 4 hours; the **intravenous dose** is 0.125 mg every 4 hours; and the **oral dose** is 5 mg every 6 hours.

        (2) Side effects include tachycardia, palpitations, shortness of breath, pulmonary edema, hyperglycemia, hypokalemia, and tachyphylaxis.

3. **Indomethacin.** This nonsteroidal anti-inflammatory medication inhibits the synthesis of prostaglandins, which are involved in the biochemical process of labor.

    a. Indomethacin, 50 to 100 mg, is initially given rectally. Remaining doses are given orally, 25 to 50 mg every 6 hours. This agent is usually given for no longer than 48 hours.

    b. Maternal side effects include nausea, vomiting, and gastrointestinal bleeding.

    c. A main **neonatal side effect** is **constriction of the ductus arteriosus.**

        (1) Such constriction in a fetus causes tricuspid regurgitation and eventual right heart failure. Ductal constriction is usually transient and responds to discontinuation of the drug. Prior to 32 weeks' gestation, the incidence of ductal constriction is 5 to 10%. **From 32 to 35 weeks' gestation, the incidence of ductal constriction is 50%.**

        (2) Because of this significant side effect, indomethacin is **uncommonly used as a tocolytic after 32 weeks' gestation.**

    d. Other significant neonatal complications include oligohydramnios, pulmonary hypertension, and (possibly) necrotizing enterocolitis.

4. **Nifedipine.** This calcium channel blocker decreases smooth muscle contractions.

    a. Nifedipine is administered orally, 10 to 20 mg every 8 hours.

    b. Maternal side effects include a decrease in blood pressure and tachycardia.

B **Contraindications to tocolytic therapy**

1. Preeclampsia-eclampsia

2. Antepartum hemorrhage

3. Maternal cardiac disease

4. Chorioamnionitis

5. Lethal fetal anomaly

6. In utero fetal compromise

    a. Nonreassuring fetal heart rate

    b. Significant fetal growth restriction

C **Refractory preterm labor.** This condition is defined as persistent uterine contractions and cervical change despite maximal tocolytic therapy. Management may include **amniocentesis,** which can be performed to rule out an intra-amniotic infection.

1. A Gram stain is positive for intra-amniotic infection if bacteria are present.

2. A glucose level of less than 14 mg/dL may be a sign of intra-amniotic infection.

3. A positive amniotic fluid culture signals intra-amniotic infection.

D **Adjunctive therapy**

1. Corticosteroids
   a. Corticosteroids are given to women in preterm labor at 24 to 34 weeks' gestation.
   b. This medication induces fetal lung maturity, and optimal benefit begins 24 hours after initiation of therapy. Corticosteroids accelerate pulmonary maturity by stimulating the synthesis and release of surfactant from type II pneumocytes.
   c. Corticosteroids decrease mortality, respiratory distress syndrome, and intraventricular hemorrhage.

2. **Antibiotics.** These agents are given as prophylaxis for neonatal group B streptococcal infection.
   a. Antibiotics are started on admission and continued if the group B *Streptococcus* culture is positive. Affected women are treated for 7 days and then retreated during labor and delivery if the latency period is longer than 7 days.
   b. Antibiotics are discontinued if the group B *Streptococcus* culture is negative.

E **Fetal assessment**

1. Ultrasound
   a. An ultrasound is performed on admission to assess the estimated fetal weight and fetal presentation.
      (1) The estimated fetal weight can indicate whether the fetus has grown appropriately.
      (2) The fetal presentation is important when making a delivery plan. A fetus in breech presentation usually requires a cesarean section.

2. **Fetal well-being.** The fetal heart rate testing should be reassuring before starting tocolytic therapy. If the fetal heart rate is a concern, a biophysical profile should be performed before starting tocolytic therapy.

V PRETERM PREMATURE RUPTURE OF MEMBRANES

A **Definition.** Preterm premature rupture of membranes (PPROM) is rupture of fetal membranes prior to 37 weeks' gestation.

B **Epidemiology**

1. PPROM is responsible for 25 to 33% of all of preterm births each year.
2. Between 13 and 60% of patients with PPROM have an intra-amniotic infection.
3. Between 2 and 13% of patients with PPROM have postpartum endometritis.
4. The earlier the gestational age, the greater the potential for pregnancy prolongation; 75% of patients deliver within 1 week.

C **Etiology**

1. **Intrauterine infection is the major causal factor.**
2. Associated etiologic factors include low socioeconomic status, STDs, prior PPROM and preterm delivery, vaginal bleeding, cervical conization, tobacco smoking, uterine overdistention, and emergency cerclage.

D **Evaluation.** A sterile **speculum examination** is performed to evaluate the fetal membrane status and to inspect the cervix.

1. Membrane rupture is confirmed by visualization of amniotic fluid in the posterior fornix or by passing of amniotic fluid from the cervical canal.

2. The vaginal pH is normally 4.5 to 6.0, and the pH of amniotic fluid is 7.1 to 7.3. Nitrazine paper turns blue with a pH above 6.0 to 6.5.

    a. False-positive Nitrazine tests result from semen, alkaline antiseptics, bacterial vaginosis, and blood.

    b. Amniotic fluid from the vaginal pool produces a fernlike pattern on a microscope slide when allowed to dry.

    c. If the patient's history is suggestive of PPROM but the sterile speculum examination is equivocal, an amniocentesis can be performed. Amniotic fluid can be sent for Gram stain and culture. In addition, dilute indigo carmine can be instilled into the amniotic fluid. A tampon is then placed in the patient's vagina. After a few hours it is removed. If the tampon is blue, PPROM has been confirmed. If the tampon is white, the patient does not have PPROM.

3. Once membrane rupture has been confirmed, **digital examination of the cervix should be avoided** until labor or induction of labor.

4. Endocervical samples are obtained for gonorrhea and chlamydia testing.

5. Group B *Streptococcus* cultures are obtained.

6. A urine specimen is sent for culture.

7. Fetal heart rate and uterine activity monitoring are used to assess fetal well-being and uterine contraction pattern.

8. An ultrasound is performed on admission to assess the estimated fetal weight and fetal presentation.

D Management

1. In the **absence of labor, chorioamnionitis, or nonreassuring fetal heart rate testing,** patients with PPROM can be **expectantly** managed **until 34 to 36 weeks' gestation** with the following medications:

    a. Corticosteroids. A complete course is given from 24 to 34 weeks' gestation.

    b. Broad-spectrum antibiotics. A 7-day course (2 days intravenous, 5 days oral) is given.

2. Fetal well-being is assessed daily with a nonstress test and a follow-up biophysical profile as needed.

3. Chorioamnionitis, labor, or nonreassuring fetal heart rate testing mandates delivery at any gestational age.

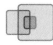

Study Questions for Chapter 15

Directions: Each of the numbered items or incomplete statements in this section is followed by answers or by completions of the statement. Select the ONE lettered answer or completion that is BEST in each case.

1. A 25-year-old gravida 1, para 0, at 10 weeks of gestation is coming to see you for a prenatal visit. She has osteogenesis imperfecta. She has no other medical problems other than a history of multiple fractures and bruises as a child. She takes no medication and denies drug allergies. During pregnancy, she is at risk for

   A Preeclampsia
   B Kidney disease
   C Premature delivery
   D Placenta previa
   E A single umbilical artery in the umbilical cord

2. A 28-year-old gravida 3, para 2, at 28 weeks of gestation has been admitted to the hospital for several days to treat her preterm labor. Her cervix was dilated to 3 cm and 100% effaced when $MgSO_4$ was started at 2.5 g/hr after a bolus over 30 minutes. An entire workup for preterm labor was done, and she received antibiotics and steroids. Currently, she has three to four contractions per minute that she barely feels on 2 g/hr. Treatment with $MgSO_4$ is most likely to

   A Reduce rate of preterm birth
   B Reduce morbidity associated with preterm delivery
   C Reduce mortality associated with preterm delivery
   D Stop contractions
   E Delay delivery for 2 days

QUESTIONS 3–4

A 22-year-old gravida 1, para 0 at 33 weeks of gestation presents to labor and delivery and reports cramping and lower back pain. She denies leaking of fluid from the vagina. You perform a speculum examination that shows no pooling, and Nitrazine paper stays yellow after contact with the secretions in the posterior fornix. Cervical cultures are taken. She is placed on fetal heart rate and uterine contraction monitoring, which shows a baseline heart rate of 155 bpm and three uterine contractions per a 10-minute period. Her cervix is dilated to 2 to 3 cm and 80% effaced. She also tells you that she has diabetes mellitus that has not been well controlled throughout pregnancy.

3. The next best step in management of this patient is

   A Antibiotics
   B $MgSO_4$
   C Terbutaline
   D Corticosteroids
   E Ultrasound

4. Management of this patient should also include

   A Culture for bacterial vaginosis
   B Urine culture
   C Avoidance of digital examinations
   D Fetal fibronectin
   E Assessment of ferning pattern on microscope slide

5. A 29-year-old gravida 3, para 1, sab 1 at 30 weeks of gestation is in preterm labor. She has received an initial bolus of 6 gm of $MgSO_4$ over 30 minutes, and she is placed on a maintenance rate of 4 g/hr for the last 2 days to reduce her contraction pattern to 1 every 15 minutes (her contractions are barely noticeable to her). Currently, her vitals are as follows: P = 88, BP = 90/50, R = 9, SaO_2 = 95% on room air. Her deep tendon reflexes are 0 bilaterally. She has crackles on her lung bases on deep inspiration. The next best step in management is

- A Serum magnesium level
- B Calcium gluconate
- C Switch to terbutaline
- D Discontinue MgSO4
- E Reevaluate her cervix

Answers and Explanations

1. The answer is C [II B 3]. Osteogenesis imperfecta is an inherited disorder of connective tissue matrix which makes tissue weak and susceptible to trauma. These individuals may have multiple fractures with minimal trauma; blue sclerae; hearing problems; the tendency to bleed from capillaries; unstable joints; and problems during pregnancy, such as preterm rupture of membranes and preterm labor.

2. The answer is E [IV A]. Treatment with tocolytic medications may not reduce the rate of preterm birth, but it may delay delivery for 48 hours and reduce the associated complications. The time gained allows for transfer to a tertiary center or corticosteroid administration.

3. The answer is E [IV B]. The patient is in preterm labor. Antibiotics and corticosteroids are given after initiation of tocolytic therapy, since tocolysis buys time (at least 48 hours) for the steroid to take effect on the fetal lung tissue and the antibiotics to treat an occult infection. Terbutaline is contraindicated in uncontrolled diabetes mellitus because it causes hyperglycemia. An ultrasound is indicated prior to inception of tocolytic therapy because a lethal fetal anomaly, in utero fetal compromise, and significant fetal growth restriction are all contraindications to tocolytic therapy. This is especially important in someone with diabetes mellitus who has not been under strict control.

4. The answer is B [V D 6]. A urine culture is an important step in the workup of preterm labor because advanced urinary tract infections are associated with preterm labor. We do not take cultures for bacterial vaginosis (a wet mount will suffice). You do not have to avoid doing more digital examinations because the patient's membranes are not ruptured (Nitrazine negative, pooling negative, and no loss of fluid from vagina per history). Fetal fibronectin is of no use because you have already diagnosed preterm labor. Looking for ferning on microscope slide is important when you want to confirm whether her amniotic membranes are ruptured.

5. The answer is A. This patient is probably becoming toxic on $MgSO_4$. Her reflexes are gone, she is lethargic, her respirations are slow, but she is oxygenating well. Check her serum magnesium level and turn it down (decrease $MgSO_4$ to 2 g/hr). It is also wise to monitor urinary output because magnesium is cleared by the kidneys. Calcium gluconate is given when magnesium levels are too high. (NOTE: Therapeutic serum magnesium levels are 4 to 7 mEq/L. Patellar reflex is lost at 7 to 10 mEq/L. Levels higher than 10 to 15 mEq/L cause pulmonary to cardiac toxicity. Also know this conversion: 1 mEq/L = 2 mM = 1.2 mg/dL.) There is no need to completely discontinue $MgSO_4$ without turning it down first (if the patient is in preterm labor). It is unnecessary to reevaluate her cervix because she is contracting only once every 15 minutes and barely feels the contractions. There is no need to switch to terbutaline, which is arguably less effective than magnesium at this point.

chapter 16

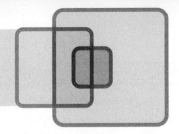

Hypertension in Pregnancy

DOMINIC MARCHIANO AND SAMUEL PARRY

I INTRODUCTION

Hypertensive disease complicates 8 to 11% of all pregnancies. It ranks second only to pulmonary embolism as a cause of maternal mortality in developed countries and accounts for 15% of maternal deaths in the United States.

II DEFINITIONS

A Chronic hypertension

1. Persistent **blood pressure greater than 140/90 mmHg before the twentieth week** of pregnancy
   a. **Mild:** Over 140/90 mmHg
   b. **Moderate:** Over 150/100 to 170/110 mmHg
   c. **Severe:** Over 170/110 mmHg

2. Hypertension initially diagnosed any time during pregnancy that persists for more than 12 weeks postpartum

B Gestational hypertension (pregnancy-induced hypertension, or PIH). Definitions of hypertension based on **incremental increases** in blood pressure over baseline (e.g., diastolic blood pressure at 24 weeks that is 15 mmHg higher than a reading from before 20 weeks) are **no longer used.**

1. **Diagnostic criterion:** onset of hypertension after 20 weeks' gestation
   a. Absolute blood pressure of 140/90 mmHg twice over 6 hours, without prior comparison
   b. Absolute mean arterial pressure of 105 mmHg without prior comparison
   c. Blood pressure returns to normal by 12 weeks postpartum

C Preeclampsia: Gestational hypertension with proteinuria

a. **Proteinuria** is defined by
   (1) 30 mg/dL on dipstick (1+) on repeated samples **or**
   (2) 300 mg on 24-hour urine collection
b. **Preeclampsia** may be **mild or severe** (Table 16-1). Criteria for **severe preeclampsia** suggest end-organ involvement (Table 16-2). After a **grand mal seizure,** preeclampsia is termed **eclampsia.**
c. **HELLP syndrome** (hemolysis, elevated liver enzymes, low platelets). This **variant of severe preeclampsia** develops in 10% of women with severe preeclampsia. However, approximately 10% of women with HELLP syndrome are normotensive, which is classified as atypical HELLP syndrome.
d. Superimposed preeclampsia on chronic hypertension
   (1) New onset proteinuria after 20 weeks in a woman with chronic hypertension
   (2) Sudden increase in proteinuria or blood pressure or a platelet count less than $100,000/mm^3$ in a woman with chronic hypertension and proteinuria before 20 weeks' gestation

TABLE 16-1 Hypertensive Disorders During Pregnancy: Indications of Severity

Abnormality	Mild	Severe
Diastolic blood pressure	<100 mgHg	≥110 mmHg
Proteinuria	Trace to +1	Persistent 2+ or more
Headache	Absent	Present
Visual disturbance	Absent	Present
Upper abdominal pain	Absent	Present
Oliguria	Absent	Present
Convulsion	Absent	Present (eclampsia)
Serum creatinine	Normal	Elevated
Thrombocytopenia	Absent	Present
Liver enzyme elevation	Minimal	Marked
Fetal growth restriction	Absent	Obvious
Pulmonary edema	Absent	Present

Reprinted with permission from Cunningham FG, MacDonald PC, Gant NF. Williams Obstetrics. 21st Ed. New York: McGraw-Hill, 2001:570, Figure Table 24-2.

III CHRONIC HYPERTENSION

A Effects on mother

1. Mild chronic hypertension is unlikely to adversely affect pregnancy. Pregnancy is unlikely to hasten the progression of maternal hypertensive end-organ disease.

2. Morbidity is increased over de novo preeclampsia.

B Effects on fetus

1. **Abruptio placentae** is four to eight times more likely in pregnancies complicated by chronic hypertension.

2. When preeclampsia is superimposed on chronic hypertension, preeclampsia occurs earlier and is associated with more pronounced **decreases in uteroplacental perfusion.** Intrauterine growth retardation (IUGR) may result from decreased uteroplacental perfusion.
   a. However, IUGR is not more frequent in cases of mild chronic hypertension.
   b. When preeclampsia is superimposed on chronic hypertension, the incidence of IUGR is 30 to 40%.

TABLE 16-2 Criteria for Severe Preeclampsia

Systolic hypertension >160 mmHg
Diastolic hypertension >110 mmHg
Proteinuria >5 g/24 hr
Oliguria <500 mL/24 hr
Cerebral or visual disturbances
Epigastric pain
Pulmonary edema
Evidence of microangiopathic hemolysis
Hepatocellular dysfunction
Thrombocytopenia
Intrauterine growth restriction
Oligohydramnios

3. **Prematurity is more common** with severe chronic hypertension.

4. **Perinatal mortality** approaches 25% in severe chronic hypertension.

C **Antihypertensive management**

1. Treatment reduces the risk of maternal morbidity. Whether it reduces perinatal morbidity and mortality remains controversial.

2. Existing antihypertensive therapy should be continued on diagnosis of pregnancy.

3. **Antihypertensive agents**
   a. α-**Methyldopa** is most used frequently and has been studied the most. There is **no evidence of fetal or maternal adverse events.**
   b. **Labetalol** (α- and β-blockade) is associated with a possible increase in growth restriction.
   c. **Nifedipine** has limited data, but it rapidly reduces blood pressure.
   d. β-**antagonists** have been associated with low birth weight.
   e. **Angiotensin-converting enzyme inhibitors are contraindicated** in pregnancy because of adverse effects on fetal renal function.

E **Antepartum management**

1. **Baseline evaluation for end-organ disease**
   a. Renal function tests
   b. Ophthalmologic examination
   c. Electrocardiogram

2. Antihypertensive therapy is unlikely to benefit a pregnancy complicated by mild hypertension. It should be reserved for pregnancies complicated by moderate or severe hypertension (diastolic blood pressure more than 100 to 110 mmHg), where it reduces the incidence of cardiovascular and cerebrovascular events.

3. Ultrasound should be used to determine specific gestational age. Serial ultrasound surveillance should be reserved for clinical suspicion of IUGR or superimposed preeclampsia.

4. Nonstress testing and amniotic fluid assessment should be started at 32 to 34 weeks' gestation.

5. Labor induction by 40 weeks' gestation can be considered.

IV **PREECLAMPSIA: EPIDEMIOLOGY**

A **Rate of occurrence:** 7% of pregnancies, excluding first-trimester losses

B **Risk factors**

1. **Pregnancy history.** Primigravidas constitute 65% of cases.
   a. Multiple gestation: 30% incidence
   b. Gestational trophoblastic disease: 70% incidence

2. **Maternal age.** Preeclampsia occurs at extremes of maternal age. However, the association with young age is confounded by the association with primigravidity. However, **maternal age of more than 40 years** is an independent risk factor.

3. **Family history.** Evidence for a genetic contribution includes a 37% incidence in sisters and a 26% incidence in daughters. This pattern is consistent with a dominant gene with reduced penetrance.

4. **Obesity.** Incidence is directly related to degree of obesity.

5. **Chronic hypertension.** Preeclampsia occurs in approximately 25% of women with chronic hypertension.

V PREECLAMPSIA: PATHOPHYSIOLOGY

A Pathophysiologic changes

1. **Cardiovascular system**

   a. Cardiac output remains normal, and increased total peripheral vascular resistance accounts for the hypertension.

   b. Preeclamptic endothelial cells generate less prostacyclin, a vasodilator, than normal endothelial cells. Less prostacyclin allows greater vascular sensitivity to angiotensin II, thus promoting vasospasm and increasing peripheral vascular resistance.

2. **Coagulation system**

   a. Disseminated intravascular coagulation occurs in 10% of patients with preeclampsia.

   b. Because of endothelial damage, most of these patients have mild procoagulant consumption and elevated fibrin degradation products.

   c. Diffuse intravascular coagulation may arise from vascular damage sustained during vasospasm.

3. **Renal function**

   a. **Glomerular changes**

      (1) Glomerular filtration rate (GFR) is usually decreased in preeclampsia. Deceased renal plasma flow and **glomeruloendotheliosis,** which occludes the capillary lumen, account for the lower GFR.

      (2) Protein leaks into urine. The glomerulus, which is normally impermeable to large proteins, becomes more permeable. In part, glomerular damage results from both vasospasm and endothelial damage. This leakage exceeds the tubules' ability to reabsorb proteins.

   b. **Tubular changes,** which affect the clearance of uric acid

      (1) Uric acid is normally completely filtered at the glomerulus, secreted, and mostly reabsorbed by the proximal tubules.

      (2) Uric acid clearance is 10% of creatinine clearance.

      (3) Decreased uric acid clearance is observed prior to a GFR disturbance, suggesting a tubal etiology in which the mechanism remains unknown.

      (4) Increased production by hypoxic tissues contributes to increased serum uric acid.

   c. **Renin-angiotensin-aldosterone system**

      (1) Levels of the following components are increased:

         (a) Plasma renin activity and plasma renin concentration

         (b) Angiotensinogen

         (c) Angiotensin II

         (d) Aldosterone

      (2) The theory that the renin-angiotensin system mediates the pathophysiologic alterations of preeclampsia is suggested by three factors:

         (a) Potent vasoconstrictor effect of angiotensin II

         (b) Stimulation of aldosterone by angiotensin II and consequent sodium retention

         (c) The finding that large doses of angiotensin II can cause proteinuria

      (3) It is possible that, despite decreased intravascular volume, preeclamptic vasoconstriction results in a physiologic perception of overfill, which suppresses renin release.

4. **Other signs of end-organ disease**

   a. Visual disturbances result from papilledema and suggest cerebral involvement.

   b. Epigastric pain suggests hepatocellular dysfunction and edema and liver capsule distention.

   c. Intrauterine growth retardation and oligohydramnios suggest placental vasculopathy and uteroplacental insufficiency.

B **Pathologic findings**

1. **Liver**

    a. Initially, arteriolar vasodilation results in hemorrhage into the hepatocellular columns. This condition is found on liver biopsy in 66% of patients with eclampsia.

    b. Hepatic infarction occurs later and is found on liver biopsy in 40% of patients with eclampsia.

2. **Kidney**

    a. **Glomerular endotheliosis** is the characteristic renal lesion of preeclampsia.

    (1) Endothelial cells enlarge and may occlude the capillary lumen.

    (2) Podocytes are not altered.

    (3) Changes are completely reversible with resolution of preeclampsia.

    b. Nonglomerular changes such as tubular alterations are less common.

3. **Placenta and placental site**

    a. The syncytiotrophoblast is abnormal, containing areas of cell death and degeneration, syncytial knots, and decreased density of microvilli.

    b. Cytotrophoblastic cells proliferate in placental villi.

    c. Placental vascular pathology

    (1) In normal pregnancy, the spiral artery endothelium, elastic lamina, and smooth muscle are replaced by trophoblast. This creates a low-resistance, high-flow system. These changes affect both the decidual and myometrial vessels.

    (2) In preeclampsia, these changes do not uniformly occur or are limited to decidual vessels.

    (3) These observations can be made on first-trimester abortion specimens, suggesting that pathologic change precedes the clinical presentation.

VI PREECLAMPSIA: CLINICAL MANIFESTATIONS

A **Clinical signs**

1. **Hypertension** is required for diagnosis.

2. **Edema** is related to sodium retention, not limited to dependent edema.

3. **Hyperreflexia** is common.

C **Laboratory findings**

1. **Renal function**

    a. Proteinuria

    b. Hyperuricemia is likely caused by both altered renal function and increased production of uric acid.

    c. Increased serum creatinine is inversely correlated with creatinine clearance.

2. **Hematology findings**

    a. Hemoconcentration as reflected by an increased hematocrit

    b. Thrombocytopenia

3. **Hepatic findings.** Increased transaminases, when associated with microangiopathic hemolysis and coagulopathy, suggest HELLP syndrome.

VII PREECLAMPSIA: MANAGEMENT

A Delivery is the only known treatment. At term (37 weeks' gestation), delivery is recommended.

B **Route of delivery**

1. **Vaginal delivery is preferable** to cesarean delivery, which should be reserved for the usual obstetric indications.

2. Cesarean delivery may be preferred in cases of severe preeclampsia remote from term with an unfavorable cervix.

3. Some evidence suggests that preeclampsia may expedite cervical ripening and labor induction.

C **Antepartum treatment (before 37 weeks)**

1. **Mild preeclampsia** may be managed expectantly using the following interventions. It is controversial whether in- or outpatient management is preferable.
    (1) Bed rest
    (2) Blood pressure and urinary protein monitoring
    (3) Twice-weekly nonstress tests
    (4) Laboratory surveillance

2. **Stable severe preeclampsia**
    a. **Before 24 weeks.** Pregnancy termination should be offered.
    b. **Before 32 weeks.** Delivery is always a legitimate course of action, but expectant management with blood pressure control is an option.
        (1) Expectant management requires intensive fetal and maternal surveillance.
        (2) Antenatal corticosteroids are recommended.
        (3) Delivery is mandatory if the patient develops thrombocytopenia, abnormal liver function tests, uncontrollable hypertension, pulmonary edema, oligohydramnios, or abnormal fetal testing.
        (4) Presence of proteinuria or controllable hypertension does not require immediate delivery.
    c. **After 32 weeks.** Delivery is appropriate after documentation of fetal lung maturity.
        (1) If fetal lung maturity is negative, antenatal steroids should be given before 34 weeks.
        (2) Alternatively, steroids can be given to all patients between 32 and 34 weeks. Delivery may be effected 48 hours later without documenting fetal lung maturity.

3. **Unstable severe preeclampsia.** Treatment **at any gestational age** involves prompt delivery.

E **Intrapartum management**

1. **Seizure prophylaxis.** Because there are no signs that accurately predict seizures, **prophylaxis is most effective if all women with preeclampsia are treated.**
    a. **Magnesium sulfate** is superior to other antiepileptic medications for preventing eclampsia-related seizures and seizure-related morbidity and mortality.
        (1) An intravenous loading dose of 6 g is usually followed by a maintenance infusion of 2 to 4 g per hour.
        (2) Patients must be monitored for signs of magnesium toxicity, such as hyporeflexia and respiratory depression.
        (3) Magnesium toxicity may be confirmed by testing serum levels (Table 16-3). It can be reversed with 1 g of calcium gluconate.
        (4) In instances in which magnesium sulfate cannot be used (e.g., myasthenia gravis, end-stage renal disease [because of impaired magnesium clearance]), phenytoin is safe.

TABLE 16-3 Effects of Magnesium at Different Serum Levels	
Effect	**Level (mEq/L)**
Seizure prophylaxis	4–6
Loss of deep tendon reflexes	10
Respiratory depression	15
General anesthesia	15
Cardiac arrest	25

2. Antihypertensive therapy
   a. Indications
      (1) Persistent diastolic blood pressure of over 105 mmHg
      (2) Isolated diastolic blood pressure of over 110 mmHg
   b. Pharmacologic agents
      (1) **Hydralazine** (preferred agent) reduces afterload but compensates by increasing heart rate; therefore, uterine perfusion is not usually compromised.
      (2) **Labetalol** does not reduce afterload.
   c. **Invasive cardiac monitoring** should be considered in the presence of oliguria or pulmonary edema.
3. Type of anesthesia
   a. **Epidural anesthesia** is safe for patients with normal clotting ability and no thrombocytopenia. It can be used for either vaginal or cesarean deliveries.
   b. **General anesthesia** should be used with caution because the stimulation of intubation may exacerbate hypertension.

F **Postpartum management**

1. Magnesium sulfate should be continued for 24 hours but may be discontinued earlier in the presence of pronounced diuresis, because therapeutic levels are not likely attainable.
2. Indications for acute antihypertensive therapy are the same as for the antepartum or intrapartum period.
3. Women who continue to have hypertension but have a persistent diastolic blood pressure of less than 100 mmHg may be discharged on oral therapy.
4. Pregnancy-induced hypertension usually disappears completely by 2 weeks postpartum.

VIII PREECLAMPSIA: PREVENTION

There is no reliable method for preventing preeclampsia. Low-dose aspirin, calcium, antioxidants, low sodium diet, and fish oil have all been shown to be ineffective.

IX ECLAMPSIA

Eclampsia is preeclampsia complicated by generalized tonic-clonic seizures. Pathophysiology of the convulsions is unknown.

A May occur **before, during, or after labor and delivery**

B May cause maternal death

C Consider cerebral imaging, especially if the seizures occur more than 24 hours postpartum

D **Treatment** includes **magnesium sulfate** to control seizures; **antihypertensive therapy** with hydralazine, labetalol, or nifedipine; **prevention** of aspiration and hypoxia; and **delivery** when the mother is stabilized

X PREECLAMPSIA: PROGNOSIS

With **timely delivery and magnesium sulfate,** the maternal mortality rate should be virtually zero.

A **Recurrence.** The risk is 40% for severe preeclampsia and increases with earlier diagnosis of the index case.

B **Future hypertension.** Preeclampsia does not accelerate hypertension but seems to unmask existing, yet undiagnosed, chronic hypertension.

1. Women with preeclampsia in a first pregnancy are no more likely to develop hypertension than controls.

2. Multiparous women are more likely to develop hypertension, but this is confounded because preeclampsia is unlikely to develop de novo in multiparas. Many of these women had underlying hypertension.

Study Questions for Chapter 16

Directions: Each of the numbered items or incomplete statements in this section is followed by answers or by completions of the statement. Select the ONE lettered answer or completion that is BEST in each case.

1. You have been seeing a 23-year-old woman, gravida 1, para 0 at 28 weeks of gestation throughout her pregnancy. She has no known medical history. She denies blurry vision, epigastric or right upper quadrant pain, severe headache, or trouble breathing. Her blood pressure (BP) and urine protein dipstick results for the past three visits are as follows: visit 1, BP = 105/60, U_{dip} = 0; visit 2, BP = 110/65, U_{dip} = 1+; visit 3, BP = 115/68, U_{dip} = 1+. Today her BP = 120/75 and U_{dip} = trace. She reports lots of fetal movement. Her fundus measures 25 cm. Lungs are clear to auscultation bilaterally. Deep tendon reflexes are 2+ symmetric. Results from laboratory studies you sent on visit three are the following:

> Platelet count = $130 \times 10^3/mm^3$
> Leukocytes = 10,400/mL
> Peripheral blood smear = no hemolysis
> Aspartate aminotransferase = 340 U/l
> Alanine aminotransferase = 200 U/l
> Blood Urea Nitrogen = 12 mg/dL
> Creatinine = 0.6 mg/dL
> Uric Acid = 6.0 mg/dL
> Glucose = 105 mg/dL

The most accurate diagnosis for this patient is

- **A** Chronic hypertension
- **B** Gestational hypertension
- **C** Mild preeclampsia
- **D** Severe preeclampsia
- **E** Superimposed preeclampsia on chronic hypertension

2. A 20-year-old primigravid woman at 37 weeks of gestation (confirmed by a first trimester ultrasound) presents to the clinic for routine prenatal care. She reports active fetal movement and abdominal pain. Her blood pressure is 162/103 initially and she has 2+ protein on the urine dipstick. Her physical examination is unremarkable except for diffuse tenderness on the abdomen; however, there is no rebound tenderness. Her fundus measures 36 cm above the symphysis pubis. You send her to labor and delivery where a complete blood cell count, liver enzymes, electrolytes, uric acid, urinalysis, and coagulation profile are drawn. On L&D, her blood pressure is 166/104 and there is 3+ proteinuria on urine dipstick. Her cervix is closed, long, firm, and posterior, and fetal vertex is high. What is the best next step in management?

- **A** Oxytocin
- **B** Prostaglandin analogue and magnesium sulfate
- **C** Magnesium sulfate
- **D** Methyldopa
- **E** Hydralazine

QUESTIONS 3–6

For the next few questions, match the description below with the organ or structure above that is affected during preeclampsia. You may use the above answers once, more than once, or not at all.

[A] Kidney
[B] Liver
[C] Brain
[D] Retina
[E] Placenta

3. Increasing levels of uric acid

4. Growth retardation measured by ultrasound

5. Epigastric pain

6. Blurry vision

7. A 26-year-old nurse, gravida 2, para 1 at 32 weeks of gestation presents to L&D because of elevated blood pressures. She says her systolic blood pressures have been in the high 170s and her diastolic blood pressures have been in the low 110s. She denies abdominal pain, visual disturbances, or severe headache. Her blood pressure at L&D is 150/98 and she has 1+ proteinuria. You send off appropriate labs, admit the patient to the hospital, and keep her in bedrest. Which of the following is an appropriate next step in management?

[A] Induce labor–vaginal delivery
[B] Cesarean section
[C] Phenytoin
[D] Labetalol
[E] Betamethasone

8. A 35-year-old woman, gravida 5, para 1, at 6 weeks of gestation is seeing you because she just found out she is pregnant. She has a 6-year history of essential hypertension controlled on a diuretic agent. After you perform a routine prenatal examination, you change her blood pressure medication to methyldopa and ask her to use it throughout the entire pregnancy. Which of the following is the best reason for using methyldopa in a patient with chronic hypertension during pregnancy?

[A] It is the best antihypertensive during pregnancy
[B] It decreases the risk of IUGR in the fetus
[C] It decreases the risk of abruption placentae
[D] It decreases the risk of maternal end-organ damage
[E] It increases uteroplacental perfusion

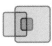

Answers and Explanations

1. The answer is D [II C c and Table 16-1]. Although this patient has normal blood pressures and only mild proteinuria, her blood pressure measurements have been rising steadily over the last few visits. This is the opposite of what happens in normal pregnancy. The most important feature that makes this clinical scenario "severe" is the elevated liver enzymes. Both AST and ALT are more than three times normal. [Note: you should have a sense of normal and abnormal laboratory values for common electrolytes, liver enzymes, and cell counts. However, the exact range of normal values will be provided to you in your examination booklet.] This patient has severe preeclampsia, and the clinician should send the patient to the hospital for admission. Gestational hypertension is not a diagnosis and it is an uncommon term. Chronic hypertension is defined as blood pressure greater than 140/90 before week 20 of pregnancy or hypertension that is diagnosed at any time during pregnancy and persists for more than 12 weeks postpartum.

2. The answer is B [VII A and VII E 1]. This clinical scenario is describing severe preeclampsia based on her elevated systolic blood pressure (>160 mmHg) and persistent elevated proteinuria (≥2+). She also has abdominal pain, which is a sign of severe preeclampsia. While awaiting her labs, you should start the delivery process by inducing her with a prostaglandin agent and put her on magnesium sulfate for seizure prophylaxis. It may sound counterintuitive to place someone on magnesium (which is also a tocolytic agent) while attempting to deliver. However, in the management of preeclampsia, magnesium sulfate is used for seizure prophylaxis, and another agent such as a prostaglandin analogue or oxytocin (if cervix is favorable; high Bishop score) is used to achieve delivery. Remember, delivery is the only true cure for preeclampsia. Using oxytocin to induce this patient would be unsuccessful because her cervix is unfavorable (low Bishop score). Methyldopa is used for patients with chronic hypertension during pregnancy. Hydralazine is used for persistently high diastolic blood pressure, usually diastolic of over 105 mmHg.

3. A [V A 3 b] **4. E** [V A 4 c] **5. B** [V A 4 b] **6. C** [V A 4 a]. Elevated uric acid levels in preeclampsia represent decreased uric acid clearance, suggesting tubal etiology. This mechanism is unknown. Epigastric pain suggests hepatocellular dysfunction and edema and liver capsule distension. IUGR and oligohydramnios suggest placental vasculopathy and uteroplacental insufficiency. Visual disturbances result from papilledema and suggest cerebral involvement.

7. The answer is E [VII C 1 and C 2 c 1]. According to criteria discussed in this chapter, this patient represents mild preeclampsia. Management of this case is more complicated because she is preterm (32 weeks). Because definitive management of preeclampsia is delivery, you must weigh the risks of premature delivery for the fetus against the benefits of delivery to the mother. Mild preeclampsia may be managed expectantly (by bedrest, blood pressure and urine protein monitoring, twice weekly NST, and lab evaluations) before 37 weeks of gestation. The best course of action (given the above answer choices) is to give antenatal steroids to try to effect fetal lung maturity. Delivery by cesarean section or vaginal birth is not appropriate in someone less than 37 weeks with mild preeclampsia. Anyone who has the diagnosis of preeclampsia needs to be on seizure prophylaxis. The best agent is magnesium sulfate, not phenytoin. Labetalol is used to treat persistently elevated diastolic blood pressure of over 105 mmHg.

8. The answer is D [III C 1]. Treatment of hypertension during pregnancy reduces the risk of **maternal** morbidity probably by preventing end-organ damage. Whether therapy reduces perinatal morbidity and mortality remains controversial. Methyldopa is the most commonly used anti-hypertensive medication but it is not necessarily the best. There is evidence that labetalol is as good, if not better, then methyldopa during pregnancy. Methyldopa does not increase uteroplacental perfusion.

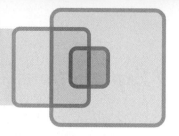

chapter 17

Medical Complications of Pregnancy

HARISH M. SEHDEV

I DIABETES

Diabetes affects 2 to 3% of all pregnancies. **Gestational diabetes,** which is diabetes diagnosed during pregnancy, accounts for 90% of these cases.

A Effect of pregnancy on glucose metabolism

1. **Maternal metabolism adjusts** to provide nutrition for both the fetus and the mother.
   a. Increased insulin secretion occurs as a result of β-cell hyperplasia from the increased levels of estrogen and progesterone.
   b. Insulin antagonism results from the increase in human somatomammotropin (produced by syncytiotrophoblasts).
   c. Increased insulin degradation by placental insulinase occurs.
2. A more than 40% **decrease in insulin sensitivity** normally occurs by late in pregnancy, and maintenance of glucose homeostasis results from exaggeration in both the rate and amount of insulin release.
3. Therefore, as pregnancy progresses, women with marginal pancreatic reserve may be unable to meet insulin demands, especially in late pregnancy, and those with preexisting diabetes will need more insulin.
4. **Fetal glucose levels are directly proportional to maternal glucose concentrations.**
   a. Insulin **does not cross** the placenta.
   b. After delivery, insulin requirements for patients with underlying diabetes **decrease** because of the decrease in estrogen, progesterone, placental insulinase, and human somatomammotropin.

B Effects of preexisting diabetes on pregnancy.
Before the use of insulin therapy, complications of diabetes for both the mother and fetus were extremely high. Although insulin therapy has lowered the risk of complications, pregnancies in women with diabetes are still associated with an increased risk of adverse events.

1. Maternal complications
   a. Preeclampsia and eclampsia
   b. Diabetic ketoacidosis
   c. Worsening preexisting nephropathy
   d. Worsening preexisting retinopathy
   e. Infection

   f. Polyhydramnios
   g. Cesarean delivery
   h. Postpartum hemorrhage
   i. Mortality

2. **Fetal complications**
   a. Miscarriage
   b. Unexplained stillbirth
   c. **Perinatal mortality** of approximately 2 to 5% (significantly lower than the risk of approximately 65% before insulin therapy)
   d. **Congenital malformations,** which account for up to 50% of associated perinatal mortality. Anomalies can affect most organ systems, in particular anencephaly and spina bifida in the **central nervous system,** ventricular septal defect, situs inversus in the **cardiac system,** and a characteristic embryopathy called sacral agenesis or **caudal regression.** These usually occur by **7 weeks' gestation** (see Chapter 7).
   e. Abnormal fetal intrauterine growth (both macrosomia and growth restriction)
   f. Neonatal complications, including respiratory distress syndrome, hypoglycemia, hypocalcemia, polycythemia, and hyperbilirubinemia

C **Management**

1. **Prior to conception.** Appropriate prenatal care for women with **preexisting diabetes** should begin before conception. Such care may decrease the risk of congenital malformations.
   a. Adjust insulin to normalize glucose levels.
   b. Provide **folic acid** supplementation.
   c. Provide nutrition counseling.

2. **First trimester**
   a. Obtain ultrasound between 6 and 8 weeks' gestation if possible for accurate dating.
   b. Order **hemoglobin A1C** to assess glycemic control and determine the risk of congenital abnormalities.
   c. Assess overall health for effects of background vascular involvement (e.g., renal, ophthalmologic, or cardiac).
   d. **Multiple** daily injections of insulin (or an insulin pump) may be needed to maintain the **goal** of a fasting glucose **less than 95 mg/dL** and 2-hour postprandial glucose less than **120 mg/dL**

3. **Second trimester: screening for malformations**
   a. Maternal serum α-fetoprotein (AFP) screening at 15 to 20 weeks to assess the risk of fetal neural tube abnormalities
   b. Ultrasound at 16 to 20 weeks to check fetal anatomy
   c. Fetal echocardiography at 20 to 22 weeks to help screen for fetal cardiac abnormalities

4. **Third trimester: assessment of fetal well-being**
   a. Surveillance of fetal well-being should begin at **28 weeks** with maternal fetal activity assessment (kick counts) because the risk of unexplained stillbirth has increased. **Nonstress testing or biophysical profiles** should begin at 32 weeks or earlier if significant maternal vascular disease exists or evidence of fetal growth restriction.
   b. Ultrasound every 4 to 6 weeks to assess fetal growth

5. **Timing of delivery.** The time at which delivery occurs depends on both maternal glycemic control and the health and maturity of the fetus.
   a. In patients with good glycemic control and reassuring fetal testing, the physician can wait for the onset of labor until 40 weeks' gestation.
   b. If induction of labor is considered before 39 weeks, assessment of fetal lung maturity by amniocentesis should be performed to assess the lecithin/sphingomyelin (**L/S**) ratio and the presence of **phosphatidylglycerol** in the amniotic fluid. If testing does not reveal an L/S ratio

of at least 2:1 or the presence of phosphatidylglycerol, delivery should be delayed until after 39 weeks as long as fetal testing remains reassuring.

6. **Method of delivery.** The mode of delivery should be individualized. In patients with diabetes, fetal growth can increase the risk of **shoulder dystocia** (entrapment of the shoulder after delivery of the head). However, many cases still occur in fetuses that weigh less than 4000 g. Ultrasound assessment of fetal weight is helpful but not completely accurate.
   a. If the suspected weight of the fetus does not exceed 4000 g, vaginal delivery (including induction of labor) can be attempted.
   b. If the suspected weight of the fetus exceeds 4000 g (macrosomia), elective cesarean delivery can be offered.
   c. For all deliveries, euglycemia should be maintained and ketosis avoided.

D **Gestational diabetes**

1. **Effect of gestational diabetes on pregnancy**
   a. Increased risk of macrosomia
   b. Increased risk of preeclampsia
   c. Increased rate of stillbirth if fasting glucose elevated
   d. **Fetal anomalies are not increased.**

2. **Screening** for gestational diabetes may be needed based on the following **risk factors:**
   a. Strong family history
   b. Persistent glucosuria
   c. History of unexplained stillbirth or miscarriage
   d. Prior macrosomic fetus
   e. Obesity
   f. Age older than 25 years

3. **Universal screening is recommended** because selective screening may miss up to 50% of cases of gestational diabetes.
   a. The **1-hour glucose tolerance test** consists of a 50-g glucose load. There is no set abnormal value, and the threshold value may be 130, 135, or 140 mg/dL. The lower the threshold, the greater the screen positive rate with a greater sensitivity. An abnormal value requires a standard glucose tolerance test.
   b. The **standard glucose tolerance test is a 3-hour test** consisting of a 100-g glucose load and four serum glucose determinations. Gestational diabetes is diagnosed if there are at least two abnormal values.
      (1) Fasting value: 95 mg/dL
      (2) 1-hour value: 180 mg/dL
      (3) 2-hour value: 155 mg/dL
      (4) 3-hour value: 140 mg/dL

4. **Management**
   a. Provide nutritional counseling and dietary adjustment. If the disease can be controlled by diet alone, patients can be followed similarly to those without diabetes. No evidence supports early delivery.
   b. Monitor fasting and 2-hour postprandial glucose values.
   c. Give insulin if fasting glucose values are greater than 105 mg/dL and 2-hour postprandial values are greater than 120 mg/dL.
   d. Patients who require insulin or are unable to maintain glycemic control should be followed similarly to patients with preexisting diabetes.

5. **Follow-up.** After the postpartum visit, patients with gestational diabetes should be screened routinely for diabetes.

II THYROID DISEASE

Thyroid disease affects up to 0.2% of all pregnancies.

A Effects of pregnancy on thyroid function.

1. Plasma inorganic iodine concentration decreases because of increased renal excretion and increased glomerular filtration.

2. Enlargement of the thyroid gland occurs.

3. Increased serum thyroxine (T_4)-binding globulin.

4. Laboratory assessment of thyroid function is altered.
   a. Increased total T_4
   b. Increased total triiodothyronine (T_3)
   c. Increased radioiodine uptake
   d. Decreased T_3 resin uptake
   e. Unchanged free T_4, free T_3, thyroid-stimulating hormone (TSH) levels

B Hyperthyroidism. This condition occurs in approximately 1 in 200 pregnancies.

1. **Effects on pregnancy.** The signs and symptoms of normal pregnancy can mimic signs of hyperthyroidism. If hyperthyroidism is untreated, the risk of complications (e.g., preeclampsia, preterm delivery congestive heart disease, and adverse perinatal outcome) is increased.

2. **Causes**
   a. **Graves disease,** an autoimmune process, is the most common cause. This condition is associated with an increase in thyroid-stimulating antibodies that stimulate the TSH receptors; these antibodies can cross the placenta, resulting in fetal thyrotoxicosis.
   b. **Gestational trophoblastic disease** (see Chapter 18) should be considered, especially if hyperthyroidism occurs early in gestation and a pelvic ultrasound should be ordered.

3. **Diagnosis**
   a. Tachycardia
   b. Thyromegaly
   c. Exophthalmos
   d. Poor maternal weight gain
   e. Severe hyperemesis gravidarum
   f. Onycholysis (separation of nail from the nail bed)
   g. Decreased TSH with increased free T_4

4. **Management.** Therapy can be either medical or surgical with minimal risk to mother and fetus.
   a. **Medical therapy**
      (1) **Propylthiouracil** prevents both the synthesis of thyroid hormone in the thyroid gland and the peripheral conversion of T_4 to T_3. The drug readily crosses the placenta and may induce **fetal hypothyroidism** and goiter, although this is rare. The goal of treatment is to maintain a maternal high-normal level of free T_4.
      (2) **Methimazole** prevents only the release of thyroid hormone and has been associated with **aplasia cutis**, a reversible developmental disorder of the fetal scalp.
      (3) β-blockers may be used to control symptoms of hyperthyroidism.
      (4) **Radioactive iodine is contraindicated** in pregnancy because it crosses the placenta and can ablate the fetal thyroid gland.
   b. **Surgical therapy.** In cases that are refractory to medical therapy, thyroidectomy may be necessary.

5. **Thyroid storm** is a rare complication of hyperthyroidism that can be associated with heart failure. Treatment includes propylthiouracil, potassium iodide, β-blockers, hydration, and control of body temperature.

C **Hypothyroidism**

1. **Effects on pregnancy**
   a. Often associated with decreased fertility
   b. Increased risk of miscarriage, preeclampsia, abruptio placentae, stillbirth, and intrauterine growth restriction (IUGR).
   c. Infants of untreated women with significantly increased TSH levels may be at risk for **decreased performance on IQ tests.**

2. **Diagnosis.** Increased TSH and decreased free T_4 are the basis of diagnosis.

3. **Management.** Hypothyroidism is treated with supplemental thyroid hormone. Infants of treated mothers are healthy.

III URINARY TRACT INFECTION

Women are at greater risk for urinary tract infections during pregnancy because of the anatomic and physiologic changes that occur with pregnancy. **A urine culture should be obtained in all women at their first prenatal visit,** and urine dipstick analysis should be performed at all subsequent visits.

A **Asymptomatic bacteriuria.** This condition is defined as the presence of bacteria within the urinary tract without symptoms.

1. Asymptomatic bacteriuria is present in 5 to 10% of all pregnant women. The incidence is highest in black multiparas with sickle cell trait.

2. **Treatment** requires administration of an antibiotic (e.g., ampicillin or nitrofurantoin) to which the causal organism is sensitive.

3. **Consequences of lack of treatment**
   a. Pyelonephritis in up to 40% of affected women
   b. Risk factor for low birth weight

4. **A follow-up culture** is necessary after treatment has been completed.

B **Acute urethritis**

1. Usually, the **etiologic agents** are *Escherichia coli, Chlamydia trachomatis,* and *Neisseria gonorrhoeae.*

2. **Signs and symptoms** include frequency, dysuria, and urgency. Mucopurulent discharge from the urethra may be present.

3. **Urinalysis** reveals white blood cells without bacteria.

4. **Urine culture** and urethral culture for gonorrhea and chlamydia should be performed.

5. **Treatment** is based on the causal agent.

C **Cystitis**

1. **Etiologic agents**
   a. The most common pathogen is *E. coli* (80 to 90% of cases).
   b. Other causal pathogens include *Klebsiella pneumoniae, Proteus* species, and gram-positive organisms such as enterococci and group B streptococci.

2. **Symptoms** include frequency, urgency, suprapubic pain, dysuria, and hesitancy. Hematuria may be present. Fever is uncommon.

3. **Diagnosis** is made by using a clean catch specimen or one obtained by midstream urine collection or bladder catheterization.

4. **Treatment** involves a short course of antibiotics to which the organism is sensitive. Inadequate treatment may lead to pyelonephritis.

5. **A follow-up culture** is necessary after treatment is complete.

D **Acute pyelonephritis.** This condition affects 1 to 2% of all pregnancies. It usually results from lower tract infection. Up to 90% of cases are unilateral and usually affect the right side.

1. **Predisposing factors unique to pregnancy**
   a. Ureteral compression at the pelvic brim caused by the enlarging uterus
   b. Decreased tone and peristalsis of the ureters resulting from increased progesterone levels
   c. Decreased bladder sensitivity, which may result in overdistention and the need for catheterization

2. The **most common causative agent** is *E. coli.*

3. **Signs and symptoms** may include:
   a. Fever, chills, and back pain
   b. Nausea or vomiting
   c. Anorexia
   d. Preterm contractions and preterm labor

4. **Complications** may include:
   a. Bacteremia and septic shock
   b. Pulmonary edema and respiratory distress syndrome
   c. Renal dysfunction
   d. Preterm labor

5. **Treatment**
   a. Inpatient therapy is preferred.
   b. Hydration is useful.
   c. Intravenous antibiotics are used until the patient is afebrile for 24 to 48 hours; they are followed by oral antibiotics with appropriate sensitivity to complete a 7- to 10-day course of treatment.
   d. Lack of response to treatment should prompt radiologic evaluation for an abscess or renal calculi.
   e. Follow-up therapy includes daily antibiotic suppression for the remainder of the pregnancy.
   f. Up to 30% of patients may develop recurrent urinary tract infections during pregnancy.

IV ANEMIA

Anemia has been defined by the Centers for Disease Control and Prevention as a hemoglobin concentration of less than 11 g/dL in the first and third trimester of pregnancy and less than 10.5 g/dL in the second trimester. Anemia is broadly classified as acquired or hereditary.

A **Acquired anemias**
1. **Iron-deficiency anemia.** The most common cause of anemia in pregnancy is **iron deficiency.** The iron requirements of pregnancy are considerable, and most women enter pregnancy with low iron stores.
   a. In pregnancy, a woman needs an additional 1000 mg of elemental iron.
      (1) 300 mg goes to the fetus.
      (2) 500 mg is used to expand the maternal red cell mass.
      (3) 200 mg is shed through the gut and skin.
   b. The level of **hematocrit naturally decreases** during the second trimester of pregnancy, because of the greater expansion of maternal plasma volume compared with the increase in red cell mass and hemoglobin mass.
   c. Late in pregnancy, hemoglobin mass continues to increase while plasma volume remains steady.

   d. Because of the normal transfer of iron from the mother to the fetus, the **fetus does not suffer from iron-deficiency anemia.**

   e. While maternal absorption of iron is increased in pregnancy, treatment involves additional daily elemental iron (200 mg in divided doses) to correct the anemia and maintain adequate stores.

2. **Megaloblastic anemia.** This condition, which is rare in the United States, is characterized by impaired DNA synthesis. It occurs in pregnant women who consume neither fresh vegetables nor foods with a high content of animal protein.

   a. **Folic acid deficiency** is the most common form.

   b. Many women also have iron deficiency.

   c. **Vitamin B_{12} deficiency is rare** but should be checked for in women with a gastrectomy, Crohn's disease, or ileal resection.

   d. Ethanol consumption may be a contributing factor.

   e. Symptoms and signs of megaloblastic anemia during pregnancy include nausea, vomiting, and anorexia.

   f. Treatment includes a well-balanced diet, oral iron, and folic acid (1 mg per day).

B **Hereditary anemias,** which are characterized by the hemoglobinopathies, result in increases in maternal morbidity and mortality, spontaneous abortion, and perinatal mortality.

1. **Sickle cell anemia** (hemoglobin SS disease; SS disease). This condition occurs when an individual receives the gene for the production of hemoglobin S, an abnormal variant of hemoglobin, from both parents.

   a. The incidence of sickle cell trait in black adults is 1 in 12; therefore, the theoretical incidence of SS disease is 1 in 576 in the United States. The actual incidence in pregnant women is somewhat lower because of the higher mortality rate in individuals with SS disease. Pregnancy poses an increased risk of adverse outcome for both mother and fetus.

   b. Infectious complications, such as pyelonephritis, cholecystitis, pneumonia, and skin infections, are increased in SS disease.

   c. Complications of pregnancy increase. These include:

   (1) Spontaneous abortion

   (2) Preeclampsia

   (3) Preterm labor and delivery

   (4) IUGR

   (5) Unexplained fetal demise

   d. The number of **vaso-occlusive** crises increases in pregnancy. Treatment includes:

   (1) Hydration

   (2) Analgesics

   (3) Oxygen

   (4) Transfusion

   (5) Screening and therapy for infections

   e. Treatment during pregnancy includes:

   (1) Screening and treatment of asymptomatic bacteriuria

   (2) Urine culture every trimester

   (3) Pneumococcal vaccine (recommended)

   (4) Serial ultrasound to assess fetal growth

   (5) Antepartum fetal surveillance

   (6) Folic acid supplementation

   e. Treatment during labor includes:

   (1) Adequate hydration and oxygen to prevent sickling

   (2) Analgesia

   (3) Packed red blood cell transfusion if a cesarean section is considered and the hemoglobin level is very low.

f. Although prophylactic transfusions may decrease the number of vaso-occlusive crises, they do not improve perinatal outcome.

2. **Sickle cell–hemoglobin C disease** (SC disease). Hemoglobin C, like hemoglobin S, results from a change in the sixth position of the β chain and may be seen in patients of West African or Sicilian descent.
   a. The incidence in the United States is 1 in 823 adult African Americans.
   b. This disease is associated with less morbidity than SS disease but still carries an increased risk of pregnancy loss and pregnancy-induced hypertension.
   c. Affected patients may experience pain crises that are marked by splenic sequestration and that can be associated with thrombocytopenia.
   d. Treatment and follow-up are the same as that for patients with SS disease. The resulting anemia may require transfusion; such treatment is uncommon in the nonpregnant state.

3. **Sickle cell–β-thalassemia disease.** This condition has a perinatal mortality and morbidity rate similar to that of SC disease, with somewhat less maternal morbidity and mortality.

4. **Sickle cell trait** is inheritance of the gene for the production of hemoglobin S from one parent and hemoglobin A from the other. This condition occurs in 8.5% of African Americans, and it occurs in individuals of Mediterranean, Caribbean, Latin American, North African, Indian, and Southeast Asian descent.
   a. The anemia in most patients is only mild.
   b. Sickle cell trait does not appear to increase the risk of miscarriage, stillbirth, IUGR, or pregnancy-induced hypertension.
   c. There is an **increased risk for asymptomatic bacteriuria and urinary tract infections.** Therefore, women with the trait should have frequent urine cultures during pregnancy.
   d. Paternal testing may be important because prenatal diagnosis of SS disease is available.

5. **Thalassemias.** The normal adult hemoglobins are A, A_2, and F. Ninety-five percent of adult hemoglobin is hemoglobin A (made by two α-chains and two β-chains). Most individuals also have small amounts of hemoglobin A_2 (two α-chains and two Δ-chains). The remainder is made up of hemoglobin F (two α-chains and two γ-chains). Patients with thalassemias have a **microcytic anemia** that can be found on their screening complete blood count.
   a. **α-Thalassemia.** The α-thalassemias are characterized by a deletion of one or more of the four genes from the α-chain.
      (1) Deletion of one α-gene does not cause anemia.
      (2) Deletion of two genes causes α-thalassemia trait, characterized by mild anemia.
      (3) Deletion of three genes (hemoglobin H) causes moderate anemia; transfusion or splenectomy is rare.
      (4) Deletion of four genes (Bart hemoglobin) causes severe intrauterine anemia with fetal hydrops and death, as well as maternal preeclampsia and postpartum hemorrhage.
   b. **β-Thalassemia.** The β-thalassemias occur because of point mutations in the genes for β-chain production, leading to a decrease in β-chain formation. This decrease leads to a decrease in hemoglobin A production and a relative increase in the percentage of hemoglobin A_2 (more than 4.0%), which is evident on hemoglobin electrophoresis.
      (1) β-thalassemia trait occurs when β-globin production is decreased by 50%, causing a mild anemia with hypochromic microcytosis and occasional hepatosplenomegaly.
      (2) β-thalassemia intermedia occurs when production is decreased by 75%, leading to moderate anemia with occasional need for transfusion, hepatosplenomegaly, and iron overload.
      (3) β-thalassemia major occurs with no production of the β-chain, causing severe anemia, transfusion dependency, iron overload, bone deformities, and death in early adulthood. (Fetuses and newborns with β-thalassemia are not anemic because of the presence of hemoglobin F.)

c. Women with the most severe forms of α- or β-thalassemia do not usually survive until child-bearing age. During pregnancy, women with β-thalassemia intermedia may experience a drop in hemoglobin and hematocrit levels. The red blood cell mass does not expand normally because of deficient hemoglobin production.

(1) Folic acid supplementation is recommended to keep up with the accelerated red blood cell turnover.

(2) Iron therapy is indicated only for patients with demonstrable iron deficiency because of the risk of iron overload and hepatotoxicity.

(3) Pregnancy is well tolerated in patients with α- or β-thalassemia trait.

(4) Paternal testing may be important because **prenatal diagnosis is available.**

V HEART DISEASE

A Incidence of heart disease in pregnancy

1. **Approximately 1% of pregnancies are complicated by maternal heart disease.** Today, fewer women are seen with heart disease because of the decreased incidence of rheumatic fever and rheumatic heart disease. Because of advances in corrective heart surgery, more women with congenital cardiac abnormalities reach childbearing age.

2. Women with severe heart disease are **at greater risk for pregnancy complications:**
   a. Miscarriage
   b. IUGR
   c. Preterm delivery
   d. Intrauterine demise

3. **Maternal mortality** with pregnancy depends on the specific lesion. All women with cardiac disease should seek preconceptual counseling with cardiac and perinatal specialists.
   a. The **highest risk** (maternal mortality as high as 50%) is associated with **pulmonary hypertension,** Marfan syndrome with aortic involvement, complicated coarctation of the aorta, and Eisenmenger syndrome.
   b. The **lowest risk** (less than 1%) is associated corrected tetralogy of Fallot, small atrial and ventricular septal defects, and patent ductus arteriosus.

B Diagnosis of heart disease during pregnancy

1. **Changes associated with normal pregnancy that may place an extra burden on women with heart disease include:**
   a. **Expansion of plasma volume** by as much as 50%
   b. **Increased cardiac output** (30 to 50%)
   c. **Drop in systemic vascular resistance** up to 28 weeks' gestation
   d. **Changes specific to labor**
      (1) Pain, which can increase heart rate and blood pressure
      (2) Shift into the intravascular compartment of as much as 500 mL of plasma with each uterine contraction
      (3) Regional anesthesia, which can decrease cardiac output and blood pressure
      (4) Postpartum increase in blood volume and cardiac output by 10 to 20%. Initially, cardiac output and blood pressure may fall after delivery.

2. **Symptoms of normal pregnancy that can be confused with symptoms of heart disease**
   a. Functional systolic murmurs
   b. Fatigue, dyspnea, and palpitations
   c. Edema, especially in the lower extremities
   d. Enlarged cardiac silhouette on chest radiograph

3. **Signs and symptoms that should lead to suspicion of heart disease**
    a. Progressive limitation of physical activity
    b. Chest pain
    c. Syncope with exertion
    d. Severe dyspnea
    e. Diastolic murmur
    f. Loud systolic murmur
    g. Cyanosis or clubbing
    h. Abnormal heart rhythm on electrocardiography
    i. Abnormal echocardiography

C Management

1. **Preconception**
    a. Counseling about risks
    b. Reviewing current medical regimen

2. **During pregnancy**
    a. Close follow-up with a cardiologist
    b. Frequent maternal echocardiography
    c. Fetal echocardiography at 20 to 22 weeks' gestation (A woman with a congenital cardiac abnormality is at greater risk for having a fetus with a congenital cardiac lesion.)
    d. Careful evaluation of any change in maternal symptoms
    e. Evaluation and treatment for infection and anemia, which could worsen the maternal condition
    f. Anticoagulation, with heparin if appropriate
    g. Hospitalization for signs of deterioration

3. **In labor and postpartum**
    a. Team management, involving cardiology, anesthesiology, and nursing
    b. Invasive monitoring, if necessary
    c. Antibiotic prophylaxis, if necessary
    d. Avoidance of rapid changes in blood pressure and heart rate
    e. **Forceps or vacuum-assisted** delivery in some cases
    f. Continued close observation in the postpartum period

VI   PULMONARY DISEASE

A Physiologic changes associated with pregnancy

1. **Mechanical changes of chest cavity**
    a. Upward displacement of diaphragm (as much as 4 cm)
    b. Increase in transverse diameter of chest (2 cm)
    c. Increase in chest circumference (5 to 7 cm)
    d. Increased diaphragmatic excursion
    e. Increase in subcostal angle

2. **Changes in pulmonary function**
    a. Increased tidal volume (30 to 40%)
    b. Decrease in expiratory reserve
    c. Increase in minute ventilation
    d. Decreased lung volume caused by displacement of diaphragm. (Total lung volume decreases 5%, and residual volume decreases 20%.)
    e. No change in forced expiratory volume in 1 second

B **Dyspnea of pregnancy.**   As many as 70% of pregnant women report dyspnea, and the etiology is not understood.

C **Asthma.**   This condition complicates approximately 1% of all pregnancies and worsens about one third of cases.

1. Pregnancy complications
   a. If asthma is poorly controlled, it may be associated with increased risk of preterm delivery, IUGR, and perinatal morbidity and mortality.
   b. Use of steroids can be associated with increased risk of gestational diabetes and postpartum hemorrhage.

2. Goals of treatment
   a. Reduce the number of flare-ups.
   b. Prevent severe attacks (status asthmaticus; see VI C 4).
   c. Ensure adequate oxygenation.

3. Treatment
   a. **β-agonists,** the primary treatment for acute exacerbations and chronic therapy
      (1) No increase in the incidence of congenital malformations
      (2) Side effects such as tachyphylaxis and arrhythmias
   b. Glucocorticoids
      (1) Inhaled for chronic therapy
      (2) Intravenous and oral therapy for acute exacerbations
      (3) Safe in pregnancy
   c. **Aminophylline,** which has declined in use
      (1) This drug **crosses the placenta** and has no demonstrable effects on the fetus.
      (2) Levels must be adjusted in pregnancy.
      (3) Side effects are common and include:
         (a) Nausea and vomiting
         (b) Tachycardia
         (c) Arrhythmias

4. Status asthmaticus. Provide immediate treatment using the following interventions:
   a. Oxygenation
   b. Hydration
   c. Subcutaneous catecholamines
   d. Intravenous steroids
   e. Nebulized β-agonists
   f. Intubation, if necessary

D **Pneumonia.**   In addition to being life-threatening to the mother when severe, pneumonia is also associated with preterm birth.

1. *Streptococcus pneumoniae*: most common bacterial pathogen
   a. Associated with **smoking**
   b. **Sudden onset** is characteristic. **Signs and symptoms** include:
      (1) Tachypnea
      (2) Fever
      (3) Shaking chills
      (4) Productive cough
      (5) Purulent sputum
   c. **Diagnosis**
      (1) Lobar consolidation on chest radiograph
      (2) Sputum culture and Gram stain
      (3) Blood culture

    d. Treatment

        (1) Hospitalization

        (2) Intravenous penicillin followed by oral penicillin for 10 to 14 days

  2. Other pathogens that cause pneumonia

    a. *Mycoplasma pneumoniae*

        (1) Common in young adults

        (2) Slow onset of symptoms with nonproductive cough

        (3) Clinical diagnosis, with a chest radiograph that reveals patchy infiltrates

        (4) Not responsive to penicillin and should be treated with erythromycin

    b. *Klebsiella pneumoniae* and *Haemophilus influenzae*

        (1) Usually occurs in heavy smokers, alcoholics, and immunocompromised patients

        (2) Requires immediate hospitalization and appropriate antibiotics

    c. Influenza A

        (1) Characterized by sparse sputum production and interstitial infiltrates

        (2) Usually self-limited but can be complicated by secondary bacterial pneumonia

    d. Varicella (chickenpox)

        (1) Has mortality as high as 30%. The risk of pneumonia with primary varicella infection increases in smokers and in pregnant women in the third trimester.

        (2) Requires treatment with intravenous acyclovir. Varicella-zoster immune globulin can be given as prophylaxis to a susceptible woman exposed to the virus.

        (3) The **varicella vaccine** is a live virus and is **contraindicated** in pregnancy.

E **Sarcoidosis.**　The etiology of this granulomatous disease is unknown. Sarcoidosis can affect many organ systems.

  1. Most commonly, affected individuals are 20 to 40 years of age.

  2. The condition is most commonly diagnosed by evidence of **bilateral hilar adenopathy** on routine chest radiography. Definitive diagnosis is made by histology.

  3. Most patients are asymptomatic and require no treatment. If therapy is necessary, glucocorticoids are the primary treatment.

  4. Pregnancy has no long-term side effects. Sarcoidosis does not appear to affect pregnancy outcome adversely. **Most patients improve** as the pregnancy progresses.

  5. In pregnant women, it is necessary to assess renal and hepatic involvement and test pulmonary function.

F **Tuberculosis.**　This condition, which is caused by *Mycobacterium tuberculosis,* is unfortunately becoming more common because of HIV infection and increasing immigration from developing countries. Congenital tuberculosis is rare, and most cases of perinatal infection result from horizontal transmission.

  1. Symptoms

    a. Lethargy

    b. Cough

    c. Dyspnea

    d. Night sweats

  2. Diagnosis

    a. Skin testing with subcutaneous dose of intermediate strength purified protein derivative (PPD)

    b. Chest radiograph

    c. Culture and identification of acid-fast bacilli or fluorescent stain of sputum

  3. Treatment. The risk of adverse outcome in pregnancy does not appear to increase if treatment is adequate. Therapy has become more complex with the emergence of resistant strains of *M. tuberculosis.*

    a. Isoniazid for 9 months: standard therapy
      (1) Side effects: peripheral neuropathy, toxic hepatitis (especially if older than 35 years)
      (2) Prophylactic use in recent PPD converters without active disease
    b. Ethambutol: added for resistant strains
      (1) Safe in pregnancy
      (2) Side effect with higher doses: optic neuritis in the mother
    c. Streptomycin
      (1) Avoid in pregnancy
      (2) Associated with damage to cranial nerve VIII and renal damage in fetus
    d. Rifampin
      (1) Crosses the placenta
      (2) May increase the risk of congenital malformations

VII THROMBOEMBOLIC DISEASE

A Epidemiology and etiology

1. Thromboembolic disease is **the leading cause of death in pregnant and postpartum women.**

2. Thromboembolic disease occurs in 0.02 to 0.3% of pregnant patients and in 0.1 to 1.0% of postpartum patients.

3. Untreated deep vein thrombosis (DVT) in pregnancy causes pulmonary embolism (PE) in as many as 24% of patients.
    a. The mortality rate is 15%.
    b. If patients are treated adequately, the risk of PE is 4.5%, with a risk of mortality of less than 1%.

4. Most cases of thromboembolic disease in pregnancy are associated with a hereditary thrombotic disorder. These disorders may also be associated with an increased risk in adverse second- and third-trimester outcome. The risk of thromboembolic disease increases significantly with the presence of more than one of the following abnormalities:
    a. Factor V Leiden mutation
    b. Prothrombin mutation
    c. Antiphospholipid antibody
    d. Protein C or protein S deficiency
    e. Antithrombin III deficiency
    f. Homocystinemia

B Pathophysiology

1. Pregnancy is a hypercoagulable state. Increased estrogen production is associated with increases in clotting factors.

2. The gravid uterus may cause venous stasis.

C Diagnosis

1. Deep vein thrombosis
    a. Signs and symptoms
      (1) Calf pain
      (2) Palpable cord
      (3) Tenderness
      (4) Unilateral edema of the leg
      (5) Homans sign
      (6) Dilated superficial veins

    b. Real time ultrasonography with duplex and color Doppler ultrasound is the **procedure of choice** to detect proximal DVT. Although it is highly sensitive and specific for femoral and popliteal thrombosis, real time ultrasonography **does not detect pelvic vein thrombosis,** which may be responsible for pulmonary embolism.

    c. Venography. This procedure is considered the gold standard for diagnosis of DVT.

        (1) Radiation is minimal, and the fetus can be protected by abdominal shielding.

        (2) This procedure is invasive and expensive.

    d. ^{125}**I radioisotope scanning** should **not** be used in pregnancy.

    e. Impedance plethysmography is safe, but its sensitivity and specificity have not been well studied in pregnancy.

  2. Pulmonary embolism

    a. Clinical findings

        (1) Tachypnea

        (2) Dyspnea

        (3) Pleuritic pain

        (4) Apprehension

        (5) Cough

        (6) Tachycardia

        (7) Hemoptysis

    b. Arterial blood gas analysis

        (1) A PaO_2 of more than 80 mmHg on room air makes the diagnosis unlikely. If signs and symptoms persist, further evaluation is recommended.

        (2) An increased alveolar-arterial gradient may indicate PE.

    c. Ventilation-perfusion scan

        (1) Most patients with a PE have an abnormal ventilation-perfusion scan (sensitivity, 98%).

        (2) Many patients without emboli also have an abnormal scan (specificity, 10%).

        (3) The degree of abnormality is graded low, intermediate, or high probability, with further intervention and therapy guided by clinical suspicion.

    d. Pulmonary angiogram. This technique is the gold standard for diagnosis of PE.

        (1) It is indicated for anticoagulation failures when caval interruption is considered, to distinguish between recurrent embolization and fragmentation of the original clot.

        (2) It is associated with minimal risk to the fetus.

    e. Spiral computed tomography (CT) scan. This is replacing the angiogram as the gold standard, but it may miss small emboli.

D **Management**

  1. Deep vein thrombosis

    a. Bed rest with extremity elevation

    b. Therapeutic anticoagulation with heparin or low-molecular-weight heparin. Both forms of heparin **do not cross the placenta** and are safe when breastfeeding.

    c. Warfarin is a known **teratogen** and should be avoided in pregnancy. It may be used postpartum, even if the mother is nursing.

  2. Pulmonary embolism

    a. Oxygen to maintain maternal PaO_2 more than 70 mmHg

    b. Bed rest for 5 to 7 days

    c. Therapeutic anticoagulation with heparin until 3 to 6 months postpartum

E **Management of women who have experienced a prior thromboembolic event.** The management of women with a prior history of a DVT or PE is controversial. Evaluation for a hereditary thrombotic abnormality should be pursued, and consideration should be made for prophylactic anticoagulation with either heparin or low-molecular-weight heparin.

VIII SEIZURE DISORDERS

Seizure disorders affect approximately 1% of the population and 1 in 200 pregnancies. Fifteen percent of these cases result from infection, injury, intracranial processes, and metabolic disorders. The remaining 85% are idiopathic (no inciting incident or etiology). Patients with seizure disorders may have reduced fertility.

A Effects of pregnancy on seizure disorders

1. Seizure activity may increase. Increased seizure activity can be controlled with appropriate medication and compliance.
2. Pregnancy can affect medication levels.

B Effects of seizure disorders on pregnancy

1. **Maternal complications.** No increase in the risk of maternal complications usually results.
2. Fetal complications
   a. Increased risk of stillbirth
   b. Decreased birth weight
   c. Increased risk of epilepsy in life
   d. Increased risk of hemorrhagic complications in newborns exposed to anticonvulsants in utero
   e. Increased risk of congenital abnormalities
      (1) Anticonvulsants are associated with increased risk.
         (a) Carbamazepine: neural tube defects, craniofacial defects, and nail hypoplasia
         (b) Phenytoin: microcephaly, dysmorphic facies
         (c) Trimethadione: multiple malformations and mental retardation
         (d) Valproic acid: neural tube defects
      (2) The risk increases with the number of anticonvulsants used in the first trimester.
      (3) It is unclear whether a maternal seizure disorder itself may be a risk factor for fetal anomalies.

C Management of pregnant women with a seizure disorder

1. Preconception
   a. If the patient is seizure-free, consider stopping medications under supervision of a neurologist.
   b. Monotherapy should be used, if possible.
   c. Folic acid supplementation may decrease risk of neural tube abnormalities.
2. During pregnancy
   a. Early ultrasound to establish correct gestational age
   b. Monitoring of medication levels
   c. Compliance with medication regimen
   d. Second-trimester screening for congenital abnormalities, including maternal serum AFP, ultrasound, and fetal echocardiography
   e. Serial ultrasound examinations to check for fetal growth restriction
   f. Vitamin K supplementation late in the third trimester (controversial)

IX Rh ISOIMMUNIZATION

A Definitions

1. **Isoimmunization (sensitization)** is caused by maternal antibody production in response to exposure to red blood cell antigens. If these antibodies are directed against fetal red cell antigens, the antibodies can cross the placenta and cause fetal hemolytic disease.

2. **Rh isoimmunization,** a leading cause of hemolytic disease, specifically refers to antibodies against the Rh group, C, c, E, e, and D (the most commonly encountered). Rh antigens are present on fetal cells by the 38th day postconception.

B **Epidemiology**

1. Approximately 1% of all pregnancies are complicated by red blood cell sensitization. The incidence of Rh isoimmunization in the United States has fallen since the 1960s because of anti-D immune globulin.

2. Fifteen percent of Caucasians, 5 to 8% of African Americans, and 1% of Native Americans and Asians are Rh negative (absence of D antigen).

C **Criteria** (all factors must be present in an Rh-negative pregnant woman)

1. The fetus must be Rh positive.

2. Enough fetal cells must reach the maternal circulation (fetomaternal bleed).

3. The mother must make antibody to D antigen.
   a. Some women are immunogenic nonresponders (as many as 30%).
   b. ABO incompatibility with the fetus can be protective.
   c. The amount of antigen necessary to generate an immune response with anti-D antibody is different for each woman.

D **Prevention of Rh isoimmunization** (anti-D immunoglobulin)

1. Anti-D immunoglobulin can prevent Rh-negative women from mounting an immune response (producing anti-D antibodies) when exposed to Rh-positive (D-positive) blood.

2. A dose of 300 µg of Rh immune globulin (RhoGAM) can protect (prevent immune response) from an exposure of up to 30 mL of fetal blood

3. To prevent immunologic response, the patient must:
   a. Not yet be sensitized to the D antigen
   b. Be given enough immune globulin
   c. Be treated in a timely fashion

4. Treatment of Rh-negative women within 72 hours of delivery decreases immunization to less than 1.5%.

5. Treatment of all Rh-negative women at 28 weeks' gestation further decreases risk of sensitization to less than 0.2%.

6. Other indications for use in pregnant Rh-negative, unsensitized women include:
   a. Abortion (spontaneous or elective)
   b. Ectopic pregnancy
   c. Antepartum bleeding
   d. Abdominal trauma
   e. After amniocentesis or chorionic villus sampling
   f. After external cephalic version

7. Failure to prevent sensitization may occur in the following conditions:
   a. Inadequate dose (maternal exposure to more than 30 mL of fetal Rh-positive blood)
   b. Treatment delay
   c. Previously sensitized patient

E **Management of the Rh-negative, unsensitized pregnant woman**

1. Type and screen at initial visit.

2. Treat with Rh-immune globulin at 28 weeks (it is usual, although not necessary, to confirm that the patient is unsensitized prior to treatment).

3. Treat with Rh-immune globulin after delivery (within 72 hours) if the fetus is Rh-positive.

4. After delivery, check for "excessive" fetomaternal hemorrhage and treat with additional doses of Rh-immune globulin if exposure is greater than 30 mL of fetal Rh-positive blood.

5. The amount of fetal-maternal hemorrhage can be estimated by the **Kleihauer-Betke** test. Treatment of maternal blood with acid elutes the adult hemoglobin from red cells, and only fetal hemoglobin remains. A smear is made and treated with a special stain that detects the red cells with fetal hemoglobin and the **volume of fetal red cells in the maternal circulation can be estimated.**

F **Management of the Rh-negative, sensitized pregnant woman**

1. Accurately assess gestational age with early ultrasound.

2. Determine **paternal blood type.**
   a. If the partner is **Rh-negative, there is no need for further evaluation and intervention.**
   b. If the partner is homozygous for D, the fetus is D-positive.
   c. If the partner is heterozygous for D, the fetus has a 50% chance of being Rh-negative and not at risk for anemia.
   d. In amniocentesis or chorionic villus sampling, DNA analysis can be performed to evaluate whether the fetus is Rh-positive.

3. **Assess prior obstetrical history.**
   a. The risk of hemolytic disease tends to be as severe (or more severe) in subsequent pregnancies.
   b. If the mother had a previous hydropic fetus, the risk that the next Rh-positive fetus will become hydropic is 80%.
   c. Hemolysis and hydropic changes usually develop at earlier gestational ages with each successive pregnancy. In general, the risk of severe fetal hemolysis and hydropic changes in the first sensitized pregnancy is low.

4. **Assess antibody titer.**
   a. In the first sensitized pregnancy, titers should be drawn every 2 to 4 weeks to assess need for amniocentesis. Amniocentesis should be offered when the "critical titer" is reached. In general, the critical titer is 1:16; at that titer, a fetus has been severely anemic. The critical titer is laboratory specific.
   b. In subsequent sensitized pregnancies, antibody titer is not as useful as a guide to the timing of amniocentesis. The patient's history should be used to guide the timing of invasive testing and intervention.

5. **Use amniocentesis** to assess degree of hemolysis and risk for fetal death. Once invasive testing is initiated, further assessment of antibody titers is not indicated.
   a. **Bilirubin in amniotic fluid** is a byproduct of fetal hemolysis.
   b. Bilirubin enters the amniotic fluid from fetal secretions, and the level of bilirubin in amniotic fluid correlates with fetal hemolysis.
   c. **Spectrophotometry** is used to assess the level bilirubin in amniotic fluid.
      (1) Bilirubin causes a shift in optical density away from linearity.
      (2) Shift is greatest at a wavelength of 450 nm.
      (3) Degree of **shift at 450 nm (ΔOD450) is used to estimate degree of hemolysis.**
   d. In the early 1960s, Liley devised a chart based on the natural history of Rh-sensitized pregnancies from **27 to 41 weeks'** gestation. The chart compares gestational age (x axis) versus assessment of ΔOD450 (y axis). Use of the **Liley curve** (Figure 17-1) is associated with less iatrogenic premature delivery for those pregnancies at low risk of severe fetal anemia.
      (1) The chart is divided into three zones (marked by downsloping lines to reflect increased ability of the fetus to metabolize bilirubin with advancing gestational age).
         (a) Zone I is associated with mild anemia or unaffected fetuses.
         (b) Zone II is associated with mild-to-severe anemia.
         (c) Zone III is associated with severe fetal anemia and fetal death within 7 to 10 days.

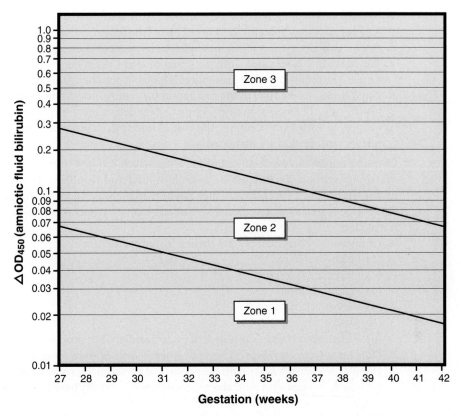

FIGURE 17-1 Liley graph. (From Pritchard JA, MacDonald PC, Gant NF. Williams Obstetrics. 21st Ed. New York: McGraw-Hill, 2001.)

(2) Management of results in upper zone II or zone III includes cordocentesis to assess fetal hemoglobin, fetal transfusion, or delivery (depending on gestational age).

   e. Prior to 27 weeks, assessment of $\Delta OD450$ values is unclear and debatable. Past obstetric history and ultrasound findings may dictate cordocentesis to assess fetal hemoglobin and need for transfusion.

   f. **Amniocentesis** is associated with an **increased risk of sensitization, infection, rupture of membranes, and fetal loss.**

6. **Perform cordocentesis** when it is believed that the fetus is at risk for severe anemia.

   a. This technique should be performed with a 22-gauge spinal needle under ultrasound guidance.

   b. This technique may be performed along any portion of umbilical cord, preferably in the umbilical vein (if transfusion is planned).

   c. The initial sample should assess fetal hemoglobin and hematocrit, platelet count, reticulocyte count, and blood type.

   d. Transfusion should occur if fetal hematocrit is less than 30%.

7. If necessary, **perform fetal transfusion** either **intraperitoneally or intravascularly** (through fetal umbilical vein). Intravascular transfusion instantly increases fetal hematocrit, whereas intraperitoneal transfusion requires the fetus to absorb transfused blood through the lymphatic system (severely anemic or hydropic fetuses may due so very poorly). The goal is to raise fetal hematocrit.

   a. Donor cells are matched with the mother and fetus (if available from prior cordocentesis).

   b. Donor cells are buffy-coat poor, washed irradiated, filtered, and resuspended in normal saline to a hematocrit of 70 to 75%.

    c. Nomograms exist to determine the amount to be transfused at one time based on donor and fetal hematocrit and on the gestational age of the fetus.

    d. Once transfusion is complete, the final fetal hematocrit is assessed.

    e. The procedure is repeated until the gestational age when the risks of prematurity are minimized. The timing of repeat procedures is based on fetal hematocrit and usually occurs within 2 to 3 weeks. At the time of the first repeat procedure, initial fetal hematocrit can help identify the rate of hemoglobin degradation to help determine the time of future procedures.

    f. Compared with amniocentesis, the **risk** of infection, rupture of membranes, fetal loss, and further sensitization are **increased.**

8. Consider noninvasive assessment of the fetus, which can be extremely useful in helping guide initial intervention. Techniques include ultrasound and Doppler velocimetry. Although these modalities are still investigational, they can be extremely useful for guiding timing of initial cordocentesis, especially at gestational ages of less than 27 weeks, when assessment of $\Delta OD450$ is not as clear.

    a. Ultrasound. Assessment of fetal anemia includes evidence of:

        (1) Polyhydramnios

        (2) Placental thickening

        (3) Pleural effusions

        (4) Pericardial effusions

        (5) Ascites

        (6) Increased liver size (suggestive of extramedullary hematopoiesis)

    b. Doppler velocimetry. Not all severely anemic fetuses show evidence of hydropic changes. Doppler assessment is based on the premise that fetal anemia is associated with abnormal vascular flow. Fetuses with mild and moderate anemia usually have flow velocities in the normal range.

        (1) Assess for increased peak velocity in the fetal middle cerebellar artery.

        (2) Abnormal velocities in fetal aorta, inferior vena cava, or umbilical vein.

G **Management of maternal sensitization for other antigens.** In addition to the D antigen, red cells have hundreds of other antigens. The frequencies of these antigens depend on the population; fortunately, antibodies to many of these antigens do not place the fetus at risk for severe hemolytic disease. Other antigens that can pose a risk to the fetus by maternal antibody production include the other antigens in the Rh locus (c, C, e, and E), Kell, and Duffy. When a pregnant woman is sensitized to these antigens, the pregnancy is usually managed as outlined above for anti-D.

Study Questions for Chapter 17

Directions: *Each of the numbered items or incomplete statements in this section is followed by answers or by completions of the statement. Select the ONE lettered answer or completion that is BEST in each case.*

1. A 24-year-old primigravid who just discovered via a home pregnancy kit that she is pregnant is seeing you for her first prenatal visit. After confirming her pregnancy, you take a complete history and perform a physical examination. She has had type 2 diabetes for 6 years now and has been on oral medications for blood sugar control. Her capillary blood glucose level is 110 mg/dL today. After delivery, her newborn will be at risk for

- [A] Elevated blood glucose
- [B] Low hematocrit
- [C] Low calcium
- [D] Elevated potassium
- [E] Low bilirubin

2. A 22-year-old woman, gravida 2, para 0 at 22 weeks of gestation presents to you for routine prenatal care. She has been seeing you throughout her pregnancy. You review her chart and notice that she had diabetes prior to becoming pregnant and was taking an oral hypoglycemic agent to control her blood sugars. Today, she reports lower back discomfort. Her fundus measures 21 cm and she has 1+ glucose on urine dipstick. She has been self-administering daily regular and NPH (neutral protamine Hagedorn's) insulin. Her average fasting blood sugar is 93 mg/dL, and her 2-hour post-prandial sugar is 119 mg/dL. What is the next best step in management of this patient?

- [A] Adjust her insulin
- [B] Measure maternal serum AFP
- [C] Perform fetal ultrasound
- [D] Perform fetal echocardiograph
- [E] Perform magnetic resonance imaging (MRI) of the spine

3. A 28-year-old woman, gravida 2, para 1 at 20 weeks of gestation who has increased levels of total T_4, total T_3, and free T_4 is seeing you prior to her next scheduled prenatal visit because she has been sweating frequently and has palpitations. Her fundus measures 17 cm. Her vitals are as follows: T = 98.8, BP = 115/80, P = 132, R = 16. What is the initial step in management of this patient's problems?

- [A] Propranolol
- [B] Methimazole
- [C] Propylthiouracil
- [D] Potassium iodide
- [E] Fetal ultrasound

4. An 18-year-old woman, gravida 3, para 2 at 28 weeks of gestation has been hospitalized because she presented with right-sided back pain, fever, chills, and severe nausea. Her physical examination was remarkable for bilateral costovertebral angle tenderness, with greater discomfort on the right side. Her temperature on admissions was 102.6°F, and the results of her CBC and Chem-7 were unremarkable. However, her urinalysis was significantly abnormal. Her urine culture is still pending. She has been in the hospital for the last 3 days on intravenous antibiotics; however, despite initial improvement, her temperature is now 103°F. What is the next best step in management?

- [A] Repeat urine culture
- [B] Repeat CBC
- [C] Change antibiotics

    D Perform an ultrasound

    E Perform an intravenous pyelogram (IVP)

5. A 20-year-old woman who just delivered a viable male neonate was recently involved in a car accident where she was a restrained passenger. She was at 38 weeks of gestation when she arrived at the emergency department. She was "cleared" by the trauma and orthopedic teams and sent to the labor and delivery floor. There she began having vaginal bleeding and then went into labor spontaneously. The estimated blood loss with delivery was 900 mL, and now she is stable. After obtaining her prenatal information you realize she is Rh negative and antibody D negative. You immediately give her one shot of Rh immune globulin. What is the next best step in management?

    A Perform a CBC

    B Transfuse packed red blood cells

    C Perform a Kleihauer-Betke test

    D Give additional Rh immune globulin

    E Assess neonatal Rh antigen status

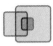

Answers and Explanations

1. The answer is C [I B 2]. A diabetic woman is at higher risk for delivering a baby with respiratory distress, hypoglycemia (low glucose), hypocalcemia (low calcium), polycythemia (high hematocrit), and hyperbilirubinemia (high bilirubin). Potassium levels are usually not affected.

2. The answer is D [I C 3 b]. Women with preexisting diabetes are at higher risk for congenital anomalies, especially cardiac anomalies such as ventricular septal defect and situs inversus. Thus, a fetal echocardiograph should be performed, and the best time to perform one is between 20 and 22 weeks of gestation. Her insulin does not need to be changed because she is below the goals for fasting and 2-hour blood glucose levels. Maternal serum AFP is useful only during weeks 15 through 20. Fetal ultrasound should have already been performed if this is a patient you have been seeing throughout her pregnancy (the optimal time to perform a fetal ultrasound is between 16 weeks and 20 weeks of gestation). The MRI of the maternal spine is unnecessary for her back discomfort, which is a common problem during pregnancy. Further evaluation of her back would be needed if more information in the clinical scenario made you suspicious of a more significant problem.

3. The answer is A [II B 4 a 3]. This patient has hyperthyroidism based on her elevated free T_4 levels. Therefore, β-blockers are the initial treatment of choice for her symptoms of tachycardia and occasional palpitations. For this patient, propylthiouracil is also necessary to maintain her free T4 levels near high-normal; however, PTU is not the initial treatment to control her symptoms. Methimazole is not used often because if is associated with aplasia cutis and the alternative agent, PTU, is safer. Potassium iodide is one of the agents used to treat a thyroid storm. A fetal ultrasound would be appropriate given the disparity between the gestational age and the fundal height. However, an ultrasound is not the initial step, nor is it a step that will solve this patient's problems.

4. The answer is D [III D 5 d]. The clinical scenario presented is that of pyelonephritis that is not responding to treatment. This finding should always prompt radiologic evaluation to rule out an abscess or a renal calculi. The least invasive initial procedure is a renal ultrasound, not an intravenous pyelogram. There is no need to repeat the urine culture or to change her antibiotics until results of her initial urine culture and sensitivity returns. Repeating CBC is fine, but it will not tell you why there is lack of response to treatment.

5. The answer is E [IX D 3]. In the management of an Rh-negative, unsensitized (i.e., antibody-negative) patient, you should know the Rh antigen status of the baby. If the baby is Rh negative, then there is no need for Rh immune globulin because the maternal immune system would not form any antibodies directed toward fetal red blood cells. Had the baby been Rh positive, the next step would be to quantitate the amount of fetomaternal blood transfusion by performing a Kleihauer-Betke test. Then, based on those results, you may give additional Rh immune globulin. A CBC or transfusion is not necessary in this scenario because this patient stopped bleeding and is "stable." A CBC or capillary hemoglobin concentration test is appropriate during the first postpartum day for all postpartum patients.

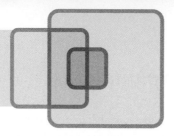

chapter 18

Gestational Trophoblastic Disease

CHRISTINA BANDERA

I   INTRODUCTION

Gestational trophoblastic disease (GTD) is the general term for a spectrum of proliferative abnormalities originating from the trophoblast of the placenta.

A   Classification (Table 18-1)

1. **Hydatidiform mole.** Benign GTD is also referred to as a hydatidiform mole, or more commonly a "**molar pregnancy.**" It is characterized by abnormal proliferation of the placental trophoblastic cells. These abnormal cells distend the uterus and secrete the polypeptide hormone **human chorionic gonadotropin (hCG)**, mimicking a normal pregnancy. Hydatidiform moles may be **complete (classic)** or **partial (incomplete).**

2. **Gestational trophoblastic tumor (GTT).** This malignant form of GTD, which arises from the trophoblastic elements of the developing blastocyst, retains the invasive tendencies of the normal placenta and remains able to secrete hCG. GTT can be either **metastatic** or **nonmetastatic.**

B   Incidence

1. **Hydatidiform mole.** Benign GTD occurs in 1 of 1500 pregnancies in the United States and in as many as 1 of 125 pregnancies in other parts of eastern Asia.
   a. **Complete moles** are the most commonly identified type of molar pregnancy. They are 5 to 10 times more common in pregnancies in women older than 40 years of age. Dietary factors, such as low intake of vitamin A and animal fat intake, are associated with this condition.
   b. **Partial moles** are associated with oral contraceptive use and irregular menses.

2. **GTT.** Malignant GTD is identified in 1 of 20,000 pregnancies in the United States and can occur after any type of pregnancy.
   a. Hydatidiform mole precedes GTT in 50% of cases.
   b. Normal pregnancy precedes GTT in 25% of cases.
   c. Abortion or ectopic pregnancy precedes GTT in 25% of cases.

II   HYDATIDIFORM MOLE (Table 18-2)

A   Complete mole

1. **Origin.** In 90% of cases, an "**empty**" ovum containing no genomic DNA is fertilized by one **sperm,** which duplicates its DNA, leading to an abnormal 46,XX karyotype. In the remaining 10% of cases, the "empty" ovum is fertilized by two sperm, resulting in an abnormal 46,XX or 46,XY karyotype. In a complete mole, all the **chromosomes are paternally derived** (Fig. 18-1).

TABLE 18-1   Clinical Classification of Gestational Trophoblastic Disease

Hydatidiform mole (molar pregnancy)
    Complete, or classic
    Incomplete, or partial
Gestational trophoblastic neoplasia
    Nonmetastatic
    Metastatic
        Low risk (good prognosis)
        High risk (poor prognosis)

TABLE 18-2   Comparison of Complete and Partial Mole

Feature	Complete Mole	Partial Mole
Age	Greater risk (5–10×) >40 years	Not age-related
Karyotype	90% XX, 10%XY	XXX or XXY
	All chromosomes paternally derived	1 chromosome set maternal; 2 chromosome sets paternal
Fetus	Absent	Present
hCG	Often >100,000 mIU/mL	Rarely elevated above normal levels for pregnancy
Primary symptom	Bleeding	Bleeding
Secondary symptoms	Large uterine size for gestational age	Rare
	Hyperemesis	
	Theca lutein cysts	
	Preeclampsia	
	Hyperthyroidism	
Risk of persistence (GTT)	20%	4%

Adapted from Lu KH, Goldstein DP, Bernstein MR, Berkowitz RS. Managing molar pregnancy. O G B Management 1999,11:67–76.
hCG, human chorionic gonadotropin; GTT, gestational trophoblastic tumor.

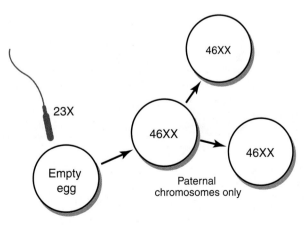

FIGURE 18-1   Chromosomal origin of a diploid complete hydatidiform mole. (Adapted from Kurman RJ. Blaustein's Pathology of the Female Genital Tract. 4th Ed. New York: Springer-Verlag, 1994:1051.)

2. Histologic features
   a. Marked edema and enlargement of the villi
   b. Disappearance of the villous blood vessels
   c. Proliferation of the trophoblastic lining of the villi
   d. Absence of fetus, cord, or amniotic membrane
3. Clinical features
   a. **Abnormal uterine bleeding** is the most common presenting symptom in the first trimester of pregnancy.
   b. **"Classic symptoms"** occurring later in pregnancy include heavy bleeding, uterine size greater than expected for gestational age, and lack of fetal heart tones. Additional classic symptoms that probably arise from stimulation by excessive hCG are hyperemesis gravidarum (nausea and vomiting), **theca lutein cysts** within the ovaries, preeclampsia, and hyperthyroidism. *(tachycar*
   c. A **diagnosis of complete molar pregnancy** rather than miscarriage is suspected when the **hCG level is greater than 100,000 mIU/mL** and when **ultrasound reveals vesicles** within the uterus. Pathologic correlation and cytogenetic analysis for DNA content confirm the diagnosis.

Snowstorm app?
on Ultrasound

B Partial or incomplete mole

1. **Origin.** A partial mole (see Table 18-2) is a normal ovum that is fertilized by two sperm. The resulting karyotype is 69,XXX or 69,XXY (Fig. 18-2).
2. **Histologic features**
   a. Marked swelling of the villi with **atrophic trophoblastic cells**
   b. Presence of normal villi
   c. Presence of an **umbilical cord, amniotic membrane, and fetus** that is usually not viable and has features of a triploid gestation
3. **Clinical features**
   a. **Abnormal uterine bleeding** is the most common presenting symptom in the first trimester of a pregnancy, as with complete moles.

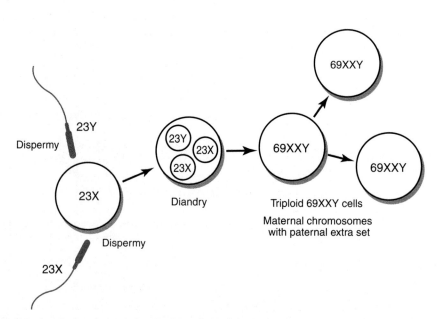

FIGURE 18-2 Chromosomal origin of a triploid partial hydatidiform mole. (Adapted from Kurman RJ. Blaustein's Pathology of the Female Genital Tract. 4th Ed. New York: Springer-Verlag, 1994:1052.)

b. Excessive vaginal bleeding, hyperemesis, preeclampsia, hyperthyroidism, and ovarian cysts are rare.

c. hCG is generally **not significantly elevated,** and ultrasound may show a fetus as well as hydropic villi. Pathologic correlation and cytogenetic analysis for DNA content confirms the diagnosis.

d. Many spontaneous abortions may represent undiagnosed partial moles.

e. Case reports indicate that normal pregnancies coincident with partial moles have proceeded to term without adverse sequelae.

C Management of molar pregnancies (complete and partial)

1. **Diagnostic studies**
   a. **Laboratory tests** include a complete blood count with platelets, quantitative hCG, coagulation studies, type and screen, baseline renal function and liver function studies, and thyroid function tests.
   b. **Imaging studies** include chest radiograph and ultrasound.

2. **Dilation and suction curettage** of the uterus is the primary tool for evacuating a molar pregnancy even when the uterus has enlarged beyond the size expected for a pregnancy of 20 weeks.
   a. **Intravenous oxytocin** should be given to enhance uterine involution after the procedure to minimize blood loss.
   b. **Respiratory distress** resulting from fluid overload, emboli of trophoblastic tissue, and thyroid storm may occur in as many as 2% of patients in the perioperative period.
   c. Even large **theca lutein cysts** of the ovaries associated with molar gestation resolve as hCG levels drop. These cysts are not an indication for surgical intervention.

3. The **risk of developing GTT** after evacuation is 20% for a complete mole and 4% for a partial mole. **High-risk factors** associated with persistent disease include pretreatment hCG greater than 100,000 mIU/mL, theca lutein cysts greater than 6 cm, age older than 40 years, and previous molar pregnancy.

4. **Hysterectomy** is a treatment option for patients who do not desire future fertility.

D Follow-up of a molar pregnancy.
After evacuation, the expected average time to complete elimination of hCG is 9 to 11 weeks. This period depends on the initial level of hCG, the amount of viable trophoblastic tissue remaining after evacuation, and the half-life of hCG. Follow-up of a molar pregnancy should include:

1. **Determinations of hCG** made at 48 hours postevacuation, then weekly until the results are negative for 3 consecutive weeks, then every month for 6 months, and then yearly. An increase or plateau in hCG indicates the development of **GTT** and necessitates the initiation of chemotherapy.

2. **Physical examination,** including a pelvic examination, at regular intervals until remission to ensure adequate involution of pelvic organs.

3. **Birth control** (recommended for 1 year). Oral contraceptives or medroxyprogesterone (Depo-Provera) injections are recommended.

4. **Prophylactic chemotherapy is rarely recommended.** Most patients with molar pregnancies are cured with evacuation and do not require any therapy. Serial hCG determinations identify patients who develop GTT (20% of complete moles and 4% of partial moles). The toxicity from prophylactic chemotherapy can be severe, even leading to death.

E Future fertility

1. **Normal pregnancy** is the most likely result of future gestations.

2. **Risk of a second molar pregnancy** is 1%; risk of a third molar pregnancy is 33%; and risk of a fourth molar pregnancy is 100%. Subsequent molar pregnancies may be complete or partial, regardless of the type of initial molar pregnancy.

| **III** | **GESTATIONAL TROPHOBLASTIC TUMOR** |

A **Characteristics.** The occurrence of GTT (Table 18-3) after a molar pregnancy may have the **histologic appearance of a mole or choriocarcinoma.** After a normal pregnancy, abortion, or ectopic pregnancy, GTT always has the appearance of **choriocarcinoma,** or occasionally the aggressive **placental site trophoblastic tumor** variant of choriocarcinoma.

1. **Nonmetastatic GTT (persistent or invasive mole)** is molar tissue that invades the uterine wall, produces persistent hCG elevation, and potentially causes bleeding. It is confined to the uterus and is the most common form of GTT.

2. **Metastatic disease** (disease outside the uterus) may be found most commonly in the vagina and lung but may also affect the gastrointestinal (GI) system, liver, and brain. Patients have various symptoms, such as **vaginal bleeding (vaginal metastasis), hemoptysis (pulmonary metastases),** or **neurologic symptoms (brain metastases).** The disease is often associated with hemorrhage because of the propensity of trophoblastic tissue to invade vessels.

B **Diagnosis**

1. **After evacuation of a molar pregnancy,** GTT is diagnosed when there hCG increases, the value of hCG reaches a plateau for 3 weeks, or metastatic disease is identified.

2. Weeks or years **after an abortion or ectopic pregnancy,** elevated hCG may indicate GTT or another pregnancy.

C **Management**

1. **Workup of patients with GTT** should include the following:
   a. Complete history and physical examination
   b. Pretreatment hCG titer, hematologic survey, serum chemistries, and liver function studies
   c. Pelvic ultrasound
   d. Computed tomography (CT) scan of the abdomen and pelvis
   e. Chest radiograph or chest CT
   f. CT or magnetic resonance imaging of the brain in high-risk patients

2. **Nonmetastatic GTT is almost 100% curable.**
   a. **Single-agent chemotherapy** cures more than 90% of patients. Hysterectomy may be offered to decrease the number of treatments required for the patient who does not desire future fertility.
      (1) **Methotrexate** is the most commonly used treatment agent. This **antimetabolite** inhibits purine synthesis by blocking the dihydrofolate reductase enzyme required to process folic acid. This results in arrested synthesis of DNA, RNA, and proteins.
         (a) **Common side effects** include ulcerations of the mouth and GI tract mucosa, as well as nausea. **Less common side effects,** seen when multiple or high doses are used, include myelosuppression, hepatotoxicity, nephrotoxicity, alopecia, and pneumonitis.

TABLE 18-3 Classification of Gestational Trophoblastic Neoplasia

Nonmetastatic: disease confined to the uterus
Metastatic: disease spread outside the uterus

Good prognosis (low risk)	Poor prognosis (high risk)
Short duration: disease present <4 months	Long duration: disease present >4 months
Pretreatment hCG titer: <40,000 mIU/mL	Pretreatment hCG titer: >40,000 mIU/mL
No previous chemotherapy	Brain or liver metastases
	Failure of previous chemotherapy
	Disease after term pregnancy

hCG, human chorionic gonadotropin.

> **(b) Leucovorin** is folinic acid and is administered 24 hours after methotrexate treatment to rescue normal cells from methotrexate toxicity.

(2) Actinomycin D is an antibiotic that intercalates DNA strands. It is also effective single-agent treatment for nonmetastatic GTT.

(3) Failure of single-agent treatment is rare. Most patients are still curable by switching to another agent or switching to a multidrug regimen.

b. Follow-up

(1) hCG titers should be followed carefully.

(2) Contraception, preferably with oral contraceptives or medroxyprogesterone (Depo-Provera), should be used for at least 1 year.

3. Metastatic GTT

a. Good-prognosis metastatic GTT

(1) The following factors are associated with a **good prognosis:**

(a) Short duration (less than 4 months)

(b) Low pretreatment hCG titer (less than 40,000 mIU/mL)

(c) No metastatic spread to the brain or liver

(d) No previous chemotherapy

(2) Single-agent chemotherapy with methotrexate or actinomycin D can be used to treat good-prognosis metastatic GTT. However, more courses of chemotherapy are usually required, and alternative therapy is needed more frequently.

(3) Follow-up is similar to that for nonmetastatic GTT (see III C 2 b).

b. Poor-prognosis metastatic GTT

(1) The following factors are **associated with a poor prognosis:**

(a) Long duration (more than 4 months)

(b) High pretreatment hCG titer (more than 40,000 mIU/mL)

(c) Liver or brain metastases

(d) Failure of previous chemotherapy

(e) Disease after a term pregnancy

(2) Treatment

(a) Affected patients are treated with **multiagent chemotherapy** such as EMA-CO (Etoposide, Methotrexate, Actinomycin D, Cyclophosphamide, and vincristine [Oncovin]) and a multiple modality approach (i.e., chemotherapy, surgery, and radiation).

(b) High-risk patients should be treated in centers that have a special interest and expertise in this disease, especially when life-threatening toxicity from therapy is a factor.

(c) The survival rate is approximately 80%.

(d) Hysterectomy usually does not improve the outcome.

(3) Follow-up

(a) Three additional courses of chemotherapy after a negative hCG titer

(b) Monitoring of hCG levels (similar to that for nonmetastatic GTT)

(c) Contraception for at least 1 year after negative levels of hCG

D Recurrence rates

1. Nonmetastatic GTT: 1%

2. Good-prognosis metastatic GTT: 5%

3. Poor-prognosis metastatic GTT: up to 20%

E Future fertility. Fertility after chemotherapy for GTT is usually retained. Women who choose to become pregnant should be monitored carefully. A normal intrauterine pregnancy should be documented in the first trimester, the placenta should be histologically evaluated after delivery, and hCG titers should be followed to zero postpartum.

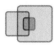

Study Questions for Chapter 18

Directions: *Each of the numbered items or incomplete statements in this section is followed by answers or by completions of the statement. Select the ONE lettered answer or completion that is BEST in each case.*

QUESTIONS 1 AND 2 ARE BASED ON THE CLINICAL SCENARIO DESCRIBED BELOW.

A 24-year-old woman, gravida 1, para 0 at 24 weeks of gestation by her last menstrual period presents to the emergency department because of vaginal bleeding. Her vitals are as follows: T = 97.8, BP = 135/88, P = 105, R = 16. Her fundus is below the umbilicus. On speculum examination you see blood emerging from an undilated external os, but no lesions are seen on the cervix or the vaginal walls. Her quantitative hCG level is 85,000 mIU/mL. You are awaiting a formal ultrasound by a radiologist.

1. What is the most likely explanation for this scenario?
   - A. Maternal 0 + Paternal Y (which duplicates)
   - B. Maternal 0 + Paternal X (which duplicates)
   - C. Maternal Y + Paternal X (which duplicates)
   - D. Maternal X + Paternal X + Paternal X
   - E. Maternal X + Paternal Y + Paternal Y

2. Which of the following findings is the most likely on pelvic ultrasound examination?
   - A. A fetus with biparietal diameter consistent with 22 weeks
   - B. Two-vessel umbilical cord
   - C. Two separate placentas
   - D. Left ovary 6 cm and right ovary 3 cm
   - E. Left ovary 6 cm and right ovary 6cm

3. A 33-year-old gravida 4, para 3 at 16 weeks of gestation by her last menstrual period presents to labor and delivery complaining of vaginal bleeding. Her vital signs are as follows: T = 98.9, BP = 150/94, P = 103. Fundal height measures 23 cm. A pelvic ultrasound examination reveals a uterus with a diffuse indistinct mass, and no fetal parts are seen. A dilatation and suction curettage is performed and 10 minutes afterwards she is placed on a dilute intravenous oxytocin drip. Complications involving which of the following organs are most likely to occur at this time?
   - A. Liver
   - B. Kidney
   - C. Vagina
   - D. Lung
   - E. Brain

4. A 27-year-old nulliparous woman presents to the emergency room reporting hemoptysis. She has no medical history other than a pregnancy 3 months ago that resulted in spontaneous abortion (SAB). She also has had intermittent vaginal spotting since the miscarriage. Her BP = 110/70 and P = 88. Significant labs are hemoglobin = 9.6 mg/dL and quantitative β-hCG = 35,000 mIU/mL. Her chest radiograph shows several masses in the right middle lobe. Which of the following is the best treatment option for her?

A Dilation and curettage
B Hysterectomy
C Methotrexate and leucovorin
D Actinomycin D
E Methotrexate, Actinomycin D, and etoposide

5. A 36-year-old multiparous woman just underwent a hysterectomy because of a molar pregnancy. Other than her treatment for gestational trophoblastic disease, she has no medical problems. She had an appendectomy 3 years ago. She is allergic to penicillin and, although she does not smoke, she admits to drinking at least 3 to 4 alcoholic beverages per day. You obtain a β-hCG 2 days after the operation. What is the next best step in management of this patient?

A β-hCG in 1 week
B β-hCG in 1 month
C Methotrexate
D Levonorgestrel plus ethinyl estradiol
E Chest radiograph in 1 month

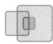

Answers and Explanations

1. The answer is D [I B 1] 2. **The answer is B** [I B 2 c]. The clinical scenario is consistent with a partial or incomplete mole because the uterus is smaller than dates (uterus below umbilicus is less than 20 weeks) and an hCG level lower than 100,000 mIU/mL. In a partial mole, the ovum is normal and thus contributes only one of its chromosomes. The normal ovum is fertilized by two sperm (each with one sex chromosome). The result is a triploid fetus (69 chromosomes) that usually has the karyotype XXX. Also, a partial mole will have an umbilical cord (two or three vessel), an amniotic membrane, and a fetus. The ovaries usually are not enlarged because the hCG levels are not high. Furthermore, even in a complete mole where theca lutein cysts form, the ovaries are usually equally enlarged. Two separate placentas suggest twins.

3. The answer is D [II C 2 b]. After a dilatation and suction curettage of the uterus after a molar pregnancy (especially when there is delay in the inception of oxytocin infusion), respiratory distress is a possible complication. The lungs can be injured because of embolic events from trophoblastic tissue at time of D&C, from fluid overload, or as a result of thyroid storm.

4. The answer is C [III C 3 a 2]. This patient has metastatic disease (lung metastasis) with a good prognosis (β-hCG less than 40,000 mIU/mL, no brain or liver metastasis, last pregnancy not normal [spontaneous abortion], disease occurred less than 4 months from the last pregnancy, and no previous chemotherapy). Thus, the best treatment for her is single-agent chemotherapy; usually, methotrexate is the first choice. Note: Leucovorin is not considered multiagent chemotherapy because it is folic acid added to methotrexate to rescue normal cells from methotrexate toxicity. There is no regimen that consists of only methotrexate, Actinomycin D, and etoposide.

5. The answer is A [II D]. The most important step after treatment of a molar pregnancy is to ensure that the patient does not get pregnant within the next year because it would confound follow-up with hCG levels. Had the patient not had a hysterectomy, the next step would be to place her on birth control pills (levonorgestrel plus ethinyl estradiol). Because this patient has had the 48 hour "postevacuation" hCG levels, the next step is to do a weekly hCG until the results are negative three times, then every month for 6 months, and then annually.

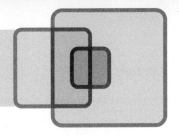

chapter 19

The Menstrual Cycle

PETER J. CHEN

I INTRODUCTION

The menstrual cycle is characterized by the regular occurrence of ovulation throughout a woman's reproductive life. The development of predictable, regular cyclic, and spontaneous ovulatory menstrual cycles is regulated by complex interactions of the hypothalamic-pituitary axis, the ovaries, and the genital tract. The menstrual cycle is divided into two phases: the follicular (or proliferative) phase and the luteal (or secretory) phase.

A Length of the cycle

1. The **mean duration** of the cycle is **28 days,** plus or minus 7 days.
   a. **Polymenorrhea** is defined as menstrual cycles that occur at short intervals (less than 21 days).
   b. **Oligomenorrhea** is defined as menstrual cycles that occur at long intervals (more than 35 days).
2. Menstrual cycles are the most irregular during the 2 years after menarche (i.e., the first menses) and during the 3 years before menopause. At both times, **anovulation** (i.e., absent ovulation) is most common.

B Follicular or proliferative phase.
This phase lasts from the first day of menses until ovulation, during which time the **endometrial glands** proliferate under the influence of **estrogen,** primarily **estradiol.** The follicular phase is characterized by:

1. Variable length
2. Low basal body temperature
3. Development of ovarian follicles
4. Vascular growth of the endometrium
5. Secretion of estrogen from the ovary

C Luteal or secretory phase.
The second part of the cycle extends from ovulation until the onset of menses. Under the influence of progesterone, the endometrial glands develop the secretory status necessary for implantation of the embryo. The luteal phase is characterized by:

1. A fairly constant duration of 12 to 16 days
2. An elevated basal body temperature (higher than 98°F)
3. The formation of the **corpus luteum** in the ovary, with the secretion of progesterone and estrogen
4. An endometrium that reveals gland tortuosity and secretion, stromal edema, and a decidual reaction

D Cycle integration.
The integration of the menstrual cycle involves the interaction among **gonadotropin-releasing hormone** (GnRH), the **gonadotropins** (i.e., follicle-stimulating hormone [FSH] and [LH]), and the **sex steroids** (i.e., androstenedione, estradiol, estrone, and progesterone).

II GONADOTROPIN-RELEASING HORMONE

GnRH is the hypothalamic hormone that controls gonadotropin release.

A Characteristics
1. This hormone, a decapeptide, is produced by hypothalamic neurons, principally from the arcuate nucleus, and is transported along axons that terminate in the median eminence around capillaries of the primary portal plexus.
2. It is secreted into the portal circulation, which carries it to the anterior lobe of the pituitary gland.

B Secretion
1. Gonadotropin-releasing hormone is secreted in a **pulsatile manner;** the amplitude and frequency of the secretions vary throughout the cycle.
   a. One pulse every hour is typical of the follicular phase.
   b. One pulse every 2 to 3 hours is typical of the luteal phase.
2. The **amplitude and frequency** are regulated by:
   a. Feedback of estrogen and progesterone
   b. Neurotransmitters within the brain, mainly the catecholamines dopamine (inhibitory) and norepinephrine (facilitatory)

C Action of GnRH on gonadotropin production
1. When GnRH binds to specific receptors on the surface membrane of target cells, it:
   a. Activates a second messenger, **adenyl cyclase**
   b. Changes the concentration of **cyclic adenosine monophosphate (cAMP)**
2. This stimulates the synthesis and storage of both FSH and LH from the same cell.
3. Gonadotropin-releasing hormone activates and moves gonadotropins from the reserve pool to a pool ready for secretion, which leads to their immediate release.
4. High, prolonged GnRH exposure saturates the GnRH receptors and inhibits FSH and LH secretion. This is desensitization or **downregulation.**

III GONADOTROPINS: FOLLICLE-STIMULATING HORMONE AND LUTEINIZING HORMONE

A Follicle-stimulating hormone receptors exist primarily on the granulosa cell membrane.
1. Follicle-stimulating hormone acts primarily on the granulosa cells, where it stimulates follicular growth.
2. It stimulates formation of LH receptors.
3. It activates the aromatase and 3-hydroxysteroid dehydrogenase enzymes.
4. It stimulates follicular growth by increasing both FSH and LH receptors in granulosa cells. The estradiol produced by the granulosa cells enhances this action.

B Luteinizing hormone receptors exist on theca cells at all stages of the cycle and on granulosa cells after the follicle matures under the influence of FSH and estradiol.
1. Luteinizing hormone stimulates **androgen synthesis** by the theca cells.
2. With a sufficient number of LH receptors on the granulosa cells, LH acts directly on the granulosa cells to cause **luteinization** (i.e., the formation of the corpus luteum) and the production of progesterone.

C Two-cell hypothesis of estrogen production (Fig. 19-1)
1. Luteinizing hormone acts on the theca cells to produce androgens (i.e., androstenedione and testosterone).

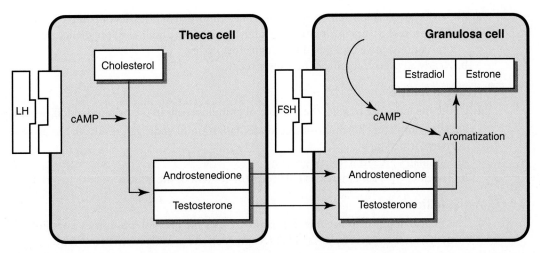

FIGURE 19-1 Two-cell hypothesis of estrogen production. cAMP, cyclic adenosine monophosphate; FSH, follicle-stimulating hormone; LH, luteinizing hormone. (Reprinted with permission from Speroff L, Glass RH, Kase NG. Regulation of the menstrual cycle. In Speroff L, Glass RH, Kase NG, eds. Clinical Gynecologic Endocrinology and Infertility. 4th Ed. Baltimore: Williams & Wilkins, 1999:207.)

2. Androgens are transported from the theca cells to the granulosa cells.

3. Androgens are aromatized to estrogens (i.e., estradiol and estrone) by the action of FSH on the enzyme aromatase in the granulosa cells.

IV OOGENESIS

A Primordial follicle

1. The primordial follicle is covered by a single layer of granulosa cells (Fig. 19-2).

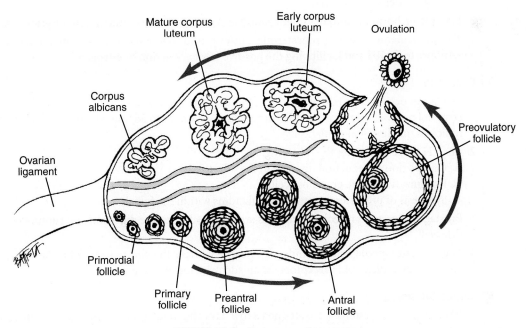

FIGURE 19-2 The process of oogenesis.

2. Even without gonadotropin stimulation, some primordial follicles develop into preantral follicles.
    a. This process occurs during times of anovulation (i.e., childhood, pregnancy, and periods of oral contraceptive use) and during ovulatory cycles.
    b. Nearly all preantral follicles become atretic.

B | Preantral follicle

1. Under the influence of FSH, the number of granulosa cells in the primordial follicle increases.
2. Follicle-stimulating hormone–induced aromatization of androgen results in the production of **estrogen**, which then:
    a. Stimulates preantral follicle growth
    b. Together with FSH increases FSH receptor content of the follicle

C | Antral follicle

1. The follicle destined to become dominant secretes the greatest amount of estradiol, which, in turn, increases the density of the FSH receptors on the granulosa cell membrane.
2. Rising estradiol levels result in negative feedback and suppression of FSH release; this halts the development of other follicles, which then become atretic.
3. The follicular rise of estradiol exerts a positive feedback on LH secretion.
    a. LH levels rise steadily during the late follicular phase.
    b. LH stimulates androgen production in the theca.
    c. The dominant follicle uses the androgen as substrate and further accelerates estrogen output.
4. FSH induces the appearance of LH receptors on granulosa cells.
5. Follicular response to the gonadotropins is modulated by a variety of growth factors.
6. Inhibin, secreted by the granulosa cells in response to FSH, directly suppresses pituitary FSH secretion.

D | Preovulatory follicle

1. Estrogens rise rapidly, reaching a peak approximately 24 to 36 hours before ovulation.
2. Luteinizing hormone increases steadily until midcycle, when there is a surge, which is accompanied by a lesser surge of FSH.
3. Luteinizing hormone initiates luteinization and progesterone production in the granulosa layer.
4. The preovulatory rise in progesterone causes a midcycle FSH surge by enhancing pituitary response to GnRH and facilitating the positive feedback action of estrogen.

E | Ovulation (Fig. 19-3)

1. Ovulation occurs approximately 10 to 12 hours after the LH peak and 24 to 36 hours after the estradiol peak. The **onset of the LH surge,** which occurs 34 to 36 hours before ovulation, reliably indicates the timing of ovulation.
2. The **LH surge** stimulates the following:
    a. Completion of reduction division in the oocyte
    b. Luteinization of the granulosa cells
    c. Synthesis of progesterone and prostaglandins within the follicle
3. Prostaglandins and proteolytic enzymes are responsible for the digestion and rupture of the follicle wall.
4. The progesterone-dependent midcycle rise in FSH frees the oocyte from follicular attachments and ensures sufficient LH receptors for an adequate luteal phase.

F | Corpus luteum

1. Peak levels of progesterone are attained 8 to 9 days after ovulation, which approximates the time of implantation of the embryo.

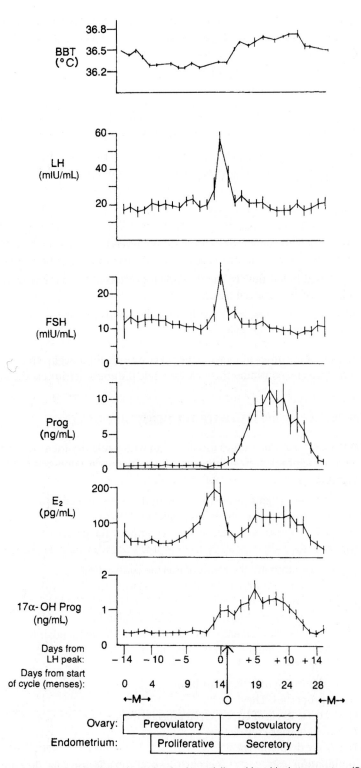

FIGURE 19-3 Hormonal (ovarian and pituitary), uterine (endometrial), and basal body temperature (BBT) correlates of the normal menstrual cycle. Mean plasma concentrations (±SEM) of luteinizing hormone (LH), follicle-stimulating hormone (FSH), progesterone (Prog), estradiol (E₂) [day +1], and 17 α-hydroxyprogesterone (17 α-OH Prog) are shown as a function of time. Ovulation occurs on day 15 (day +1) after the LH surge, which occurs at midcycle on day 14 (day 0). M, menses; 0, ovulation. (Adapted from Thorneycroft IA, Mishell DR Jr, Stone SC, et al. The relation of serum 17-hydroxyprogesterone and estradiol 17-β levels during the human menstrual cycle. Am J Obstet Gynecol 1971, 111:947–951.)

2. Normal luteal function requires optimal preovulatory follicular development.
   a. Suppression of FSH during the follicular phase is associated with:
      (1) Low preovulatory estradiol levels
      (2) Depressed midluteal progesterone production
      (3) Small luteal cell mass
   b. The accumulation of LH receptors during the follicular phase sets the stage for the extent of luteinization and the functional capacity of the corpus luteum.
   c. A defective luteal phase can contribute to both infertility and early pregnancy wastage.

3. In early pregnancy, human chorionic gonadotropin maintains luteal function, with secretion of progesterone, until placental steroidogenesis (production of progesterone) is established.

V MENSTRUATION

A In the absence of a pregnancy, decreasing steroid levels lead to increased coiling and constriction of the spiral arteries, which supply the upper two thirds of the functional endometrium.

1. The decreased blood flow to the functional portion of the endometrium causes **ischemia** and degradation of endometrial tissue.

2. The bleeding, or **menses,** is the result of the degraded endometrial tissue, which is desquamated, or shed, into the uterine cavity.

B Within 2 days of the onset of menses, the surface epithelium begins to regenerate under the influence of estrogen and continues this process while the endometrium is shedding.

VI CLINICAL PROBLEMS ASSOCIATED WITH THE MENSTRUAL CYCLE

A **Dysmenorrhea.** Painful menses usually begin with ovulatory menstrual periods and are the most common medical problem in young women. Dysmenorrhea does not occur in anovulatory cycles.

1. Clinical aspects
   a. Dysmenorrhea begins just before or with the onset of menses and lasts 24 to 48 hours.
   b. The pain is suprapubic, sharp, and colicky.
   c. Nausea, diarrhea, and headache may accompany the pain.

2. Physiology
   a. Menstrual cramps are the result of **uterine contractions.**
   b. **Prostaglandins** are potent **stimulators** of uterine contractions.
      (1) Endometrial prostaglandins are produced during the luteal phase. If ovulation does not occur, there is no luteal increase in prostaglandins.
      (2) In the first-day menstrual endometrium, the prostaglandin level increases until it is several times higher than its concentration in the luteal phase.

3. Management
   a. **Prostaglandin synthetase inhibitors** (e.g., nonsteroidal anti-inflammatory drugs) have certain properties. They:
      (1) Decrease levels of endometrial prostaglandin
      (2) Lessen uterine contractions
      (3) Relieve dysmenorrhea
   b. **Combination** (estrogen plus progestin) **oral contraceptive agents** eliminate ovulation.
      (1) Estrogen followed by progesterone (in ovulatory cycles) is necessary to produce high menstrual levels of prostaglandin in the endometrium.
      (2) Combination oral contraceptives prevent dysmenorrhea by eliminating the natural estrogen-progesterone progression found only in ovulatory cycles.

B **Premenstrual syndrome**

1. **Definition.** Premenstrual syndrome (PMS) is a group of disorders and symptoms related to the menstrual cycle that include **premenstrual dysphoric disorder (PDD)**. Symptoms must be:
   a. Cyclic
   b. Sufficiently severe to interfere with some aspects of life
   c. Have a consistent and predictable relationship to the menstrual cycle

2. **Epidemiology**
   a. Eighty percent of women report premenstrual symptoms, and 5 to 10% of women experience PMS that is severe enough to interfere with normal activities, such as work, study, parenting, or relationships.
   b. As many as 50 to 60% of women with severe PMS have an underlying psychiatric disorder.

3. **Etiology**
   a. The causes of PMS are not completely understood but involve fluctuation of ovarian steroids, central nervous system neurotransmitters, genetic predisposition, and psychosocial expectations.
   b. Causal factors include estrogen, progesterone, testosterone, and neurosteroids.
      (1) Symptoms are temporally associated with luteal phase fluctuations in ovarian hormones. Serum levels of estrogen and progesterone are not diagnostic or predictive of PMS.
      (2) Cyclic ovarian hormone fluctuations are associated with changes in brain neurotransmitters and neurosteroids. Changes in brain chemistry may result in PMS symptoms in biologically susceptible women.

4. **Clinical manifestations.** The most commonly occurring symptoms of PMS are:
   a. Bloating or weight gain
   b. Breast tenderness
   c. Anxiety
   d. Irritability
   e. Food cravings or changes in appetite
   f. Poor concentration
   g. Sleep disturbances
   h. Depressive symptoms or dysphoria
   i. Affective lability
   j. Feeling overwhelmed

5. **Management** (based on the guidelines of the American College of Obstetricians and Gynecologists). Both the physiologic and the psychosocial aspects of PMS must be considered when designing a therapeutic program. Most treatments for PMS are aimed at alleviating symptoms. They include:
   a. **Lifestyle changes** (i.e., regular exercise and a balanced diet)
   b. **Calcium supplementation**
   c. **Oral contraceptives** for physical symptoms. These should not be used if mood symptoms are primary.
   d. **Long-acting GnRH agonists.** These agents should be limited to short-term use because of long-term effects of hypoestrogenism and the resultant osteoporosis.
   e. **Fluoxetine,** a serotonin reuptake inhibitor. This agent can help relieve symptoms of PMS when it is taken continuously throughout the menstrual cycle.
   f. **Alprazolam,** a benzodiazepine that acts on the γ-aminobutyric acid receptor complex. This agent has been reported to be beneficial. Because of the addictive potential of alprazolam, it should be reserved for patients who can be monitored reliably and should be restricted to the luteal phase of the menstrual cycle.

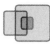

Study Questions for Chapter 19

Directions: Each of the numbered items or incomplete statements in this section is followed by answers or by completions of the statement. Select the ONE lettered answer or completion that is BEST in each case.

1. A 24-year-old woman, gravida 1, para 1 is seeing you because every month since age 19 she has had severe lower pelvic pain during her periods. She says the pain is similar to "labor pains" and it interferes with her ability to concentrate at work and during leisure activities on the weekends. Her pain has also caused her to become extremely anxious and irritable. She denies having a depressed mood or changes in sleep, energy, or eating patterns. Her past medical history is remarkable for mild asthma controlled with albuterol. She is sexually active, is in a monogamous relationship, and uses condoms for contraception. She has no known drug allergies but admits to drinking a few alcoholic beverages every day. The best next step for this woman is

- [A] Ibuprofen
- [B] Norgestimate plus ethinyl estradiol
- [C] Fluoxetine
- [D] Calcium
- [E] Leuprolide

2. Two female medical students are having a discussion about ovarian reserve. Medical student #1 claims that because women are born with a finite number of follicles and because she has been taking birth control pills since age 16, she has slowed down loss of her follicles every month by inhibiting ovulation. Medical student #2 claims that because she has been pregnant more times than medical student #1, she has a higher ovarian follicle reserve. Which of the following statements is true?

- [A] Medical student #1 has slowed down depletion of her eggs
- [B] Medical student #2 has slowed down depletion of her eggs
- [C] Medical student #1 has higher ovarian reserve than medical student #2
- [D] Both students have slowed down depletion of their eggs
- [E] There is no way to slow down depletion of eggs

3. Hormone X is secreted before ovulation and is responsible for enhancement of pituitary response to GnRH and facilitation of the positive feedback action of estrogen. Hormone X causes midcycle surge in hormone Y, which also frees the oocyte from its follicular attachments. What are hormones X and Y, respectively?

- [A] Estrogen and LH
- [B] Estrogen and FSH
- [C] Progesterone and LH
- [D] Progesterone and FSH
- [E] Prostaglandin and LH

4. Many infertility patients undergo in vitro fertilization (IVF) and embryo transfer (ET) in order to become pregnant. IVF-ET uses many of the principles of the normal menstrual cycle to achieve pregnancy. The patient begins taking one birth control pill (BCP) per day starting on a chosen Sunday for 2 weeks to regulate her cycle. On the 10th day of BCP, she also begins to take hormone Y for the next 20 days so that the hypothalamic-pituitary axis is "shut off," and the cycle is completely under the control of the physician. On the 11th day of hormone Y, hormone XX is added to promote development of several ovarian follicles. On the final day of hormone Y, another hormone, hCG (an LH analogue) is given

to induce ovulation so that the patient's eggs can be harvested and fertilized in the laboratory. The name of hormone Y is

- [A] Ethinyl estradiol
- [B] Progesterone derivative
- [C] FSH
- [D] Luteinizing hormone
- [E] Leuprolide (GnRH analogue)

Answers and Explanations

1. The answer is B [VI A 3 b]. The clinical scenario presented here is describing dysmenorrhea (pain only during menses) and not premenstrual syndrome. The best treatment for this woman would be birth control pills (norgestimate plus ethinyl estradiol), which would not only treat her dysmenorrhea, but would also allow her have intercourse without using condoms if she wishes. However, use of birth control pills alone does not protect her against sexually transmitted diseases. NSAIDs, such as ibuprofen, are also useful. The other choices mentioned are useful for premenstrual syndrome, not dysmenorrheal.

2. The answer is E [IV A 2 a]. Even without gonadotropin (LH and FSH) stimulation, several primordial follicles develop into preantral follicles (which undergo atresia automatically). Pregnancy and oral contraception (i.e., anovulation) do not stop this process. Therefore, women lose a certain number of their follicles every month whether they ovulate or not.

3. The answer is D [IV D 4 and IV E 4]. The onset of LH initiates luteinization and progesterone production by the granulosa layer. The rise in progesterone is responsible for the midcycle FSH surge, which enhances pituitary response to GnRH, facilitates positive feedback action of estrogen, frees the oocyte from follicular attachments, and ensures sufficient LH receptors for an adequate luteal phase.

4. The answer is E [II C 4]. Leuprolide is a GnRH analogue (i.e., has the same effects as GnRH). When GnRH is given for prolonged periods (20 days), it saturates the GnRH receptors and inhibits FSH and LH secretion (in essence it "shuts off" the anterior pituitary). Hormone XX represents FSH, which is given to stimulate the granulosa cells and to promote development of several follicles simultaneously without interference from signals sent by the pituitary.

chapter 20

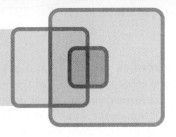

Amenorrhea

MELISSA ESPOSITO AND KURT BARNHART

I INTRODUCTION

A **Definitions.** Amenorrhea is the absence of menses for 6 months or longer and can be primary or secondary.

1. **Primary amenorrhea** is the absence of menses by 14 years of age in girls without appropriate development of secondary sexual characteristics or by 16 years of age regardless of secondary sex characteristic development.

2. **Secondary amenorrhea** is the cessation of menses for a period of 6 months or a three-cycle interval in women who have been menstruating regularly (most common presentation). Amenorrhea, or anovulatory cycles, is common in pregnancy, during the 5 to 7 years after menarche, and in women approaching menopause.

B **Normal menstrual cycle physiology**

1. Pulsatile gonadotropin-releasing hormone (GnRH) secretion stimulates secretion of follicle-stimulating hormone (FSH) and luteinizing hormone (LH) from the anterior pituitary.

2. FSH stimulates ovarian follicular growth and development.

3. Androgens produced in theca cells are converted to estrogens in granulosa cells (aromatase enzyme).

4. Increasing estradiol levels exert negative feedback on FSH, and the follicle with the most FSH receptors becomes dominant. Other follicles undergo atresia.

5. Increasing levels of estradiol exert positive feedback on LH secretion from the pituitary. Shortly after LH levels peak, ovulation occurs.

6. Granulosa cells produce progesterone during the luteal phase, and if pregnancy is not established, the corpus luteum regresses and menses ensue.

C **Normal menstruation: anatomic requirements**

1. Nonobstructed outflow tract

2. Appropriately primed endometrium

3. Ovaries that are able to respond to FSH and LH

4. Secretion of FSH and LH under the stimulation of GnRH, which is essential to ensure adequate development of a dominant follicle each month

II CLASSIFICATION AND ETIOLOGY

A **Categories**

1. **Hypergonadotropic:** FSH more than 20 IU/l; LH more than 40 IU/l

2. **Hypogonadotropic:** FSH and LH less than 5 IU/l

3. **Eugonadotropic:** FSH and LH 5 to 20 IU/l

B **Hypergonadotropic amenorrhea** commonly, but not always, results from a chromosomal anomaly. The most common genotype is 45,XO. Mosaicism (45,X/46,XX) may be seen, and structural aberrations of the X chromosome, including deletions of the short (p) or long (q) arms, isochromosomes, or ring chromosomes may occur. For patients with Y-bearing cell lines, gonadectomy should be performed to decrease the risk of future malignancy (e.g., dysgerminoma, gonadoblastoma, and choriocarcinoma). Menopause and premature ovarian failure also manifest as hypergonadotropic amenorrhea.

1. Turner syndrome
   a. The most common genotype is 45,XO. Mosaicism (45,X/46,XX), with existence of functional tissue, may also occur.
   b. Phenotypic characteristics include short stature, webbed neck, shield chest, and increased carrying angle at the elbow. It is essential to rule out cardiovascular and renal anomalies in suspected cases.
   c. Other developmental characteristics include spontaneous puberty (10 to 20% of cases) and spontaneous menses (2 to 5% of cases).

2. Premature ovarian failure
   a. This condition is defined as ovarian failure before 40 years of age.
   b. Causes include:
      (1) Genetic (45X; 45,X/46,XX; 47,XXY)
      (2) Autoimmune disease. If coexisting autoimmune disease is present, it is necessary to obtain the following laboratory studies: calcium, phosphorous, thyroid-stimulating hormone (TSH), free thyroxine (T_4), AM cortisol, antinuclear antibody, thyroid antibodies, fasting glucose, rheumatoid factor, complete blood count (CBC), and erythrocyte sedimentation rate (ESR).
      (3) Infectious (e.g., mumps)
      (4) Chemotherapy or radiation therapy

3. Gonadal dysgenesis (XY genotype, Swyer syndrome)
   a. The genotype is XY, and the phenotype is female.
   b. Symptoms and signs include lack of sexual development, a normal female testosterone level, and a palpable müllerian system.

4. Gonadal agenesis: development into prepubertal female

5. Resistant ovary syndrome
   a. This condition represents amenorrhea with normal growth and development.
   b. Signs include absent or defective gonadotropin receptors or a postreceptor signaling defect and unstimulated ovarian follicles.

6. Perimenopause
   a. This condition is marked by cycle irregularity that occurs during the 2 to 8 years preceding menopause.
   b. Etiology involves elevated FSH secondary to decreased inhibin levels.

7. Galactosemia
   a. This condition is an autosomal recessive deficiency in galactose-1-phosphate uridyltransferase activity.
   b. Decreased numbers of oogonia secondary to the toxic effects of galactose metabolites are characteristic.

8. Enzyme deficiencies
   a. 17 α-Hydroxylase deficiency
      (1) The ovaries and adrenal glands are affected.
      (2) Presenting signs include absent secondary sex characteristics, hypertension, hypokalemia, and elevated progesterone levels.
   b. Decreased aromatase enzymes

C **Hypogonadotropic amenorrhea** is usually a result of a deficiency in GnRH pulsatile secretion from the hypothalamus. It is a diagnosis of exclusion after pituitary tumors have been evaluated and ruled out. Hypogonadotropic amenorrhea may be secondary to stress, less-than-normal weight, or an eating disorder. Stress leads to an increased output of corticotropin-releasing hormone, which subsequently results in decreased GnRH pulsatile secretion and thus decreased secretion of FSH and LH.

1. **Anorexia**
   a. Anorexia occurs in 1% of all young women. It may identify a dysfunctional family unit.
   b. Signs and symptoms include amenorrhea, bradycardia, dry skin, hypothermia, lanugo hair, constipation, and edema. Bulimia (binging and purging with vomiting, laxatives, or diuretics) may be seen in 50% of patients.
   c. Laboratory markers include decreased FSH, LH, and triiodothyronine (T_3); increased cortisol and reverse T_3 and normal prolactin levels; TSH; and T_4.

2. **Exercise.** Important influential factors include the critical level of body fat and stress.
   a. Body fat
      (1) About 17% is necessary for initiating menarche.
      (2) About 22% is necessary for maintaining menstrual regularity.
   b. Hypothalamic suppression
   c. Laboratory results associated with acute exercise
      (1) Decreased FSH and LH
      (2) Increased prolactin, growth hormone, testosterone, adrenocorticotropic hormone (ACTH), adrenal steroids, and endorphins

3. **Kallmann syndrome**
   a. Deficient secretion of GnRH is associated anosmia or hyposmia. Kallmann syndrome involves the failure of olfactory axonal and GnRH neuronal migration from the olfactory placode in the nose.
   b. Inheritance is either X-linked, autosomal dominant, or autosomal recessive.
   c. Symptoms and signs include primary amenorrhea, normal karyotype, infantile sexual development, and the inability to perceive odors.
   d. Possible coexisting features include bone and renal anomalies, cleft lip and palate, color blindness, or hearing deficit.

4. **Postpill amenorrhea**
   a. Amenorrhea may occur 6 or more months after patients stop taking oral contraceptive pills or 12 months after they stop taking medroxyprogesterone (Depo-Provera).
   b. Workup of patients with suspected postpill amenorrhea should be pursued.

5. **Medications or drugs**
   a. Birth control pills may cause amenorrhea.
   b. Drugs such as phenothiazine derivatives, reserpine, and ganglia blockers likely interfere with the levels of dopamine and norepinephrine; these agents are also associated with galactorrhea.

6. **Pituitary diseases.** Evaluation of the sella turcica using magnetic resonance imaging (MRI) with gadolinium or radiography is necessary. Pituitary tumors may be associated with visual changes; galactorrhea; and other hormone deficiencies, including hypothyroidism, amenorrhea, and Addison disease.
   a. Craniopharyngioma
      (1) Calcifications may be apparent on radiography of the sella turcica.
      (2) Frequent manifestations include visual field defects and blurry vision.
   b. Adenomas
      (1) These tumors vary in size.
         (a) Microadenomas (less than 10 mm)
         (b) Macroadenomas (more than 10 mm)

(2) The most common are prolactinomas and nonfunctioning tumors.

(a) Elevated prolactin levels cause amenorrhea by suppressing GnRH secretion.

(b) Treatment may involve dopamine agonist therapy, surgery, or, in severe cases, radiation therapy.

D **Eugonadotropic amenorrhea** is a subgroup of amenorrhea that includes disorders of androgen excess and of the outflow tract or uterus.

1. **Disorders of androgen excess: polycystic ovary syndrome**

   a. The triad of anovulation, or oligo-ovulation, obesity, and hirsutism (androgen excess), is characteristic.

   b. Tonically elevated LH and low normal FSH result in the following events:

   (1) Prevention of dominant follicle emergence

   (2) Absence of ovulatory cycles

   (3) Elevated levels of androgens produced from the theca cells

   c. Sex hormone–binding globulin levels are decreased because of elevated levels of androgens.

   d. Patients are at increased risk of endometrial hyperplasia secondary to higher levels of free estrogens, primarily estrone (a weakly active estrogen).

   e. Evidence suggests that these patients are hyperinsulinemic; as such, they are at increased risk for diabetes mellitus, obesity, and cardiovascular disease. They must be observed closely throughout their lives.

   f. A loss of only 5 to 10% of body weight may help patients reestablish ovulatory cycles.

2. **Disorders of the outflow tract or uterus**

   a. Müllerian agenesis (also known as Mayer-Rokitansky-Küster-Hauser syndrome)

   (1) The most common congenital anomaly of the uterus, müllerian agenesis occurs in 1 in 4000 births.

   (2) The underlying mechanism involves unwanted exposure to anti-müllerian hormone activity with failed fusion of the müllerian ducts.

   (3) Absence or hypoplasia of the vagina, uterus, and tubes is characteristic. Thirty-three percent of patients may have urinary tract abnormalities, and another 12% may have skeletal anomalies.

   (4) A karyotype should be obtained.

   b. Androgen insensitivity (also known as testicular feminization)

   (1) Inheritance is X-linked recessive.

   (2) Patients have male gonads, a normal male karyotype with normal male levels of testosterone, and elevated LH.

   (3) The defect is in the androgen receptor. Affected patients have androgen receptors and male levels of testosterone, but the receptors cannot respond to androgen.

   (4) Patients have a blind vaginal canal and an absent uterus. (The condition should be suspected in a female with bilateral inguinal hernias.)

   (5) Primary amenorrhea, absent uterus, and normal growth and development are evident. Unlike patients with müllerian agenesis, these patients have an absence of body hair. Breasts are usually small, and the testes are not capable of spermatogenesis.

   (6) This condition is one of the only cases in which gonadectomy may be deferred until after puberty because the incidence of malignant transformation is low.

   c. Asherman syndrome

   (1) Intrauterine scarring, usually a result of vigorous curettage during a hypoestrogenic state (e.g., postpartum curettage for retained products of conception) may occur. However, it may be secondary to other uterine surgical procedures or intrauterine infection.

   (2) Cyclic pain and bloating, with absent or scant menses, may also occur.

   (3) A high degree of suspicion, with appropriate history, should be maintained.

d. Infection. Tuberculosis and schistosomiasis may cause amenorrhea, usually secondary to intrauterine scarring and adhesions.

III CLINICAL EVALUATION (Fig. 20-1)

A History

1. Review pediatric growth and development charts.
2. Take a careful and comprehensive menstrual history.
3. Inquire about childhood or chronic illnesses and medication use.
4. Ask about sexual history and use of illegal drugs.
5. Ask about eating habits, exercise patterns, and self-image concerns.
6. Perform a detailed review of systems, checking for the following conditions:
   a. Hyperprolactinemia: galactorrhea and amenorrhea
   b. Hyperthyroidism: nervousness, heart palpitations, weight loss, and heat intolerance
   c. Hypothyroidism: fatigue, weight gain, and cold intolerance
   d. Hypothalamic dysfunction or tumor: visual changes or hearing loss
   e. Outlet obstruction: cyclic pain or bloating
   f. Ovarian follicle depletion or dysfunction: vasomotor symptoms

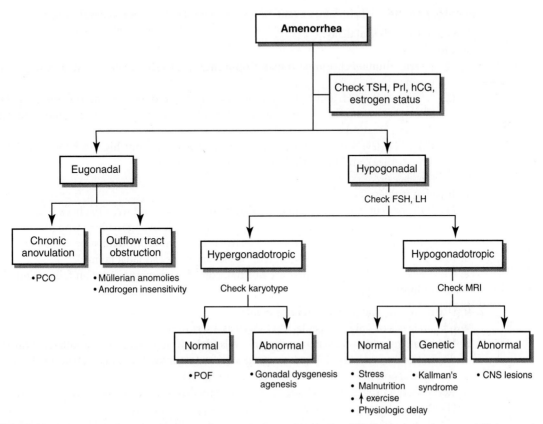

FIGURE 20-1 Clinical evaluation of amenorrhea. CNS, central nervous system; FSH, follicle-stimulating hormone; hCG, human chorionic gonadotropin; LH, luteinizing hormone; MRI, magnetic resonance imaging; PCO, polycystic ovary syndrome; POF, premature ovary failure; TSH, thyroid-stimulating hormone.

g. Hyperandrogenic states: hirsutism or signs of virilization (e.g., clitoromegaly, deepening voice, and increased muscle mass)

B **Physical examination**

1. Determine height and weight, calculate the body mass index, assess body habitus, and take vital signs (Cushing disease or steroid use).

2. Check for cachexia, hypotension, hypothermia, or bradycardia (anorexia).

3. Palpate thyroid gland.

4. Assess visual fields and cranial nerves, and perform a funduscopic examination (Kallmann syndrome or pituitary tumor).

5. Use the Tanner staging of breast and pubic hair development to assess galactorrhea or androgen excess.

6. Perform an abdominal examination to check for masses (e.g., pregnancy or ovarian masses).

7. Examine the genitals and perianal area. (Clitoromegaly may signify androgen excess.)

8. Check for Turner stigmata (e.g., short stature, webbed neck, or shield chest).

9. Perform a pelvic examination.
   a. Check for normal anatomic structures (i.e., presence of vagina and uterus).
   b. Rule out ovarian masses. If pelvic examination is not sufficient, pelvic ultrasound or a rectoabdominal examination may be necessary.

C **Laboratory studies.** Laboratory evaluation may be guided by pubertal development.

1. If patient has **pubertal delay:**
   a. Blood work
      (1) A serum human chorionic gonadotropin (hCG) level should be obtained. Always suspect pregnancy.
      (2) A CBC, ESR, TSH, and T_4 (to test for anorexia, thyroid disease, and inflammatory bowel disease) should be obtained, as well as electrolytes, liver function tests, blood urea nitrogen, and creatinine.
      (3) FSH, LH (levels low in hypogonadotropic amenorrhea but high in hypergonadotropic amenorrhea), and prolactin levels are also necessary.
   b. Urinalysis
   c. Imaging studies
      (1) If the patient is short, obtain a radiograph of the hand and wrist to check bone age.
      (2) Use MRI imaging in patients with hypogonadotropic hypogonadism who otherwise have a normal workup. Cranial masses, destruction, or infiltration must be ruled out.
   d. Karyotype. If FSH and LH are elevated, check karyotype (gonadal failure).
   e. Chromosomes. If chromosomes are normal, consider premature ovarian failure and obtain an autoimmune panel.

2. **If patient has normal puberty development:**
   a. Obtain levels of TSH and prolactin, as well as a serum hCG.
   b. If the patient is hirsute, check androgen levels (dehydroepiandrosterone sulfate, androstenedione, testosterone, and 17-hydroxyprogesterone [a marker for congenital adrenal hyperplasia, which should be checked in the follicular phase]).
   c. Administer a progesterone challenge test. Give medroxyprogesterone acetate for 10 days.
      (1) If a bleed ensues, then the endometrium is appropriately stimulated.
      (2) If no bleed ensues, a disorder of the uterus or outflow tract should be considered.
      (3) Obtain FSH and LH measurements once a hypoestrogenic state has been diagnosed.
      (4) Obtain a pelvic ultrasound to check for normal anatomic structures.

IV MANAGEMENT

A **Hypergonadotropic amenorrhea**

1. **Hormone replacement therapy.** This treatment aims to prevent development of bone loss, vasomotor symptoms, urogenital atrophy, and cardiovascular disease.
   a. **Estrogen replacement therapy**
      (1) Conjugated estrogens or estradiol may be used.
      (2) Estrogen therapy is appropriate for women without a uterus; unopposed estrogen therapy in women with a uterus may lead to endometrial hyperplasia or cancer.
      (3) Administration is daily.
   b. **Combined hormone replacement therapy**
      (1) Agents
         (a) Conjugated estrogens or estradiol in combination with medroxyprogesterone acetate or a 19-nortestosterone derivative may be used.
         (b) Oral contraceptive pills may be used in women who do not desire pregnancy (patients with hypergonadotropic amenorrhea may have transient ovarian function).
      (2) Combined hormone therapy is appropriate for women with a uterus to protect against endometrial hyperplasia or cancer.
      (3) Administration is cyclic or continuous (younger patients are usually treated with the cyclic regimen to establish monthly bleeding).

2. **Removal of Y-containing gonads**
   a. In women with a Y-containing gonad, gonadectomy should be performed to prevent increased transformation into malignant tissue (e.g., gonadoblastoma, dysgerminoma, yolk sac tumor, or choriocarcinoma).
   b. The gonad should be removed as soon as it is detected, except in the case of androgen insensitivity, where gonadectomy should occur after completion of puberty.

3. **Pregnancy.** Although it is unlikely (but not impossible) that these women will become pregnant with their own oocytes, oocyte donation is a viable option for these patients. The ultimate success rate depends on the age of the donor (younger age generally means healthier oocytes).

B **Hypogonadotropic amenorrhea.** The mainstay of therapy is hormone replacement. In the case of intracranial tumors or adenomas, medical or surgical measures may be necessary.

1. **Hormone replacement therapy (IV A 1 a–b)**
   a. Therapeutic hormones are essential in cases of anorexia or exercise-induced amenorrhea where gonadotropin and estradiol levels are excessively low.
   b. Oral contraceptives are a good option. Patients are protected against unwanted pregnancy and obtain the benefits of hormone therapy.

2. **Pregnancy.** Patients who want to become pregnant may be given injectable recombinant gonadotropins combined with either intrauterine insemination or in vitro fertilization. They may receive treatment with the GnRH pump; this option is less popular because it is difficult to use and maintain.

3. **Pituitary tumors**
   a. Asymptomatic nonfunctioning adenoma
      (1) Close surveillance is usually sufficient.
      (2) Treatment with surgery is necessary with symptom occurrence or growth of the adenoma.
   b. Prolactinoma (microadenoma or macroadenoma)
      (1) Medical therapy with a dopamine agonist (bromocriptine) or surgery is appropriate if prolactin levels are high and symptoms bothersome.
      (2) In rare cases, surgery may be combined with radiation therapy. Usually, the symptoms can be well controlled

    c. Craniopharyngiomas and other central nervous system tumors are usually amenable to surgical resection.

    4. Hypothyroidism. Hypothyroidism is easily treated with T_4 replacement, which reestablishes ovulatory cycles.

C **Eugonadotropic amenorrhea.** Treatment of disorders of androgen synthesis involves managing the symptoms primarily. The occurrence of a congenital anomaly of the outflow tract usually requires surgery.

    1. Disorders of androgen synthesis (e.g., polycystic ovary syndrome)
      a. Oral contraceptive pills are useful for anovulatory or oligo-ovulatory patients.
        (1) The progestin component suppresses endogenously elevated LH levels, thereby decreasing androgen overproduction.
        (2) The estrogen component of the pill increases the sex hormone–binding globulin level, thereby decreasing the amounts of free estrogens and androgens.
        (3) The pills also provide contraception.
      b. Cyclic progestins are useful for patients who cannot tolerate or who have contraindications to oral contraceptives.
        (1) Cyclic progestins reestablish monthly bleeding, thereby protecting the endometrium against hyperplasia or cancer.
        (2) Administration is for at least 10 to 12 days each month for maximal endometrial protection.

    2. Treatment of related infertility
      a. Clomiphene. Ovulation induction is used to establish ovulatory cycles.
        (1) The drug may be used with timed intercourse or intrauterine insemination for up to six ovulatory cycles.
        (2) In cases of clomiphene resistance, insulin-sensitizing medications may be used concomitantly, often improving the response to the drug.
        (3) In hyperandrogenic women who respond poorly to clomiphene, some experts advocate the use of dexamethasone at bedtime to decrease the endogenous androgen levels.
        (4) If patients do not respond to clomiphene or dexamethasone, injectable recombinant gonadotropin medications are often used, either in combination with intrauterine insemination or in vitro fertilization.
      b. Ovarian drilling. In refractory cases, multiple holes may be drilled into the ovary with electrocautery or laser at laparoscopic surgery to decrease the amount of androgen-producing tissue. However, excessive scar tissue may form after this procedure. Scar tissue may result in blockage of the fallopian tube or pelvic pain.
      c. Hirsutism. Several medications can be used to treat hirsutism. These medications serve as androgen receptor blockers or 5α-reductase inhibitors. In these cases, preexisting hair growth is not removed, but new hair growth is inhibited. In the most severe cases, patients may resort to electrolysis, shaving, or depilatory creams.

    3. Asherman syndrome or intrauterine adhesions
      a. Adhesiolysis may be performed hysteroscopically under direct visualization.
      b. After the adhesiolysis, patients are placed on estrogens postoperatively for 3 to 4 weeks, ending with a course of progestin to promote re-epithelialization of the cavity and subsequent menses.
      c. Other experts advocate intrauterine placement of a Foley balloon to prevent reapposition of the uterine cavity.

    4. Congenital anomalies
      a. In the absence of a uterus and vagina, a neovagina may be created with either a surgical procedure or the use of graduated dilators. This requires motivation on the part of the patient.

b. Patients with no uterus and vagina have ovaries because the ovaries are not part of the müllerian system. Therefore, pregnancy is possible. Patients who are 46,XX can be stimulated to produce multiple follicles, undergo oocyte retrieval, and have a gestational carrier carry the pregnancy to term.

c. Patients with androgen insensitivity have no ovaries, and a neovagina may be created; the Y-containing gonads must be removed after pubertal development. These patients should be placed on lifelong estrogen replacement therapy (see IV A 1).

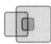

Study Questions for Chapter 20

Directions: *Each of the numbered items or incomplete statements in this section is followed by answers or by completions of the statement. Select the ONE lettered answer or completion that is BEST in each case.*

1. A 24-year-old nulligravid woman and her husband have been trying to get pregnant for 3 years and have been unsuccessful. She tells you that she has periods only a few times each year. She has no past medical or surgical history. She has never had a major illness. Her pelvic examination reveals a normal-sized vagina and a small palpable uterus. There are no adnexal masses palpated. All of her labs are negative except for elevated TSH and low free T_4. An in-office transvaginal ultrasound reveals a small anteflexed, anteverted uterus with normal stripe. The best treatment to induce ovulation and to achieve pregnancy in this patient is

- [A] clomiphene
- [B] follicle-stimulating hormone
- [C] thyroid hormone
- [D] clomiphene with intrauterine insemination
- [E] follicle-stimulating hormone and in vitro fertilization

2. An 18-year-old nulligravid is seeing you because she has not had a period for the last 8 months. She is a freshman in college majoring in dance. She enjoys hiking to relieve stress. She is sexually active. She began her menses at age 13 and had irregular periods for the first 2 years and then became regular. She is 5 foot 8 inches tall and weighs 90 lbs. Her vitals are as follows: T = 96.6, BP = 108/60, P = 52. On examination, she has a normal-appearing vulva and appropriate-sized vagina without any lesions. Her cervix and uterus are unremarkable. You do not appreciate any adnexal masses or tenderness. The rest of her physical examination is unremarkable other than her teeth, on which you see erosion of the upper and lower incisors, especially posteriorly. The most likely hormone abnormality in this patient is

- [A] increased T_4
- [B] decreased T_3
- [C] increased TSH
- [D] decreased cortisol
- [E] increased prolactin

QUESTIONS 3–4

A 25-year-old nulligravid presents to your office because she has not had a period for the last year. She didn't think too much of it initially due to her hectic schedule but is concerned now because she recently started a serious relationship. Although she admits she is not yet ready to become pregnant, she wants to have regular periods. She has no significant medical or surgical history. She started her periods at age 12 and they became regular at age 14 until last year. She has never had a major illness. She has no known allergies to medications. She is a major bank executive who travels across the United States and Europe often. She runs 5 miles a day and uses a Jacuzzi often to relax. Her vital signs are as follows: T = 98.9, BP = 135/86, P = 100. Her physical examination is unremarkable.

3. Abnormality of which structure may account for her amenorrhea?

- [A] Hypothalamus
- [B] Pituitary
- [C] Ovaries
- [D] Uterus
- [E] Vagina

4. The best next step in management of this patient is

    [A] norgestimate and ethinyl estradiol
    [B] conjugated estrogen and medroxyprogesterone acetate
    [C] clomiphene
    [D] GnRH pump
    [E] buspirone

QUESTIONS 5–6

A 16-year-old presents to you because she has never had a period. She has no past medical or surgical history. She has never had a major illness. She has no known drug allergies. She is a senior in high school has been accepted to an Ivy League university. In addition to her excellent academic performance, she is active as a volunteer in the community and enjoys tennis and volleyball. She is 5 feet 7 inches tall and weighs 125 lbs. Her vital signs are as follows: T = 98.7, BP = 110/70, P = 70. Her abdomen is unremarkable. She has Tanner stage 4 breast development, axillary hair growth, and pubic hair growth onto her thighs. On sterile speculum examination you discover a short vagina that ends blindly. Therefore, there is no cervix.

5. The diagnosis is

    [A] Testicular feminization
    [B] Swyer syndrome
    [C] 17 α-hydroxylase deficiency
    [D] Mayer-Rokitansky-Küster-Hauser syndrome
    [E] Kallmann syndrome

6. Based on the diagnosis, which of the following is the best <u>initial</u> test to order?

    [A] Radiograph of hand
    [B] Intravenous pyelogram
    [C] MRI of spine
    [D] Total testosterone levels
    [E] Karyotype

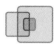

Answers and Explanations

1. The answer is C [IV B 4]. You should always start with the least invasive treatment first. Keeping that in mind, hypothyroidism is the cause of this patient's anovulation. Thyroid hormone replacement reestablishes ovulatory cycles and therefore allows her to get pregnant on her own without the use of fertility drugs (clomiphene or follicle stimulating hormone) or complex procedures (intrauterine insemination or in vitro fertilization).

2. The answer is B [II C 1 d]. The clinical scenario described in this question is anorexia nervosa (binging type). She is below ideal body weight for her height. She has many classic features (amenorrhea, bradycardia, hypothermia, dry skin, and erosion of her teeth from stomach acid caused by repetitive induced vomiting). Patients with anorexia nervosa have decreased gonadotropins (low LH and FSH), which causes amenorrhea. They also have low free T_3 but normal levels of free T_4, TSH, and prolactin. They also have elevated cortisol (because it is a "stress"-related hormone).

3. The answer is A [II C 1 and 2] **4. The answer is A** [IV B 1 b]. Any type of excessive stress in the form of lifestyle (e.g., busy executive), exercise (e.g., ballet dancer or marathon runner), or major illness (e.g., chronic kidney or lung disease) changes neurotransmitter function within the hypothalamus. Therefore, stress causes hypothalamic dysfunction resulting in changes in the GnRH pulse, which results in low levels of LH and FSH. The optimal treatment of hypogonadotropic amenorrhea is either hormone replacement therapy (e.g., conjugated estrogen with medroxyprogesterone acetate) or birth control pills (e.g., norgestimate and ethinyl estradiol). Because this patient is not ready for pregnancy, the latter treatment is more reasonable. Buspirone can be given to a young patient with general anxiety disorder. Clomiphene is used to stimulate follicle development and is therefore not necessary for this patient. A GnRH pump, which is difficult to administer and maintain, is not useful for this patient because she is not trying to become pregnant.

5. The answer is D [II D 2 a] **6. The answer is B** [II D 2 and 3]. The most common disorder of the outflow tract and the second most common cause of primary amenorrhea is called Mayer-Rokitansky-Küster-Hauser syndrome. Patients with this syndrome have a normal female karyotype with normal ovarian function; therefore, growth and development is normal. Because of exposure to müllerian inhibiting substance/factor, there is lack of development and failure of fusion of the müllerian ducts. These patients usually have an absent or very short vagina. They lack a uterus and fallopian tubes or can have rudimentary uterine cords that do not connect to the introitus. There is a 33% association with urinary tract abnormalities and only a 12% association with skeletal abnormalities. An intravenous pyelogram (IVP) is essential to characterize the urinary tract, especially to ensure that there are two functioning kidneys. A karyotype should also be obtained to rule out other causes, but this is not as urgent as an IVP. An MRI of the spine can also be obtained to rule out skeletal abnormalities in the spine. MRI can also be obtained when there is suspicion of a rudimentary uterine structure. A radiograph of the hand is not necessary here because it is used for bone age determination when there is abnormal growth. The total testosterone levels are in the normal female range in these patients because they have axillary and pubic hair growth. This is in contrast to androgen insensitivity or testicular feminization, which involves normal or slightly elevated male levels of testosterone and elevated LH. In Swyer syndrome, a phenotypic female patient with an XY karyotype has a palpable müllerian system, normal female testosterone levels, and lack of sexual development. The syndrome characterized by 17 α-hydroxylase deficiency is marked by hypertension, hypokalemia, and elevated progesterone levels in addition to absent sexual development. Kallmann syndrome is amenorrhea caused by hypothalamic dysfunction along with anosmia.

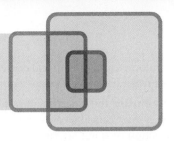

chapter **21**

Dysfunctional Uterine Bleeding
SAMANTHA BUTTS

I   DEFINITIONS

A **Dysfunctional uterine bleeding (DUB).** This **abnormal bleeding,** which is usually excessive, reflects a disturbance in normal ovulatory function. It is a manifestation of **abnormal hormonal stimulation** of the endometrial lining.

1. DUB may be **infrequent or chronic.**

2. DUB results from **abnormalities of endocrine origin** with no demonstrable organic or anatomic cause.

3. DUB is **most often associated with anovulation** and **estrogen breakthrough bleeding.** However, it may occur in women with ovulatory cycles that have inadequate luteal or follicular phases.

B **Menstrual cycle characteristics** (see Chapter 19)

1. **Cycle length.** Most reproductive cycles range in length from 24 to 35 days. Fewer than 2% of women have menstrual periods more often than every 21 days or less often than every 35 days.
   a. **Polymenorrhea** is bleeding that occurs more often than every 21 days.
   b. **Oligomenorrhea** is bleeding that occurs less often than every 35 days.

2. **Cycle regularity.** Although the length of the menstrual cycle may vary from woman to woman, it usually remains the same in a particular individual.
   a. The **follicular phase,** the first half of the cycle, is the **source of the person-to-person variation** in cycle length. The follicular phase begins with the onset of menses; it then produces a mature follicle and culminates in ovulation.
   b. The **luteal phase,** the second half of the cycle, is more consistent in length, lasting **14 days in most individuals.** If a woman has a 28-day cycle, she tends to ovulate on or about day 14; if a woman has 30-day cycle, she tends to ovulate on or about day 16.
   c. **Metrorrhagia** refers to bleeding at irregular intervals. When irregular bleeding is excessive, it is termed **menometrorrhagia.**

3. **Volume and duration of menstrual bleeding.** The normal amount of menstrual blood produced per cycle is 30 to 50 mL. More than 80 mL is considered abnormal. The average duration of menstrual bleeding is 4 to 6 days. **Menorrhagia** is prolonged and excessive bleeding that occurs at regular intervals.

II   PHYSIOLOGY OF NORMAL MENSTRUAL BLEEDING

A **Postovulatory estrogen-progesterone withdrawal bleeding.** This bleeding occurs in a normal menstrual cycle.

1. During the follicular phase of the cycle, the ovary elaborates **estrogen,** which results in **endometrial proliferation.** After ovulation, the **corpus luteum** develops from the remnant of the ovulatory follicle. The main function of the corpus luteum is to secrete progesterone (it also produces

estrogen), which limits endometrium growth and causes it to differentiate. If pregnancy does not occur, the corpus luteum regresses and hormonal support of the endometrium ceases.

2. **Regression of the corpus luteum** and a **decline in estrogen and progesterone** initiate a cascade of events that culminates in menstrual bleeding.

   a. Rhythmic **vasoconstriction** of spiral arterioles leads to ischemia, necrosis, and **sloughing of the surface endometrium.** In addition to playing a key role in the onset of menses, this vasoconstriction helps limit the amount of blood lost during the process. Thrombin and platelet plugging of spiral arterioles also promotes hemostasis.

   b. **Lytic enzymes** are released from intracellular lysosomes, and matrix metalloproteinases are upregulated. This results in **breakdown of endometrial tissue** via degradation of extracellular matrix components and the basement membrane. Endometrial breakdown also leads to the release of significant quantities of prostaglandins (particularly PGF_{2a}), which are potent mediators of myometrial contractions and vasoconstriction.

   c. **Estrogen stimulation** at the beginning of a new menstrual cycle helps control bleeding by healing the raw surface of the endometrium.

III PATHOPHYSIOLOGY OF DYSFUNCTIONAL UTERINE BLEEDING

A **Anovulatory cycles.** As previously stated, DUB most often occurs in the absence of the cyclic hormonal changes that regulate the menstrual cycle.

B **Estrogen breakthrough bleeding.** Approximately 90% of all DUB is a manifestation of estrogen breakthrough bleeding.

1. In the absence of ovulation, **estrogen stimulates the endometrium** without the production of progesterone by the corpus luteum.

2. This **unopposed estrogen stimulation** leads to excessive glandular proliferation with lack of differentiation or development of stromal support. The result is an unstable, fragile, and heterogeneous endometrium that is prone to superficial breakdown and bleeding.

3. As this pattern of unopposed estrogen stimulation continues, the **endometrium sloughs off in isolated locations.** The remaining raw surface is restimulated by estrogen and heals as another part of endometrium is sloughed off. Prolonged and excessive bleeding results.

4. The **duration and level of unopposed estrogen** stimulation directly affect the amount and duration of bleeding.

5. Estrogen breakthrough bleeding is **unpredictable.** In the absence of estrogen-progesterone withdrawal, there is loss of rhythmic, progressive, vasoconstriction of the **spiral arteries.** Without this, there is no periodic, orderly, self-limited shedding of the endometrium.

IV ETIOLOGY OF DYSFUNCTIONAL UTERINE BLEEDING

A **Causes of anovulation or oligo-ovulation.** Anovulatory cycles are a symptom of a disruption of the normal regulatory mechanisms that control the menstrual cycle. Ovulatory cycles result from a complex interaction of factors involving the hypothalamic-pituitary-ovarian axis. Abnormalities at any of these sites interfere with normal ovulation; a loss of normal ovulatory function occurs because of several causes. Anovulatory, estrogen breakthrough bleeding is **most common** during the **postmenarchal and premenopausal periods,** although the underlying mechanism may be different in each case.

1. **Immaturity of the hypothalamic-pituitary-ovarian axis.** Anovulation and DUB are often seen in postpubertal adolescents shortly after menarche. The onset of the first menstrual period may occur before the hypothalamic control mechanisms of ovulation are fully mature. Gonadotropin-releasing hormone (GnRH) secretion has not yet attained the pulsatile nature characteristic of ovulatory cycles.

2. **Dysfunction of the hypothalamic-pituitary-ovarian axis.** Any factor that interferes with the normal pulsatile secretion of GnRH leads to anovulation. Prolonged insults lead to progressive dysfunction and, ultimately, to amenorrhea.

   a. **Hyperprolactinemia.** Elevation of circulating prolactin may be caused by pituitary adenomas or a side effect of medications, most notably psychotropic drugs. Elevated prolactin inhibits normal GnRH pulsatility and results in anovulation.

   b. **Stress and anxiety.** Anovulation and menstrual irregularities often occur during times of stress and major life changes. Loss of pulsatile GnRH secretion may occur as a result.

   c. **Rapid weight loss.** Sudden and rapid weight loss from crash dieting may also interfere with normal GnRH secretion.

   d. **Borderline anorexia nervosa.** Anovulation occurs early in the course of this disorder. If the anorexia increases in severity, complete loss of ovarian function may occur, resulting in amenorrhea and hypoestrogenism.

   e. **Hypothyroidism.** This condition may also cause anovulation through dysregulation of a feedback loop that results in increased prolactin levels. Normal GnRH pulsatility is suppressed, as it is in primary hyperprolactinemia.

   f. **Perimenopause.** This stage includes the years leading up to menopause, when complete cessation of menses occurs secondary to loss of ovarian function. During this period, menstrual cycles begin to lengthen because of accelerated follicular atresia, erratic ovulation, and prolongation of follicular phases.

3. **Abnormalities of normal feedback signals.** Estradiol levels play a critical role in controlling the sequence of events during the normal ovulatory cycle. The rise and fall of estradiol at critical points in the cycle are important feedback mechanisms of cycle control. **Estradiol primarily exerts a negative feedback effect on follicle-stimulating hormone (FSH) secretion and must decrease appropriately before menses to allow the increase in FSH necessary for initiation of a new cycle. Sustained estradiol levels at this time prevent normal cycling. Elevated estradiol levels can result from persistent secretion, abnormal clearance and metabolism, and production by extragonadal sources.

   a. Certain medical conditions, most notably **hepatic disease or thyroid abnormalities**, may affect the metabolism and clearance of estradiol. The fluctuation in circulating estrogen levels seen in these conditions may cause ovulatory and menstrual dysfunction.

   b. Conditions that lead to an increase in the production or conversion of estrogen precursors result in extragonadal production of estrogen. **Adipose tissue**, which contains aromatase, is capable of converting peripheral androgens to estrogens. This process increases with increasing body weight.

4. **Luteinizing hormone (LH) surge.** Ovulation depends on a midcycle LH surge that is induced by a concomitant estradiol surge.

   a. If estrogen levels fail to reach a critical value, LH levels do not peak, and ovulation fails to occur.

   b. This condition most commonly occurs in perimenopausal women. Failure of ovarian follicles to produce sufficient estradiol necessary for induction of the LH surge leads to the anovulatory cycles common in these women.

5. **Polycystic ovary syndrome (PCOS).** This condition involves a complex set of endocrine derangements, including anovulation. PCOS is associated with hyperandrogenism, glucose intolerance, and often obesity, each playing a role in the evolution of an anovulatory state. Women with PCOS are at risk for cardiovascular illness and diabetes mellitus.

B **Causes with ovulation.** DUB secondary to hormonal causes may occur during ovulatory cycles, although it is more common during anovulatory cycles. Abnormal bleeding may occur at any age but is most likely to occur in association with the declining ovarian function characteristic of the years preceding menopause.

V OTHER PATTERNS OF ABNORMAL UTERINE BLEEDING

Other types of bleeding are abnormal, but they do not constitute DUB. These patterns are commonly seen and may be confused with DUB.

A Hormonally related bleeding

1. **Estrogen withdrawal bleeding.** This bleeding may occur at **midcycle** when estrogen levels decline briefly just before ovulation. Estrogen withdrawal also causes bleeding that occurs after bilateral oophorectomy, radiation of mature follicles, or cessation of hormone replacement therapy in menopausal women.

2. **Progesterone breakthrough bleeding.** In the setting of prolonged progesterone administration, the endometrium receives relatively little estrogenic support. This occurs most often when women use progestin-only contraceptives for extended periods. The antimitotic effect of progesterone on the endometrium combined with inadequate estrogen stimulation results in atrophy. As a result, the endometrial surface bleeds irregularly, varying in amount and duration.

B Organic causes of uterine bleeding.
Abnormal uterine bleeding may also be associated with conditions that are not endocrine in nature (Table 21-1). Organic conditions, such as polyps, uterine fibroids, endometritis, endometrial hyperplasia, pregnancy, and blood dyscrasias must be considered as possible causes of the bleeding.

VI EVALUATION AND DIAGNOSIS OF DYSFUNCTIONAL UTERINE BLEEDING

A History.
Most often, a presumptive diagnosis of DUB can be made or ruled out based on history alone, with examination and diagnostic tests used to confirm the diagnosis.

1. **Current bleeding history.** It is critical to describe the current pattern of bleeding accurately and to determine to what extent it differs from previous bleeding patterns. Variations from normal cyclic patterns may be a sign of DUB.

2. **Menstrual history.** Although women with DUB may present with any of the previously described abnormal bleeding patterns, DUB is most commonly associated with either oligomenorrhea or metrorrhagia. Age at menarche, cycle frequency and duration, and presence of cyclically occurring symptoms establish the presence or absence of ovulatory cycles. A history of prolonged anovulation identifies women at risk for endometrial hyperplasia, requiring endometrial sampling.

3. **Contraceptive use.** Pregnancy should always be ruled out in women of reproductive age even if they use contraception. All methods of contraception have small, inherent failure rates when used properly. This rate increases with faulty or erratic use. Moreover, some patients on hormonal contraception experience abnormal bleeding (e.g., progesterone breakthrough bleeding) that either resolves spontaneously or can be remedied with estrogen therapy. Intrauterine devices (IUDs) may also be associated with abnormal bleeding.

4. **Medical history.** The presence of a medical condition associated with abnormal bleeding (e.g., coagulation disorders with or without liver disease) should be considered. Thirty percent of adolescents who present with severe blood loss have an associated coagulopathy, such as **von Willebrand disease**, in which platelets are dysfunctional. In addition, thyroid disease and pituitary adenomas may be the underlying cause of bleeding associated with anovulatory cycles.

5. **Medication history.** Certain medications may be associated with abnormal uterine bleeding (e.g., anticoagulants). Psychotropic medications may secondarily cause DUB through an elevation of prolactin.

TABLE 21-1   Differential Diagnosis of Abnormal Uterine Bleeding

Reproductive tract pathology	**Endocrine gland dysfunction**
Cervicitis	Hypothyroidism
Cervical neoplasia	Hyperthyroidism
Endometritis	Pituitary adenoma
Endometrial polyps	
Endometrial hyperplasia	**Ovulatory dysfunction**
Uterine leiomyomas	Anovulation
Adenomyosis	Shortened follicular phase
Uterine sarcomas	Luteal phase deficiency
Ovarian neoplasms (estrogen producing)	Prolonged corpus luteum function
Medications	**Pregnancy-related conditions**
Estrogen administration	Threatened abortion
Oral contraceptives	Spontaneous abortion
Progesterone-only contraceptives	Ectopic pregnancy
Aspirin	Gestational trophoblastic neoplasm
Anticoagulants	
Psychotropic medications	**Systemic disease**
	Hematologic disorders
Trauma	von Willebrand disease
Foreign body	Thrombocytopenia
Lacerations	Hepatic disease
Intrauterine device	Renal disease

B **Physical examination.** A complete physical examination detects organic causes of abnormal uterine bleeding and signs associated with causes of anovulation and DUB.

1. **General physical examination.** Thyroid enlargement, galactorrhea (prolactinoma), ecchymosis, and purpura may be apparent. Pallor or vital sign instability suggests either brisk bleeding or long-standing bleeding with associated anemia. Such information helps guide the method and acuity of treatment.

2. **Gynecologic examination.** A complete gynecologic examination, including a Papanicolaou smear, detects organic causes of abnormal uterine bleeding. Elimination of anatomic or structural causes of abnormal bleeding is the first step in the diagnosis of DUB.

C **Laboratory studies.** The history and physical examination determine the need for additional laboratory studies. Not all tests are necessary in all patients.

1. **Pregnancy test.** Modern urine pregnancy tests are highly sensitive, inexpensive, and easy to perform. Such tests should be performed in all premenopausal women with abnormal bleeding.

2. **Complete blood count.** A hemoglobin and hematocrit should be obtained in women with heavy or prolonged bleeding. A white blood cell count may be useful in the diagnosis of endometritis or rare conditions such as leukemia. A platelet count detects thrombocytopenia.

3. **Thyroid-stimulating hormone and prolactin.** Levels of these hormones should be obtained whenever bleeding is associated with anovulation.

4. **Coagulation profile.** Prothrombin time, partial thromboplastin time, and a workup for von Willebrand disease should be performed when an associated coagulation disorder is suspected.

5. **Androgen profile.** Testosterone, dehydroepiandrosterone, and 17 OH-hydroxyprogesterone should be obtained whenever evidence of **hyperandrogenism and anovulation** is present. PCOS, late-onset congenital adrenal hyperplasia, and androgen-producing tumors are among the conditions that can cause hyperandrogenism and anovulation.

D **Diagnostic procedures.**   The need for additional diagnostic testing is determined on an individual basis.

1. **Ultrasonography and sonohysterography.** Ultrasound evaluation of the uterus can often isolate intrauterine polyps or submucosal fibroids that lead to heavy bleeding. The transvaginal approach is often more sensitive than the transabdominal approach. Sonohysterography, in which saline is instilled into the uterine cavity during transvaginal sonography, can often delineate intracavitary lesions even better than traditional ultrasound. Once the cavity is distended with saline, intracavitary polyps and fibroids can be localized and measured.

2. **Endometrial biopsy.** To rule out endometrial carcinoma, a sample of the endometrial lining should be obtained in the following groups of women: those at risk for endometrial hyperplasia or carcinoma, those older than 40 years of age, and those younger than 40 years of age who have chronic unopposed estrogen breakthrough bleeding. Atypical endometrial hyperplasia, which is believed to be a precursor of endometrial carcinoma, can be treated medically or surgically. Endometrial biopsy is performed as an office procedure using a small catheter to obtain the specimen.

3. **Dilation and curettage (D&C).** This procedure is warranted in those women who have DUB and do not respond to medical management with hormonal manipulation. D&C is also required when an endometrial biopsy cannot be performed in the office; this is usually the case if a woman has a stenotic cervical os, making it impossible to pass the biopsy catheter.

4. **Hysteroscopy or direct visualization of the endometrial cavity.** Hysteroscopy and D&C are routinely performed at the same time. Hysteroscopy is particularly useful when a polyp or submucosal fibroid is suspected, because these lesions can be confirmed and resected hysteroscopically. After hysteroscopy, a D&C is performed to rule out coincident endometrial pathology whether a cavitary lesion is visualized or not.

VII TREATMENT OF DYSFUNCTIONAL UTERINE BLEEDING

A **Hormonal therapy.**   The treatment of anovulatory DUB is hormonal therapy with a progestin, estrogen, or combination of the two. The choice of therapy is based on the duration of bleeding, age of the patient, and preference of the patient.

1. **Progestins. Progesterone supplementation** is the treatment of choice because most women with DUB are anovulatory. The bleeding represents estrogen breakthrough bleeding that is a manifestation of unopposed estrogen stimulation of the endometrial lining. Addition of progesterone restores the normal controlling influences to the endometrium.
   a. **Progestins act as antiestrogens.** The **antimitotic, antigrowth effect of progestins** supports their use in the treatment of endometrial hyperplasia.
      (1) They enhance the conversion of estradiol to estrone, which is then displaced from the cell.
      (2) They diminish the effect of estrogen on target cells by inhibiting estrogen receptor replenishment in the cell.
      (3) They **support and stabilize the endometrium** so that an organized sloughing of the endometrium occurs after its withdrawal.
   b. **Medroxyprogesterone** (10 mg/day for 10 days) produces regular withdrawal bleeding in patients with adequate amounts of endogenous estrogen.
   c. Progestins may not stop an acute episode of DUB as effectively as estrogen, especially if bleeding has been prolonged. However, **progestin, either alone or in combination with estrogen,** is warranted for long-term control after the acute episode of DUB is controlled.
   d. The **levonorgestrel IUD** (see Chapter 24, III B 2) can reduce menstrual bleeding and is an excellent treatment option for women interested in long-term contraception. It requires replacement every 5 years.

2. **Oral contraceptive therapy.** Frequently, DUB is associated with prolonged endometrial buildup and heavy bleeding in younger women. Combined estrogen-progestin therapy in the form of

oral contraceptives is used to treat episodes of acute bleeding. Combined oral contraceptives convert a fragile, overgrown endometrium into a pseudodecidualized, structurally stable lining. Bleeding usually is controlled within 24 hours of initiation of therapy. If no response has occurred by this time, another treatment for the DUB should be pursued.

  a. Any low-dose combination oral contraceptive can be used. The pill is administered two or three times a day for 5 to 7 days.

  b. A heavy withdrawal bleed is expected after cessation of therapy.

  c. After the withdrawal bleed, cyclic therapy with once-a-day administration is continued for 3 months to reduce the endometrial lining to baseline levels. The oral contraceptive can be continued if birth control is desired.

3. Estrogens. High-dose estrogen therapy rapidly stops bleeding within 12 to 24 hours. The acute mechanism of action is thought to be **initiation of clotting at the capillary level.** Proliferation of the endometrial surface is a later effect. It is especially useful when bleeding has been **prolonged or** is secondary to **progesterone breakthrough bleeding.**

  a. Conjugated estrogens (1.25 mg) or estradiol (2 mg) are administered daily for 7 to 10 days. If bleeding is moderately heavy, the same doses are administered every 4 hours during the first 24 hours of therapy. Treatment is continued for another 10 days, with the daily dose of estrogen combined with 10 mg medroxyprogesterone. A withdrawal bleed is expected after cessation of therapy.

  b. Parenteral estrogen is effective in treating **acute profuse DUB.** Estrogen (25 mg) is administered intravenously every 4 hours until the bleeding lessens, or up to 12 hours. A progestin must be started at the same time.

  c. After the acute episode is controlled, **chronic therapy** is initiated with the oral contraceptive or periodic progesterone for at least 3 months.

B Medical therapy

1. Nonsteroidal anti-inflammatory agents (NSAIDS)

  a. NSAIDS inhibit the synthesis of prostaglandins, which are substances that have important pharmacologic actions on the endometrial vasculature and on endometrial hemostasis. The concentration of endometrial prostaglandins, including thromboxane and prostacyclin, increases progressively during the menstrual cycle.

  b. NSAIDS may work by altering the balance between thromboxane and prostacyclin.

  c. NSAIDS are primarily effective in limiting menstrual blood loss in women who ovulate, and they reduce excessive blood flow by as much as 50%.

2. GnRH agonists. After control of an episode of acute bleeding, GnRH agonists may help achieve amenorrhea in chronically ill patients. Expense and the long-term effects of hypoestrogenism limit therapy. If long-term therapy is chosen, hormone replacement therapy with estrogen and progestin is advised.

3. Desmopressin. A synthetic analog of arginine vasopressin, desmopressin is used as a treatment of last resort in patients with coagulation disorders.

C Surgical therapy

1. D&C with or without hysteroscopy. This procedure is not the treatment of first choice in DUB. It is undertaken in patients who have bleeding refractory to medical therapy or who are not candidates for hormonal manipulation. It can be a diagnostic and therapeutic modality.

2. Hysterectomy. This procedure is a realistic treatment option in the following situations:

  a. For women who have completed childbearing in whom persistent abnormal bleeding is often worrisome and bothersome

  b. For women who do not tolerate medical management

  c. For women diagnosed with atypical endometrial hyperplasia and with an increased risk of endometrial cancer, who may opt for surgical as opposed to medical management

3. Endometrial ablation. Ablation of the endometrium is a surgical option for women who are not candidates for hysterectomy because of medical conditions or who wish to avoid hysterectomy but choose not to pursue hormonal therapy.

  a. Ablation of the endometrium is performed using laser, electrocautery, or thermal destructive techniques.

  b. Fifty percent of women achieve amenorrhea; 90% achieve a decrease in bleeding.

  c. The long-term risk of the occurrence of undetectable endometrial carcinoma in isolated segments of endometrium has yet to be defined.

Study Questions for Chapter 21

Directions: *Each of the numbered items or incomplete statements in this section is followed by answers or by completions of the statement. Select the ONE lettered answer or completion that is BEST in each case.*

1. A 50-year-old woman, gravida 3, para 2, SAB 1 presents to you reporting vaginal bleeding. Her menstrual cycles used to occur regularly every 30 days and lasted 3 to 4 days. She has periods every 20 to 22 days and they last for 6 to 7 days for the last 6 months. She denies any past medical or surgical history. Review of systems is negative, including denial of lightheadedness. Her speculum examination is unremarkable. The bimanual examination reveals a slightly enlarged, regular contour, anteverted uterus that is nontender to palpation. The next best step in management is

- A Low-dose oral contraceptive pills
- B Endometrial biopsy
- C Dilatation and curettage
- D Endometrial ablation
- E Levonorgestrel IUD

2. A 16-year-old nulligravid girl reports cycles every 45 to 50 days and bleeds a moderate amount for 4 days. She is not sexually active. Her physical examination is unremarkable, and her serum pregnancy test is negative. The next best step in management is

- A Reassurance
- B Low-dose birth control pills
- C Non-steroidal anti-inflammatory drugs (NSAIDs)
- D Hysteroscopy and dilatation and curettage
- E Coagulation profile

3. A 27-year-old woman gravida 1, para 1 presents to you reporting bleeding between her periods and slight lengthening in the duration of her periods. Review of systems is unremarkable, including denial of galactorrhea, acne, hirsutism, or clitoromegaly. She denies any medical problems. She is 5 feet 4 inches tall and weighs 130 lbs. Her physical examination is also unremarkable. Her serum TSH is elevated, Hg = 11 g/dL, and WBC = 4K. The most likely explanation for her bleeding is

- A Increased GnRH pulse amplitude
- B Decreased GnRH pulse frequency
- C Increased prolactin levels
- D Psychotropic medication
- E Exogenous estrogen supplementation

QUESTIONS 4–5

A 15-year-old nulligravid girl presents to the emergency department by ambulance because she passed out on the floor of her house in a pool of blood. She is now conscious and has brisk bleeding from the vagina. Her BP = 88/48, P = 140, R = 16, T = 96.2. Her speculum examination reveals blood emerging from the cervical os. There are no lesions in the vagina or cervix. The bimanual examination is unremarkable. Serum hCG is negative, and her hemoglobin is 7 g/dL. An intravenous line is placed and a blood transfusion is begun.

4. The next best step in management of this patient is
   - A Low-dose combination oral contraceptive pills
   - B Conjugated estrogen
   - C Intravenous estrogen
   - D Depot-medroxyprogesterone acetate
   - E Packed red blood cell transfusion

5. In this scenario, the mechanism by which treatment given acutely stops bleeding from the uterus is by
   - A Initiating clotting
   - B Vasoconstriction of capillaries
   - C Rapid proliferation of endometrium
   - D Making endometrial lining atrophic
   - E Increasing oxygen carrying capacity

Answers and Explanations

1. The answer is B [VI D 2]. The risk of endometrial carcinoma increases with age and should be ruled out in patients with abnormal bleeding who are over age 40 years. In addition, endometrial hyperplasia often develops in women with a history of chronic anovulation and unopposed estrogen stimulation of the endometrium (most likely in this perimenopausal patient). When a woman is diagnosed with endometrial hyperplasia with atypia, she has an increased risk of endometrial carcinoma. Endometrial hyperplasia can be treated with progestin therapy. Many women who are perimenopausal have erratic bleeding because of the transition from regular ovarian folliculogenesis and hormone production to relative ovarian quiescence. An office endometrial biopsy must be performed. Birth control pills will regulate her bleeding but will not tell you about the endometrium. Dilatation and curettage is the next step after an endometrial biopsy if the results are not satisfactory (e.g., cervical stenosis and inability to obtain biopsy in the office or no tissue obtained on biopsy) or if the patient is refractory to agents aimed at stopping the bleeding. Endometrial ablation should not be done until you know the endometrium is completely normal. Levonorgestrel IUD is a good treatment option after biopsy of the endometrium.

2. The answer is A [IV A 1, 2]. The pattern of bleeding demonstrated by this patient is characteristic of the early menses. Unless it is prolonged and very heavy (not the case in this patient), it should evolve into a pattern of regular estrogen-progesterone withdrawal bleeding with time. The chance that an anatomic lesion such as a polyp or a fibroid would be the cause of her bleeding is unlikely given her age and pattern of bleeding. Therefore, hysteroscopy with dilatation and curettage would not help. Oral contraception and NSAIDs are not indicated at this point unless she desires contraception. Coagulopathy is an unlikely cause of her bleeding because the timing, not the volume, is problematic for this patient.

3. The answer is C [IV A 2 e]. Elevated TSH means that she has hypothyroidism. This condition may also cause abnormal bleeding through dysregulation of a feedback loop that results in elevation of prolactin levels. Normal GnRH pulsatility is suppressed. There is no mention of medications (she denies medical problems) or exogenous estrogen used in the clinical scenario.

4. The answer is C [VII A 3 b]. Parenteral estrogen is effective in treating acute profuse dysfunctional uterine bleeding (DUB). Estrogen (25 mg) is administered intravenously every 4 hours until the bleeding lessens. Although a transfusion is among the first management steps, it is more important to treat the source of bleeding first before giving packed red blood cells. The other answer choices are also correct in situations where the DUB is not as severe and life threatening as it is in this case (unstable vital signs and low hemoglobin).

5. The answer is A [VII A 3]. The acute mechanism of action is thought to be initiation of clotting at the capillary level. Proliferation of the endometrium is a later effect. DUB leads to loss of the rhythmic, progressive, vasoconstriction of the spiral arteries, which causes uniform shedding and bleeding. Contraction of the myometrium is important in stopping bleeding immediately postpartum. Medroxyprogesterone makes the endometrial lining atrophic. Transfusion of packed red blood cells increases the oxygen-carrying capacity.

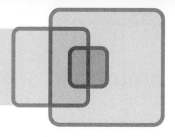

chapter 22

Pediatric and Adolescent Gynecology

SAMANTHA F. BUTTS AND SAMANTHA M. PFEIFER

I INTRODUCTION

An awareness of the problems that are unique to pediatric and adolescent gynecology is invaluable for proper management of the young patient. Particular care is essential in addressing gynecologic concerns in this age group because both physical and emotional trauma may be inadvertently inflicted. Often, performing a complete physical examination before the pelvic examination can help establish rapport and reassurance in a patient unaccustomed to pelvic examinations. A female adolescent does not need a pelvic examination unless she is experiencing abnormal symptoms; even then, noninvasive imaging (e.g., pelvic ultrasound and magnetic resonance imaging [MRI]) can be performed instead of a pelvic examination. Once an adolescent is sexually active or is at an age when this is likely to occur, a regular pelvic examination is indicated.

A **Pelvic examination of a pediatric patient** may reveal the following:

1. A mucoid vaginal discharge and even vaginal bleeding in an infant for up to 2 weeks after birth; caused by maternal estrogens
2. An introitus that is located more anteriorly than normal and a clitoris that is more prominent than normal (1 to 2 cm)
3. A redundant hymen that may protrude on straining and that remains essentially the same size until 10 years of age
4. A vaginal epithelium that is uncornified and erythematous with an alkaline pH
5. A small uterus (2.5 to 3 cm in length), with the cervix comprising two thirds of the organ (the reverse of adult proportions)
6. A cervical os that is covered with glandular epithelium and normally appears red (ectropion)

B **Visualization of the vagina.** Instruments for visualizing the vagina include the vaginoscope, the urethroscope, and the pediatric speculum. Stirrups are usually not necessary for the preadolescent; a simple "frog-leg" position is usually sufficient. Occasionally, intravenous sedation may be necessary to accomplish a thorough genital examination. To determine the presence or absence of internal genitalia, ultrasound and MRI are helpful.

C **Rectal examination** is often more informative than a vaginal examination because the short posterior vaginal fornix cannot be distended and a cul-de-sac does not exist.

II VULVOVAGINAL LESIONS

A Lichen sclerosus et atrophicus

1. **Clinical picture.** A white, papular lesion resembling leukoplakia may cover the vulva and perianal regions. As the disease progresses, there may be loss of normal architecture, including loss of demarcation of the labia and scarring of the clitoral hood.

2. **Etiology.** Causes are unknown.

3. **Diagnosis.** Biopsy, which shows superficial hyperkeratosis with basal atrophic and sclerotic changes, should be performed to clarify the diagnosis.

4. **Management.** This condition is benign and can be self-limiting. Improved hygiene is the first line of therapy. Low-potency topical steroid cream is usually effective, and high-potency topical steroids may be necessary in severe cases. Progesterone cream has been used with variable success. Testosterone, used in the treatment of adults with this condition, should be avoided. The condition may resolve at puberty but is usually chronic.

B Trauma

1. **Clinical picture**
   a. **Tears, abrasions, ecchymoses, and hematomas** are common in preadolescent girls. The incidence is highest in children between 4 and 12 years of age. The most common mechanisms of injury are sexual abuse, straddle injuries, accidental penetration, sudden abduction of the extremities, and pelvic fractures. Most genital trauma results from straddle injuries, such as a child landing on the center bar of a boy's bicycle. The injury may appear as a small ecchymotic area or a large vulvar hematoma. The clinician must always suspect sexual abuse when a child presents with genital trauma.
   b. **Sexual abuse** necessitates immediate medical attention, including a complete physical examination, cervical and rectal smears, serologic tests, and psychological evaluation and follow-up. Genital findings, when present, should be recorded very carefully because of their importance in supporting allegations of abuse in court proceedings. The colposcope is used to document specific normal and abnormal findings. However, in cases of sexual abuse, 96% of patient abnormalities are detected with the unaided eye.

2. **Management**
   a. When vaginal bleeding occurs because of pelvic trauma, **a complete and thorough examination is mandatory.** This includes evaluation of the urinary system and rectum. A vaginoscope is used to visualize the vagina to locate sources of bleeding. A large vaginal laceration may result in an expanding hematoma in the retroperitoneal space. Superficial abrasions and lacerations of the vulva, if not actively bleeding, can be cleaned and left alone.
   b. **Conservative therapy** for most trauma consists of rest, ice, and analgesics.
   c. In sexual abuse, **antibiotic therapy** is advised as prophylaxis against some sexually transmitted diseases.

C Labial agglutination

1. **Clinical picture.** Adhesion of the labia minora in the midline is the usual presentation. This vertical line of fusion distinguishes labial agglutination from imperforate hymen or vaginal atresia. The agglutination encourages retention of urine and vaginal secretions and can lead to vulvovaginitis or a urinary tract infection. Labial agglutination is believed to result from vulvar inflammation or skin disease.

2. **Management**
   a. If asymptomatic, **improved hygiene** may be all that is necessary. Treatment is indicated if there is a chronic vulvovaginitis or difficulty urinating.
   b. **Lubrication of the labia** with a bland ointment and **gentle separation** over several weeks may be effective.

    c. Topical estrogen, applied twice daily, induces cornification of the epithelium and promotes spontaneous separation. The use of estrogen in the prepubertal female, if prolonged, may stimulate breast growth and vaginal bleeding. Therapy must be limited to 2 weeks.

    d. Surgical separation is rarely necessary.

D Prolapsed urethra

1. **Clinical picture.** A small, hemorrhagic, friable mass surrounding the urethra is the most common presentation. The average age at diagnosis is 5 years. The bleeding is usually painless. The prolapse is thought to result from increased intra-abdominal pressure. The lesion can easily be confused with a condyloma but can be distinguished by applying a dilute acetic acid solution: a condyloma turns white, whereas a prolapsed urethra remains pink and fleshy.

2. **Management**
   a. If voiding is uninhibited, **local therapy** may be all that is needed. Topical estrogen and sitz baths are the mainstays of therapy. The prolapse usually resolves after 4 weeks of therapy.
   b. If urinary retention or necrosis is present, **surgical repair** and catheterization are necessary.

E Vaginal discharge

1. **Clinical picture**
   a. A **mucoid discharge** is common in infants for up to 2 weeks after birth; it results from maternal estrogen. It is also a common finding in prepubertal and postpubertal girls, who experience increased estrogen production by maturing ovaries.
   b. **Pathologic discharge** may result from any of the following conditions:
      (1) **Infections with organisms,** such as *Escherichia coli*, *Proteus*, *Pseudomonas*, yeast, *Gardnerella*, *Neisseria gonorrhoeae*, *Chlamydia*, and *Trichomonas*
      (2) **Hemolytic streptococcal vaginitis,** which results in a bloody or serosanguineous discharge, usually after a streptococcal infection elsewhere (e.g., skin or throat)
      (3) **Monilial vaginitis,** which is common in children with diabetes or after antibiotic therapy
      (4) **A foreign body,** which can cause persistent vaginal discharge, sometimes with pain and bleeding
      (5) **Nonspecific vaginitis** from local irritation, scratching, manipulation, or poor hygiene

2. **Management.** Conservative management is advisable, as follows:
   a. **Culture** to identify causative organisms. Preliminary search for *Monilia*, nonspecific bacteria, and *Trichomonas* can be accomplished by examining the discharge on a laboratory slide with saline and sodium hydroxide (20%) preparations added.
   b. **Urinalysis** to rule out cystitis
   c. **Review proper hygiene.** Instruct the child's mother to avoid tight clothing, perfume soaps, bubble bath, and powders. The child should avoid prolonged periods in moist clothing.
   d. **Perianal examination** with transparent tape to test for pinworms

III NEOPLASMS

A Tumors of the vagina, although uncommon, are most often malignant. Sarcoma botryoides is the most common malignant vaginal tumor.

1. **Clinical picture**
   a. Sarcoma botryoides arises from mesenchymal tissue of the cervix or vagina, usually on the anterior wall of the upper vagina. It grows rapidly, fills the vagina, and then protrudes through the introitus.
   b. It appears as an edematous, grapelike mass that bleeds readily on touch. It is usually multicentric and extension is usually local, with rare instances of distant metastases.

2. **Management.** A combination of surgery and chemotherapy is most commonly used.

B **Ovarian tumors**

1. **Clinical picture.** Although uncommon in children, ovarian tumors may present as torsion (twisting) of the ovaries. Among ovarian neoplasms, 40% are of non–germ cell origin (coelomic epithelium), and 60% are of germ cell origin. Most ovarian neoplasms in adolescents are also endocrine secreting regardless of origin.

   a. **Non–germ cell origin**
      (1) Lipoid cell tumors (feminizing)
      (2) Granulosa-theca cell tumors (feminizing), of which approximately 20% are malignant

   b. **Germ cell origin**
      (1) Benign cystic teratomas
      (2) Benign cysts
      (3) Arrhenoblastomas (virilizing)
      (4) Dysgerminomas and gonadoblastomas (tumors of dysgenetic gonads)
      (5) Endodermal sinus tumors
      (6) Embryonal carcinomas (gonadotropin-secreting tumors)
      (7) Immature teratomas, which account for 20% of malignant germ cell tumors

2. **Therapy. Treatment is surgical,** alone or in combination with chemotherapy, depending on the tumor. Radiation is sometimes used to treat dysgerminomas.

IV CONGENITAL ANOMALIES IN THE PEDIATRIC PATIENT

A **Vaginal agenesis.** Vaginal agenesis (atresia) represents a failure of the caudal müllerian duct to fuse with the urogenital sinus.

1. **Clinical picture**
   a. This condition most often is diagnosed at the time of puberty because of the resulting amenorrhea. **Ovarian development is normal,** but the **uterus is usually absent or fails to develop** beyond a rudimentary structure.
   b. Vaginal agenesis must be distinguished from androgen insensitivity syndrome, which is also associated with an absent vagina (see V, E).

2. **Management. Surgical creation** of a neovagina and nonsurgical dilation techniques both successfully create a vagina. However, treatment should be deferred until after puberty, when the patient has a good understanding of the condition and is emotionally ready to consider treatment.

B **Ectopic ureter with vaginal terminus**

1. **Clinical picture**
   a. Ectopic ureter, the most common cause of vaginal cysts in infants, presents as a **ureterocele,** which appears as a cystic mass protruding from the vagina. If the ureter is patent, constant irritation and vaginitis may be presenting signs.
   b. The ectopic ureter is usually one of a pair to a single kidney, and it usually drains the rudimentary upper renal pole of the kidney.
   c. **Hydroureter** and **hydronephrosis** may develop.

2. **Diagnosis.** The existence of an ectopic ureter is made using **intravenous pyelography,** which allows visualization of the entire urinary tract.

3. **Management.** It is preferable to **resect the lowest portion of the ureter** and **implant it into the bladder** rather than remove the ureter and the associated portion of the kidney.

C **Vaginal ectopic anus**

1. **Clinical picture.** Vaginal ectopic anus is an **imperforate anus associated with rectovaginal communication.** Only a skin dimple is found at the normal anal site.

2. **Management. Surgical correction** is indicated.

V   DEVELOPMENTAL DEFECTS OF THE GENITALIA (AMBIGUOUS GENITALIA)

Early diagnosis is important to guarantee proper assignment of sex during the neonatal period. The management plan should be established at that time to minimize psychological problems and to help establish the gender role.

A **Congenital adrenal hyperplasia.**   This condition results when enzymatic regulation of the biosynthesis of cortisol and aldosterone is impaired at various steps in the pathway. Adrenocorticotropic hormone (ACTH) secretion by the pituitary is increased because of low levels of blood cortisol. Both the precursors immediately preceding the impaired step and the byproducts have biologic activity that can lead to the clinical and biochemical features observed. The 21-hydroxylase defect is the most common cause of distinct virilization of the female newborn. Its incidence is 1 in 5000 births, and it accounts for 95% of all cases of congenital adrenal hyperplasia, which is inherited as an autosomal recessive trait.

1. **Clinical picture.** The chromosomes, gonads, and internal genitalia are female, and the degree of closure of the urogenital orifice varies. Clitoral enlargement and accentuation of labial folds are characteristic. The disorder is progressive if untreated.

2. **Diagnosis.** Serum 17-hydroxyprogesterone and dehydroepiandrosterone (DHEA) obtained after 24 hours of life are both elevated. A blood karyotype should be obtained. Serum electrolytes should be followed because salt wasting may occur.

3. **Management.** Hydrocortisone is administered indefinitely to all patients.

B **Adrenal tumors.**   These tumors, which may cause virilization of the external genitalia after infancy, should be suspected in children with high levels of dehydroepiandrosterone sulfate (DHEAS).

C **Maternal ingestion of androgenic substances.**   This condition can result in **masculinization of the female fetus.** Causal agents identified include androgens, danazol, and synthetic progestins (in doses much higher than in oral contraceptive pills).

1. **Clinical picture.** Masculinization is limited to the external genitalia. The clitoris is enlarged and the labia may be fused, but the vagina, tubes, and uterus are normal. Growth and development are normal, and progressive virilization does not occur.

2. **Diagnosis.** The condition can be diagnosed based on a positive history and on exclusion.

3. **Management.** Clitoral reduction and surgical correction of the fused labia may be necessary.

D **Childhood ingestion of androgens.**   This condition usually involves preparations that have androgenic activity.

1. **Clinical picture.** Clinical manifestations are the same as those resulting from maternal ingestion of androgenic substances (i.e., masculinization; see V C 1).

2. **Management.** Therapy involves clitoral reduction and surgical correction of the fused labia, if necessary.

E **Androgen insensitivity syndrome (testicular feminization)**

1. **Clinical picture.** A 46, XY genotype is present, but a female phenotype develops.
   a. Androgens are produced by the testes (which develop in the presence of a Y chromosome) and by the adrenal glands. A defect in the androgen receptor prevents normally androgen-sensitive tissue from responding to androgen stimulation.
   b. External genitalia are feminized because normal development of these structures depends on their ability to be stimulated by the androgen dihydrotestosterone. Patients are ultimately reared as girls.

    c. The testes produce müllerian inhibitory substance; as a result, there is no uterine, cervical, upper vaginal, or fallopian tube development. A short vagina that ends in a blind pouch and labia, which often contain testes, develops in these patients.

    d. Lack of responsiveness to testosterone during embryonic sexual differentiation affects development of internal genitalia. Normal male internal genitalia do not develop because testosterone is required for that process to occur.

    e. An incomplete form (Reifenstein syndrome) occurs in which external genitalia appear virilized.

  2. Diagnosis. Patients with this androgen insensitivity syndrome are usually diagnosed at puberty with primary amenorrhea and a blind or absent vagina. Because of the inability to respond to androgens, there is lack of pubic and axillary hair development. Breast development does occur because estrogen concentration is high because of conversion of testosterone produced after puberty.

  3. Management. The gonads should be removed because of an increased risk of malignancy (3 to 4% before 25 years of age). However, removal is usually performed after puberty.

F **True hermaphroditism**

  1. Clinical picture. The genotype of most true hermaphrodites is 46,XX. The external genitalia may appear male, female, or ambiguous. Both male and female internal genitalia may be present. Sex assignment and rearing should be consistent with the dominant appearance of the external genitalia and with surgical correctability.

  2. Management. The genitalia that are inconsistent with sex assignment should be surgically removed or modified.

G **Maternal virilizing tumor during pregnancy** (luteoma of pregnancy).   This condition may result in masculinization of the female fetus. The clinical picture and therapy are similar to those for the maternal ingestion of androgenic substances (see V C). Psychological development and mental capacity are consistent with chronologic age. Reproductive potential is not adversely affected, and the patient can become pregnant.

VI   NORMAL AND ABNORMAL PUBERTAL DEVELOPMENT

A **Normal puberty.**   Puberty encompasses the psychological, physical, and endocrinologic changes beginning in late childhood that ultimately allow for reproductive capacity. In North America, the average age of puberty in girls is 9 years. Once initiated, it proceeds over an average of 4 to 5 years and culminates in the onset of menses. Increased production of luteinizing hormone and follicle-stimulating hormone, as well as other factors (such as leptin), is responsible for the initiation of the pubertal process.

B   The normal physical changes associated with puberty were studied and outlined in detail by two British physicians in the late 1960s, Marshall and Tanner. Their work resulted in the Tanner stages of breast and pubic hair development. Tanner stages are currently used to evaluate pubertal development in children (Table 22-1). Components of the normal puberty include the following:

  1. Growth spurt. The growth spurt begins before the onset of other signs of puberty. The peak growth velocity occurs at an average age of 11 to 12 years, usually 1 year before menarche.

  2. Thelarche. The onset of breast development usually begins between 9 and 11 years of age. It is a sign of ovarian estrogen production and is completed over approximately 3 years. Tanner stages describe the normal changes in the transition from the prepubertal to the mature breast contour (Fig. 22-1).

  3. Adrenarche and pubarche. Adrenarche refers to the production of androgens from the adrenal gland, and pubarche is the development of axillary and pubic hair that results from the adrenal

TABLE 22-1   Tanner Staging

	Breast	Pubic Hair
Stage 1 (prepubertal)	Elevation of papilla only	No pubic hair
Stage 2	Elevation of breast and papilla as small mound; areola diameter enlarged; median age: 9.8 years	Sparse, long, pigmented hair chiefly along labia majora; median age: 10.5 years
Stage 3	Further enlargement without separation of breast and areola; median age: 11.2 years	Dark, coarse curled hair sparsely spread over mons; median age 11.4 years
Stage 4	Secondary mound of areola and papilla above the breast; age: 12.1 years	Adult-type hair, abundant but limited to mons; median age: 12 years
Stage 5	Recession of areola to contour of breast; median age: 14.6 years	Adult-type spread in quantity and distribution; median age: 13.7 years

Adapted with permission from Speroff L, Glass RH, Kase NG. Clinical Gynecologic Endocrinology and Infertility. 6th Ed. Philadelphia: Lippincott Williams & Wilkins, 1999:397.

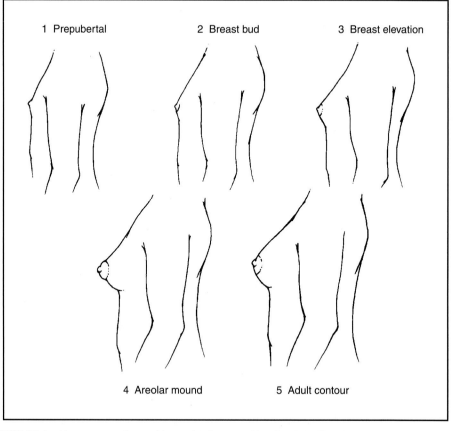

FIGURE 22-1   Tanner stages of normal breast development. (Based on Speroff L, Glass RH, Kase NG. Clinical Gynecologic Endocrinology and Infertility. 6th Ed. Philadelphia: Lippincott Williams & Wilkins, 1999:398.)

and gonadal androgens. Adrenarche is not regulated by the same hypothalamic-pituitary process that governs the rest of puberty. Pubarche usually follows thelarche in the pubertal sequence but can be the first sign of puberty in up to 20% of girls. Again, Tanner stages are used to describe normal pubic hair development (Fig. 22-2).

4. **Menarche.** In menarche, vaginal bleeding occurs in response to hormonal changes, specifically production of estrogen by the ovary, for the first time. The average age of the first menses is 12 to 13 years. For the first 2 years following menarche, menses are often irregular because of anovulation or sporadic ovulation.

C **Precocious puberty.** This condition is characterized by the onset of secondary sexual characteristics before 8 years of age (less than 2.5 standard deviations below the average age) in girls who have exhibited thelarche, adrenarche, and menarche. Beside the psychological ramifications inherent in this syndrome, there exists the risk of short stature from early epiphyseal closure. Most cases of precocious puberty are idiopathic.

1. **Forms of precocious puberty**
   a. **Central precocious puberty.** This type of precocious puberty is caused by early activation of the hypothalamic-pituitary-gonadal axis, leading to the onset of hormonal secretion from the ovaries. The most common cause is idiopathic (74%). Other causes are rare and include central nervous system lesions such as infection, craniopharyngioma, astrocytoma, neurofibroma, hemangioma of the hypothalamus, hydrocephalus, and neoplasm of the floor of the third ventricle.

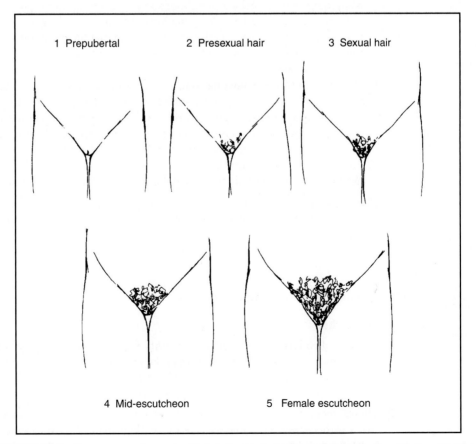

FIGURE 22-2 Tanner stages of normal pubic hair development. (Based on Speroff L, Glass RH, Kase NG. Clinical Gynecologic Endocrinology and Infertility. 6th Ed. Philadelphia: Lippincott Williams & Wilkins, 1999:399.)

b. **Peripheral precocious puberty.** This type of precocious puberty is caused by secretion of sex steroids from the ovary or exogenous hormone ingestion. These include hormone-producing ovarian or adrenal tumor, McCune-Albright syndrome, ectopic gonadotropin production, and primary hypothyroidism.

2. **Diagnosis.** Physical and radiologic signs are the basis of diagnosis. Assessment of bone age is critical, usually with a plain film of the wrist of the nondominant hand. An endocrine profile including gonadotropin levels and thyroid function tests must be evaluated. In addition, imaging of the brain with computed tomography (CT) or MRI is essential to rule out an intracranial mass.

3. **Management.** Therapy is aimed at slowing down accelerated growth; reducing pituitary, ovarian, and adrenal function; and inducing regression of secondary sex characteristics. For idiopathic precocious puberty, the treatment of choice is gonadotropin-releasing hormone (GnRH) agonists, which suppress the pituitary and halts the progression through puberty. The treatment is continued until an appropriate age has been reached; when treatment is stopped, pubertal development resumes. In cases of known etiology, recommended therapy is with surgery, chemotherapy, or radiation therapy as indicated.

D **Delayed puberty.** Delayed puberty is characterized by the absence of breast development by age 14 years or the absence of menses by age 16 years (see Chapter 20).

1. **Categories**
   a. **Hypergonadotropic hypogonadism.** This condition affects almost 50% of all patients with delayed puberty. It includes conditions in which the ovaries or gonads are not functioning and are unable to respond to gonadotropins; as a result, gonadotropin levels are high. Examples include Turner syndrome (45,XO); idiopathic premature ovarian failure; autoimmune ovarian failure; gonadal dysgenesis; and ovarian failure secondary to radiation therapy or chemotherapy.
   b. **Hypogonadotropic hypogonadism.** This condition accounts for 10 to 15% of patients with pubertal delay. The ovary is normal; however, the signal from the hypothalamus is not. Hypogonadotropic hypogonadism includes Kallmann syndrome (isolated GnRH deficiency), hypothalamic suppression by stress, severe disease or malnutrition, and tumor invasion of the pituitary (prolactinoma or craniopharyngioma).
   c. **Eugonadotropic.** Constitutional delay accounts for 10 to 20% of cases. These patients have normal progression of the stages of puberty; the initiation of the process is simply delayed.

2. **Management.** Treatment is based on the etiology of the delay. In cases of gonadal dysgenesis, the gonads should be removed at diagnosis because of the risk of neoplastic degeneration. Otherwise, hormone replacement with estrogen, and subsequently both estrogen and progesterone, is required to promote sexual development and menarche.

VII **SPECIAL PROBLEMS OF THE ADOLESCENT**

A **Dysmenorrhea**

1. **Etiology.** Primary dysmenorrhea accounts for most cases and is attributed to increased prostaglandin production with menses in the presence of normal anatomy. Secondary dysmenorrhea results from conditions such as endometriosis and müllerian anomalies with an obstruction in the outflow tract (vagina, cervix, or uterus).

2. **Clinical picture.** Severe, cyclic, cramplike pain located in the lower abdomen and pelvis is associated with menses. Pain may radiate to the thighs and back and be accompanied by nausea, vomiting, and diarrhea.

3. **Management.** First-line therapy is prostaglandin inhibitors followed by combined oral contraceptive pills. If medical management fails to control the symptoms, then pelvic ultrasound and laparoscopy are recommended for definitive diagnosis.

B **Dysfunctional uterine bleeding (DUB)** (see Chapter 21).   This excessive, prolonged, or irregular bleeding is not associated with an anatomic lesion. Most adolescent girls have anovulatory menstrual periods for the first 2 to 3 years following menarche. Approximately 2% of adolescents ovulate regularly in the first 6 months after menarche, and 18% by the end of the first year, making DUB common in this age group.

1. **Etiology.** The cause of DUB in 75% of cases is an immature hypothalamic-pituitary axis, resulting in anovulation. Other causes include psychogenic factors, juvenile hypothyroidism, and coagulation disorders (von Willebrand disease).

2. **Clinical picture**
   a. **Menometrorrhagia** (irregular, heavy bleeding) is the most characteristic symptom.
   b. Bleeding can be prolonged and heavy, in some cases leading to severe anemia.
   c. The condition is usually self-limited.

3. **Management.** Therapy involves the use of cyclic hormonal manipulation with progestins or combined oral contraceptive pills.

C **Amenorrhea** (see Chapter 20).   Primary amenorrhea is menarche that has not yet occurred; evaluation is indicated if menarche is delayed beyond 16 years of age. Chromosomal abnormalities account for approximately 30 to 40% of all cases of primary amenorrhea. Secondary amenorrhea is menstruation that ceases for more than 6 months.

1. **Müllerian anomalies** and **vaginal agenesis** cause amenorrhea in 20% of cases. The incidence of renal or urinary tract anomalies in patients with müllerian anomalies is approximately 45%. Treatment is usually surgical.
   a. **Mayer-Rokitansky-Küster-Hauser syndrome** involves vaginal agenesis with or without uterine agenesis. Adolescents may present with cyclic abdominal pain and amenorrhea when a partial endometrial cavity is present (see Chapter 20).
   b. **Imperforate hymen** results in obstructed outflow of menstrual blood. Affected patients present with amenorrhea and cyclic abdominal pain, and a bulging introitus is present on examination. An imperforate hymen is not a müllerian anomaly because the hymen is derived from the urogenital sinus.

2. **Hypogonadotropic hypogonadism.** This condition is characterized by a deficiency of pituitary or hypothalamic hormone secretion (particularly gonadotropin). It accounts for 40 to 50% of all cases of amenorrhea. The resulting hypoestrogenism in this form of amenorrhea may lead to the development of osteoporosis.
   a. **Kallmann syndrome** is a rare autosomal-dominant disorder that involves a deficiency of GnRH. It is associated with anosmia.
   b. **Central nervous system lesions,** including craniopharyngioma and pituitary adenoma, may cause hypogonadotropic amenorrhea.
   c. **Anorexia nervosa,** a condition characterized by extreme weight loss with no known organic cause, can affect adolescent development and result in amenorrhea. Psychiatric symptoms may be present, and occasionally the outcome is fatal.
   d. **Female athlete triad** is a syndrome defined by amenorrhea, an eating disorder, and osteoporosis. Typically, this condition is seen in athletes whose performance is enhanced by a lean physique, such as ballet dancers, ice skaters, and long-distance runners. The etiology most likely involves an inadequate caloric intake for the level of energy expended, which leads to hypoestrogenism and amenorrhea.

3. **Gonadal dysgenesis** (hypergonadotropic hypogonadism). This condition is characterized by absence of secondary sex characteristics, infantile but normal genitalia, and streaklike gonads that are devoid of germ cells and appear as fibrous white streaks. The presence of a Y chromosome dictates early removal of the gonads because of their propensity for malignancy (25% of cases occur by the age of 15 years). The different forms of gonadal dysgenesis are as follows:

   a. **Turner syndrome** (45,X) is characterized at birth by low weight, short stature, edema of the hands and feet, and loose skin folds on the neck. Adolescent patients have short stature, lack of sexual maturation, low posterior hairline, prominent ears, a broad chest, and epicanthal folds.

   b. **Swyer syndrome** (46,XY) is characterized by a female phenotype with amenorrhea and lack of secondary sex characteristics. Growth is usually normal, and some virilization may occur after puberty, especially when gonadal tumors are present. Swyer syndrome is inherited as an X-linked recessive trait. The clinical picture without virilization and tumor propensity may also occur in 46,XX individuals. This condition is termed pure gonadal dysgenesis and is an autosomal-recessive inheritance.

   c. **Mixed gonadal dysgenesis** (45,X/46,XY mosaicism) is characterized by sexual ambiguity in newborns. Internal structures include müllerian and wolffian derivatives. Asymmetric development of the gonads is expressed as a testis or gonadal tumor on one side with a streaklike, rudimentary gonad or no gonad on the other side.

   d. **Abnormalities of the X chromosome** (e.g., mosaicism, isochromosome, short-arm X deletion, long-arm X deletion, and translocation) result in amenorrhea and varying degrees of Turner syndrome.

4. **Ovarian failure.** This condition, which is rare in adolescents, is usually attributed to genetic defects (e.g., deletion of the long arm of the X chromosome), autoimmune conditions, radiation or chemotherapy for cancers, or galactosemia. Treatment involves estrogen and progesterone replacement; this condition is not usually reversible.

5. **Polycystic ovary syndrome.** This condition is the **most common cause of anovulation** and secondary amenorrhea in the adolescent age group. This syndrome is characterized by oligomenorrhea, hirsutism, and obesity, and it is associated with insulin resistance and the development of diabetes. Oral contraceptives are the mainstay of therapy for menstrual cycle regulation and control of hirsutism. In addition, weight loss effectively improves symptoms.

6. **Systemic illnesses.** Renal failure, diabetes mellitus, cystic fibrosis, and hemoglobinopathies (sickle cell anemia and thalassemia) may cause amenorrhea.

7. **Other endocrine gland disorders.** Thyroid disease, late-onset congenital adrenal hyperplasia, Cushing syndrome, and pituitary adenomas may all cause amenorrhea.

D **Contraception.** Most sexually active adolescents do not use contraception, especially at the time of the first sexual act. Because younger patients probably do not mention contraception, a discussion about the use of contraceptives and preventing the transmission of sexually transmitted diseases should follow a physical examination, regardless of whether the patient is sexually active.

E **Sexual abuse.** Defined as sexual touch by someone at least **5 years older than the adolescent,** sexual abuse incorporates a wide range of behavior, from coerced seduction to violent assault. Rape is a form of sexual abuse. Seven percent of American men and women between 18 and 22 years of age have experienced at least one episode of nonvoluntary sexual intercourse.

1. Lack of findings on examination does not mean that abuse did not occur. A thorough history, assessment of family and environment, and laboratory studies should accompany the examination to establish the diagnosis.

2. Follow-up studies suggest that many people, particularly adolescents, may remain disabled long after the abuse had ended.

Study Questions for Chapter 22

Directions: Each of the numbered items or incomplete statements in this section is followed by answers or by completions of the statement. Select the ONE lettered answer or completion that is BEST in each case.

1. Which of the following statements about the examination of a pediatric patient is true?

- **A** An adolescent female should have a pelvic examination for abnormal symptoms
- **B** Pediatric stirrups are useful during vaginoscopic examination
- **C** Sedation is rarely necessary to accomplish a genital examination
- **D** Rectal examination is more informative than a pelvic exam
- **E** Rapport can be established while performing a pelvic examination

2. An 8-year-old girl is brought to your office by her mother because of occasionally bloody vaginal discharge. Her mother suspects sexual abuse because she doesn't "know of any other way why a little girl should be bleeding from her vagina." She has no other medical history except for a throat infection a few weeks ago, which was treated with penicillin. On physical examination, she is has enlargement of both breasts and enlarged areola. There is no axillary hair growth. No pubic hair is apparent. The external genitalia have an age-appropriate clitoris and normal labia minora. There are no bruises, hematomas, or lacerations. You take a culture of the vaginal discharge, which is pink to red colored and not foul-smelling. You are not able to perform a more through examination. The most likely cause of her vaginal bleeding is

- **A** Precocious puberty
- **B** Sexual abuse
- **C** Foreign body
- **D** Bacterial infection
- **E** Pinworm

3. A 6-year-old girl is brought to your office because she has had four urinary tract infections within the last 3 months. While the mother is holding her, you examine her genitalia. There is lack of pubic hair. The labia minora are in apposition but are easily separable with gentle traction. You note a 1-cm sized clitoris. There is a 0.3 cm cystic structure in the inferior aspect of the urethra, which is nontender to cotton swab palpation; however, it has left a red hue on your cotton swab. You order a urinalysis and a urine culture and sensitivity. The safest and next best step in management is

- **A** Estrogen cream
- **B** Sitz baths
- **C** Intravenous pyelography
- **D** Low-potency steroid cream
- **E** Surgical repair

4. A 24-year-old gravida 1, para 1 just delivered a live female infant by natural birth. The infant weighed 3990 g and had APGARs of 8 and 9 at 1 and 5 minutes, respectively. Upon inspection of the neonate, the pediatricians are unable to assign a gender because there is clitoral hypertrophy and the labia majora are partially fused. You do not palpate any masses within them. The most important next step in management of this condition is

- **A** 17-OH-progesterone level
- **B** Dehydroepiandrosterone level
- **C** Serum sodium level
- **D** Tell the parents they have a baby girl
- **E** Karyotype

5. You are a world-renowned reproductive endocrinologist and are asked to make a diagnosis for a patient who has ambiguous genitalia. Here is the data:

Karyotype	XY
Spermatogenesis	absent
Müllerian structures	absent
Wolffian structures	present
External genitalia	male hypospadias
Breast	gynecomastia

The diagnosis is

A True hermaphroditism
B Mixed gonadal dysgenesis
C Swyer syndrome
D Complete androgen insensitivity
E Reifenstein syndrome

Answers and Explanations

1. The answer is D [I C]. The rectal examination is often more informative than a vaginal examination because the short posterior vaginal fornix cannot be distended and a cul-de-sac does not exist. A complete physical examination before a pelvic examination can help establish rapport. There is no need for a female adolescent to have a pelvic examination if noninvasive imaging (MRI or ultrasound) can elucidate the problem. Stirrups are not necessary, and the simple "frog-leg" position will suffice when examining the preadolescent patient. Frequently, intravenous sedation or examination under general anesthesia is necessary to accomplish a thorough genital examination.

2. The answer is D [II E 1 b 2]. Given the clinical scenario, the only cause that is consistent is hemolytic streptococcal throat infection which has translated into vaginitis weeks later. Although sexual abuse should always be suspected with bloody vaginal discharge, the evidence is lacking, and the mother has no good reason to believe that her daughter has been sexually abused. Precocious puberty is unlikely in an 8-year-old girl with isolated development of the breast (thelarche) without pubarche. Pinworm would present with intense vaginal and perianal itching, especially at night. Given her older age and lack of information in the clinical scenario (especially because the discharge is not foul-smelling), foreign body is less likely.

3. The answer is B [II D 2 a]. The diagnosis is prolapsed urethra, characterized by a small, hemorrhagic, friable (blood on cotton swab), painless mass surrounding the urethra. The safest and least expensive initial therapy is sitz baths. The bathtub is filled with lukewarm water with or without Epsom salt, and the patient sits in the bathtub a few times each day. Estrogen cream may stimulate breast growth and vaginal bleeding. Intravenous pyelography would be useful if the diagnosis was ectopic ureter. Low-potency steroid creams are useful for lichen sclerosus. Surgical repair of prolapsed urethra is not necessary unless the patient has urinary retention or necrosis is present.

4. The answer is C [V A 2]. Because congenital adrenal hyperplasia (CAH), especially 21-hydroxylase deficiency, is the most common cause of distinct virilization of the female newborn, efforts should be made to obtain serum electrolytes immediately because the salt-wasting type of CAH can be life-threatening. Diagnosis of CAH is best accomplished by finding elevated levels of 17-OH-progesterone. A karyotype can be ordered later to rule out other causes of ambiguous genitalia, such as hermaphroditism and mixed gonadal dysgenesis. You should not assign a gender until you have all of the information.

5. The answer is E [V E 1 e]. This is a difficult question! The two most important syndromes that have an XY karyotype are the androgen insensitivity syndromes (AIS) [incomplete, Reifenstein, 5 α-reductase] and Swyer syndrome. Complete androgen insensitivity syndrome (CAIS) has the following features: XY, no spermatogenesis, absent Müllerian structures, absent Wolffian structures, *female external genitalia*, and female breast development. Reifenstein syndrome is exactly the same as CAIS except for more "male influence": Wolffian structures are present, external genitalia are male (male hypospadias) and breasts are not as well developed (gynecomastia). Swyer syndrome is different from the AIS in that there is more of a "female influence." This syndrome is characterized by the *presence of Müllerian structures, absence of Wolffian structures*, infantile female external genitalia, and lack of breast development. Mixed gonadal dysgenesis is characterized by mosaicism for 45 X/46 XY. There is usually a streak gonad on one side and a functioning testis on the other side. Both Wolffian and Müllerian structures are present and the external genitalia are ambiguous (although a wide range of phenotypes is possible). A true hermaphrodite has both testicular tissue (XY genotype plus testicular tissue histology) and ovarian tissue (XX genotype plus ovarian tissue histology). One gonad can be a testis and the other an ovary, or one gonad can have both tissue types ("ovotestis"). True hermaphrodites have ambiguous external genitalia, which are most often more in the male spectrum than in the female. They also have gynecomastia.

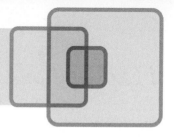

chapter 23

Hirsutism

BETH W. RACKOW AND SAMANTHA M. PFEIFER

I   INTRODUCTION

Increased hair growth in women may be associated with normal or increased levels of **circulating androgens.** It is important to view hirsutism as a potential endocrine abnormality as well as a psychological and cosmetic problem.

A Definitions

1. **Types of hair**
   a. **Lanugo** is soft, short hair covering the fetus that is shed in late gestation and during the neonatal period.
   b. **Vellus** is soft, fine, unpigmented hair that covers apparently hairless areas of the body.
   c. **Terminal** is longer, coarse, pigmented hair that may grow in response to sex hormones (e.g., over the chin and abdomen of men) or may be sex hormone–independent (e.g., eyebrows and eyelashes).
2. **Hypertrichosis** is excessive growth of androgen-independent hair in nonsexual areas, such as forearms and legs.
3. **Hirsutism** is the presence of terminal hair in androgen-dependent sites where hair does not normally grow in women. This hair growth is located predominantly on midline portions of the body, including the face, chest, abdomen, and inner thigh.
4. **Virilization** is hirsutism associated with other signs of hyperandrogenism, such as increased muscle mass, clitorimegaly, temporal balding, voice deepening, and increased libido. It can also be associated with signs of defeminization, such as decreased breast size and loss of vaginal lubrication.

B Etiology.   Hair growth, and thus hirsutism, is regulated by:

1. **Number and concentration of hair follicles.** This varies according to racial and ethnic background but not gender. For example, Asian women generally have low concentrations of hair follicles, and hirsutism is rarely seen in these individuals.
2. Degree to which hair follicles are sensitive to androgens and able to convert vellus hairs to terminal hairs
3. **Degree of 5α-reductase activity** in the skin, which determines local androgen activity
4. Ratio of growth to resting phases in affected hair follicles
5. Thickness and degree to which individual hairs are pigmented

II   ANDROGENS

These steroids promote the development of male secondary sexual characteristics. In women, androgens are mainly produced by the adrenal gland, the ovary, and peripheral transformation. Testosterone is the most potent androgen; androstenedione, dehydroepiandrosterone (DHEA), and DHEA sulfate (DHEAS) are less potent.

A **Testosterone.** Blood testosterone levels are a function of blood production rates and metabolic clearance rates; thus, these levels may not represent the actual state of androgenicity.

1. **Total testosterone** levels in women are usually less than 70 ng/dL.

2. Sources:
   a. Ovarian 25% (in stroma and follicles)
   b. Adrenal origin 25%
   c. Peripheral transformation of androstenedione to testosterone 50%

3. Free testosterone
   a. Most testosterone in the blood circulates bound to **albumin** (19%) or to **sex hormone– binding globulin (SHBG)** (80%).
      (1) Normal women (1%)
      (2) Hirsute women (2%)
      (3) Men (2 to 3%)
   b. Androgenicity depends mainly on the unbound fraction of testosterone because this represents the active form of the hormone.

B **Sex hormone–binding globulin**

1. An inverse relationship exists between SHBG and the percentage of free testosterone. As SHBG decreases, the percentage of free testosterone increases; as SHBG increases, the percentage of free testosterone decreases. However, the total testosterone level may remain normal.
   a. Factors that decrease plasma SHBG
      (1) Obesity
      (2) Increased androgen production
      (3) Hyperinsulinemia
      (4) Corticosteroid therapy
      (5) Hypothyroidism
      (6) Acromegaly
   b. Factors that increase plasma SHBG
      (1) Estrogen therapy
      (2) Pregnancy
      (3) Hyperthyroidism
      (4) Cirrhosis

2. In general, hirsute women have reduced serum concentrations of SHBG.

C **5α-Reductase**

1. 5α-Reductase converts testosterone to **dihydrotestosterone (DHT)** in androgen-sensitive tissues such as hair follicles and skin. Levels of this enzyme are significantly elevated in the skin of hirsute women compared with control subjects. The enzyme activity is partly stimulated by elevated circulating testosterone levels.

2. Dihydrotestosterone is responsible for stimulating hair growth and is two to three times as potent as testosterone.

3. **3α-androstanediol glucuronide (3α-AG)** is the peripheral tissue metabolite of DHT. Although it has been used as a marker of target tissue cellular action, it is not often used clinically.

D **Pathophysiology of androgens in hirsutism.** A combination of the following factors results in hirsutism:

1. Increased concentration of serum androgens, especially free testosterone

2. Decreased levels of SHBG, resulting in increased bioavailable androgen

3. Increased activity of 5α-reductase

III DIAGNOSIS

A **History.** Several factors are important.

1. **Onset of hirsutism**
   a. **Gradual onset** of hirsutism is associated with acne, oily skin, weight gain, and irregular menstrual cycles. This suggests an underlying endocrine condition, such as polycystic ovary syndrome (PCOS).
   b. **Abrupt onset** or rapidly worsening hirsutism with signs of virilization should prompt concern for an androgen-producing tumor.

2. Presence or absence of **virilization**

3. **Drug ingestion.** Drugs are usually associated with hypertrichosis, but androgenic drugs (e.g., steroids and phenytoin) may cause hirsutism.

4. **Family history.** A family history of hirsutism may indicate an inherited disorder (i.e., familial hypertrichosis).

5. **Ethnic background.** The pattern of hair growth is genetically predetermined and is associated with differences in 5α-reductase activity at hair follicles.

6. **Local trauma.** Changes in skin and hair growth may occur.

7. **Regularity of menstrual cycles**
   a. Patients with regular menstrual cycles and hirsutism often have idiopathic, ethnic, or familial hirsutism.
   b. Some anovulatory hirsute patients (as many as 40%) appear to have regular menstrual cycles; thus, testing is necessary to determine whether ovulation is occurring.

8. **History of infertility**

B **Differential diagnosis**

1. **Polycystic ovary syndrome** (see Chapter 20, IID1). This heterogeneous endocrine, metabolic, and genetic disorder is seen in 5 to 10% of the general population and is the cause of androgen excess in 65 to 85% of hirsute patients. This syndrome is characterized by hyperandrogenism, oligomenorrhea or amenorrhea (caused by chronic anovulation), and obesity. It is associated with insulin resistance. Patients usually present with hirsutism, menstrual irregularity, and infertility.
   a. The fundamental pathophysiologic defect is not known.
   b. Increased production of androgens may result in:
      (1) Increased secretion of luteinizing hormone (LH) from the anterior pituitary, leading to increased ovarian androgen production
      (2) Insulin resistance and compensatory hyperinsulinemia, stimulating ovarian and adrenal androgen production by direct and indirect mechanisms
   c. Gonadotropin regulation of the menstrual cycle is disrupted, leading to oligo-ovulation or anovulation and menstrual irregularity.
   d. Increased androgen levels inhibit follicular development in the ovary; thus, multiple small atretic follicles are produced. These "polycystic ovaries" are therefore a reflection of the hormonal environment within the ovary rather than the cause of the disorder.
   e. Affected patients are at increased risk for endometrial hyperplasia or cancer, glucose intolerance, type 2 diabetes mellitus, hyperlipidemia, and cardiovascular disease.

2. **HAIR-AN syndrome** (hyperandrogenism, insulin resistance, and acanthosis nigricans syndrome)
   a. This condition is similar to PCOS, but patients have a greater degree of insulin resistance and hyperinsulinemia.
   b. This disorder is often inherited.
   c. Severe abnormalities of insulin action cause hyperinsulinemia, which stimulates excess ovarian androgen secretion.

3. **Idiopathic hirsutism.** This condition, which accounts for 15 to 30% of hirsute women, is caused by end-organ (skin) hypersensitivity to androgens. Characteristics include:
   a. Regular ovulatory menstrual cycles
   b. Normal circulating androgen levels
   c. Increased peripheral conversion of androgens caused by **increased skin 5α-reductase activity**

4. **Nonclassical (adult-onset) adrenal hyperplasia.** This condition is present in approximately 1% of hyperandrogenic women.
   a. **Deficiency in activity of adrenal enzymes** and thus formation of excess cortisol precursors (e.g., 17-hydroxyprogesterone [17-OHP] and androstenedione) leads to increased production of androgens. The most common enzyme deficiency is 21-hydroxylase.
   b. Inheritance is autosomal recessive, and occurrence is increased in Ashkenazi Jews.
   c. Deficiencies of adrenal enzymes 11β-hydroxylase and 3β-hydroxysteroid dehydrogenase are less common.

5. **Cushing syndrome**
   a. **Adrenocortical hyperfunction** leads to excess production of corticosteroids as well as hyperandrogenism, menstrual irregularities, glucose intolerance, and obesity.
   b. Causes are multiple and include adrenal neoplasm, ectopic adrenocorticotropic hormone (ACTH)–producing tumor, and pituitary tumor or Cushing disease.

6. **Androgen-producing tumors** are associated with sudden-onset hyperandrogenic state, rapid progression, and frank virilization.
   a. **Ovarian tumors** (e.g., Sertoli-Leydig cell tumor, granulosa-theca cell tumor, thecoma, luteoma of pregnancy)
   b. **Adrenal tumors**

7. **Disorders of pituitary origin**
   a. Hyperprolactinemia
   b. Acromegaly

8. **Androgenic drug exposure**
   a. **Without virilization:** phenytoin, diazoxide, minoxidil, danazol, corticosteroids, cyclosporin
   b. **With potential virilization:** anabolic steroids, androgen therapy, or supplements

9. **Y-containing mosaics** and **incomplete androgen insensitivity.** These patients show signs of androgen stimulation at puberty.

C **Laboratory evaluation**

1. **Serum testosterone** (see II A) is a marker of ovarian and adrenal activity.
   a. **Total testosterone levels greater than 200 ng/dL** suggest an androgen-producing tumor. However, 10 to 20% of patients with androgen-producing tumors may have low testosterone levels. Imaging is warranted.
      (1) **Pelvic ultrasound** is best to provide an image of the ovaries.
      (2) **Computed tomography or magnetic resonance imaging** views the adrenal glands.
   b. **Total testosterone levels less than 200 ng/dL** are associated with anovulation and hirsutism. The most likely diagnosis is PCOS.

2. **Serum DHEAS** is almost exclusively produced by the adrenal glands and reflects adrenal androgen activity.
   a. **Levels greater than 700 μg/dl** suggest an adrenal tumor.
   b. Moderately elevated DHEAS levels may occur with anovulation, PCOS, or adrenal hyperplasia.
   c. Normal DHEAS levels indicate that adrenal disease is less probable and that ovarian androgen production is more likely.

3. Elevated levels of **serum androstenedione** suggest ovarian disease.

4. Serum 17-OHP

    a. 17-OHP is elevated in 21-hydroxylase deficiency, the most common form of nonclassical adrenal hyperplasia. Normal values should be less than 200 ng/dL.

    b. Circumstances under which 17-OHP must be measured:

        (1) Early in the morning because of diurnal variation of adrenal secretion

        (2) In the follicular phase of the menstrual cycle in ovulatory women to avoid confusion with ovarian production of this hormone

    c. Baseline values greater than 200 ng/dL are abnormal and should be further evaluated with the ACTH stimulation test to confirm the diagnosis of nonclassical adrenal hyperplasia.

5. Increased production of **cortisol** is associated with Cushing syndrome. Diagnosis is made by:

    a. 1-mg overnight dexamethasone suppression test

    b. 24-hour urinary-free cortisol excretion

6. Gonadotropins may be useful. An elevated LH:follicle-stimulating hormone (FSH) ratio (2–3:1) suggests PCOS. However, this finding is not present in approximately 40% of patients with PCOS.

7. Serum 3α-AG is rarely measured. Increased levels of 3α-AG indicate an increased activity of 5α-reductase in the periphery and measure peripheral target tissue activity.

8. The evaluation of irregular menstrual cycles and hirsutism also includes **thyroid-stimulating hormone and prolactin.**

IV TREATMENT

A combination of hormonal suppression of hair growth and mechanical hair removal offers the most complete and effective treatment for patients with hirsutism.

A Goals

1. The major goal is **arresting the virilizing process**, not removing hair. Once terminal hair has been established, withdrawal of androgens does not affect the established hair pattern.

2. Amelioration of a specific disease state helps slow the rate of growth by **preventing the establishment of new hair follicles.**

3. Results may not be apparent for 6 to 12 months. Treatment of hirsutism is a **long-term process.**

B Elimination of specific causes

1. Removal of ovarian or adrenal tumors

2. Elimination of drugs suspected to contribute to the abnormal hair growth

3. Treatment of Cushing syndrome, thyroid disease, or hyperprolactinemia

4. Bilateral salpingo-oophorectomy with or without hysterectomy. This procedure is an option for women who have persistent or progressive hirsutism or who have a contraindication to hormones or other medications and do not desire fertility.

C Suppression of androgen synthesis

1. In most **idiopathic or ovarian-related hirsutism**, suppression of ovarian steroidogenesis is the goal.

2. Combination oral contraceptives have a potent negative feedback effect on the pituitary and other effects that ameliorate peripheral androgen stimulation. Low-dose formulations (less than 50 μg estrogen) are effective in treating hirsutism, and a demonstrated benefit has been shown with 20-μg preparations.

    a. Both **estrogen** and **progestin** in the oral contraceptives cause a decrease in gonadotropin secretion with a consequent decrease in ovarian androgen production.

        (1) Estrogen also stimulates an increase in SHBG, causing increased binding of testosterone and decreased free testosterone levels.

(2) **Progestin** also may displace active androgens at the hair follicle and may inhibit 5α-reductase activity.

b. Blood testosterone levels are effectively suppressed within 1 to 3 months of therapy. This reduction has been associated with a clinical improvement in the progression of hirsutism.

3. **Medroxyprogesterone acetate** (150 mg intramuscularly every 3 months or 10 to 20 mg orally per day) is effective in suppressing gonadotropin secretion in patients for whom oral contraceptives are contraindicated. It results in:
   a. Decreased production of androgens caused by suppression of LH and FSH
   b. Increased clearance of testosterone from the circulation caused by induction of liver enzymes

4. **Gonadotropin-releasing hormone (GnRH) agonists** suppress the hypothalamic-pituitary-ovarian axis, thereby decreasing ovarian steroidogenesis.
   a. Uses
      (1) In severely androgenized patients refractory to other therapies
      (2) With estrogen and progesterone replacement, and calcium supplements
   b. Side effects include hot flashes, vaginal dryness, and bone loss.

5. **Corticosteroid** suppression of adrenal androgen production is useful in more severe cases of congenital adrenal hyperplasia (CAH). For mild cases of nonclassical CAH, patients can instead be managed effectively with oral contraceptives and antiandrogen therapy. Long-term side effects include osteoporosis, diabetes mellitus, and avascular necrosis of the hip, which dictate careful use of this medication.

D Androgen-receptor blockers. These medications inhibit binding of DHT to the androgen receptor, thus directly inhibiting hair growth. When combined with oral contraceptives, progestins, or GnRH agonists, further benefit may be obtained.

1. **Spironolactone** is an aldosterone antagonist and diuretic.
   a. This agent also inhibits 5α-reductase and variably suppresses the ovarian and adrenal synthesis of androgens.
   c. Side effects include initial diuresis and fatigue. Hyperkalemia and hypotension may also occur.

2. **Flutamide** is a nonsteroidal antiandrogen.
   a. Side effects include hepatotoxicity; liver enzymes must be monitored.
   b. Contraception must be used with this medication because flutamide may be teratogenic to a male fetus.

3. **Cyproterone acetate** is a potent progestin and antiandrogen.
   a. This agent inhibits gonadotropin secretion (primarily LH), which leads to decreased androgen levels.
   b. It is not currently available in the United States. It is used as a progestin in oral contraceptives.

E Other medications

1. **Finasteride** inhibits 5α-reductase activity with negligible side effects.
   a. This agent blocks the conversion of testosterone to DHT.
   b. Contraception must be used with this medication because DHT is necessary in the development of genitalia in a male fetus.

2. **Cimetidine** is a less potent androgen-receptor blocker.

3. **Ketoconazole** blocks ovarian and adrenal androgen synthesis by inhibition of the cytochrome P450 system. This agent has multiple side effects, including the potential for hepatotoxicity and adrenal insufficiency. Therefore, it is rarely used for hirsutism.

4. **Insulin-sensitizing agents.** Metformin and thiazolidinediones are being used in patients with PCOS to improve insulin sensitivity, thus decreasing hyperinsulinemia and androgen levels.

Improvement in menstrual cyclicity has been demonstrated, but there is little information regarding the effect on hirsutism. These agents are not approved by the U.S. Food and Drug Administration for treatment of hirsutism.

5. **Eflornithine hydrochloride** is a new topical cream that decreases or arrests facial hair growth through inhibition of the enzyme ornithine decarboxylase at the hair follicle.

F **Supportive measures**

1. **Shaving, tweezing, waxing,** and use of **depilatories** are temporary measures, which may need to be repeated daily. These methods neither stimulate hair growth nor increase the rate of hair growth.

2. **Bleaching** is effective for mild hair growth.

3. **Electrolysis** involves the permanent destruction of hair follicles. Multiple treatments are necessary, and scarring may occur. This method should be used after 6 months of hormonal therapy when new hair growth has ceased.

4. **Laser epilation** provides directed damage to hair follicles, which temporarily or permanently removes terminal hair. This method can be used over a larger area than electrolysis, but it is not yet perfected for the treatment of hirsutism.

Study Questions for Chapter 23

Directions: *Match the appropriate hormone(s), substance, or enzyme (which you could measure) with the description that is most likely to account for excessive hair growth in a woman. Each answer may be used once, more than once, or not at all.*

QUESTIONS 1–3

[A] Androstenedione
[B] 3α-androstanediol glucuronide
[C] Dehydroepiandrosterone sulfate (DHEA-S)
[D] 5α-reductase
[E] 17-hydroxyprogesterone

1. Hypertrichosis in skin of legs and forearms of Mediterranean women

2. Ovary as a potential source of androgen excess

3. Hyperplasia of adrenal gland as source of androgen excess

Directions: *Each of the numbered items or incomplete statements in this section is followed by answers or by completions of the statement. Select the ONE lettered answer or completion that is BEST in each case.*

QUESTIONS 4–6

4. A 33-year-old woman, gravida 2, para 1, SAB 1 presents to your office reporting increasing dark hair growth on her chin, upper lip, and lower abdomen. This growth has occurred over many years and has forced her to wax and bleach more often. She denies changes in her voice, size of her clitoris, reduction in breast size, or acne. During her early teen years, she had regular menstrual periods that lasted 4 to 5 days. Now, however, she has to take birth control pills to regulate her cycles. Her past medical history is significant for hepatitis C, which she acquired from a blood transfusion to treat postpartum hemorrhage with her first pregnancy. The next best step in the management of hirsutism in this patient is

[A] Depo-medroxyprogesterone acetate
[B] Flutamide
[C] Spironolactone
[D] Dexamethasone
[E] Leuprolide

5. A 23-year-old woman, gravida 1, para 0, tab 1 has irregular, unpredictable menstrual periods every 30 to 90 days. Physical examination reveals acne on her face and back and several dark, coarse hairs on her chin and lower abdomen. The initial step in diagnosis of androgen excess in this woman is to measure which of the following?

[A] Androstenedione
[B] Dehydroepiandrosterone sulfate
[C] LH and FSH
[D] Free testosterone
[E] 5α-reductase

6. A 20-year-old woman is given depot-medroxyprogesterone acetate every 3 months as a means of birth control. After 8 months, she notices decrease in hair growth in her upper lip, chin, and lower abdomen. The primary mechanism shared by depot-medroxyprogesterone acetate and combination oral contraceptive pills that is responsible for this occurrence involves

- A Increase in sex hormone binding globulin (SHBG)
- B Decrease in gonadotropin release
- C Displacement of androgen molecules at the hair follicle
- D Inhibition of 5α-reductase
- E Induction of liver enzymes

Answers and Explanations

1. D [I A 2 and II C 1 and 3] **2. A** [III C 3] **3. E** [III C 4]. Excessive hair growth is caused by the concentration of hair follicles in the skin (which is genetically determined), degree of 5α-reductase activity, and the sensitivity or response of hair follicles to DHT. 3α-androstanediol glucuronide is the peripheral tissue metabolite of DHT. It is rarely measured for clinical purposes. Androstenedione is an androgen that is secreted chiefly by the ovary. Thus, measurement of androstenedione levels is a good screening test when the ovary is suspected of being the source of excess androgen. 21-hydroxylase deficiency is the cause of the most common form of non-classical adrenal hyperplasia (CAH). Although moderately elevated DHEA-S may occur with adrenal hyperplasia, measurement of 17-OHP is diagnostic for CAH. The diagnosis can be made by measuring 17-OHP.

4. The answer is C [IV D 1]. The best complement to oral contraceptive pills in the treatment of hirsutism is spironolactone. The mechanism is as follows: it binds to the androgen receptor, preventing the binding of DHT and thus inhibiting hair growth; it also inhibits 5α-reductase and thus the production of DHT. Depo-medroxyprogesterone acetate works similarly to oral contraceptive pills (OCPs) in that it suppresses gonadotropins, which decrease ovarian androgen production. Flutamide, another androgen receptor blocker, is contraindicated because of hepatotoxicity. Dexamethasone, a glucocorticoid, suppresses pituitary corticotrophin and thus adrenal androgen production, but this drug is used only in patients with elevated adrenal androgen production. GnRH agonists suppress the hypothalamic-pituitary-ovarian axis, which decreases ovarian stimulation and steroidogenesis. This medication is used infrequently for this indication and is not added to OCPs.

5. The answer is D [II A 3]. Free testosterone is the biologically active form of testosterone and is thus the best marker of androgen excess. However, this test does not indicate the source of the excess androgens. The LH to FSH ratio may suggest the diagnosis of polycystic ovary syndrome (PCOS) in some patients. Elevated androstenedione indicates the ovary as the source of androgens. Serum DHEAS reflects adrenal androgen production. 5α-reductase activity reflects levels of DHT at the skin and can be evaluated by measuring levels of the 3α-androstanediol glucuronide.

6. The answer is B [IV C 2 a and IV C 3]. Both medroxyprogesterone acetate and combination OCPs suppress gonadotropin release with consequent decrease in ovarian androgen production. Only OCPs cause an increase in SHBG, which binds free testosterone, leaving less available to interact at its target sites. The progestin component of combination OCPs displaces active androgens at the hair follicle and inhibits 5α-reductase. Medroxyprogesterone acetate increases clearance of testosterone from the circulation by inducing liver enzymes.

chapter 24

Family Planning: Contraception and Complications

MOLINA B. DAYAL AND STEVEN SONDHEIMER

I CONTRACEPTIVE EFFICACY

This value is the number of pregnancies per 100 women-years or the number of pregnancies in 100 sexually active, fertile women who use a given method of contraception for 1 year. The expected pregnancy rate in women using no method of contraception is 85 pregnancies per 100 women-years.

II BARRIER METHODS

A **Condoms.** One of the oldest surviving forms of birth control, condoms are effective, safe, and relatively inexpensive. Moreover, their effects are reversible. Condoms are highly effective when used consistently.

1. **Mode of action.** Both female and male condoms act as physical barriers to semen.

2. **Advantages**
   a. **Protection from sexually transmitted diseases (STDs)**
      (1) **Latex condoms protect against STDs** caused by herpes simplex virus, *Neisseria gonorrhoeae*, *Chlamydia trachomatis*, *Ureaplasma urealyticum*, *Mycoplasma hominis*, *Trichomonas vaginalis*, *Treponema pallidum*, and HIV, but not human papilloma virus.
      (2) **Natural, or nonlatex, condoms do not protect against most STDs** because they contain small pores that allow passage of microbes.
   b. **Easy accessibility**
   c. **Few side effects**

3. **Disadvantages**
   a. Must be used in each act of intercourse
   b. Unacceptability by some partners

4. **Types of condoms**
   a. **Female condoms** line the entire surface of the vagina and partially shield the perineum. They can be inserted up to 8 hours in advance but should be removed immediately after each act of intercourse. Female condoms should not be used in conjunction with male condoms.
   b. **Male condoms** cover the glans and the shaft of the penis and must be used from the beginning to the end of each act of intercourse to be effective. Some condoms contain spermicidal agents. **Condoms impregnated with spermicide are no more effective than condoms alone.**

5. **Efficacy.** Pregnancy rate is 3–21:100 women-years of use.

B **Spermicides.**   Creams, jellies, aerosol foams, nonfoaming and foaming suppositories, and vaginal films are commonly used with other forms of contraception, such as diaphragms, sponges, and condoms. Only about 3% of women use spermicides alone.

1. **Mode of action.** Spermicides serve as a **chemical barrier** to sperm. The **active agents** in spermicides (e.g., nonoxynol 9) disrupt the outer lipoprotein surface layer of spermatozoa, killing the sperm, decreasing their motility, or inactivating the enzymes needed to penetrate the ova.

2. **Advantages**
   a. Increased efficacy of vaginal sponges, diaphragms, and cervical caps
   b. Easy accessibility
   c. No need for medical consultation
   d. Few side effects

3. **Disadvantages**
   a. Need for insertion with each act of intercourse
   b. Limited time of effectiveness
   c. Possible increase in the risk of HIV transmission caused by disruption of vaginal epithelium. Well-designed studies are needed to address this issue in normal use.

4. **Efficacy. Pregnancy rate** is as much as 26 in 100 women-years of use. Efficacy depends on the couple's motivation to use spermicides correctly with every act of intercourse.

C **Vaginal sponges**

1. **Mode of action.** Vaginal sponges release spermicide during coitus, absorb ejaculate, and physically block the entrance to the cervical canal.

2. **Advantages**
   a. Use for as long as 24 hours regardless of frequency of sexual intercourse
   b. Few systemic side effects

3. **Efficacy. Pregnancy rate** is 40 in 100 women-years of use in parous women, and 20 in 100 women-years of use in nulliparous women.

D **Diaphragms.**   These dome-shaped shaped contraceptives are 50 to 105 mm in diameter and are made of latex rubber. They rest between the posterior aspect of the symphysis pubis and the posterior fornix of the vagina, thus covering the anterior vaginal wall and the cervix.

1. **Mode of action.** Diaphragms act as physical barriers to sperm and are effective vehicles for holding spermicide over the cervix.

2. **Advantages**
   a. Contraception for up to 6 hours after placement
   b. Some protection against cervical dysplasia
   c. Few side effects

3. **Disadvantages**
   a. Need to keep in place for at least 6 hours after intercourse to ensure that no motile sperm are left in the vagina
   b. Requirement for use with a spermicidal agent
   c. Need to replace spermicide with each act of intercourse
   d. Twice the incidence of urinary tract infections
   e. Needs to be fit by a clinician

4. **Efficacy. Pregnancy rate** is reported to be 5 to 10 in 100 woman-years of use.

E **Cervical caps.**   These contraceptives are as effective as diaphragms but are more difficult to fit.

1. **Mode of action.** The cervical cap has the same mode of action as the diaphragm.

2. Advantages

a. Ability to leave in place up to 48 hours (compared to 6 hours with the diaphragm), regardless of number of acts of intercourse

b. Effectiveness without the addition of a spermicidal agent

3. Disadvantages

a. Need to keep in place for at least 6 hours after intercourse (same as the diaphragm)

b. Few physicians are trained in the placement and use of the cervical cap.

4. Efficacy. Pregnancy rate is reported to be about 5 to 10 in 100 woman-years of use.

III INTRAUTERINE DEVICES (IUDs)

These reversible methods of contraception are one of the most widely used throughout the world. IUDs are extremely effective in reducing the risk of pregnancy. The copper IUD (ParaGard) and the progestin-only IUD (Mirena) are currently available in the United States. Both IUDs have multiple mechanisms of action but primarily act by preventing sperm mobility and oocyte fertilization. Evidence does not support the claim that IUDs are abortifacients.

A Types

1. The **copper-impregnated IUD** is approved for 10 continuous years of use.

2. The **progestin-only IUD,** with levonorgestrel 20, is approved for 5 years and then must be replaced.

B Mode of action

1. **Copper-impregnated IUD**

   a. This IUD causes a local, sterile inflammatory reaction in the uterus, and the intrauterine environment becomes spermicidal.

   b. The copper intensifies the inflammation in the uterine cavity, producing a lining that is unfavorable for implantation.

2. **Progestin-only IUD**

   a. This IUD exerts its contraceptive effect locally on the endometrium and the cervix. Progestin alters the endometrium, rendering it unfavorable for implantation.

   b. In addition, both uterine and tubal motility are impaired, thereby impairing sperm-egg interaction. Thickening of the cervical mucus makes the passage of sperm difficult.

C Advantages. These IUDs do not interfere with lactation and are independent of sexual intercourse.

1. **Copper-impregnated IUD**

   a. As many as 10 years of contraceptive efficacy from one IUD

   b. Can be inserted at any time during the menstrual cycle

   c. Resumption of fertility on removal

2. **Progestin-only IUD**

   a. As many as 5 years of contraceptive efficacy from one IUD

   b. Useful for treatment of menorrhagia (heavy menstrual bleeding) and dysmenorrhea (painful menses)

   c. Resumption of fertility on removal of the IUD

D Disadvantages

1. **Insertion.** Although the copper-impregnated IUD may be inserted at any time during the menstrual cycle, the progestin-only IUD should be inserted within the first 7 days.

2. **Uterine perforation.** This complication occurs in about 1 in 1000 insertions and should be suspected if the patient can no longer feel the string.

3. **Infection.** Risk is highest in the first 2 weeks after insertion because of possible introduction of bacteria into uterine cavity at the time of insertion. The risk of infection increases in women with a history of recent pelvic infection and multiple sexual partners.

E **Efficacy.** **Pregnancy rate** among users of either type of IUD is less than 2 to 3 in 100 women-years of use.

F **Contraindications**

1. Having multiple sexual partners or having a partner who has other partners at risk for STDs
2. Recent (less than 3 month) history of endometritis or purulent cervicitis
3. Known or suspected pregnancy
4. Distorted uterine cavity (increases expulsion rate)

G **Pregnancy-related issues.** If a woman becomes pregnant with an IUD in place, it should be removed immediately because the IUD increases the risk of pregnancy loss and preterm labor. In addition, the risk of increased infection necessitates the removal of the IUD early in pregnancy.

1. The **spontaneous abortion rate** is about 50% if an IUD remains in place. The risk of miscarriage after removal in early pregnancy is about 20 to 30%.
2. In general, **ectopic pregnancy** is prevented by both the progestin-only and copper-impregnated IUDs. If a pregnancy does occur with an IUD in place, about 5% of women have an ectopic pregnancy.
3. The chance of a **premature birth** is 12 to 15% in pregnancies when an IUD is left in place. This is thought to occur because of IUD irritation of the myometrium during the third trimester.

IV **PROGESTIN-ONLY METHODS**

A **Mode of action**

1. Diminishing and thickening cervical mucus, thereby preventing sperm penetration
2. Inhibiting ovulation by suppressing the midcycle peaks of luteinizing hormone (LH) and follicle-stimulating hormone (FSH)
3. Producing a thin, atrophic endometrium, precluding implantation
4. Reducing the ciliary action of the fallopian tube, preventing sperm and egg transport
5. Diminishing the function of the corpus luteum

B **"Minipill"** (Micronor, others). Less than 1% of oral contraceptive prescriptions in the United States are for this progestin-only oral contraceptive, which is generally less effective than the combined oral contraceptives.

1. Advantages
   a. No alteration of milk production and nearly 100% effectiveness in breastfeeding women
   b. Tolerance in women who are unable to take estrogen
   c. Independent of sexual intercourse
2. Disadvantages
   a. Irregular vaginal bleeding
   b. No protection against STDs
   c. Need for daily administration
      (1) Progestin-only pills are taken continuously for 28 days without a pill-free interval. Because these pills have a dose of progestin that is very close to the threshold of contraceptive efficacy, they must be taken at approximately the same time each day.

(2) Suppressed ovulation occurs in approximately one half of cycles, and contraceptive efficacy depends on the other progestin-related mechanisms previously listed (see IV A).

3. Efficacy. Pregnancy rate is 5 in 100 woman-years of use. Consistent administration is necessary. A difference of a few hours may contribute to reduced contraceptive protection.[pa

C **Injectable progestin.** Medroxyprogesterone (Depo-Provera), the most commonly used injectable form of contraception, is given as a deep intramuscular injection every 12 weeks. Menstrual patterns may be irregular during the first year of use; this is a common reason for discontinuation. Fifty percent of women develop amenorrhea within 1 year of use.

1. Advantages
   a. Effectiveness for 12 weeks
   b. Independent of sexual intercourse
   c. Safe for use during breastfeeding
   d. Women on antiepileptic medications may have fewer seizures, and those with sickle cell disease may have fewer sickle cell crises.

2. Disadvantages
   a. No protection against STDs
   b. Irregular bleeding and spotting
   c. Weight gain (year one, 5 lb; year two, 16 lb)
   d. Prolonged return of fertility (median time from discontinuation to return of fertility, 8.5 months)

3. Efficacy. Pregnancy rate is less than 1 in 100 women-years of use.

D **Implantable progestin.** Implantable progestin-containing rods release hormones at a low but constant rate.

1. Advantages
   a. Effectiveness for up to 3 to 5 years
   b. Independent of sexual intercourse
   c. Almost immediate return of fertility after removal

2. Disadvantages
   a. Menstrual irregularity
   b. No protection against STDs
   c. Weight gain
   d. Higher rate of failure with high patient weight
   e. Need for surgical placement and removal
   f. Less effective in women who take antiseizure medications or rifampin

3. Efficacy. Pregnancy rate is less than 1 in 100 women-years of use.

4. Specific types of implants
   a. Original form (Norplant) is no longer manufactured. Six implants each contain levonorgestrel and are effective for up to 5 years.
   b. Implanon
      (1) This single implantable rod contains 3-keto-desogestrel, a progestin that is more potent than levonorgestrel. Studies have shown that serum hormone concentrations remain adequate for at least 3 years. Implanon users have a lower incidence of prolonged or irregular menstrual bleeding compared with users of Norplant; however, the incidence of oligomenorrhea (infrequent menses) and amenorrhea is higher.
      (2) Implanon is currently available in Europe.

E **Progestin-only IUD** (see III B)

V   COMBINATION ORAL CONTRACEPTIVE PILLS

A **Composition.**   Combination oral contraceptive pills (OCPs) contain various amounts of estrogen (ethinyl estradiol) and one of a variety of progestins. The current preparations contain low doses of estrogen (usually 20 to 50 μg per pill). Most are taken for 21 days, with 1 week between pill packs, in either monophasic or triphasic combinations.

B **Mode of action.**   The primary mechanism is inhibition of the LH surge.

1. Suppression of ovulation
2. Thickening of the cervical mucus, resulting in ineffective sperm migration
3. Alteration of tubal motility
4. Alteration of endometrium to make it thin and inactive, thus hampering implantation

C **Efficacy.**   **Pregnancy rate** is five pregnancies in 100 women-years.

D **Current controversies regarding complications**

1. Venous thromboembolism
   a. Estrogen causes an increase in serum levels of several clotting factors, especially factor VII. Antithrombin III levels fall within 10 days of starting OCPs.
   b. The incidence of both superficial and deep vein thromboses is increased in OCP users. Risk increases as estrogen dose increases.
   c. Despite these risks, it is still safer for a woman to use OCPs than to become pregnant. The **attributable risk**, or the number of venous thromboembolic events attributable to estrogen in OCPs, is approximately 6 in 100,000 woman-years. The estimated risk in pregnant women is 20 in 100,000 woman-years.
   d. Initial epidemiologic studies reported that women using **third-generation** (those that contain gestodene or desogestrel) OCPs have increased rates of venous thromboembolism compared with those using **second-generation** (containing norethindrone and levonorgestrel) OCPs. Additional studies demonstrated an inconsistent and weak association between OCPs and venous thromboembolism (strength of association, 0.7 to 2.3).
   e. Women with **inherited thrombophilias** who take OCPs have an increased risk of thromboembolism. The risk of thrombosis with OCP use is six times higher in **carriers of antithrombin and protein C and protein S defects**. The odds of having a venous thromboembolism event are 10 times higher in OCP users than in nonusers in carriers of the **factor V Leiden** mutation and seven times higher in carriers of the **prothrombin G20210A mutation.**

2. Cardiovascular disease
   a. There is no evidence to support an increased or decreased risk of **myocardial infarction** resulting from past or current use of OCPs. The strength of association between OCP use and **stroke** is weak, with an odds ratio of 1.1:1.8 (most 95% confidence intervals cross 1.0).
   b. However, a **synergistic effect** exists **between OCPs and smoking** as causes of cardiovascular events. **Heavy smoking, hypertension, severe diabetes mellitus with vascular complications,** and **obesity** (more than 50% above ideal body weight) are independent risk factors for cardiovascular disease. Women older than 35 years of age are at the highest risk for a cardiovascular event. However, women older than 35 years with no risk factors can safely use OCPs.

3. Hypertension. Plasma renin activity, angiotensin levels, aldosterone section, and renal retention of sodium are all increased in OCP users. The resulting hypertension in a small number of OCP users may represent the failed suppression of plasma renin activity that occurs with elevated levels of angiotensin. The length of OCP use appears to relate to the development of hypertension, which develops in approximately 5% of users after 5 years of use. Normotensive levels return in almost all women who developed hypertension while taking OCPs when the contraception is discontinued.

4. **Liver tumor.** An association between the use of OCPs and the subsequent development of a rare liver tumor, **hepatocellular adenoma,** has been reported. The associated risk increases when OCPs have been used for 5 years or more. Tumor development occurs at a rate of 3 in 100,000 woman-years of use.

5. **Neoplasia**
    a. **Breast cancer**
        (1) Progestins antagonize the stimulating effect of estrogen on breast tissue. The incidence of breast cancer has remained fairly constant during the past 15 to 20 years despite widespread use of OCPs.
        (2) A **small but statistically significant increase in risk of breast carcinoma exists in current** (relative risk, 1.24) **and recent users** (relative risk, 1.16) of OCPs, but not in past users.
            (a) This increased risk equates to a small increase in the actual number of new cases of breast cancer, and it disappears after 10 years of use.
            (b) **Cancers diagnosed** in recent or current OCP users **are not advanced and tend to be localized** compared with OCP nonusers.
        (3) Patients with a **family history of breast cancer have no additional risk.**
    b. **Cervical cancer.** Although this finding is controversial, there may be a small increased risk of cancer the cervix. This may be especially true with use of more than 5 years and in women who test positive for human papillomavirus. Cervical hypertrophy and eversion are seen in OCP users.
    c. **Endometrial cancer.** Progestins reduce the stimulating effect of estrogen and prevent the normal proliferative endometrium from progressing to hyperplasia, thus **decreasing the risk of endometrial cancer by 50%.**
    d. **Ovarian cancer** (see I E 1)

E **Noncontraceptive benefits**

1. **Ovarian cancer.** OCPs suppress ovarian activity and inhibit ovulation; the interruption of a significant number of ovulatory cycles in oral contraceptive users may lead to a decreased incidence of ovarian cancer.
    a. Users of OCPs are less likely to develop ovarian cancer than those who have never used OCPs. An average decrease of 40% in the likelihood of ovarian cancer is seen in women who have taken OCPs at some time. Protection is provided after as little as 3 to 6 months of use and persists for at least 15 years after discontinuation. Recent data also suggests that OCPs serve as primary prevention for women at risk for hereditary ovarian cancer.
    b. In particular, the risk of ovarian cancer is **significantly reduced in current and past users** of OCPs. This risk reduction increases as the period of OCP use increases. Women at increased risk for epithelial ovarian cancer may benefit from OCP use.

2. **Endometrial cancer.** Users of OCPs have a 50% reduction in endometrial cancer compared with those who have never used OCPs. Risk is reduced with longer use of pills. The actual duration of protection is unknown but lasts for a minimum of 15 years.

3. **Benign breast disease.** Fibrocystic change and fibroadenoma development are significantly reduced with OCP use. Larger amounts of progestin and longer periods of use decrease the risk of benign breast disease. The risk is lowest in current OCP users.

4. **Ectopic pregnancy.** The contraceptive effect of OCPs prevents ectopic pregnancy. The protection rate is 90% in current OCP users.

5. **Iron deficiency anemia.** OCPs decrease menstrual blood loss and regulate menstrual bleeding, thus decreasing likelihood of iron deficiency anemia. This action benefits both past and current OCP users.

6. **Pelvic inflammatory disease (PID).** OCPs protect against only those patients with PID who require hospitalization. At least 12 months of OCP use is necessary, and protection is limited to current users. No protection against lower genital tract infections (e.g., cervicitis) and tubal infertility is evident.

F New combination OCPs

1. One new combined OCP (Seasonale) maintains the level of estrogen for the entire 28 days.

2. Another new combined OCP (Yasmin) contains ethinyl estradiol with drospirenone, an analog of spironolactone, as the progestin. Premenstrual symptoms may be improved with this formulation.

VI OTHER COMBINATION HORMONAL METHODS

A Injection (Lunelle). This injectable form of combined hormonal contraception contains 5 mg of estradiol cypionate and 25 mg of medroxyprogesterone acetate. After injection, the cypionate ester is cleaved so that the circulating estrogen is similar to the ethinyl estradiol found in oral contraceptives.

1. **Use.** The monthly injectable is administered during the first 5 days of a woman's cycle and reinjected every 28 days with a margin of error of 5 days.

2. **Mode of action** is similar to that of combined OCPs (see V B).

3. **Advantages**
   a. Given at monthly intervals
   b. Independent of sexual intercourse
   c. Rapid resumption of fertility on discontinuation
   d. Fewer side effects (e.g., weight gain, acne, bleeding irregularities, and breast tenderness) than combined OCPs

4. **Disadvantages** include no protection against STDs.

5. **Efficacy** is similar to that of combined OCPs.

B Transdermal patch (Ortho Evra). The once-weekly contraceptive patch releases norelgestromin, the active metabolite of norgestimate, and ethinyl estradiol daily to the systemic circulation.

1. **Use.** Typical use includes placement of the patch on the same day of each week for 3 consecutive weeks followed by a patch-free week.

2. **Mode of action** is similar to that of combined OCPs (see V B).

3. **Advantages**
   a. Maintenance of normal activity, including bathing, swimming, and heavy exercise while using the patch
   b. Noncontraceptive benefits. The noncontraceptive effects of transdermal administration have not yet been studied but are expected to be similar to those of combined OCPs.
   c. Independent of sexual intercourse
   d. Rapidly reversible on discontinuation

4. **Disadvantages** include no protection from STDs.

5. **Efficacy** is similar to that of combined OCPs.

C Vaginal ring. This hormonal contraceptive contains ethinyl estradiol and etonogestrel (3-keto-desogestrel).

1. **Use.** The vaginal ring is worn continuously for 3 weeks and then discarded; a new ring is inserted into the vagina 1 week later. If the ring is left in place for more than 4 weeks, its contraceptive efficacy may be reduced.

2. Mode of action and **efficacy** are similar to combined OCPs.

3. Advantages
   a. Contraceptive effect of 3 weeks
   b. Beginning of contraceptive effect within the first day of use
   c. Independent of sexual intercourse
   d. Rapid resumption of fertility on discontinuation

4. Disadvantages include lack of protection from STDs.

VII EMERGENCY CONTRACEPTION

The primary **advantage** of this type of contraception is that it has no medical contraindications except previously established pregnancy. Its primary **disadvantage** is lack of protection against STDs. Methods of emergency contraception include the OCP, copper-impregnated IUD, and mifepristone (RU486).

A **Overall mode of action.** A single mechanism of action has not yet been established. Emergency contraception probably prevents pregnancy by causing anovulation or delaying ovulation, not by disrupting an existing pregnancy.

B **Overall efficacy.** Effectiveness declines with increasing delay between unprotected intercourse and initiation of treatment. Among the oral contraceptives, the progestin-only method is more effective in preventing pregnancy than the combination-pill method (85% effective versus 57%). The copper-impregnated IUD is significantly more effective than the use of hormonal emergency contraception, which has a failure rate of 0.1%.

C **"Morning-after pill"**
   1. Combination method. The most common regimen involves four tablets that are a combination of ethinyl estradiol and norgestrel, given as two tablets twice over 12 hours. The necessary **minimum effective dose** of ethinyl estradiol and norgestrel is 100 μg and 1.0 mg, respectively (**Yuzpe method**).
   2. Progestin-only method. The most common regimen is levonorgestrel, 0.75 mg, taken 12 hours apart. The necessary **minimum dose** of levonorgestrel is 1 mg. A single dose of 1.5 mg may be as effective.
   3. Prepackaged, commercially available emergency hormonal contraception
      a. Plan B is a **progestin-only method** that consists of two tablets, each containing 0.75 mg of levonorgestrel, and detailed instructions for both physicians and patients.
      b. The **Preven** Emergency Contraceptive Kit, **a combination hormonal method,** consists of four pills, each containing 0.25 mg of levonorgestrel and 0.05 mg of ethinyl estradiol, a urine pregnancy kit, and a patient information book.
   4. Use. The "morning-after pill" is best taken within 72 hours of unprotected coitus; use within 24 hours increases efficacy.
   5. Side effects. Most common side effects include nausea (about 50% of women) and vomiting (about 20% of women). An antiemetic is often needed with combination pills but not with progestin-only pills.

D The **copper-impregnated IUD** can be used as an alternative method. It should be inserted up to 5 to 7 days after ovulation to prevent pregnancy. The copper IUD is significantly more effective than the use of hormonal emergency contraception; the failure rate is 0.1%.

E **Mifepristone (RU486)** is a progestational antagonist that binds to the progesterone receptor and prevents or interrupts progestational action. A single oral dose (600 mg) is associated with an efficacy rate of nearly 100%.

VIII   NATURAL FAMILY PLANNING

This contraceptive method entails planning or avoiding pregnancies by abstaining from sexual intercourse during the fertile phase of the menstrual cycle. Drugs, devices, and surgical procedures are not used. Coitus is limited to before and after the fertile period each month.

A **Fertility awareness.**   Women are most fertile several days around the time of ovulation.

1. Fertility status can be determined by charting basal body temperature, maintaining a menstrual calendar, and monitoring changes in cervical mucus.

2. Fertility determination depends on a couple's ability to identify and interpret signs of fertility.

B **Basal body temperature** is the temperature of the body at complete rest after a period of sleep and before normal activity, including eating.

1. The basal body temperature exhibits a biphasic pattern during an ovulatory cycle (i.e., it is lower in the first half of the cycle, increases at the time of ovulation, and remains higher for the rest of the cycle).

2. The basal body temperature **increases 0.4 to 1.0°F during the postovulatory phase** of the cycle because the secretion of progesterone has a thermogenic effect.

3. **As an indicator of fertility,** the basal body temperature can detect only the end of the fertile phase because the temperature remains elevated for 3 days after the shift.

4. **To avoid pregnancy,** a couple must restrict sexual intercourse from the end of menses to 1 to 2 days after the temperature elevation.

C **Menstrual calendar calculations**

1. Calculations are based on the following assumptions:
   a. Ovulation occurs on day 14 (plus or minus 2 days) before the onset of menses.
   b. Sperm remain viable for about 5 days.
   c. The ovum survives for about 1 day.

2. Lengths of previous cycles give an estimate of when to avoid intercourse during a current cycle.

D **Cervical secretions**

1. Varying concentrations of estrogen and progesterone affect the quantity and quality of cervical mucus.

2. Secretions **during the fertile period are abundant, clear or white, slippery, and stretchy.** Ovulation occurs within 1 day before to 1 day after the appearance of this discharge.

3. **After ovulation,** as progesterone levels increase, cervical secretions become **thick, cloudy, and sticky.**

4. It is presumed that the **fertile period** begins when cervical secretions are first noted until 4 days past the peak of the slippery discharge. **To avoid pregnancy, couples should abstain from intercourse during the fertile period.**

E **Advantages**

1. Acceptance by some religions that disapprove of other methods of contraception

2. Involvement of both partners

3. Minimal cost

4. No medical consultation needed

F **Disadvantages**

1. No protection against STDs

2. Difficulty of use with irregular menses

G **Efficacy.** **Pregnancy rate** among women using natural family planning is 10 to 23 in 100 woman-years of use.

IX SURGICAL STERILIZATION

These procedures have become one of the most widely used methods of contraception. Both tubal ligation and vasectomy are designed to be permanent. Depending on the technique used, tubal sterilization has a failure rate during the first year of 0.7 to 5.4%. Counseling is essential; nearly 6% of women regret their decision. Vasectomy has a failure rate during the first year of 0.1%.

Study Questions for Chapter 24

Directions: *Match the description below with the best method of contraception above. Each answer may be used once, more than once, or not at all.*

QUESTIONS 1–4

[A] Depot-medroxyprogesterone acetate
[B] Progestin-only pill (minipill)
[C] Combination birth control pill
[D] Progesterone IUD
[E] Weekly combination transdermal patch

1. A 24-year-old woman, gravida 3, para 3 who just delivered a healthy boy and is breastfeeding him. She is a successful model and cannot tolerate excessive weight gain.

2. A 29-year-nulliparous woman who has factor V Leiden deficiency. She is a librarian who exercises 6 days a week in order to maintain her physique. She has had several tumultuous relationships this year. She tries to use condoms in addition to this contraceptive method to prevent STDs.

3. A 28-year-old nulliparous physician who has a history of major depression. She is on call in the hospital every 4 days and sometimes forgets to take her antidepressant medication. She has been in a new relationship for the past 2 months. She always uses condoms in addition to this contraceptive method to prevent STDs.

4. A 26-year-old gravida 4, para 4 who is happily married for 14 years. She has regular periods which last 9 to 10 days and are associated with severe cramping.

Directions: *Each of the numbered items or incomplete statements in this section is followed by answers or by completions of the statement. Select the ONE lettered answer or completion that is BEST in each case.*

5. The contraceptive method currently available in the United States that has the lowest reported failure rate is (in x/100 woman-years of use)

[A] Copper IUD
[B] Progestin IUD (Mirena)
[C] Depot medroxyprogesterone acetate injection (Depo Provera)
[D] Implantable progestin (Norplant)
[E] Cervical caps

6. A 25-year-old gravida 1, para 0, tab 1 presents to the emergency department and is being evaluated for date rape, which occurred 12 hours ago. She says that the rapist forced himself onto her and had time to ejaculate inside her. She has no past medical history. In addition to prophylactic treatment for STDs, complete rape evaluation, and counseling, the most effective and widely available management to prevent pregnancy is

[A] Ethinyl estradiol and norgestrel, 2 tabs now and 2 in 12 hours
[B] Ethinyl estradiol and norgestrel, 2 tabs now and 2 in 12 hours and prochlorperazine
[C] Ethinyl estradiol and norgestrel, 4 tabs now and 4 in 12 hours and prochlorperazine
[D] Levonorgestrel, 0.75 mg now and another in 12 hours
[E] Mifepristone (RU-486)

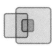

Answers and Explanations

1. B [IV B] **2. B** [IV B] **3. E** [VI B] **4. D** [III C 2]. Women who are breastfeeding should use progestin-only contraceptive methods so as to not affect their quantity and quality of breast milk. This first patient cannot tolerate depot-medroxyprogesterone acetate because it is associated with 5-pound-per-year weight gain. The second patient would also benefit from the minipill because 1) she should avoid estrogen-containing contraceptive methods (combination pills or patch) because of her inherited thrombophilia; 2) she should avoid depot-medroxyprogesterone acetate because she is concerned with weight loss; and 3) she should avoid IUDs because multiple sexual partners is a contraindication. For the third patient, IUD is not a good choice because nulliparity is a relative contraindication. The third patient has depression, and depot-medroxyprogesterone acetate has been associated with major depression. She may forget to take any form of daily (pill) contraceptive because of her busy schedule. Therefore, the transdermal combination patch is the best option for the third patient. The fourth patient would benefit from the progestin-releasing IUD because her dysmenorrheal and menorrhagia would improve. She is also in a monogamous relationship, which makes her the perfect candidate for this form of contraception.

5. The answer is C [IV C 3]. The pregnancy rate with each of the methods of contraception presented in this question is as follows: depo-medroxyprogesterone acetate <1/100 woman-years; Norplant <1/100 woman-years (but it is no longer manufactured); progestin IUD = copper IUD = 2 to 3/100 woman-years; cervical caps = 5 to 10/100 woman-years.

6. The answer is D [VII B and VII C 3 a]. The progestin method is more effective in preventing pregnancy than the combination pill method. The copper IUD is even more effective than the progestin method, but it is not in the answer choices. The combination method should be used with anti-nausea medication. Although RU-486 has a nearly 100% efficacy rate, it is not widely available in the United States.

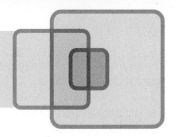

chapter 25

Benign Breast Disease
MICHELLE BERLIN

I   INTRODUCTION

Most women who present with breast pain, nipple discharge, or breast masses are primarily concerned about the possibility of breast cancer. A careful, thorough history and physical examination are essential to evaluate these conditions. The role of the health care provider must include not only providing evaluation and treatment (if warranted), but also appropriately communicating the findings and treatment plan to the patient. This includes ensuring that the patient's questions and concerns are addressed. Documentation of these discussions is important.

A **History.**   Pertinent aspects of the patient's history include age; age at menarche; parity, including age at first delivery; occurrence of breastfeeding after each delivery and for how long; method of birth control and duration of use; and personal and family history of cancer, particularly breast, ovarian, and colon, including age at diagnosis. Questions about the types and duration of medications and procedures used are appropriate in women with a history of infertility. Questions about the use of postmenopausal hormone replacement therapy (HRT) are warranted in postmenopausal women.

B **Physical examination.**   Particular attention should be paid not only to palpable lumps, but also to skin changes (such as **dimpling**) and nipple direction, which may be altered, to **retraction** from an underlying carcinoma. Women with breast implants may be difficult to examine. If clinical evaluation is at all unclear, women with breast implants should be referred to a breast surgeon.

C **Clinical findings.**   Women with benign breast conditions generally present with one of three signs or symptoms: **breast pain, nipple discharge,** or **breast mass.**

II   BREAST PAIN

Women commonly seek advice from physicians for breast pain (also known as **mastalgia** or **mastodynia**). Breast pain most often occurs in women in the reproductive years (i.e., before menopause). Of the three clinical findings (see I C), breast pain is the least likely to be associated with breast cancer.

A **Types of breast pain**
1. **Cyclic mastalgia.** Symptoms of breast pain often occur during the premenstrual or menstrual phases of the menstrual cycle.
    a. **Etiology.** Although this cyclic pattern suggests hormonal involvement, no laboratory tests have confirmed that hormonal variation plays a causal role.
    b. **Treatment**
        (1) **Analgesics,** especially nonsteroidal anti-inflammatory drugs (NSAIDs), are useful in many patients.

(2) Vitamin E supplementation and a reduction or elimination of caffeine consumption is commonly suggested, although evidence in support of these treatments is inconsistent at best.

(3) Evening primrose oil has been used with some success and continues to be evaluated.

(4) Danazol (Danocrine) should be reserved for only the most severe cases because of its marked side-effect profile and inconsistent success in reducing symptoms.

(5) Bromocriptine (Parlodel) is also of limited usefulness because of its inconsistent efficacy and potential negative side effects.

(6) Tamoxifen has been used with minimal success; the long-term consequences of its use for breast pain are not clear.

2. **Noncyclic mastalgia.** This breast pain does not vary with the menstrual cycle.

   a. **Etiology.** Common noncyclic causes of breast pain are chest wall pain, including costochondritis; trauma; and sclerosing adenosis.

   b. **Treatment.** In postmenopausal women who take HRT, reducing the amount of estrogen or discontinuing HRT often remedies breast pain.

3. **Breast pain associated with cancer.** This type of breast pain is uncommon, although not unknown, and it is more likely to be unilateral, localized, unremitting, and constant.

III NIPPLE DISCHARGE

A Approximately 3 to 10% of breast complaints involve nipple discharge.

B Etiology

1. **Premenopausal women.** Nipple discharge is most likely the result of **benign causes.**

   a. **Galactorrhea** (milk production in a woman who is not breastfeeding) is the usual cause of noncancerous nipple discharge.

   b. **Most commonly,** galactorrhea is **endocrinologic or medication-induced.** Several medications can cause hyperprolactinemia and associated galactorrhea, including psychotropic medications (e.g., phenothiazines, tricyclic antidepressants); oral contraceptives; some gastrointestinal preparations (e.g., cimetidine, metoclopramide); calcium channel blockers; and methyldopa.

2. **Postmenopausal women.** Nipple discharge is more likely to result from malignancy.

C Appearance and types of discharge

1. Nipple discharge resulting from noncancerous causes is more likely to be bilateral and to be milky.

2. One common type of benign nipple discharge is generally bilateral and yellow or green. It is apparent at several ducts and rather than being spontaneously evident, it can be elicited with breast manipulation.

3. Nipple discharge **associated with malignancy is more likely to be unilateral.** It is likely to be **pink, bloody, and nonmilky,** and it is frequently associated with a breast mass.

4. **Ductal papilloma** is characterized by **bloodstained secretion from the nipple.** Although in most instances this is a benign condition, as many as 20 to 30% of cases are malignant. By stroking the areola to center, it is often possible to distinguish which duct is affected. Biopsy is required for diagnosis.

D Evaluation and treatment

1. Prolactin and thyroid-stimulating hormone (TSH) levels should be evaluated.

   a. If the TSH is in the normal range (0.4 to 5 mU/L), then hypothyroidism is not the cause of galactorrhea.

   b. If the prolactin level is less than 100 ng/mL (which suggests the presence of a microadenoma), then magnetic resonance imaging (MRI) is the evaluation of choice. If the prolactin level is greater than 100 ng/mL (which suggests the presence of a macroadenoma), then computed tomography or MRI may be used.

  c. If the prolactin level is high and medication-induced galactorrhea is unlikely, then the patient requires radiologic imaging studies to determine whether an abnormality of the pituitary gland is present.

2. A careful evaluation of the patient's **medications** and the side-effect profile of each medication are necessary. If the prolactin level is high (or normal), either substituting a drug that does not induce galactorrhea or discontinuing a medication that may be causing galactorrhea should be attempted, if possible.

3. If galactorrhea is not the result of thyroid disease or pituitary adenoma, galactorrhea may respond to treatment with either bromocriptine or cabergoline. If galactorrhea is accompanied by anovulation and infertility and the patient is interested in actively attempting pregnancy, bromocriptine is preferable.

IV BREAST MASS

A **Benign breast masses** are more likely to be soft or cystic, have regular borders, and be freely mobile.

B **Malignant breast masses** are more likely to be asymptomatic early in the course of breast cancer; however, later in the disease they often exhibit distinct, irregular, and hard edges.

C **Types of breast masses**

1. **Fibrocystic disease or fibrocystic change** (currently the preferred term for this condition). The greatest incidence of fibrocystic change is among women in their 30s and 40s.

   a. **Clinical manifestations.** Fibrocystic change is characterized by palpable areas of fibrosis and cysts within the breast. Although fibrocystic change was once thought to be a precursor of carcinoma, this belief has been dispelled in the literature. The only risk associated with fibrocystic change is the difficulty that may occur on clinical examination, because carcinomatous lesions may be more difficult to distinguish from the surrounding tissue.

   b. **Treatment.** Vitamin E supplementation, reduced caffeine intake, and other therapies have been used (see II A 1 b). No randomized trials have confirmed the efficacy of these treatment methods. If concomitant discomfort is severe, physicians may consider the use of androgenic hormonal treatment.

2. **Cysts**

   a. **Clinical manifestations.** On clinical examination, cysts generally feel rubbery, firm, round, and distinct. Cysts can be tender, especially at the time of menses.

   b. **Evaluation and treatment.** When a breast cyst is palpated on clinical examination, cyst aspiration or ultrasound should be performed.

      (1) **Aspiration.** Aspiration of cystic fluid provides information about whether the cyst is likely to be benign or malignant. It also provides the patient with relief from discomfort (if present).

      (a) Fluid aspirated from a benign cyst is likely to be **clear or brown-green.** If such fluid is obtained, it **does not require submission** for cytologic evaluation.

      (b) However, if the fluid obtained is **bloody,** the possibility of carcinoma increases, and the fluid **must be sent for cytopathologic evaluation.**

      (c) If the cyst recurs, then a second aspiration may be attempted. If the cyst recurs a third time, however, surgical removal is recommended. If a clinically suspected breast cyst does not yield fluid on aspiration, then the lesion should be evaluated as a breast mass. A mammogram should be obtained, and a biopsy (fine needle aspiration, core biopsy, or surgical excision) should be performed.

      (2) Ultrasound. Ultrasonic evaluation is useful to confirm that a palpable lesion is cystic or solid.

      (3) Mammography. Mammography should be considered if a breast mass is found or if a cystic-appearing lesion yields no fluid on aspiration and is not cystic on ultrasound. In these instances, mammography is being used as a diagnostic test because the lesion of concern has been identified (as opposed to mammographic screening, which is conducted in women without symptoms or known or suspected lesions).

3. **Fibroadenoma.** These benign lesions, most common among women in their 20s and 30s, tend to feel lobular, smooth (not serrated), firm, and distinct. Once they are identified, no further evaluation is needed.

4. **Sclerosing adenitis.** Sclerosing adenitis is a type of fibrosis. This condition is benign, but biopsy is required to distinguish it from carcinoma.

5. **Fat necrosis.** This condition is often identified as an irregular, tender firm mass, without increase in size over time. The cause of fat necrosis is trauma (usually direct injury to the breast). Fat necrosis may mimic carcinoma on mammography because of the presence of calcifications. Surgical excision may be required to confirm diagnosis.

6. **Mondor's disease.** This disease represents thrombophlebitis of the breast and is most likely to be apparent in lactating women. Breast lesions generally appear firm and tube-like. The condition is benign and self-limited, although treatment with heat and analgesics is helpful.

7. **Duct ectasia.** This condition is seen primarily in perimenopausal and postmenopausal women. Patients report burning, itching, or existence of a pulling sensation in the nipple area, with or without a thick, greenish-black nipple discharge. On examination, a tender, hard, erythematous mass is palpated next to areola. In most cases, this condition is benign, but further evaluation is necessary.

Study Questions for Chapter 25

Directions: *Each of the numbered items or incomplete statements in this section is followed by answers or by completions of the statement. Select the ONE lettered answer or completion that is BEST in each case.*

1. A 36-year-old woman, gravida 4, para 4 presents to your clinic because she has had bilateral white-colored nipple discharge for the last 3 months. She breast fed her last baby, but that ended almost 2 years ago. She has no past medical history other than recently diagnosed hypertension for which she takes oral nifedipine. She is married and uses birth control pills for contraception. She has no known drug allergies. Examination of the breasts reveals no discrete masses. When the nipple discharge is placed on a slide and viewed under a light microscope, fat globules are seen that are reminiscent of milk. Which of the following is the next best step in management?

    A Obtain a TSH level
    B Schedule a follow-up in 6 weeks
    C Collect discharge for cytopathology
    D Discontinue nifedipine
    E Substitute non-hormonal method of contraception

2. A 30-year-old woman, gravida 2, para 2 presents to your office reporting bilateral breast pain. The pain is constant and occurs a few days before the beginning of her periods, is of 4/10 intensity, and does not radiate. She has no history of a recent upper respiratory tract infection. Her past medical history is significant for duodenal ulcer, and she is taking a proton pump inhibitor. She has no known drug allergies. The initial pharmacologic management of this patient is

    A Aspirin
    B Ibuprofen
    C Danazol
    D Evening primrose oil
    E Tight-fitting bra

3. A 60-year-old woman, gravida 3, para 2, SAB 1 presents to your clinic reporting red-colored discharge from her left nipple. Her past medical history and medications, respectively, are as follows: diabetes, oral hypoglycemic; hypertension, angiotensin-converting enzyme inhibitor; and major depression, fluoxetine. She is also taking conjugated estrogen with medroxyprogesterone acetate daily. She is allergic to penicillin. She says her mother was diagnosed with ovarian cancer at age 71. What is the next best step in management?

    A Mammogram
    B Fine-needle aspiration (FNA)
    C Referral to breast surgeon
    D Cessation of hormone replacement therapy
    E Breast examination

4. A 28-year-old woman, gravida 2, para 2 who delivered a health female infant 10 days ago comes to labor and delivery because of tender breast mass on the right. She is breastfeeding exclusively. On examination of her breasts you note bilateral mild engorgement of the breasts and a tender, firm, linear, and slightly erythematous area in the upper outer quadrant of her right breast. What is the next best step in management?

    A Observation
    B Heat compresses
    C Mammogram
    D Biopsy
    E Dicloxacillin

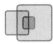

Answers and Explanations

1. The answer is E [III B 1 b]. The most likely cause of this patient's galactorrhea is medication-related. Oral contraceptives are known to cause galactorrhea. Although calcium channel blockers can cause galactorrhea (but not as often), this answer choice is not the "best" because it suggests "discontinuing" (rather than "changing") a needed therapy without offering another in its place. There is no need in sending white, yellow, or green discharge for cytopathological analysis. Simply scheduling a follow-up for this patient without taking any steps is not appropriate. Hypothyroidism and prolactinomas cause galactorrhea; therefore, prolactin and TSH levels are the second step in management of this patient.

2. The answer is D [II A 1 b 3]. Evening primrose oil has been used with some success and continues to be scientifically evaluated. Both aspirin and ibuprofen would be the initial choices had this patient not had the contraindication of duodenal ulcer. Danazol is never the initial treatment of choice because of its severe androgenic side effects. A tight-fitting bra is not "pharmacologic" management.

3. The answer is E [III B 2 and III C]. Don't jump the gun! The first step in management of any breast complaint is a clinical examination of the breast. This patient may have a common benign condition such as intraductal papilloma, which can be confirmed by expressing the bloody discharge from a discrete duct. Also, if a concomitant breast mass exists, it would increase the probability that the condition is malignant. Definitive diagnosis, however, requires biopsy.

4. The answer is B [C 6]. In a lactating woman, the most likely diagnosis is Mondor's disease, or superficial thrombophlebitis of the right thoracoepigastric vein. The key here is the linear tender mass. The best treatment is heat and analgesia. Antibiotics are not necessary because the condition is self-limited. Observation without offering a helpful suggestion is not appropriate.

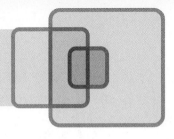

chapter 26

Vulvovaginitis

JANE HONDESHEL

I   **INTRODUCTION**

Vulvovaginitis is one of the most commonly seen gynecologic problems. A broad spectrum of disorders can produce vulvovaginal symptoms.

II   **VULVOVAGINAL ANATOMY**

A   **Vulva.** The vulva is made up of the **mons pubis, labia majora and minora, clitoris, and vestibule;** it contains the urinary meatus, vaginal orifice, Bartholin glands (major vestibular glands), ducts of the Skene glands, and minor vestibular glands (Fig. 26-1). The vulva is subject to any conditions that may affect the skin and related structures, including psoriasis, hypersensitivity reactions, and benign and malignant neoplasms.

1. Anatomy
   a. The entire vulva is covered by a **keratinized** squamous epithelium.
   b. Hair-bearing regions contain associated hair follicles, sebaceous glands, and apocrine and eccrine sweat glands.
   c. Regions without hair, such as the labia minora and prepuce, contain sebaceous glands but not hair follicles or eccrine and apocrine sweat glands.
   d. The **labia majora** are composed of skin enclosing a variable amount of fat and smooth muscle.
      (1) They extend from the mons anteriorly to the fourchette posteriorly.
      (2) The embryologic homolog in the male is the scrotum.
   e. The **labia minora** are erectile tissue, devoid of fat and composed of skin and vascular and connective tissue.
      (1) They extend from the prepuce two thirds of the distance of the perineum.
      (2) The embryologic homolog in the male is the floor of the penile urethra.
   f. The **clitoris** is a highly vascular and innervated, erectile organ located between the bifurcating folds of the labia minora.
      (1) It consists of the glans and the body, covered by the prepuce.
      (2) The embryologic homolog in the male is the penis.
   g. The **vestibule** is the space between the labia minora extending from the clitoris to the vaginal introitus. It contains the urethral meatus and the openings of the major and minor vestibular glands as well as the Skene glands.
   h. **Bartholin glands** are the major vestibular glands.
      (1) They lie posterior and lateral to the vaginal introitus.
      (2) The embryologic homolog in the male is the Cowper glands.
   i. **Ducts of the Skene glands** and **minor vestibular glands** are paraurethral structures.

2. Nerve supply. The nerve supply to the vulva includes sensory nerves, special receptors, and autonomic nerves to vessels and glands. Symptoms of vulvovaginal disorders are frequently caused

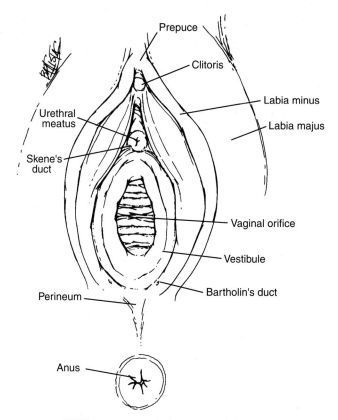

FIGURE 26-1 Anatomical structures of the vulva.

by irritation of the sensory nerves of the vulva. The major nerves supplying the vulva include those derived from the pudendal, ilioinguinal, and posterior femoral cutaneous nerves.

    a. The **pudendal nerve** gives rise to the inferior hemorrhoidal nerve, the perineal nerve, and the dorsal nerve of the clitoris.

    b. The **ilioinguinal nerve** gives rise to the anterior labial nerves.

    c. The **posterior femoral cutaneous nerve** gives rise to the posterior labial nerves.

  3. Vascular supply. The major blood vessels supplying the vulva derive from the internal pudendal artery, which arises from the internal iliac artery, and the superficial and deep external pudendal arteries, which arise from the femoral artery.

  4. Lymphatic supply. The femoral and inguinal lymph nodes receive the lymphatic drainage from the vulva. The superficial inguinal lymph nodes are the initial site of drainage. Many infections or inflammatory conditions of the vulva and distal vaginal wall are accompanied by an increase in lymphatic drainage, resulting in tender lymphadenopathy at this site.

B **Vagina.** This structure is a hollow cylinder approximately 9 to 10 cm in length. It extends from the introitus to the uterus and lies dorsal to the bladder and ventral to the rectum.

  1. Anatomy. The vaginal wall has three layers: the mucosa, muscularis, and adventitia.

    a. The **mucosa** is covered by a stratified, **nonkeratinized**, squamous epithelium.

      (1) It is a mucous membrane that is under the hormonal influence of the ovarian steroids. **Estrogen stimulates** the proliferation and maturation of vaginal epithelial cells, whereas progesterone is inhibitory.

      (2) There are no glandular structures. Endocervical secretions and **transudation of fluid** across the vaginal epithelium provide lubrication.

   b. The **muscularis** is composed of an outer longitudinal and inner circular layer.

   c. The **adventitia** is a strong sheet of connective tissue, condensed anteriorly to form the pubo-cervical fascia, and fused to the fascial coverings of the pelvic and urogenital diaphragms.

2. **Nerve supply.** The nerve supply is derived from the lumbar plexus and the pudendal nerve. The pudendal nerve does not have as rich a distribution of fine sensory nerves as the nerves supplying the vulva.

3. **Vascular supply.** The major vessels supplying the vagina include the vaginal artery, arising from the internal iliac or uterine artery; the azygous artery of the vagina, arising from the cervical branch of the uterine artery; and branches of the pudendal artery. Venous drainage forms a plexus surrounding the vagina, and major vessels follow the arterial course.

4. **Lymphatic supply.** The lymphatic drainage of the vagina includes a complex anastomotic plexus that involves drainage to the internal iliac, pelvic, sacral, inferior gluteal, anorectal, femoral, and inguinal nodes.

III VAGINAL PHYSIOLOGY

The vaginal ecosystem is a finely balanced environment maintained by a complex interaction among vaginal flora, microbial by-products, estrogen, and host factors. The vagina is **usually resistant to infection** for two reasons: **marked acidity** and a **thick protective epithelium.** Other host factors, such as the immune system, also play a role in vaginal defense mechanisms.

A **Microbiology.** The vaginal flora play a critical role in vaginal defenses by maintaining the normally acidic pH (3.8 to 4.2) of the vagina.

1. Normally, 5 to 15 different bacterial species (e.g., group B *Streptococcus, Escherichia coli),* both aerobic and anaerobic, inhabit the vagina. The type and number may vary in response to normal and abnormal changes in the vaginal environment.

2. *Lactobacillus acidophilus* is the dominant bacterium in a healthy vaginal ecosystem. Lactobacilli play a critical role in maintaining the normal vaginal environment.
   a. The acidic environment of the vagina is maintained through the production of lactic acid.
   b. Lactic acid and hydrogen peroxide produced by lactobacilli are toxic to anaerobic bacteria in the vagina.

3. **Insults that affect the acidic pH** and lead to a more alkaline environment result in a decrease in lactobacilli, with an overgrowth of pathogenic organisms.

B **Host factors**

1. **Normal estrogen levels** are necessary for a normal vaginal environment and resistance to infection.
   a. Estrogen stimulates proliferation and maturation of the vaginal epithelium, providing a physical barrier to infection. Conditions associated with decreased estrogen levels are associated with an increase in susceptibility to vaginal infections.
   b. Mature vaginal epithelium provides **glycogen,** necessary for lactobacillus metabolism. If glycogen levels are decreased, lactobacillus counts decrease as well.

2. **Cellular and humoral immunity** plays a role in the normal vaginal defense mechanisms.

C **Factors that alter the vaginal environment.** Insults that affect the vaginal microbiology, vaginal epithelium, or vaginal pH lead to an increased susceptibility to vaginal infections.

1. **Antibiotics** alter the microbiology of the vagina and can increase the risk of infection.

2. **Hormones** may affect the vaginal epithelium and increase the risk of infection (e.g., decreased estrogen level, increased progesterone level).

3. **Douching or intravaginal medications** can change the vaginal pH or affect the vaginal flora, altering the resistance to infection.

4. **Intercourse** affects the microenvironment of the vagina because semen has an alkaline pH. In addition, intercourse may introduce new organisms into the vagina, thus influencing the microenvironment.

5. **Sexually transmitted diseases (STDs)** affect the microbiology of the vagina, changing the resistance to infection. Other organisms may be the cause of vaginal symptomatology.

6. **Stress, poor diet, and fatigue** probably play a role by affecting microbiology, pH, and the immune system.

7. **Foreign bodies** alter the pH and microbiology of the vagina.

8. Changes in immune function associated with **HIV infection** are associated with recurrent vaginal candidiasis.

IV DIAGNOSIS

A thorough history, a physical examination, and judicious use of ancillary tests are critical to attaining the correct diagnosis. The medical history is essential in evaluating the potential causes of vulvovaginal symptoms. The patient's symptomatology is also important.

A History. Certain conditions may predispose women to certain types of vulvovaginal infections. Inciting factors may also indicate other causes, such as allergic reactions. Physicians should consider the following factors:

1. Sexual activity
   a. Are there complaints of irritation?
   b. What is the relation of the onset of symptoms to intercourse or other sexual activity?
   c. Has the patient engaged in any unusual sexual practices or had new partners?
2. Onset, intensity, and progression of symptoms
3. Recent systemic or local infection
4. Use of antibiotics
5. History of diabetes mellitus
6. Previous vulvovaginal infections
7. Vaginal hygienic practices (e.g., douching)
8. Contraceptive methods
9. Menstrual history
10. Previous treatments; use of self-prescribed medications, herbal remedies, or home remedies
11. Any other factors that may have altered the vaginal environment

B Symptomatology

1. **Vulvar symptoms.** The two **most common symptoms** are:
   a. **Burning.** Vulvar irritation or burning is a symptom associated with a variety of disorders, including vulvovaginitis, vulvovestibulitis, and vulvodynia.
   b. **Itching or pruritus.** Vulvar pruritus is a common symptom that may result from vulvovaginitis. Other possible causes include any skin disorder associated with pruritus, including allergic reactions.
2. **Vaginal discharge.** Description of the discharge is crucial to diagnosis and to the differentiation from a normal physiologic finding. Characteristics include:
   a. **Consistency (thick, watery).** A thin, white discharge is often normal.

      b. Viscosity. Cervical mucus normally changes during the menstrual cycle. Follicular mucus is normally watery and abundant; postovulatory mucus can be thick and viscous. Patients may observe such changes and report them as abnormal.

      c. Color. Normal discharges are usually white to beige. Green, yellow, or brown discharges are usually associated with an infection, a foreign body, or some other abnormality.

   3. Odor. Description of the odor is useful in establishing a differential diagnosis.

      a. An odor may be present without an associated discharge noticed by the patient.

      b. Complaints of severe, offensive odor occur most often with retained foreign bodies, such as tampons.

V   PHYSICAL EXAMINATION

A **Pelvic examination** is essential in the management of vulvovaginitis and should consist of a thorough evaluation.

   1. Inspection of the **external genitalia** detects gross lesions, edema (and discoloration) of the labia, ulceration, and condylomata. It also rules out pubic lice.

   2. The **inguinal area** should be palpated for the presence or absence of lymphadenopathy. Any discoloration should be noted.

B **Speculum examination,** using water as the only lubricant to avoid interfering with specimen collection and culturing, should reveal:

   1. Nature of the vaginal discharge (e.g., consistency, viscosity, color, and odor)

   2. Evidence of trauma, congenital abnormalities, or characteristic lesions of the vaginal walls (e.g., "strawberry spots" if *Trichomonas vaginalis* is suspected)

   3. Presence or absence of cervical abnormalities. A culture of the endocervix detects gonorrhea or chlamydial infection, and a Papanicolaou test (Pap smear) detects carcinoma or infection.

C **Laboratory tests**

   1. When an infectious vaginitis is suspected, **vaginal pH** helps differentiate the various types of infections.

   2. A specimen should be obtained for **wet mount preparation.** Microscopic inspection of the vaginal secretions in saline and a 10% potassium hydroxide (KOH) solution is pivotal when diagnosing vaginitis.

   3. Occasionally, **cultures** are useful in difficult cases.

VI   VULVOVAGINAL CONDITIONS (Table 26-1)

Vaginitis is characterized by one or more of the following symptoms: **increased volume of discharge; abnormal color (yellow or green) of discharge; vulvar itching, irritation, or burning; dyspareunia; and malodor.** Vaginitis may be caused by infectious agents (e.g., *Candida, Gardnerella,* and *Trichomonas*) or by atrophic changes. Symptoms of other vulvovaginal conditions, including vulvar dystrophies, vulvar dermatitis, and other skin conditions of the vulva, may be similar to those of vaginitis. Acute herpes simplex genitalis may cause acute vulvar symptoms, necessitating prompt evaluation and treatment.

A **Bacterial vaginosis** is the most common vaginal infection in the United States today. In the past, bacterial vaginitis was known as nonspecific vaginitis and *Gardnerella* vaginitis.

   1. Etiology

      a. Bacterial vaginosis is caused by an **overgrowth of a variety of bacterial species,** particularly anaerobes, often found normally in the vagina. Organisms most often involved include *Bacteroides, Peptostreptococcus, Gardnerella vaginalis,* and *Mycoplasma hominis.*

TABLE 26-1   Signs, Symptoms and Diagnosis of Vulvovaginitis

Etiology	Symptoms	Clinical Signs	Diagnostic Method
Monilial vaginitis	Pruritis	Thick white discharge; pH 4.0–4.7	Wet prep or KOH prep (pseudohyphae)
Trichomonas	Malodorous discharge, pruritis	Fruthy, copious yellow-green discharge; pH 5.0–7.0	Wet prep (motile trichomonads)
Bacterial vaginosis	Discharge, fishy odor	Thin, gray discharge; pH 5.0–5.5	Wet prep, sniff test (clue cells)
Chlamydia	Discharge	Mucopurulent discharge, cervical erosion	Culture; MicroTrak or Chlamydiazime
Gonorrhea	Discharge	Cervical discharge	Cervical culture; Gram stain
Genital herpes	Pain	Ulcerative, vulvar vesicles and ulcers	Virus culture, Tzanck prep
Chemical	Discharge	Erythema; may be ulcerative	History and exclusion of other causes
Physiologic	Discharge	No odor or erythema	Wet prep; history, exclusion of other causes; cervical culture

KOH, potassium hydroxide.

b. The anaerobic bacteria produce enzymes that break down peptides to amino acids and amines, resulting in compounds associated with the discharge and odor characteristic of this infection.

2. Clinical presentation. Fifty percent of women with bacterial vaginosis are asymptomatic. In symptomatic patients, the most common presentation is a malodorous, gray discharge.

3. Diagnosis. Three of the following four criteria must be present:
   a. The vaginal pH is generally between 5.0 and 5.5.
   b. Wet mount preparations with saline reveal a "clean" background with **minimal or no leukocytes**, an abundance of bacteria, and the characteristic **clue cells.** The clue cells are squamous cells in which coccobacillary bacteria have obscured the sharp borders and cytoplasm.
   c. Application of 10% KOH to the wet mount specimen produces a **fishy odor,** indicating a positive "whiff" test.
   d. A gray, homogenous, malodorous discharge is present.

4. Treatment. Therapy is based on the use of agents with anaerobic activity and involves both topical and systemic agents. The combination appears to be 90% effective.
   a. Vaginal preparations
      (1) Intravaginal 2% **clindamycin cream** is used at bedtime for 7 days.
      (2) Intravaginal **metronidazole** is applied twice a day for 5 days.
   b. Oral regimens
      (1) Metronidazole may be administered three ways: 500 mg twice daily for 7 days, 250 mg three times daily for 7 days, or a single, 2-g dose.
      (2) Clindamycin, 300 mg three times daily for 7 days (may be associated with diarrhea [especially *c.difficile*])
   c. Sexual partners should be treated in cases of repeated episodes of bacterial vaginosis. Routine treatment of partners has not been shown to improve cure rates or lower reinfection rates.
   d. Treatment during pregnancy is critical; data suggests an association of adverse maternal and fetal outcomes with bacterial vaginosis.
      (1) Clindamycin may be used throughout pregnancy.
      (2) Metronidazole may be used after the first trimester.
   e. Patients with recurrences should be screened for STDs.

B *Candida* **vaginitis** (candidiasis or moniliasis) is the second most common vaginal infection in the United States.

1. **Etiology**

   a. The etiologic agent is a yeast (fungi) organism, usually ***Candida albicans.*** The organism is a common inhabitant of the bowel and perianal region. Thirty percent of women **may have vaginal colonization and have no symptoms of infection.**

   b. Several factors may lead to symptomatic infection instead of colonization.

      (1) Contraceptive practices (e.g., birth control pills and vaginal spermicides, which influence vaginal pH)

      (2) Use of systemic steroids, which influence the immune system

      (3) Use of antibiotics, which alters the microbiology of the vagina; 25 to 70% of women report yeast infections after antibiotic use. Any antibiotic, particularly a broad-spectrum agent, may play a causative role.

      (4) Tight clothing, panty hose, and bathing suits (yeast thrives in a dark, warm, moist environment)

      (5) Undiagnosed or uncontrolled diabetes mellitus

   c. Another reason for a refractory monilial infection may be **compromised immune status;** with recurrent monilial vaginitis, an HIV test is indicated.

   d. There has been a recent **increase in the number of infections caused by non-*albicans* species.** Up to 20% of infections may be caused by organisms such as *Candida tropicalis* and *Torulopsis glabrata.* These organisms may be resistant to standard treatment regimens.

2. **Clinical presentation.** Patients with monilial vaginitis characteristically complain of a thick, white discharge and extreme vulvar pruritus. The vulva may be red and swollen.

   a. Symptoms may recur and be most prominent just before menses or in association with intercourse.

   b. Yeast infections may occur more frequently during pregnancy.

   c. Patients with infections caused by *C. tropicalis* and *T. glabrata* may have an atypical presentation. Irritation may be paramount, with little discharge or pruritus.

3. **Diagnosis.** Diagnosis is made by history, physical examination, and microscopic examination of the vaginal discharge in saline and 10% KOH.

   a. On examination, excoriations of the vulva may be noticeable; the vulva and vagina may be erythematous, with patches of adherent cottage cheese–like discharge.

   b. Infection with *C. tropicalis* and *T. glabrata* may not be associated with the classic discharge; discharge may be white-gray and thin.

   c. Vaginal pH may be normal or slightly more basic than normal (4.0 to 4.7).

   d. Wet mount microscopic examination reveals hyphae or pseudohyphae with budding yeast in 50 to 70% of women with yeast infections.

   e. Cultures are not necessary to make the diagnosis except in some cases of recurrent infections.

4. **Treatment.** Many agents are available for the treatment of vulvovaginal candidiasis. These include topical agents, which may be available over-the-counter (OTC) or by prescription, and oral agents, which are available by prescription only.

   a. **Antifungal intravaginal agents** are administered as suppositories or creams. These drugs are available in three regimens: a single dose, 3-day course, or 7-day course. Agents include butoconazole, clotrimazole, miconazole, tioconazole, and terconazole. **OTC regimens** should be used only by women who have been diagnosed with a yeast infection in the past and are experiencing identical symptoms.

   b. **Oral agents** include fluconazole and ketoconazole.

      (1) Fluconazole is available as a single-dose (150 mg) treatment for uncomplicated vaginal candidiasis.

(2) Ketoconazole is used effectively for the treatment of chronic and recurrent candidiasis; a 5% incidence of hepatotoxicity limits more widespread use. The dosing schedule is 200 mg twice a day for 5 days, then 100 to 200 mg daily for 6 months.

   c. Boric acid capsules intravaginally, 600 mg for 14 days, may be effective.

5. Chronic recurrent yeast infections (5% of women). In most cases, no exacerbating factor can be found; however, the following possibilities should be considered:

   a. Failure to complete a full course of therapy

   b. HIV infection. Recalcitrant candidiasis may be a presenting symptom in women with HIV infection. HIV testing should be considered and offered to the patient.

   c. Chronic antibiotic therapy

   d. Infection with a resistant organism such as *C. tropicalis* or *T. glabrata*

   e. Sexual transmission from the male partner

   f. Allergic reaction to partner's semen or a vaginal spermicide

C *Trichomonas vaginalis* **vaginitis (trichomoniasis)** is the third most common vaginitis, accounting for 25% of cases.

1. Etiology. The motile protozoan *T. vaginalis* is the etiologic agent. The trichomonad can be recovered from 70 to 80% of the male partners of the infected patient; therefore, *Trichomonas* vaginitis is an STD.

2. Clinical presentation. *Trichomonas* vaginitis is a multifocal infection involving the vaginal epithelium, Skene glands, Bartholin glands, and the urethra.

   a. Unless asked directly, 25 to 50% of women may not report symptoms.

   b. Most women report a discharge that is described as copious, green, and frothy. The discharge may be associated with a foul odor and vulvar irritation or pruritus.

3. Diagnosis

   a. Physical examination. Classic evidence of trichomoniasis may be seen.

     (1) The characteristic green discharge may be evident.

     (2) Punctation, described classically as the "strawberry cervix," is evident in only 25% of patients.

   b. Laboratory tests

     (1) The vaginal pH is usually between 5.0 and 7.0.

     (2) Saline wet mount of the vaginal discharge reveals **numerous leukocytes** and the highly motile, flagellated trichomonads (as many as 75% of cases).

     (3) Cultures are not usually necessary to make the diagnosis. They should be obtained when the diagnosis is suspected but cannot be confirmed by wet mount examination.

     (4) Pap smears may be positive in as many as 65% of cases. Positive Pap smears should be confirmed by wet mount examination because of the high false-positive rate.

4. Treatment. Because *Trichomonas* is sexually transmitted, **both partners require therapy;** 25% of women will be reinfected if their partner does not receive treatment.

   a. Vaginal therapy alone is ineffective because of the multiple sites of infection, and **systemic agents are necessary.**

   b. If both partners are treated simultaneously, cure rates of 90% are achieved with treatment with **metronidazole.** Patients should be warned that a disulfiram-like reaction may occur and that they should abstain from alcohol use during treatment.

     (1) The preferred regimen is 2 g in one dose because of ease of compliance. As many as 10% of patients may experience vomiting.

     (2) An alternative regimen is 500 mg twice daily for 7 days or 250 mg three times daily for 7 days.

   d. Resistant cases may require treatment with intravenous metronidazole. Because resistance is rare, other causes, such as noncompliance of the patient or partner, should be considered.

e. Metronidazole is **contraindicated for use during the first trimester of pregnancy.** After this time, it can be used to treat *Trichomonas* infections.

f. Infected patients should be screened for other STDs.

D Atrophic vaginitis

1. **Etiology.** Atrophic vaginitis, associated with decreased estradiol levels, is most often seen in postmenopausal women but also may be seen in breastfeeding women. Atrophic changes in the vulvovaginal tissues result from **estrogen withdrawal;** the normal protective thickness of the vaginal epithelium depends on estrogen stimulation.

2. **Clinical presentation**
   a. Without consistent and sufficient estrogen, the vaginal epithelium becomes thin; vulvar structures may atrophy.
   b. The amount of glycogen also decreases, and the pH becomes alkaline.
   c. The vagina is often pale with punctate hemorrhagic spots throughout the vaginal wall. There is an absence of superficial epithelial cells and a predominance of parabasal cells.

3. **Diagnosis**
   a. Atrophic vaginitis must be suspected in hypoestrogenic women who present with leukorrhea, pruritus, burning, tenderness, and dyspareunia.
   b. Physical examination of the vagina reveals atrophic, sometimes inflamed vaginal walls. A discharge may be present.
   c. Vaginal pH is usually greater than 4.5.
   d. Vaginal infection is not identified on a wet mount preparation.

4. **Treatment.** Topical administration of vaginal cream containing estrogen reverses symptoms and tissue changes.
   a. Symptoms respond to short-term therapy but recur on discontinuation.
   b. Changes in tissues require long-term therapy and may not be noticed until after 3 to 4 months of treatment. Proliferation and maturation of the vaginal epithelium, as well as compliance and elasticity of the vaginal wall, are restored.
   c. Therapeutic agents may be systemic or topical.
      (1) **Hormone replacement therapy** may be given in accordance with a standard regimen.
      (2) **Estrogen cream** is administered intravaginally every night for up to 2 weeks and then continued once or twice a week to maintain results.

E Vulvar dystrophies

1. **Etiology.** Vulvar dystrophies are dermatologic conditions of the vulvar skin of uncertain etiology. Most frequently seen in postmenopausal women, these conditions often accompany a history of chronic candidal vulvovaginitis. The dystrophies can be:
   a. Hyperplastic when the epithelium is markedly thickened
   b. Atrophic (*lichen sclerosus et atrophicus*)
   c. A mixture of both

2. **Clinical presentation**
   a. With **hyperplastic dystrophy,** the most common symptom is constant pruritus. Scratching frequently exacerbates the pruritus, creating a vicious cycle.
   b. With **lichen sclerosus,** vulvar burning, pruritus, or chronic soreness associated with "vulvar dysuria" frequently occurs.

3. **Diagnosis. Vulvar biopsy** is ultimately necessary to make the diagnosis, but a preliminary diagnosis can be made based on **physical examination.**
   a. **Hyperplastic dystrophy** presents as thickened skin ("elephant hide") accompanied by linear excoriations from scratching. Areas of leukoplakia may also be noted.

  b. Lichen sclerosus presents as extremely pale, thin skin, often with subepithelial hemorrhages. In its most severe form, painful contraction of the introitus or clitoral hood is noted. Loss of labial architecture may occur.

4. Treatment

  a. Hyperplastic dystrophy responds well to a 6- to 8-week trial of topical fluorinated steroid cream. Chronic therapy may be necessary on an intermittent basis.

  b. Lichen sclerosus responds to long-term topical testosterone preparations. If this treatment is not tolerated, a topical progesterone preparation may be helpful. Fluorinated steroid creams may also provide relief in women who cannot tolerate other preparations.

F Traumatic vaginitis

1. Etiology. Traumatic vaginitis is usually the result of injury or chemical irritation.

  a. In **adults,** the most common cause of injury to the vagina is a "lost" tampon.

  b. In **pediatric patients,** foreign bodies placed in the vagina serve as sources of infection or trauma (e.g., wads of paper, chewing gum, or paper clips).

  c. Chemical irritation can be secondary to douches, deodorants, lubricants, or topical intravaginal preparations.

2. Treatment. Vulvovaginitis resulting from foreign bodies or chemical irritants responds immediately to withdrawal of the causative agent.

G Neoplasia

1. Etiology. Malignancies can masquerade for months as vulvar lesions; thus, they are often ignored by patients or mistreated by physicians as irritations or infections.

2. Diagnosis. Patients who present with a long-term history of symptoms and treatment failures of vulvar lesions should undergo biopsy before receiving further therapy.

3. Treatment. Therapy appropriate for the condition described in the pathology report is indicated.

H Herpes simplex genitalis

1. Etiology

  a. Herpes genitalis is caused by the herpes simplex virus (HSV), a member of the Herpesviridae family of viruses, which are capable of establishing latent status and causing recurrent disease.

  b. From 70 to 90% of cases of herpes genitalis are caused by HSV type 2 (HSV-2); HSV type 1 (HSV-1) is the etiologic agent in only 13% of cases.

  c. From 60 to 85% of women with antibodies to HSV-2 have never had a recognized genital ulcer.

  d. Transmission is through direct contact with an individual who is actively shedding virus from skin or mucous membrane lesions.

2. Clinical presentation

  a. Primary infection

  (1) The infection is usually acquired from sexual contact, with symptoms appearing in 2 to 12 days

  (2) Primary infection is often associated with systemic, flulike symptoms (e.g., malaise, myalgias, and headache). Primary symptoms may last from 2 days to 3 weeks. Symptoms may be milder in women with antibodies to HSV-1.

  (3) Pain and itching may precede the development of vesicular lesions, which may appear on the labia, perineum, buttocks, urethra, vagina, cervix, and bladder. Cervical involvement is seen in 70% of women with genital involvement.

  (4) Vesicles progress to ulcers and may coalesce. Lesions are exquisitely tender. Primary lesions persist for 3 to 6 weeks and usually heal without scarring.

  (5) Local symptoms consist of hyperesthesia, burning, itching, dysuria, and (frequently) exquisite pain and tenderness of the vulva. Vulvar pain makes intercourse unbearable and may lead to urinary retention.

(6) Tender inguinal lymphadenopathy may be present.
(7) Viral shedding may persist for 12 days.
(8) Complications include sacral radiculopathy with urinary or fecal retention and aseptic meningitis (rare).

b. Recurrent infection
(1) The dormant herpesvirus resides in the neurons of the sacral ganglia, which supply the areas of cutaneous involvement.
(2) Periodic asymptomatic viral shedding occurs, particularly during the first 6 months after infection.
(3) Recurrences are most frequent during the first year. Frequency of recurrence varies. Some patients never have another outbreak; others have frequent recurrences.
(4) Many women experience prodromal symptoms of itching and burning from 30 minutes to 2 days before an outbreak. Systemic symptoms usually do not occur with recurrences.
(5) Recurrent lesions tend to be less severe and are of shorter duration (3 to 7 days).

3. Diagnosis
a. When typical lesions are present, a presumptive diagnosis of herpes genitalis can be made on physical examination. HSV-2 should be suspected when superficial ulcerations of the vulvo-vaginal tissues are identified.
b. Viral culture is the **gold standard** by which the diagnosis of HSV infection is made. It requires 48 hours for completion. **Sensitivity of cultures is 90% if vesicles are present, but only 30% if lesions are crusted.**
c. Cytologic studies and direct identification methods, such as **immunofluorescence**, offer confirmatory evidence of an HSV infection but are only **50% sensitive.**

4. Treatment
a. Local measures used for comfort during the acute outbreak include sitz baths and topical anesthetic creams. The area should be kept clean and dry to avoid secondary infection.
b. Catheterization may be necessary for acute urinary retention.
c. The **antiviral drug acyclovir**, a cyclic purine nucleoside analog, is active against herpesvirus both in vivo and in vitro. It can be applied topically or taken orally for a **primary** episode of HSV-2 infection. Other antiviral agents are being developed for this purpose.
(1) Oral acyclovir decreases the time of viral shedding, the duration of symptoms, and the time to healing in primary herpes outbreaks. The recommended dose is 200 mg five times daily for 10 days.
(2) If oral acyclovir is started when the recurrence begins, it also decreases duration of viral shedding, time to healing, and local symptoms. Recommended dose is 200 mg five times daily for 5 days.
(3) Studies have shown that oral acyclovir decreases the frequency of recurrences by as much as 75%. Suppressive therapy has been approved for up to 5 years. The recommended dose is 200 mg three times daily or 400 mg twice daily. Alternatives include famciclovir (250 mg twice daily or 500 mg once daily) and valacyclovir (500 mg twice daily or 1 g once daily). Therapy is discontinued annually, and frequency of recurrences is documented. Treatment is restarted as indicated.

Study Questions for Chapter 26

Directions: *Match each word or statement below with the most specific anatomic site above. Each answer may be used once, more than once, or not at all.*

[A] labia majora
[B] labia minora
[C] clitoris
[D] vestibule
[E] prepuce
[F] Bartholin gland
[G] Skene gland
[H] pudendal
[I] ilioinguinal
[J] posterior femoral cutaneous
[K] external pudendal
[L] cervical

1. Embryologic homolog in the male is the floor of the penile urethra

2. Embryologic homolog in the male is the Cowper's gland(s)

3. Contains sebaceous glands but not hair follicles or sweat glands; is a paired structure

4. Source of vaginal lubrication during intercourse

5. Azygous artery of the vagina

Directions: *Each of the numbered items or incomplete statements in this section is followed by answers or by completions of the statement. Select the ONE lettered answer or completion that is BEST in each case.*

6. A 23-year-old woman, gravida 2, para 1 at 10 weeks of gestation presents to your office reports increasing yellow vaginal discharge that has an odor. A vaginal smear reveals clue cells. She denies pruritus. She does not have any significant medical history or allergies to medication. The next best step in management of this patient is

[A] oral metronidazole
[B] vaginal metronidazole
[C] oral clindamycin
[D] vaginal clindamycin
[E] oral fluconazole

7. A 25-year-old woman gravida 1, para 1 presents to your office reporting four recurrent yeast infections within the last 2 months. You perform a wet mount and a 10% KOH prep and confirm presence of many pseudohyphae and absence of clue cells or leukocytes. She says she has taken every over-the-counter medication available and has been treated with oral fluconazole. She is not pregnant, is not on birth control, and has not been sexually active for 7 months. She is positive for hepatitis B surface antigen, and her liver function tests are slightly elevated. The last physician who saw her screened her for HIV and diabetes mellitus. What is the next best step in management of this patient?

[A] Long-term oral fluconazole
[B] Long-term oral ketoconazole
[C] Boric acid capsules intravaginally
[D] Oral metronidazole
[E] Oral acyclovir

Match each of the statements below with the best word(s) above. Each answer may be used once, more than once, or not at all.

A Bacterial vaginosis
B Moniliasis
C Trichomoniasis
D Herpes simplex
E Atrophic vaginitis
F Lichen sclerosus
G Hyperplastic dystrophy
H Traumatic vaginitis

8. A 19-year-old woman complains of increasing discharge and odor. Her pH is 5.5, and wet mount reveals lack of leukocytes and protozoa.

9. A 24-year-old woman who is 2 months postpartum and is breastfeeding reports itching and dyspareunia. Speculum examination reveals pale, dry vaginal walls.

10. A wet mount shows a predominance of cells with large nuclei (parabasal cells).

Answers and Explanations

1. B [II A 1 e2] 2. F [II A 1 h2] 3. B [II A 1 c] 4. L [II B 1 a2] 5. L [II B 3]. The embryologic homolog of the labia minora in the male is the floor of the penile urethra. The embryologic homolog of the Bartholin's glands in the male is the Cowper's glands. Although both the labia minora and the prepuce contain sebaceous glands but not hair follicles, only the labia minora (plural) is a paired structure (i.e., there are two labium majus [singular]). Because the vagina does not contain any glandular structures, the cervical secretions and transudation of fluid from vessels across the vaginal epithelium provide lubrication during intercourse. The azygous artery of the vagina arises from the cervical branch of the uterine artery.

6. The answer is B [VI A 4 d2]. Oral metronidazole is contraindicated in the first trimester; thus, the intravaginal preparation is preferred. Although clindamycin can be used throughout pregnancy, it is not the initial recommended agent for treatment of bacterial vaginosis because it is not as effective. Azithromycin may be used for treatment of chlamydia.

7. The answer is C [VI B 4 c]. Patients with recurrent or recalcitrant fungal infection who are negative for HIV and diabetes and who have been treated with–azole anti-fungal agents may be harboring species other than *Candida albicans* and may benefit from a trial of intravaginal boric acid (which has a different mechanism of action.) Both oral fluconazole and ketoconazole should not be used in a patient with elevated liver enzymes because of their potential hepatotoxicity. Oral metronidazole is used to treat bacterial vaginosis or trichomonas vaginalis. Oral acyclovir is used to treat herpes simplex.

8. A [VI A 3] 9. E [VI D 1] 10. E [VI D 2]. The only discharges that have a pH higher than 4.2 are bacterial vaginosis, trichomonas, and atrophic vaginitis. Trichomonas is unlikely because there are no protozoa on wet mount and there is paucity of leukocytes. Atrophic vaginitis is unlikely in a young woman who is not estrogen deprived. Absence of superficial epithelial cells and a predominance of parabasal cells are typical of atrophic vaginitis.

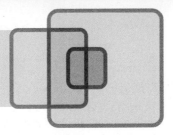

chapter **27**

Sexually Transmitted Diseases

ANN HONEBRINK

I INTRODUCTION

A **Sexually transmitted diseases (STDs)** are among the oldest described conditions in medical history. References to gonorrhea can be found in the Bible. The number of protozoan, bacterial, viral, and ectoparasitic infections that have been identified as sexually transmitted has continued to increase since biblical times.

B **Control of STDs** is currently a major public health concern, especially because there is a growing appreciation that individuals infected with other STDs are more susceptible to infection with HIV. In the developed world, the United States has the highest incidence of STDs, with an estimated cost of more than $17 billion per year.

C **Evidence-based treatment and cure** is effective for the majority of STDs. Currently accepted treatment regimens in the United States are based on recommended regimens published and regularly updated by the Centers for Disease Control and Prevention (CDC). Primary prevention of STDs focuses on counseling at-risk individuals in an attempt to control this major health problem. Because incidence rates of many STDs are highest among adolescents, it is essential that prevention counseling, screening, and treatment strategies include the special needs of this age group.

II BACTERIAL SEXUALLY TRANSMITTED DISEASES

A **Gonorrhea.** The cause of this STD is the gram-negative diplococcus *Neisseria gonorrhoeae.* Humans are the only natural host of this bacterium, which has a predilection for **columnar and transitional epithelium.** In **women,** who often have mild or no symptoms, gonorrhea may cause cervicitis, urethritis, pelvic inflammatory disease (PID), and acute pharyngitis. In **men,** who are usually symptomatic, infection causes urethritis, prostatitis, and epididymitis. Systemic sequelae (see II A 2 f, g) later develop in both men and women. In **newborns,** exposure at birth may cause blindness, infection of the joints, or even serious sepsis.

1. Epidemiology
   a. In 2001, 361,705 cases of gonorrhea were reported to the CDC; this figure is believed to represent about half of the total infections in the United States. An estimated 650,000 new cases of gonorrhea occur in the United States annually. Infection rates increased between 1997 and 1999, especially among gay and bisexual men. **Approximately 75% of reported cases occur among 15- to 29-year-old individuals.** Approximately 77% of reported cases occurred in African Americans in 1999.
   b. In annual screening programs in non-STD clinics, the average gonorrhea detection rate is 2.7%. **Transmission** from men to women by sexual contact is likely to result in infection after a **single exposure. Risk factors** include:
      (1) Young age
      (2) Multiple sexual partners

(3) Failure to use barrier contraception

(4) Early sexual activity

2. **Clinical presentation.** In both sexes, when symptoms occur, they usually appear 2 to 5 days after exposure but may not be evident for 30 days. Although women may often be initially asymptomatic, symptoms of gonococcal pelvic inflammatory disease (PID) often occur after a menstrual period. Symptoms include:

   a. Mucopurulent discharge, as occurs in acute cervicitis in women and urethritis in men

   b. Lower abdominal pain, anorexia, and fever, as is characteristic of acute PID

   c. Dysuria (men and women)

   d. Pharyngitis (in men and women after oral contact with an infected penis)

   e. Proctitis in male or female recipients of anal intercourse

   f. **Infection at other sites**

      (1) Arthritis (men and women)

      (2) Septicemia (men and women)

      (3) Perihepatitis (women)

      (4) Chorioamnionitis or endometritis (women)

      (5) Endocarditis (men and women)

   g. **Other sequelae**

      (1) Women: increased risk of infertility, chronic pelvic pain, ectopic pregnancy

      (2) Men: risk of epididymitis with subsequent infertility and urethral scarring, chronic prostatitis

      (3) Both sexes: increased susceptibility to infection with HIV exposure

3. **Diagnosis.** Exact diagnosis depends on identification of *N. gonorrhoeae* by one of several methods:

   a. **Thayer-Martin culture medium.** This technique is selective for *N. gonorrhoeae*. Culture specimens must be incubated at 35 to 36°C in a 5% CO_2 atmosphere. This culture technique is highly sensitive and specific, inexpensive, and suitable for use for specimens taken from a variety of body sites (e.g., rectum, pharynx, cervix, and urethra). In addition, it can test for antimicrobial sensitivity. Culture is preferred for children or other individuals in which the diagnosis may have legal implications.

   b. **Gram stain,** looking for gram-negative diplococci in polymorphonuclear leukocytes. This test is actually useful only in male intraurethral specimens because samples from other sites may yield results that can be confused with normal flora, decreasing both sensitivity and specificity.

   c. **Nucleic acid amplification test (NAAT).** This test, which uses nucleic acid sequences unique to a specific organism for identification, does not require viable organisms to produce a positive result. The NAAT has a sensitivity of 96.7% in endocervical specimens using culture as a standard.

4. **Treatment.** Because coinfection with *Chlamydia trachomatis* occurs often in patients infected with *N. gonorrhoeae*, consideration should be given to treatment plans that cover both organisms, especially in populations at high risk for STDs.

   a. For **uncomplicated gonococcal infection of the urethra, cervix, and rectum,** all recommended regimens involve a **single treatment,** which is important in increasing compliance. CDC-recommended regimens include:

      (1) Cephalosporins, such as cefixime 400 mg by mouth or ceftriaxone 125 mg intramuscularly. Ceftriaxone is also a recommended option for treating pharyngeal gonorrheal infection.

      (2) Quinolones, such as ciprofloxacin 500 mg orally (also recommended for pharyngeal infections), ofloxacin 400 mg orally, or levofloxacin 250 mg. Quinolones should not be used in children under 18 years of age who weigh less than 45 kg and should not be used in pregnant women. Quinolone-resistant strains have been reported in Hawaii.

      (3) Alternative regimen: spectinomycin 2 g intramuscularly

    b. When treating for presumed or proven coinfection with *C. trachomatis,* it is necessary to add either azithromycin 1 g orally (single dose) or doxycycline 100 mg orally twice daily for 7 days. (Doxycycline should not be used in pregnant women or in children.)

    c. More complex, inpatient treatment is required for patients with PID (see Chapter 28); infected infants; and individuals with disseminated gonorrhea, gonorrheal meningitis, or endocarditis.

5. Follow-up. As with any STD, patients with gonorrhea should be tested for other STDs, including HIV and hepatitis B. All sexual partners should also be evaluated and treated. Although tests of cure are no longer necessary when patients are treated successfully with the previously described regimens (see II A 4), tests for reinfection should be considered in individuals at high risk. When using **nucleic acid tests**, remember that the test **can remain positive for up to 3 weeks after treatment**; live organisms need not be present for a positive test. Repeat testing is also warranted in individuals with persistent symptoms.

B **Chlamydia.** *Chlamydia,* a genus of obligatory intracellular bacteria, is the pathogen in a broad spectrum of STDs. *C. trachomatis,* serotypes D, E, F, G, H, I, J, and K, is the obligate intracellular bacterium that causes chlamydia.

1. Epidemiology. Chlamydia is the **most commonly reported STD** in the United States; 650,000 cases were reported in 1999. The estimated annual number of actual infections in the United States is 3 million. Chlamydia is most commonly diagnosed in adolescents and young adults up to 25 years of age. By the age of 30 years, 50% of sexually active women in the United States have serologic evidence of prior chlamydial infection. However, the STD also occurs in older, at-risk individuals. Coinfection with *N. gonorrhoeae* is common, and susceptibility to HIV infection in individuals with chlamydia is estimated to be increased three- to fivefold.

2. Clinical presentation

    a. Women are asymptomatic 75% of the time.

    b. In symptomatic women, **mucopurulent cervicitis** can be demonstrated.

    c. Symptoms of **urethritis** and **pyuria** and a **negative urine culture** in sexually active women suggest a chlamydial infection.

    d. **Fever** and **lower abdominal pain** suggest PID, which occurs in as many as 40% of women with untreated chlamydia (see Chapter 28). These infections may be more insidious and protracted in duration than those associated with gonococcal PID.

    e. Although 50% of chlamydial infections in men are asymptomatic, urethritis may occur.

    f. In exposed infants, *C. trachomatis* may cause conjunctivitis and pneumonia.

3. Diagnosis

    a. Culture. This highly specific technique has been the gold standard for diagnosis of chlamydia and should be used in children and in other cases that have potential legal implications. Antimicrobial susceptibility testing can be performed on isolates. However, culture techniques are expensive and technically challenging, and the results are difficult to standardize. All of these factors limit culture sensitivity.

    b. Nucleic acid amplification test. This sensitive test amplifies organism-specific nucleic acid sequences, most commonly using either PCR or LCR. Urine testing is possible to detect genital infection in both men and women; however, endocervical sampling in women may be more sensitive. These amplified techniques have recently become the gold standard.

4. Treatment. The therapy for PID is discussed in detail in Chapter 28. Treatment for uncomplicated cases of urethritis and cervicitis includes:

    a. Doxycycline 100 mg orally twice daily for 7 days

    b. Azithromycin 1 g orally

    c. Ofloxacin 300 mg orally twice daily for 7 days

    d. Erythromycin base 500 mg orally four times daily for 7 days

    e. Levofloxacin 500 mg orally for 7 days

5. Follow-up

    a. Retesting for cure may not be necessary after treatment with single-dose azithromycin or a complete course of doxycycline. In fact, retesting using nucleic acid technology less than 3 to 6 weeks after treatment may yield false-positive results in adequately treated individuals because nucleic acid technology does not rely on live organisms to produce a positive test.

    b. However, retesting is advisable when reinfection is suspected and compliance with medication is not certain, especially in cases in which symptoms persist. Because reinfection with chlamydia is common in studies of previously infected women, the CDC recommends that rescreening be considered 3 to 4 months after treatment. In addition, test of cure at 3 or more weeks after treatment is recommended when erythromycin (commonly used in pregnancy) is used for treatment.

6. Sequelae. Complications may include PID, ectopic pregnancy, and infertility.

C **Chancroid.** The gram-negative coccobacillus *Haemophilus ducreyi* causes this genital ulcerative disease.

1. Epidemiology

    a. Chancroid is rare in the United States but common worldwide. In 1999, only 143 cases were reported in the United States, where this STD is seen most frequently in discrete outbreaks. However, it is probably underdiagnosed and underreported. Trauma facilitates entry into mucosal vulvar tissues in women. The incubation time is 3 to 5 days.

    b. Chancroid is a known cofactor in HIV transmission, and there is a high incidence of coexisting HIV infection among individuals with chancroid worldwide. Ten percent of patients in the United States with chancroid may also be infected with syphilis or herpes. Coinfection is more likely when chancroid is acquired outside the United States.

2. Clinical presentation. Lesions begin as small papules and progress to painful genital ulcers in 2 to 3 days. If the lesions are left untreated, buboes and inguinal ulcers may develop, accompanied by regional lymphadenopathy.

3. Diagnosis. Culture is not widely available and is only 80% sensitive. PCR tests are being developed, but none in the United States have yet been approved by the Food and Drug Administration. Probable diagnosis is made when painful genital ulcers are present without evidence of herpes (culture) or syphilis (darkfield examination and serologic testing). Diagnosis is supported by coexisting painful inguinal adenopathy, which occurs in up to one-third of cases.

4. Treatment. Sexual partners should receive treatment as well. Therapeutic regimens include:

    a. Azithromycin 1 g orally

    b. Ceftriaxone 250 mg intramuscularly

    c. Ciprofloxacin 500 mg orally twice daily for 3 days

    d. Erythromycin base 500 mg orally three times daily for 7 days

D **Granuloma inguinale.** This genital ulcerative disease, which is also known as donovanosis, is caused by *Calymmatobacterium granulomatis*, a gram-negative bacterium.

1. Epidemiology. This STD is rare in the United States, but it is endemic in some tropical areas. Ulcers appear after an 8 to 80-day incubation period. Coinfection of ulcers with other STDs may occur.

2. Clinical presentation. Affected individuals present with a painless, beefy red, friable ulcerative lesion with accompanying inguinal groin swelling caused by subcutaneous spread of granuloma. This condition may lead to lymphedema and elephantiasis of the external genitalia.

3. Diagnosis: Culture of *C. granulomatis* is difficult. When the diagnosis is expected based on appearance of lesions, scrapings of ulcers show pathognomonic cells—mononuclear cells with inclusion cysts containing gram-negative pleomorphic rod-like organisms, known as Donovan bodies.

4. **Treatment.** Repeat courses of treatment may be necessary. One of the following therapeutic regimens may be used:
    a. **Doxycycline** 100 mg orally twice daily for at least 3 weeks
    b. **Trimethoprim—sulfamethoxazole** 160 mg/800 mg orally twice daily for at least 3 weeks
    c. **Ciprofloxacin** 750 mg orally twice daily for at least 3 weeks
    d. **Erythromycin base** 500 mg orally four times daily for at least 3 weeks
    e. **Azithromycin** 1 g orally once a week for at least 3 weeks

E **Bacterial vaginosis (BV).** This STD results from the replacement of the normal H_2O_2-producing *Lactobacillus* with high concentrations of anaerobic bacteria, such as *Gardnerella vaginalis, Mobiluncus, Bacteroides,* and *Mycoplasma.* BV is included in this chapter, but it is not considered solely an STD.

1. **Epidemiology.** BV is the most common cause of vaginal discharge and odor, but 50% of women who meet criteria for diagnosis (see I D 2) are asymptomatic. In addition, BV has also become increasingly associated with pregnancy complications, PID, and post-procedure endometritis and cuff cellulitis.

2. **Diagnosis.** BV may be diagnosed by the use of clinical or Gram stain evidence. Clinical diagnosis requires three of the following criteria:
    a. Homogenous, grayish, noninflammatory discharge that adheres to vaginal walls
    b. Saline preparation of vaginal secretions that reveals squamous cells whose borders are obscured by coccobacillary forms, known as **clue cells**
    c. pH of secretions greater than 4.5
    d. Fishy odor after addition of **10% potassium hydroxide** ("whiff" test)

3. **Treatment.** Women with symptomatic disease who are not pregnant require treatment. Whether treatment in pregnant women reduces pregnancy-related complications, most notably preterm labor, remains controversial. Studies have shown a reduction in postoperative infections in women who received preoperative treatment. **Effective treatments** include the following:
    a. **Metronidazole** 500 mg orally twice daily for 7 days
    b. **Metronidazole gel** (0.75%) one applicator intravaginally once daily for 5 days
    c. **Clindamycin** cream (2%) one applicator intravaginally at bedtime for 7 days

F **Lymphogranuloma venereum (LGV).** *C. trachomatis,* serotypes L_1, L_2, and L_3, causes LGV, producing a wide variety of local and regional ulcerations and destruction of genital tissues.

1. **Epidemiology.** LGV rarely occurs in the United States and is more frequently seen in tropical countries.

2. **Clinical presentation.** Between 34 and 21 days after exposure, genital ulcers appear at the site of inoculation. The lesions resolve spontaneously. After this, tender, unilateral inguinal or femoral adenopathy develops. When the rectum is infected, both men and women experience proctitis with accompanying perianal inflammation and lymphatic involvement, which can lead to fistula formation and strictures.

3. **Diagnosis.** Usually, diagnosis is made serologically or by exclusion of other causes of inguinal lymphadenopathy. **Complement fixation** is the test of choice. Titers greater than 1:64 indicate active infection.

4. **Treatment**
    a. **Doxycycline** 100 mg orally twice daily for 21 days
    b. **Erythromycin** 500 mg orally four times daily for 21 days
    c. **Surgical reconstruction** may be required for patients with considerable tissue destruction in the tertiary stage.

III SYPHILIS

The cause of this systemic STD is the spirochete *Treponema pallidum*. It can be transmitted by direct sexual contact with an infected lesion, by contact with the infected blood, or by intrauterine transmission from mother to fetus (congenital syphilis). Syphilis has been called the "great imitator" because of its association with a variety of signs and symptoms.

A Epidemiology. With the introduction of penicillin treatment and public health programs in the 1940s, syphilis was nearly eliminated in the United States by 1957. Since then, national epidemics have occurred in a cyclic fashion every 7 to 10 years. Infection rates have been decreasing since 1990 with a recent slight increase in 2001, largely among gay and bisexual men. Infection rates are highest in 20- to 39-year-old individuals; the disease is currently more common among men who have sex with other men. Of the total 35,600 cases of syphilis reported in the United States in 1999, 6,650 were new cases of primary and secondary syphilis and 556 were new cases of congenital syphilis. The presence of syphilis increases the risk of acquiring HIV by a factor of two to five.

B Clinical presentation

1. The **initial lesion** of primary syphilis is a painless, ulcerated, hard **chancre,** usually on the external genitalia, although vaginal and cervical lesions may also be detected. Incubation time from exposure to first symptom is 10 to 90 days. The primary lesions resolve in 2 to 6 weeks.

2. In **untreated patients,** this chancre is followed in 6 weeks to 6 months by a **secondary or bacteremic stage** in which the skin and mucous membranes are affected. A **maculopapular rash** of the palms, soles, and mucous membranes occurs. **Condyloma latum** and **generalized lymphadenopathy** are seen as well. These lesions usually resolve within 2 to 6 weeks.

3. Approximately 33% of untreated patients progress to **tertiary syphilis** with **multiple organ involvement.** Endarteritis leads to aortic aneurysm and aortic insufficiency, tabes dorsalis, optic atrophy, and meningovascular syphilis, as well as gummatous lesions.

4. **Latent infection** occurs in infected individuals with no clinical manifestations of the disease. Latent infection is detected serologically and classified as **early latent** (infection of less than 1 year's duration) or **late latent** (infection of more than 1 year's duration) or latent syphilis of unknown duration.

5. Identification and treatment of pregnant women with diagnosed syphilis is the mainstay of prevention of **congenital syphilis.** Untreated congenital syphilis may cause stillbirth, nonimmune hydrops, jaundice, infant hepatosplenomegaly, and skin rash and pseudoparalysis of an arm or leg.

C Diagnosis. **Darkfield examination** of fresh specimens detects spirochetes in the primary and secondary stages of the disease. **Serologic tests** are helpful in diagnosing syphilis in patients who have progressed beyond primary disease. In the primary stage, infected individuals have not had sufficient time to mount an immune response that can be serologically detected. There are **two types of serologic tests.**

1. **Nontreponemal tests,** which are measured quantitatively in titers and usually correlate with disease activity. These tests usually become negative after treatment, but a low-level positive titer can persist for many years. A fourfold increase or decrease in titer using the same test is believed to be clinically significant. There are two nontreponemal tests:
   a. Rapid plasma reagin (**RPR**)
   b. Venereal Disease Research Laboratory (**VDRL**)

2. **Treponemal antibody tests,** which can remain positive for life. Early treatment of primary syphilis makes it more likely that treponemal antibody tests will become negative. Treponemal antibody titers are not used to assess treatment response because they correlate poorly with disease activity. There are two treponemal antibody tests:
   a. Fluorescent treponemal antibody absorption (**FTA-ABS**)
   b. *T. pallidum* particle agglutination (**TP-PA**)

3. Both types of serologic tests should be used to diagnose syphilis because various medical conditions can cause a false-positive RPR or VDRL.

D **Treatment**

1. **General considerations**
   a. **Need for treatment.** Individuals with a history of sexual contact with a person with documented syphilis, a positive darkfield examination, or a positive FTA-ABS test should be treated. Sexual contacts of patients receiving therapy should also be treated. Possible reinfection should also prompt treatment; a fourfold increase in a quantitative antitreponemal test implies reinfection.
   b. **Safety of therapeutic regimens.** Treatment regimens are based on duration and severity of syphilis. Alternative treatments are listed for penicillin-allergic patients, but much less objective evidence exists for optimum dosing and duration of these alternative regimens. The **Jarisch-Herxheimer reaction,** an acute febrile reaction that may be accompanied by myalgias, headache, and other systemic symptoms, can occur within 24 hours after treatment of syphilis at any stage, especially early disease.

2. **Specific regimens**
   a. **Early disease:** primary, secondary, or early latent
      (1) **Benzathine penicillin G** 2.4 million units intramuscularly in a single dose
      (2) **Doxycycline** 100 mg orally twice daily or **tetracycline** 500 mg orally four times daily for 2 weeks in nonpregnant patients with penicillin allergy
   b. **Late disease:** late latent or latent syphilis of unknown duration as well as tertiary syphilis (not including neurosyphilis)
      (1) **Benzathine penicillin G** 2.4 million units intramuscularly every week for 3 weeks
      (2) **Doxycycline** 100 mg orally twice daily or **tetracycline** 500 mg orally four times daily for 4 weeks in nonpregnant patients with penicillin allergy
   c. **Neurosyphilis**
      (1) This form of syphilis may occur at any stage of infection with *T. pallidum*. It should be suspected in patients who are HIV positive, fail initial treatment, have an initial titer in excess of 1:32, have neurologic or ophthalmic signs or symptoms, or are diagnosed with aortitis or gummas. Diagnosis is made by testing the cerebrospinal fluid (CSF).
      (2) Recommended treatment is aqueous crystalline **penicillin G** 18–24 million units per day, given 3 to 4 MU intravenously every 3 to 4 hours or by continuous infusion for 10 to 14 days. Alternatively, **procaine penicillin** 2.4 million units can be given once daily with **probenecid** 500 mg orally four times daily, both for 10 to 14 days. For penicillin-allergic patients, **ceftriaxone** 2 g per day, either intramuscularly or intravenously, for 10 to 14 days may be used. The use of ceftriaxone in penicillin-allergic patients is limited by the possibility of cross-allergy to cephalosporins. However, other treatment regimens have not been tested adequately for patients with neurosyphilis.
   d. **Penicillin-allergic pregnant patients.** These patients should undergo **skin testing** followed by **penicillin desensitization** for two reasons: tetracycline and doxycycline are contraindicated in pregnancy, and only penicillin has been proven to prevent fetal infection.
   e. **Congenital syphilis**
      (1) Treatment is recommended for infants who are strongly suspected of being born with syphilis because of specific abnormalities on physical examination, serum nontreponemal serologic titer four times greater than the maternal titer, positive darkfield examination of infant body fluid, or history of inadequately treated maternal syphilis.
      (2) The recommended regimen is aqueous crystalline **penicillin G** 100,000 to 150,000 units/kg/day, administered in divided doses of 50,000 units/kg intravenously every 12 hours for the first 7 days of life and every 8 hours after this for a total of 10 days. Alternatively, **procaine penicillin G** 50,000 units/kg/dose, intramuscularly once daily, can be given for the first 10 days of life.

E **Follow-up**

1. Patients should be tested by VDRL or RPR at 3, 6, and 12 months. Patients with early syphilis should have a fourfold decline in titer by 3 months posttreatment. Retreatment should be considered for a fourfold increase in titer, failure of an initial titer greater than 1:32 to decrease fourfold 12 to 14 months after treatment, or if symptoms or signs of disease occur after treatment. Close serologic follow-up is warranted in patients treated with alternative regimens.

2. All patients diagnosed with syphilis should be tested for HIV. When neurosyphilis has been diagnosed and treated, follow-up CSF examination should be performed every 6 months until the cell count is normal.

IV ▪ VIRAL SEXUALLY TRANSMITTED DISEASES

A **HIV.** Originally identified in 1981, this unique retrovirus is believed to be responsible for severe deficiencies in cell-mediated immunity, leading to unusual opportunistic infections, malignancy, and, eventually, death. The diseases caused by HIV are known as **AIDS.** If left untreated, AIDS develops in almost all HIV-infected individuals; 87% develop AIDS within 17 years of HIV infection.

1. **Epidemiology.** In 2001, 40 million individuals were estimated to be infected with HIV worldwide, including 950,000 individuals in the United States.
   a. Exhaustive epidemiologic studies have demonstrated that male homosexuals and bisexuals, intravenous drug users, female heterosexual consorts of infected men, recipients of tainted blood or concentrated blood products, and neonates born to infected women are the predominant populations at risk. In addition, African Americans and Hispanics are more likely than whites to become infected with HIV. Recent studies show that the most rapidly increasing subset of AIDS cases in the United States results from heterosexual transmission of HIV.
   b. Transmission is both horizontal and vertical. **Incubation or latency time** is between 2 months and 17 years. The **prevalence in the general population** is estimated to be 22 in 100,000. Men are affected more frequently than women, but the prevalence in women is increasing.
   c. Other STDs increase susceptibility to HIV infection in two ways.
      (1) Genital ulcers cause breaks in the mucosa and skin in areas exposed to HIV through sexual contact, facilitating entry of HIV.
      (2) Nonulcerative STDs, such as chlamydia and gonorrhea, increase the local concentration of immune system–mediated HIV target cells, such as CD4+ cells. In addition, when HIV-infected individuals have other STDs, HIV is more likely to be present in their genital secretions. These observations support the value of HIV testing whenever another STD is diagnosed, as well as contact tracing and treatment of sexual partners if STDs are diagnosed.
   d. Most HIV infections in the United States are caused by HIV type 1 (HIV-1). However, rare cases of HIV type 2 (HIV-2) have been documented in the United States. Epidemiologic risk factors for HIV-2 are a sex partner from western Africa, where HIV-2 is endemic, or a history of nonsterile injection or blood transfusion in West Africa.

2. **Clinical presentation.** Approximately 80 to 90% of infected individuals are asymptomatic carriers. The median time between infection with HIV and the development of AIDS in adults is 10 years; this period ranges from a few months to more than 17 years.
   a. **Initial exposure to HIV** results in a retroviral syndrome in about 70% of patients.
      (1) The **usual incubation period is 2 to 4 weeks.**
      (2) **Symptoms** include febrile pharyngitis, fever, sweats, myalgia, arthralgia, headache, and photophobia.
      (3) **Lymphadenopathy** is usually generalized and begins in the second week.

    b. Later, a **more severe form of the disease** may occur.

        (1) Symptoms are generalized lymphadenopathy, night sweats, fever, diarrhea, weight loss, and fatigue.

        (2) Infections such as **herpes zoster virus** and **oral candidiasis** may occur.

        (3) Within 4 to 5 years, 30% of cases progress to AIDS.

    c. AIDS is the final stage in HIV infection

        (1) It is manifested by **severe alterations of cell-mediated immunity** (reversal of the CD4 [helper T cell]-to-CD8 [suppressor T cell] ratio.

        (2) Lymphadenopathy, Kaposi's sarcoma, opportunistic infections, malaise, diarrhea, weight loss, and death result.

3. Diagnosis

    a. Serologic screening with **enzyme-linked immunosorbent assay (ELISA)** for individuals at risk detects more than 95% of patients within 3 months of infection.

    b. A positive ELISA is confirmed by a repeat ELISA and then a **Western blot analysis,** which is more specific.

    c. Many states require pretest and posttest counseling and written informed consent for HIV testing.

    d. If acute retroviral syndrome is suspected, viral load testing for HIV plasma RNA should be performed. If HIV is detected, another test should be performed for confirmation purposes. Current research suggests that early treatment at this time may be beneficial.

4. Treatment. Care of HIV-positive patients involves:

    a. A thorough history and physical examination, including gynecologic examination and Papanicolaou (Pap) smear

    b. Evaluation for associated diseases, such as STDs and tuberculosis (TB)

    c. Identification of patients in need of immediate medical care and antiretroviral therapy or prophylaxis for opportunistic infections

    d. Determination of need for referral

    e. Administration of recommended vaccines

        (1) Pneumococcal

        (2) Influenza

        (3) Hepatitis B if susceptible

        (4) Measles if needed

        (5) *Haemophilus influenzae* B

    f. Psychosocial and behavioral evaluation and counseling, including counseling about high-risk behaviors as well as identification of sexual partners for testing.

    g. Complete blood count and CD4+ T-lymphocyte count. The **CD4+ count** is the best laboratory indicator of clinical progression, and management strategies are stratified by CD4+ count. Patients with CD4+ counts greater than $500/\mu l$ are usually not clinically immunosuppressed.

    h. The **purified protein derivative test** and **anergy panel** should be administered to all HIV-positive patients.

        (1) HIV may cause cutaneous anergy.

        (2) An area of induration larger than 5 mm in HIV-positive patients is considered indicative of TB infection. Preventive therapy with isoniazid should be considered after excluding active TB.

    i. Additional studies may include chest radiograph, serum chemistry, antibody testing for toxoplasmosis and hepatitis B and C, and RPR.

    j. Antiretroviral therapy may delay progression to advanced disease. Several antiretroviral agents are used for highly active antiretroviral therapy (HAART). Referral for treatment should be considered for asymptomatic patients with CD4+ counts less than $300/mm^3$ or symptomatic patients with CD4+ counts less than $500/mm^3$.

    k. *Pneumocystis carinii* **pneumonia (PCP) prophylaxis** with one of the following agents should be given to patients with CD4+ counts less than 200/mm^3 or with constitutional symptoms or previous PCP infection:

        (1) Trimethoprim–sulfamethoxazole. One double-strength tablet orally daily

        (2) Aerosolized pentamidine. 300 mg once a month

    l. Nutritional evaluation and counseling

5. Pregnancy. HIV testing should be offered to all pregnant women, and those individuals who are HIV positive should be evaluated as previously described. Without treatment, the risk of transmission to the fetus is 15 to 25%. Breastfeeding increases transmission by an additional 12 to 14%. Neonatal transmission can be decreased to less than 2% with maternal treatment, cesarean delivery, and avoidance of breastfeeding.

B **Human papillomavirus (HPV).** The genital virus in this double-stranded DNA family is responsible for a variety of mucocutaneous genital lesions, affecting both men and women. It is also known to be associated with lower genital tract cancers, especially cervical intraepithelial neoplasia (CIN).

1. Epidemiology. More than 20 million people in the United States are infected with HPV. Between 50 and 75% of sexually active men and women acquire HPV at some time in their lives.

    a. The **predominant means of transmission** is through **sexual intercourse.** In women whose sexual partners have obvious genital warts, the risk of contracting warts is 60 to 85%. Incubation time is between 6 weeks and 18 months, with a mean of 3 months.

    b. Recent evidence indicates that **transmission to the fetus may occur,** occasionally causing neonatal and juvenile respiratory papillomatosis. However, the risk is low, occurring in 1 of 1000 fetuses of infected mothers. Potential routes include transplacental, intrapartum, or postnatal. The presence of HPV infection is thus not an indication for cesarean section.

    c. More than 30 types of HPV have been found in genital tract infections.

        (1) HPV types 6 and 11 are the usual causes of visible external warts.

        (2) HPV types 16, 18, 31, 33, and 35 have all been strongly associated with CIN and with external genital squamous intraepithelial neoplasia.

2. Clinical presentation. Genital HPV infections are frequently asymptomatic. Lesions include overt anogenital warts (condyloma acuminatum) and dysplastic lesions. Lesions can also be subclinical or latent (not visible to the naked eye). Visual inspection of overt warty disease of the lower genital tract detects obvious lesions, which are often multifocal in distribution.

3. Diagnosis

    a. Direct inspection discerns overt warts. Their nature can be confirmed by biopsy if any doubt exists.

    b. Approximately 2 to 4% of **Pap smears** demonstrate the pathognomonic cell—the koilocyte (or halo cell). This exfoliated squamous cell has a wrinkled, somewhat pyknotic nucleus surrounded by a perinuclear clear zone or halo. Pap smears with this change are designated as low-grade squamous intraepithelial lesions.

    c. Colposcopy, the magnified inspection of lower genital tissues after staining with a weak acetic acid solution, is helpful in detecting latent or associated precancerous lesions caused by HPV. The lesions are flat, small, and acetowhite, with vascular punctation or mosaicism. Histologically, these lesions reveal koilocytosis, acanthosis, and variable nuclear atypia.

    d. Recently, **DNA hybridization techniques** have been used not only to detect HPV but also to ascertain viral type. Viral typing is becoming an increasingly useful tool in the evaluation of Pap smears with atypical squamous cells of undetermined significance (ASCUS).

4. Treatment. Even without treatment, many warts resolve. Therapy does not necessarily eradicate the virus. Treatment of visible warts is aimed at providing symptomatic relief and may reduce, but does not entirely eliminate, the ability of an infected individual to transmit HPV through sexual contact.

a. **Patient-applied methods**
   (1) Podofilox solution or gel. Patients apply this medication to warts twice daily for 3 days followed by 4 days off for up to four cycles.
   (2) Imiquimod cream. Patients apply this mediation to warts three times a week at bedtime and wash it off after 6 to 10 hours. This cream can be used for up to 16 weeks.
b. **Provider-applied methods**
   (1) Cryotherapy with liquid nitrogen or a cryoprobe
   (2) Podophyllin resin 10 to 25%
   (3) Bichloro- or trichloroacetic acid 80 to 90%
   (4) Surgical excision or ablation
c. **Methods for HPV-related precancerous conditions**
   (1) Loop electrode excision of the transformation zone
   (2) Laser vaporization
   (3) Cryotherapy
   (4) Cone biopsy of the cervix
   (5) Surgical excision of vulvar or vaginal lesions
d. The treatment of **latent HPV infections** without dysplasia is not recommended.

C **Herpes simplex virus (HSV).** HSV-2, a double-stranded DNA virus, is the predominant genital pathogen, although HSV-1 is seen in approximately 13 to 15% of herpetic genital infections. Both these viruses have an affinity for **infecting mucocutaneous tissues of the lower genital tract** and are maintained in pelvic ganglia as a latent reservoir for recurrent herpetic genital infection.

1. **Epidemiology.** Estimates of the prevalence of HSV genital infections suggest that 50 million sexually active adults in the United States are afflicted with virus. As many as 50% of affected Americans are unaware that they have HSV. The predominant mode of transmission is sexual intercourse. HSV is responsible for the highly lethal neonatal meningitis in infants delivered through an actively infected cervix. The **incubation time** is between 3 and 7 days.

2. **Clinical presentation.** The most common signs of HSV are recurrent vesiculoulcerative genital lesions. Primary genital herpetic infections are both local and systemic. Vulvar paresthesia precedes the development of multiple crops of vesicular lesions.
   a. **Primary lesions** become shallow, coalescent, painful ulcers in a few days and may last for 2 to 3 weeks. These lesions may be accompanied by severe dysuria with urinary retention, mucopurulent vaginal discharge, painful inguinal adenopathy, generalized myalgias, headaches, and fever.
   b. **Recurrent lesions** are similar but less severe in intensity, duration, and systemic side effects. **Menses** and **stressful life situations** are associated with recurrent outbreaks. Only 60% of patients have recurrent symptoms.
   c. Infants who come in contact with maternal active infection at birth are at risk for potentially fatal systemic infections. This situation is most likely to occur in infants born to mothers who are having their initial outbreak. When maternal active herpes infection is suspected at term or at the time of labor, cesarean section is generally used as the method of delivery.

3. **Diagnosis. Herpes cultures** obtained from the vesicular fluid or the edge of the ulcerative lesion give the best results. **Cytologic demonstration** of multinucleated epithelial cells with intranuclear inclusions is helpful in the diagnosis.

4. **Treatment**
   a. **Primary herpes.** One of the following regimens is appropriate:
      (1) **Acyclovir** 400 mg orally three times daily for 7 to 10 days or 200 mg orally five times daily for 7 to 10 days
      (2) **Famciclovir** 250 mg orally three times daily for 7 to 10 days
      (3) **Valacyclovir** 1 g orally twice daily for 7 to 10 days

  b. **Recurrent herpes.** One of the following regimens is appropriate.
    (1) **Acyclovir** 400 mg orally three times daily for 5 days, 200 mg orally five times daily for 5 days, or 800 mg orally two times daily for 5days
    (2) **Famciclovir** 125 mg orally twice daily for 5 days
    (3) **Valacyclovir** 1 g orally once daily for 5 days
  c. **Frequent recurrence** (more than 6 times per year). Suppressive therapy is used to reduce recurrences by 70 to 80%. One of the following regimens is appropriate.
    (1) **Acyclovir** 400 mg orally twice daily
    (2) **Famciclovir** 250 mg orally twice daily
    (3) **Valacyclovir** 500 mg orally once daily or 1 g orally once daily

D Molluscum contagiosum

  1. **Epidemiology.** Molluscum contagiosum is mildly contagious and is caused by a double-stranded DNA poxvirus. The incubation period is several weeks.
  2. **Clinical presentation.** This virus creates small (1 to 5 mm), umbilicated papules in the cutaneous genital region of sexually active individuals. It may also affect the nongenital skin.
  3. **Diagnosis.** The lesion itself is pathognomonic, but the diagnosis can be confirmed on histologic demonstration of a papule with a hyperkeratotic plug arising from an acanthotic epidermis. There are intracytoplasmic molluscum bodies noted on Wright stain.
  4. **Treatment.** The disease is usually self-limited, with spontaneous resolution in 6 to 9 months. Local excision, cryotherapy, electrocautery, and laser vaporization are suitable treatment modalities to decrease the duration of symptoms.

E Hepatitis B virus (HBV)

  1. **Epidemiology.** There were approximately 78,000 new infections in the United States in 2001, down from an average of 260,000 in the 1980s. However, approximately 1.25 million chronically infected individuals serve as a reservoir. In the United States, HBV is most commonly transmitted sexually. The disease can also be transmitted by exposure to infected blood. The incubation period is 6 weeks to 6 months. Fifteen to twenty-five percent of those with chronic infection die of liver disease.
  2. **Clinical presentation.** HBV infection is symptomatic in adults in about 50% of cases. When symptoms are present, they include jaundice and general malaise. Only 2 to 6% of infected adults become chronically infected, but 90% of infected infants develop chronic infection.
  3. **Diagnosis.** Presence of hepatitis B surface antigen (HBsAg) indicates either acute or chronic infection. Presence of hepatitis B surface antibody (anti-HBs) is indicative of immunity, either through prior infection or immunization.
  4. **Treatment and prevention.** Supportive treatment is used for acute HBV infection, which is self-limited. Interferon alfa and lamivudine have been used in attempts to treat chronic hepatitis B. Vaccination is the mainstay of prevention. Hepatitis B immune globulin (HBIG) provides postexposure prophylaxis, and the multidose hepatitis B vaccine gives long-standing immunity.
  5. **Pregnancy.** All pregnant women are tested for HBsAg carrier status. When a pregnant woman is identified as a chronic carrier, fetal infection can be prevented by prompt infant immunization and HBIG administration.

V TRICHOMONIASIS

Of all sexually transmitted protozoal infections, *Trichomonas vaginalis* infection is the most common. This protozoan is responsible for **acute vulvovaginitis.**

A Epidemiology.

Approximately 5 million infections are caused by *T. vaginalis* annually in the United States. Infection with this organism accounts for nearly one third of all office visits for infectious vulvovaginitis. Transmission of this STD is usually by sexual intercourse. Vaginal trichomoniasis has been associated with adverse pregnancy outcomes, but there is no evidence that treatment of asymptomatic women decreases these adverse events.

B **Clinical presentation**

1. Profuse, yellow-green, malodorous, frothy discharge of low viscosity
2. Vulvar pruritus
3. Vaginal erythema and occasional intense erythematous mottling of the cervix (**strawberry cervix**)
4. Usually asymptomatic male partner
5. Appearance of symptoms usually 5 to 28 days after exposure

C **Diagnosis**

1. Vaginal pH between 5 and 6
2. Inflammatory response and motile, flagellated trichomonads on wet mount preparations. These organisms are twice the size of leukocytes.
3. Cultures for *Trichomonas* are available but are usually reserved for resistant cases in which antimicrobial testing can be used.

D **Treatment.** Therapy using metronidazole in either of the following regimens produces cure rates of greater than 95%. Sexual partners must be treated to prevent reinfection.

1. **Metronidazole** 2 g orally
2. **Metronidazole** 500 mg orally twice daily for 7 days

VI ECTOPARASITES

This group of STDs includes pediculosis pubis and scabies.

A **Pediculosis pubis** *(Phthirus pubis)*. The **crab louse** is a slow-moving insect approximately 1 mm long. It lays its eggs (**nits**) at the base of hair follicles. After 7 days, nymphs arise from the nits and progress to the adult stage in 2 to 3 weeks. Adult life expectancy of the pubic louse is 30 days.

1. **Epidemiology.** Pediculosis pubis is **highly contagious.** The crab louse can be transmitted through direct sexual contact or through fomites, such as blankets and sheets. Hard, smooth surfaces such as toilet seats are not suitable fomites for the transmission of the crab louse.
2. **Clinical presentation.** Intense vulvar pruritus secondary to an allergic sensitization is the presenting symptom.
3. **Diagnosis.** Identification of the crab louse or nits can be made with a **hand lens inspection** of the hair-bearing pubic region.
4. **Treatment.** The specific treatments listed are not recommended for use in the eye area. When eyelashes are infected, treatment involves application of an occlusive ophthalmic ointment to eyelids two times daily for 10 days.
   a. **Lindane** solution (1%), applied to the infested area for 4 minutes and washed off, is effective. Lindane is contraindicated in pregnancy and lactation and in children less than 2 years of age. **Toxicity is exhibited as seizures and aplastic anemia** and has been reported when exposures exceed 4 minutes. This treatment should be used with caution in those weighing less than 100 lbs; its use has been banned in California.
   b. **Permethrin** cream, 1%, rinse for 10 minutes
   c. **Pyrethrins with piperonyl butoxide** applied to the affected area and washed off after 10 minutes
   d. **Cleaning of all contaminated bedding and clothing** is essential. Decontamination by machine washing and heat drying or dry cleaning is warranted.

5. **Follow-up.** Infected individuals should be reevaluated 1 week after treatment for nits or lice. Retreatment with an alternative regimen is indicated for persistent infestation. All sexual partners within the past month should be treated.

B **Scabies** *(Sarcoptes scabiei)*. This mite is 0.4 mm in length. Unlike the crab louse, it can be found anywhere on the skin, where it burrows a 5-mm-long tunnel to lay its eggs. Its life span is approximately 30 days.

1. **Epidemiology.** Scabies can be transmitted by close sexual contact but also by nonsexual contact, such as sharing clothing or bedding.

2. **Clinical presentation.** The predominant symptom is severe, intermittent itching. Hands, wrists, breasts, and buttocks are the most commonly affected sites. With initial infection, sensitization to scabies must occur before pruritus begins. Therefore, it can take several weeks after exposure for symptoms to develop with initial infections. Intense itching can occur within 24 hours of exposure in subsequent infections.

3. **Diagnosis.** Linear burrows are frequently seen with a hand lens. Microscopic slides prepared from scrapings of suspected lesions in mineral oil often demonstrate adult mites, eggs, and fecal pellets.

4. **Treatment**
   a. **Permethrin** cream, 5%, applied to the body from the neck down and washed off after 8 to 14 hours
   b. **Lindane** solution, 1%, applied from the neck down and washed off after 8 hours (should not be applied after a bath, or in pregnancy or lactation) and in children younger than 2 years of age (see VI A 4 a) Lindane resistance has been reported in some areas of the world, including the United States.
   c. **Ivermectin** 200 μg/kg, given orally and repeated in 2 weeks
   d. As with pubic lice, **cleaning of all contaminated bedding and clothing** is essential. Decontamination by machine washing and heat drying or dry cleaning is warranted. All close personal or household contacts within the preceding month should be examined and treated.

5. **Follow-up.** The rash and itching associated with scabies can persist for up to 14 days after treatment. If symptoms persist after 2 weeks, reinfection could be present and retreatment should be considered, especially if live mites are observed.

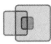

Study Questions for Chapter 27

Directions: Match each description below with the causative agent above. Each answer may be used once, more than once, or not at all.

QUESTIONS 1–5

- A Gram-negative diplococcus
- B Obligatory intracellular bacteria (subtypes D-K)
- C Obligatory intracellular bacteria (L subtypes)
- D Gram-negative coccobacillus
- E Gram-negative associated with Donovan bodies
- F Many species of anaerobic bacteria
- G Spirochete
- H Retrovirus
- I ds-DNA virus (subtypes 6/11 and 16, 18, 35, etc.)
- J ds-DNA virus (subtypes 1 and 2)
- K ds-DNA virus (poxvirus family)
- L Protozoa
- M Ectoparasite

1. Maculopapular rash, arthritis, and perihepatic "violin-string" adhesions

2. Vulvar ulcer, marked inguinal lymphadenopathy, diagnosis by complement fixation

3. Congenital infection consisting of nonimmune hydrops, skin rash, and hepatomegaly

4. 0.1% risk of respiratory papillomatosis in child born through infected genital tract

5. Infection that resolves spontaneously within 9 months but may be reduced via cryotherapy

Directions: Each of the numbered items or incomplete statements in this section is followed by answers or by completions of the statement. Select the ONE lettered answer or completion that is BEST in each case.

QUESTIONS 6–9

6. A 22-year-old nulligravid woman presents to you because of a 5-day history of frequent urination and dysuria. She was seen by a doctor 2 days ago and prescribed ampicillin. She has no remarkable medical history. She is sexually active and recently began having intercourse with a new boyfriend. She has no known drug allergies. Today her urinalysis shows the following: 2 squamous cells, 0 nitrites, 18 WBC/hpf, 0 bacteria. Her urine hCG is negative. The next best step in management is

- A Ceftriaxone
- B Trimethoprim-sulfamethoxazole
- C Spectinomycin
- D Erythromycin base
- E Doxycycline

7. A 26-year-old woman gravida 1, para 0 at 14 weeks of gestation presents to you because of increased vaginal discharge. You perform a wet mount and test for gonorrhea and chlamydia by PCR. The results of PCR are positive for chlamydia. The next best step in management is -_____. (Note: TOC = test of cure and RS = re-screen.)

[A] Azithromycin (patient and partner) + TOC 5 weeks + RS 4 months
[B] Doxycycline (patient and partner) + TOC 5 weeks + RS 5 months
[C] Ofloxacin (patient and partner) + TOC 4 weeks + RS 4 months
[D] Erythromycin (patient and partner) + TOC 3 weeks + RS 4 months
[E] Erythromycin (patient and partner) + TOC 2 weeks + RS 3 months

8. A 20-year-old presents to you with a deep, excavating, painless lesion above the clitoris, overlying the pubic bone. Her serum Venereal Disease Research Laboratory (VDRL) is positive. A lumbar puncture and analysis of her cerebrospinal fluid also yields a positive VDRL. The best term to describe her lesion is

[A] Condyloma acuminatum
[B] Condyloma latum
[C] Chancre
[D] Gumma
[E] Bubo

9. A 17-year-old adolescent presents to your office reporting intense itching "down there." You perform a wet mount and KOH prep but are unable to find anything remarkable. Examination of her pubic hair in the area of the mons with a hand lens reveals several linear lesions and adjacent erythema from self-scratching. Her pregnancy test is negative. The next best step in management is neck-down treatment with

[A] Permethrin 1% for 10 hours + wash bed sheets
[B] Permethrin 5% for 10 hours + clean toilet seats
[C] Permethrin 5% for 10 minutes + clean toilet seats
[D] Lindane 1 % for 4 minutes + wash clothing
[E] Lindane 1% for 8 hours + wash bed sheets

Answers and Explanations

1. A [II A 2 f] 2. C [II F 3] 3. G [II B 5] 4. I [IV B 1 b] 5. K [IV D 4]. Advanced disseminated gonococcal infection can give rise to septic arthritis, rash, and perihepatitis (or Fitz-Hugh-Curtis syndrome). The diagnosis is made by cervical culture for gonorrhea. Lymphogranuloma venereum (LGV) is caused by *Chlamydia trachomatis* serotypes L1–L3. It consists of genital ulcers; tender, marked inguinal lymphadenopathy (causing distortion of anatomy); and fistula formation in advanced cases. Complement fixation is the test of choice. Untreated congenital syphilis may cause stillbirth, nonimmune hydrops, jaundice, hepatosplenomegaly, and skin rash. There is a 1 in 1000 chance of respiratory papillomatosis in a child born through vaginal delivery from a patient infected with HPV. Molluscum contagiosum creates small umbilicated papules that are self limited (6 to 9 months). Duration of papules may be decreased with excision, cryotherapy, electrocautery, or laser vaporization.

6. The answer is E [II B 2]. Symptoms of urethritis (frequency and dysuria) and pyuria ("pus in urine" or many white blood cells in urine) with a negative urine culture in a sexually active woman suggest chlamydial infection. The treatment of choice in a nonpregnant patient is doxycycline. Trimethoprim-sulfamethoxazole can be used for urinary tract infections, although currently it is not the treatment of choice. This agent can also be used to treat granuloma inguinale.

7. The answer is A [II B 4 and 5 and II A 5]. Although the best management of chlamydia during pregnancy involves an erythromycin base, azithromycin may also be used and is not contraindicated. Both doxycycline and ofloxacin are contraindicated during pregnancy because the former is similar to tetracycline and causes staining of developing teeth, and the latter interferes with cartilage development. The last two answer choices are incorrect because they both perform TOC in less than 4 weeks after treatment. Because nucleic acids test do not test for live organisms, they can remain positive for up to 3 weeks after treatment. Additionally, any treatment used during pregnancy requires TOC and RS, because treatment with a first-choice agent (doxycycline) is not used.

8. The answer is D [III D 2 c]. Neurosyphilis (or tertiary syphilis) is diagnosed by ophthalmic signs in someone whose serum is VDRL +, or in someone with gummas whose CSF tests positive for VDRL. Condyloma acuminatum (warts) is caused by HPV. Condyloma latum are indicative of secondary syphilis (not tertiary). Painless chancre is a lesion of primary syphilis. Bubos are caused by *Haemophilus ducreyi*, which causes chancroid.

9. The answer is E [VI B 4]. Treatment of scabies usually consists of more potent agents, longer duration of treatment, and neck-down treatment in contrast to treatment of lice. Additionally, all bedding and clothing needs to be thoroughly washed and decontaminated. Flat, smooth surfaces such as toilet seats are not risk factors for acquisition of scabies or lice. Permethrin 1% is not powerful enough. Permethrin 5% for 10 minutes is not long enough. Lindane 1% is not long enough. Remember that a positive pregnancy test is a contraindication for treatment with Lindane.

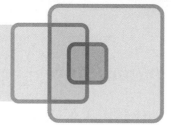

chapter 28

Pelvic Inflammatory Disease

ANN HONEBRINK

I INTRODUCTION

Pelvic inflammatory disease (PID) comprises a spectrum of inflammatory diseases of the upper genital tract of women. PID can involve infection of the endometrium (**endometritis**), the oviducts (**salpingitis**), the ovaries (**oophoritis**), the uterine wall (**myometritis**), or portions of the parietal peritoneum (**peritonitis**).

A **Acute PID** mostly involves the tubes and the sequelae of tubal infection, such as destruction of tubal architecture and function and pelvic adhesions.

B **Chronic PID** is a misnomer because the chronic problems associated with PID—hydrosalpinx, infertility, adhesions, and pain—no longer have direct bacteriologic association. True chronic PID (e.g., pelvic tuberculosis [TB] and actinomycosis) is rare.

II EPIDEMIOLOGY

A **Costs.** PID is usually the result of a sexually transmitted disease (STD), which has become a major health concern, although PID can also have iatrogenic causes.

1. Approximately 1 million cases of acute PID occur each year in the United States.
2. In the 1990s, direct and indirect costs of PID and its sequelae were greater than $4 billion annually. These costs involve 267,000 inpatient hospital admissions and 119,000 operations annually.

B **Incidence.** PID is a disease of young women. Peak incidence occurs in women in their late teens and early twenties.

1. Acute PID occurs in 1 to 2% of young, sexually active women annually and is the most common serious infection in women 16 to 25 years of age. Initiation of intercourse at age 15 years results in a one in eight chance of PID. Fifty percent of these adolescents have four or more sexual partners that first year.
2. **Medical sequelae** develop in one in four women with acute PID.
   a. **Ectopic pregnancy rate** increases six- to tenfold in women with PID. Approximately 50% of all ectopic pregnancies are thought to result from the tubal damage caused by PID.
   b. **Chronic pelvic pain** develops in 20% of women with acute PID. Both chronic pelvic pain and dyspareunia (90,000 new cases each year) are related to PID.
   c. **Infertility** results after acute PID in 6 to 60% of cases, causing more than 100,000 women per year to become infertile. The risk of **tubal obstruction** depends on the severity and the number of episodes of infection.
      (1) After one episode: 11.4%
      (2) After two episodes: 23.1%
      (3) After three episodes: 54.3%

    d. Mortality, although rare, does occur, particularly in neglected cases in which a **ruptured tubo-ovarian abscess** can lead to septic shock and death. In the United States, more than 150 deaths are attributed to PID annually.

[C] **Contraceptive use.** Women who are not sexually active and use no contraception do not contract PID. Conversely, women who are sexually active but use no contraception contract 3.42 cases of PID per 100 woman-years.

    1. Condoms, when used consistently and correctly, are very effective in preventing PID, as well as other STDs.

    2. Oral contraceptives appear to protect users against PID: only 0.91 case of PID per 100 woman-years has been reported among women using the pill. This relationship between the pill and PID may be the result of sexual factors, including:

        a. Decreased menstrual flow

        b. Decreased ability of pathogenic bacteria to attach to endometrial cells

        c. Progestin-induced changes in the cervical mucus that retard the entrance of bacteria

    3. Other barrier methods of contraception (e.g., the diaphragm, sponge, and contraceptive foam) also protect against PID. Spermicides may also be bactericidal. Any barrier to spermatozoa also acts as a barrier to pathogenic bacteria.

    4. Intrauterine devices (IUDs) have been linked to an increased risk of PID (5.21 cases per 100 woman-years). The risk is confounded by epidemiologic factors, such as history of STD and sexual promiscuity, and is lower in monogamous, healthy women. Possible mechanisms for the increased risk include:

        a. Creation of a sanctuary for bacteria from the body's defenses

        b. Establishment of a chronic anaerobic endometritis within the uterine cavity

III   BACTERIOLOGY

Acute PID is usually a **polymicrobial infection** caused by organisms that are considered normal flora of the cervix and vagina.

[A] **Organisms cultured from the fallopian tube**

    1. *Neisseria gonorrhoeae*, a gram-negative diplococcus

    2. *Chlamydia trachomatis*, an obligate intracellular organism because of its inability to produce adenosine triphosphate

    3. Endogenous aerobic bacteria, such as *Escherichia coli* and *Proteus*, *Klebsiella*, and *Streptococcus*

    4. Endogenous anaerobic bacteria, such as *Bacteroides*, *Peptostreptococcus*, and *Peptococcus*

    5. *Mycoplasma hominis*

    6. *Actinomyces israelii*, which is found in 15% of IUD-associated cases of PID, particularly in unilateral abscesses. It is rarely found in women who do not use an IUD.

[B] **Organism prevalence**

    1. *N. gonorrhoeae* is the only organism recovered by direct tubal or cul-de-sac culture in one third of women with acute PID.

    2. One third has a positive culture for *Neisseria* plus a mixture of endogenous aerobic and anaerobic flora.

    3. *C. trachomatis* alone is found in tubal cultures of approximately 20% of all women with salpingitis.

    4. *N. gonorrhoeae* and *C. trachomatis* coexist in the same individual in 25 to 40% of cases.

IV **PATHOPHYSIOLOGY**

PID has a multifactorial microbiologic etiology. Salpingo-oophoritis is usually preceded by vaginal and cervical colonization of pathologic bacteria, a state that may exist for months or years. An inciting event occurs that allows bacteria to ascend the uterus to the tubal lumen, usually bilaterally.

A **Inciting events**

1. **Menstrual periods.** Degenerating endometrium is a good culture medium. Two thirds of acute PID cases begin just after menses.

2. **Sexual intercourse.** Bacteria-laden fluids may be pushed into the uterus, and uterine contractions may assist their ascent.

3. **Iatrogenic events**
   a. Elective abortion
   b. Dilation and curettage or endometrial biopsy
   c. IUD insertion or use
   d. Hysterosalpingography
   e. Chromopertubation at laparoscopy
   f. Radium insertion into the endometrial cavity

B **Chronology of salpingo-oophoritis.** Infection is usually bilateral, but unilateral infection is possible, especially in association with an IUD. The presence of chronic anaerobic endometritis near one tubal ostium may explain this. The **clinical course** is as follows:

1. **Endosalpingitis** develops initially with edema and ultimately proceeds to destruction of luminal cells, cilia, and mucosal folds. Bacterial toxins are most likely to be responsible.

2. Infection spreads to the tubal muscularis and serosa. It then spreads by direct extension to the abdominal cavity through the fimbriated end of the tube.

3. **Oophoritis** develops over the surface of the ovaries, and microabscesses may develop within the ovaries.

4. **Peritonitis** may occur, and upper abdominal infection may result either by direct extension of infection up the abdominal gutters laterally or by lymphatic spread. Development of **perihepatitis** with adhesions and right upper quadrant abdominal pain is known as the **Fitz-Hugh–Curtis syndrome.**

5. **Low-grade, smoldering, or inadequately treated infections** allow fewer virulent bacteria to contribute to the process, resulting in mixed infections. **Anaerobes** then play a major role in the development of pelvic abscesses.

6. Sequelae of PID
   a. Pyosalpinges (tubal abscesses)
   b. Hydrosalpinges (fluid-filled, dilated, thin-walled, destroyed tubes, usually totally obstructed)
   c. Partial tubal obstruction and crypt formation, resulting in ectopic pregnancies
   d. Total tubal obstruction and infertility
   e. Tubo-ovarian abscesses
   f. Peritubular and ovarian adhesions
   g. Dense pelvic and abdominal adhesions
   h. Ruptured abscesses, resulting in sepsis and shock
   i. Chronic pelvic pain and dyspareunia

V **DIAGNOSIS**

A **Signs and symptoms of PID** are relatively nonspecific. Thus, they produce both a high false-positive rate and a high false-negative rate of diagnosis. Laparoscopic studies have revealed the inadequacy of diagnosing acute PID by means of the usual history and physical examination and laboratory studies (Table 28-1).

1. Based on symptoms, a **high degree of suspicion** is essential in making the diagnosis.

2. Sometimes, only very mild symptoms appear in spite of serious infection. Women with *C. trachomatis* infection may present with a few symptoms but then exhibit a severe inflammatory process when examined with the laparoscope.

B **Clinical criteria for diagnosis**

1. **Minimum criteria for diagnosis**
   a. Lower abdominal tenderness
   b. Uterine or adnexal tenderness
   c. Cervical motion tenderness

2. **Additional criteria.** For women with severe signs, these additional criteria are used to increase the specificity of the diagnosis:
   a. Oral temperature higher than 100.9°F (38.3°C)
   b. Abnormal cervical or vaginal discharge. Mucopurulent cervical discharge with white blood cells (WBCs) seen on wet mount is almost always seen in women with PID. If this finding is not present, other diagnoses should be seriously entertained.
   c. Elevated erythrocyte sedimentation rate (ESR)
   d. Elevated C-reactive protein
   e. Positive test for gonorrhea or chlamydia
   f. Tubo-ovarian abscess seen on ultrasound
   g. Evidence of endometritis on endometrial biopsy
   h. Laparoscopic evidence of PID

C **Differential diagnosis** for PID should include:

1. Ectopic pregnancy

2. Ruptured ovarian cyst

3. Appendicitis

TABLE 28-1 Laparoscopic Findings in Patients with False-Positive Clinical Diagnosis of Acute Pelvic Inflammatory Disease

Laparoscopic Finding	Number of Patients
Acute appendicitis	24
Endometriosis	16
Corpus luteum bleeding	12
Ectopic pregnancy	11
Pelvic adhesions only	7
Benign ovarian tumor	7
Chronic salpingitis	6
Miscellaneous	15
TOTAL	98

Reprinted with permission from Jacobson LJ. Differential diagnosis of acute pelvic inflammatory disease. Am J Obstet Gynecol 1980;138:1007.

4. Endometriosis

5. Inflammatory bowel disease

6. Degenerating fibroids

7. Spontaneous abortion

8. Diverticulitis

D Diagnostic techniques

1. **Cervical Gram stain.** If gram-negative intracellular diplococci are present, gonorrhea is the presumed diagnosis. However, Gram stain alone misses one half of the gonorrhea cases.

2. **Serum human chorionic gonadotropin.** A sensitive pregnancy test is important in the differential diagnosis of pelvic pain to rule out the possibility of ectopic pregnancy. In the past, approximately 3 to 4% of women admitted with the diagnosis of PID had an ectopic pregnancy.

3. **Ultrasound.** This technique may help define adnexal masses and intrauterine or ectopic pregnancies, especially when a patient has a tender abdomen that does not permit an adequate pelvic examination. Response to therapy can be measured objectively as pelvic masses and induration regress.

4. **Laparoscopy.** If the disease process is unclear, this technique is the ultimate way to establish the diagnosis.

5. **Culdocentesis.** If purulent fluid is obtained, a culture may assist in antibiotic selection. However, infections may be secondary to another primary process. In addition, the pain associated with this test makes limits its use.

6. **Blood studies**
   a. **Leukocytosis** is not a reliable indicator of acute PID. Less than 50% of women with acute PID have a WBC count greater than 10,000 cells/mL.
   b. An **increased ESR** is a nonspecific finding, but the ESR is elevated in approximately 75% of women with laparoscopically confirmed PID.

VI TREATMENT

A Empiric treatment of PID should be given to women with historical risk factors for PID (either sexual activity or instrumentation of the cervix and uterus) if the minimal clinical criteria are met (see V B 1) and there is no other established cause for pelvic inflammation.

B Individualized treatment and a **high index of suspicion for infection** are mandatory. Treatment should always include sexual partners. The physician must decide between outpatient management of the woman, with close follow-up in 48 to 72 hours, or hospitalization. Many experts recommend that all patients be hospitalized. **Hospitalization of PID patients** should especially be considered if:

1. The diagnosis is uncertain

2. Surgical emergencies such as appendicitis or ectopic pregnancy need to be excluded

3. A pelvic abscess is suspected

4. Severe illness (e.g., vomiting, dehydration, high fever, or signs of peritonitis) precludes outpatient management

5. The patient is pregnant

6. The patient is unlikely to comply with outpatient therapy

7. The patient has HIV infection

8. The patient has not responded to outpatient management

9. Clinical follow-up within 72 hours of beginning antibiotics cannot be arranged

C **Oral treatment regimens** provide oral coverage for organisms frequently isolated from the genital tracts of women with PID. They are generally appropriate for women who present with milder cases of PID. Select **one** of the following three regimens:

1. **Regimen A.** Use one of the following:
   a. **Ofloxacin** 400 mg orally twice daily for 14 days
   b. **Levofloxacin** 500 mg orally once daily for 14 days

2. **Regimen B.** Use one of the following:
   a. **Ceftriaxone** 250 mg intramuscular single dose
   b. **Cefoxitin** 2 g intramuscular single dose with probenecid 1 g orally at the time of infection
   c. Any **other third-generation cephalosporin** plus **doxycycline** 100 orally twice daily for 14 days with or without **metronidazole** 500 mg twice daily for 14 days

D **Parenteral regimens** are generally used in women with more severe PID. Randomized trials have demonstrated the efficacy of both oral and parenteral treatment regimens but have not compared oral and parenteral regimens objectively. Parenteral treatment is generally continued for at least 24 hours after significant clinical improvement has occurred. After this, conversion is made to an oral regimen. Regimens are designed to cover both *N. gonorrhoeae* and *C. trachomatis* as well as other commonly isolated organisms.

1. **Regimen A.** Use one of the following:
   a. **Cefotetan** 2 g intravenously every 12 hours
   b. **Cefoxitin** 2 g intravenously every 6 hours plus doxycycline 100 mg orally or intravenously every 12 hours. Both the oral and intravenous routes of doxycycline provide similar bioavailability, and considerable pain is usually associated with intravenous administration of doxycycline. Once parenteral therapy is discontinued, oral clindamycin or metronidazole may be added to doxycycline if an abscess is suspected. At least 14 days of total therapy is recommended.

2. **Regimen B.** Use one of the following:
   a. **Clindamycin** 900 mg intravenously every 8 hours plus **gentamicin** 2 mg/kg loading dose intravenously or intramuscularly followed by 1.5 mg/kg per day maintenance dose every 8 hours.
   b. When **conversion to oral therapy** takes place, doxycycline 100 mg twice daily or clindamycin 450 mg four times daily can be used. Clindamycin is usually the favored agent when a tubo-ovarian abscess is suspected.

3. **Alternative regimens.** Although less data supports the use of these regimens, they do have broad-spectrum coverage. Use one of the following:
   a. **Ofloxacin** 400 mg intravenously every 12 hours
   b. **Levofloxacin** 500 mg intravenously once daily with or without metronidazole intravenously every 8 hours
   c. **Ampicillin–sulbactam** 3 g intravenously every 6 hours plus doxycycline 100 mg intravenously or orally every 12 hours.

E **Surgical intervention.** In cases of severe PID, especially when tubo-ovarian abscess is present, consideration should be given to surgical intervention if the patient's condition worsens or fails to improve after around 72 hours of treatment.

1. **Laparoscopy** may be considered for diagnosis and may be followed by laparotomy. Unless a well-defined unilateral abscess allows a unilateral salpingo-oophorectomy, the treatment of choice is a total abdominal hysterectomy, bilateral salpingo-oophorectomy, and drainage of the pelvic cavity. The patient, regardless of age, should be prepared for this possibility before surgery.

2. If an abscess is accessible through the cul-de-sac or radiologically, **catheter drainage** may be possible.

VII OTHER CAUSES OF PELVIC INFECTION

A **Granulomatous salpingitis**

1. **Tuberculous salpingitis** almost always represents systemic TB. The incidence is high in underdeveloped countries and low in developed countries. It usually affects women in their reproductive years, but an increased incidence has been reported among postmenopausal women. Primary genital TB is extremely rare in the United States.

   a. **Physical findings** are variable. Patients usually present with adnexal masses. Induration may be noted in the paracervical, paravaginal, and parametrial tissues. The typical patient is 20 to 40 years of age with known TB and a pelvic mass. Symptoms are related to a family history of TB, low-level pelvic pain, infertility, and amenorrhea.

   b. **Pathology.** Grossly, the uterine tube has a classic "tobacco pouch" appearance—enlarged and distended. The proximal end is closed, and the fimbria are edematous and enlarged. Microscopically, tubercles show an epithelioid reaction and giant cell formation. Inflammation and scarring are intense and irreversible.

   c. **Treatment** involves the standard regimens for disseminated TB, including isoniazid, rifampin, and ethambutol. Prognosis for cure is excellent, but the outlook for fertility is dismal.

2. **Leprous salpingitis.** The histologic picture is similar to the one for TB, and the two are often difficult to distinguish on a histologic basis. Langerhans' giant cells and epithelioid cells are present. Positive cultures are necessary for a diagnosis of TB.

3. **Actinomycosis.** *A. israelii*, the causative agent, is pathogenic for humans but not for other mammals. Most gynecologic involvement is infection secondary to appendiceal infection, gastrointestinal tract disorders, or IUD use. A total of 100 cases are reported annually, and the age range of prevalence is about 20 to 40 years.

   a. **Physical findings.** Half the lesions are bilateral and are characterized by adnexal enlargement and tenderness. Presenting symptoms may be confused with those of appendicitis.

   b. **Pathology.** Grossly, there is tubo-ovarian inflammation, as well as copious necrotic material on sections of the tube. The tubal lumen may have an adenomatous appearance. Microscopically, actinomycotic "sulfur" granules are present. Clublike filaments radiate out from the center. A monocytic infiltrate is apparent, and giant cells may be present.

   c. **Treatment.** Therapy is a prolonged course of penicillin.

4. **Schistosomiasis** occurs most commonly in the Far East and Africa.

   a. **Physical findings** are pelvic pain, menstrual irregularity, and primary infertility. The diagnosis is usually made by histopathologic findings.

   b. **Pathology.** Grossly, lesions appear as a nonspecific tubo-ovarian process. Microscopically, the ova or schistosome is seen surrounded by a granulomatous reaction with giant and epidermoid cells. An egg within an inflammatory milieu is a dramatic sight.

5. **Sarcoidosis.** Although rare, sarcoidosis can lead to a granulomatous salpingitis.

6. **Foreign-body salpingitis** occurs after the use of non–water-soluble dye material for hysterosalpingography. It may also be secondary to medications placed within the vagina, such as starch, talc, and mineral oil.

B **Nongranulomatous salpingitis** refers to any other bacterial infection, usually of the peritoneal cavity, that can secondarily cause tubal infection, including:

1. Appendicitis

2. Diverticulitis

3. Crohn disease

4. Cholecystitis

5. Perinephric abscess

Study Questions for Chapter 28

Directions: *Each of the numbered items or incomplete statements in this section is followed by answers or by completions of the statement. Select the ONE lettered answer or completion that is BEST in each case.*

1. A 19-year-old woman who is sexually active presents to the emergency department reporting a 5-day history of lower abdominal pain. Her vitals are as follows: T = 101°F, BP = 110/75, P = 80, R = 16. Speculum examination reveals white exudates at the cervical os, and there is cervical motion tenderness. Bimanual examination is unremarkable for masses but produces severe discomfort. Her serum hCG is positive. Urinalysis is normal. Her white blood cell count (WBC) is 14,000. An office ultrasound shows a normal sized, normal striped uterus and no adnexal masses. The next best step in management of this patient is

- A repeat serum hCG in 48 hours
- B Penicillin G intravenously
- C Ampicillin and gentamicin intravenously
- D Clindamycin and gentamicin intravenously
- E Cefazolin and doxycycline intravenously

2. The most important reason pelvic inflammatory disease (PID) must be recognized and treated promptly is to prevent

- A Pelvic pain syndrome
- B Infertility
- C Ectopic pregnancy
- D Sepsis
- E Pelvic adhesive disease

3. A 17-year-old woman has symptoms suggestive of pelvic inflammatory disease. However, the patient is adamant that she is a virgin. If the signs of PID are present because of inflammation involving the uterus, tubes, and ovaries, the most likely diagnosis is

- A Tuberculosis
- B Endomyometritis
- C Schistosomiasis
- D Appendicitis
- E Ectopic pregnancy

A 17-year-old girl, gravida 1, para 0, TAB 1 presents to the emergency department reporting a 6-day history of lower abdominal pain and purulent vaginal discharge. She denies past medical history or surgery. Her vitals are as follow: T = 102, BP = 118/78, P = 76, R = 14. Her abdomen is without scars, bowel sounds are present, and there is tenderness in the lower pelvic region of the abdomen. However, there is no rebound tenderness or guarding. Her speculum examination reveals white exudate at the external os of the cervix. Bimanual examination reveals severe cervical motion tenderness and uterine tenderness. There is also a fullness in the left adnexa. Her urine hCG is negative. WBC = 15 K.

QUESTIONS 4–5

4. The next best step in management is

- A Pelvic ultrasound
- B Computed tomography scan
- C Quantitative serum β-hCG
- D Immediate hospitalization
- E Ceftriaxone intramuscularly plus doxycycline orally

5. The most important reason to admit this patient to the hospital is
   A WBC count
   B Temperature
   C Pelvic examination
   D Age of patient
   E Patient is unreliable

Answers and Explanations

1. The answer is D [VI D 2]. This patient has acute PID and she happens to be pregnant at the same time. Currently, there are no signs or risk factors for an ectopic pregnancy. An intrauterine pregnancy is likely, but the pregnancy is so early that it is not yet seen on ultrasound. Intravenous clindamycin and gentamicin is an appropriate combination for parenteral treatment of PID because this regimen provides anaerobic, aerobic, *Neisseria gonorrhea*, and *Chlamydia trachomatis* coverage. Penicillin resistance is common in gonorrhea, which makes penicillin alone and the ampicillin and gentamicin combination inappropriate. The use of doxycycline is contraindicated in pregnancy because, like tetracycline, it can stain developing teeth. Resistance to second-generation cephalosporins is increasingly common in endogenous bacteria found in PID as well as gonorrhea.

2. The answer is D [II B 2 d]. Untreated PID can lead to formation of tubo-ovarian abscess (TOA). Mortality, although rare, does occur, particularly in neglected cases in which a ruptured TOA can lead to septic shock and death. In the United States, more than 150 deaths annually are attributed to PID.

3. The answer is D [VII A, B and table 28-1]. Inflammation of the tubes and ovaries can be seen in conjunction with any of the conditions listed. Schistosomiasis and tuberculosis are rare in the United States. The bacterial infection involved in appendicitis can cause secondary tubal infection and is the most likely diagnosis. Patients with false-positive diagnosis of PID were found at laparoscopy to have appendicitis (#1), endometriosis (#2), corpus luteum bleeding (#3), and ectopic pregnancy (#4). Endomyometritis usually occurs postpartum, usually as a complication of cesarean section in a patient with prolonged rupture of membranes.

4. A [II B 2 d and V B 2 f and VI B3] **5. C** [II B 2 d and V B 2 f and VI B3]. Because this patient has symptoms and signs of PID along with an adnexal mass, the next few management steps all depend on an ultrasound examination. You must rule out a TOA (i.e., no adnexal mass on ultrasound) before diagnosing a patient with uncomplicated PID and sending her home on oral treatment. However, if an adnexal mass is seen on ultrasound, it could be either a mass (cyst or tumor) or a TOA. Such a patient must be admitted to the hospital and placed on intravenous antibiotics and will need to have surgical exploration. A computed tomography scan is not as useful as an ultrasound in this situation. There is no need for a quantitative hCG when the ultra-sensitive urine hCG (which can detect as low as 5 mIU/mL) is negative. A TOA or pelvic abscess may first be appreciated on pelvic examination and can be further evaluated with an ultrasound. The history does not suggest that the patient is unreliable. The other answer choices are not criteria for hospitalization (although some clinicians may consider her temperature as a reason to hospitalize).

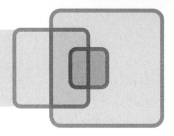

chapter 29

Pelvic Pain

SAMI I. JABARA AND RICHARD W. TURECK

I INTRODUCTION

Chronic pelvic pain syndrome is estimated to account for 10% of all visits to gynecologists. Afflicted women report continuous lower abdominal and pelvic pain that markedly hinders their daily activities. Although **acute pelvic pain may be associated with life-threatening illness,** chronic pelvic pain may also have a devastating impact on patients, and physicians should remain compassionate and empathetic. Pain is a subjective experience. The lack of physical findings does not in any way negate the significance of a patient's pain. The **psychological effects** may be considerable.

A The risk of major **depression, sexual dysfunction, and substance abuse** is increased.

B The prevalence of **childhood or adult sexual abuse** is particularly high, and the rate of marital and sexual dysfunction is greater among this cohort of patients.

C Psychological counseling and testing may be necessary to identify patients who require more extensive therapy.

II ANATOMY AND PHYSIOLOGY OF PELVIC PAIN

Pain perception involves an integration of multiple stimuli through a network of neuronal pathways. Visceral pain is more diffuse than somatic pain, probably because there is no specific identification within the cerebral sensory cortex.

A **Neuroanatomy.** The pelvic organs receive their innervation from the **autonomic nervous system,** which is composed of both sympathetic and parasympathetic fibers.

  1. **Sympathetic nerves** are used to transmit most afferent stimuli through cell bodies that lie in the **thoracolumbar** distribution. Areas that are müllerian in embryonic origin (e.g., uterus, fallopian tubes, and upper vagina) transmit impulses via sympathetic fibers into the spinal cord at the level of T10, T11, T12, and L1. Impulses from the uterus travel through the uterosacral ligaments to the uterine inferior plexus. From the uterus, they join other pelvic afferents to form the hypogastric plexus at the level of the rectum and vagina. The ovaries and distal fallopian tubes derive their nerve supply independently and enter the spinal cord at T9 and T10.

  2. **Parasympathetic nerve fibers** are also involved to a lesser extent in the transition of painful stimuli. Impulses from the upper vagina, cervix, and lower uterine segment travel through the parasympathetic system to the sacral roots S2–S4.

  3. **Both sympathetic and parasympathetic fibers** innervate the bladder, rectum, perineum, and anus, which are derived from the urogenital sinus. Fibers from the perineum and anus combine to form branches of the pudendal nerve, eventually terminating in the second and fourth sacral root.

B **Physiology.** Pelvic pain is visceral and may be either **referred** or **splanchnic.**

    1. **Splanchnic pain** occurs when an irritable stimulus is appreciated in a specific organ secondary to tension (stretching, distention, or pulling), peritoneal irritation or inflammation, hypoxia or necrosis of viscera, or production of prostanoids.

    2. **Referred pain** occurs when autonomic impulses arise from a diseased visceral organ, eliciting an irritable response within the spinal cord. Pain is sensed in the dermatomes corresponding to cells receiving those impulses.

III   EVALUATION

A **Important factors** to assess when determining the clinical significance of pelvic pain include:

    1. **Onset** of the pain

    2. **Relationship to the menstrual cycle** (is the pain constant or does it vary?)

    3. **Character** of the pain

    3. **Location** of the pain

    4. **Severity** of the pain (does it interfere with activities of daily life?)

    6. **Presence of associated symptoms** (e.g., dysmenorrhea and deep dyspareunia). Any other symptoms, such as fever, chills, nausea, vomiting, or anorexia, should also be noted.

B **Laparoscopy,** the endoscopic assessment of abdominal and pelvic pathology, is the **gold standard** for the diagnosis of pelvic pain. Approximately 40% of laparoscopies are reportedly performed in cases of chronic pelvic pain.

IV   DIFFERENTIAL DIAGNOSIS

A **Acute pelvic pain**

    1. **Ectopic pregnancy** (see Chapter 31). It is paramount to exclude the possibility of an **ectopic tubal gestation,** a life-threatening condition.

      a. Pelvic pain occurs as a result of distention of the fallopian tube caused by the growing pregnancy. The pain is usually **unilateral.** If the pregnancy ruptures through the fallopian tube, rebound tenderness may occur.

      b. Shoulder pain may develop as a result of blood in the abdomen causing diaphragmatic irritation and stimulating the phrenic nerves.

      c. A **pregnancy test** is mandated in any woman of childbearing age who presents with acute pelvic pain. If the test is positive, the presence of an ectopic pregnancy must be excluded from the differential diagnosis, particularly in patients with abnormal uterine bleeding.

    2. **Ruptured ovarian cyst.** Mid-cycle pain or **Mittelschmerz** is pain in the lower abdomen noticed at or near the time of ovulation. It is believed to be secondary to chemical irritation of the peritoneum from ovarian follicular cyst fluid after ovulation. The pain usually lasts only a few hours and usually no more than 2 days. The use of ultrasonic visualization of the ovaries most often confirms or excludes this diagnosis.

    3. **Ovarian torsion.** Acute lower abdominal pain may be the primary manifestation.

      a. The clinical presentation depends on the extent of interference with the ovarian blood supply. The more extensive the ischemia, the more severe the pelvic pain. The pain is usually paroxysmal and unilateral but becomes more constant if infarction occurs.

      b. Documentation of ovarian blood flow by **color Doppler ultrasound** is a helpful diagnostic modality in evaluating this medical emergency. Often, **laparoscopy** must be performed to confirm the diagnosis.

      c. If necrotic, the ovary and tube must usually be removed. If the ovary appears viable, it may be untwisted and a cystectomy performed.

4. Pelvic inflammatory disease (PID). Pelvic pain that is acute in onset and associated with cervical motion tenderness and febrile morbidity is characteristic of PID (see Chapter 28). Rebound tenderness and a partial ileus may result from the presence of purulent material within the pelvic and abdominal cavity.

5. Gastrointestinal disorders. Gastrointestinal causes of acute lower pelvic and abdominal pain include **appendicitis** and **diverticulitis;** the latter condition is most commonly observed in older women. In appendicitis, the pain is initially not well localized because it results from luminal distention of the appendix by inflammatory exudates. The pain eventually localizes to the right lower quadrant when the parietal peritoneum becomes locally involved in the inflammatory process.

6. Urologic causes. Conditions such as cystitis and renal lithiasis may lead to lower abdominal and pelvic pain.

B Chronic or recurrent pelvic pain.   Chronic pelvic pain may be **cyclic** or **constant. Adhesions** and **endometriosis** are the pathologic conditions most often involved.

1. Dysmenorrhea is painful menstruation. It is considered **primary** if it occurs in the absence of identifiable pathology. **Secondary dysmenorrhea** is caused by a defined pelvic abnormality, such as endometriosis or fibroids.
   a. The **pain** is usually spasmodic or throbbing. It is usually located in the lower abdomen and may radiate to the lower back and legs.
   b. Its onset is concurrent with menses, and the pain lasts for 1 to 3 days.
   c. The etiology of painful uterine contractions involves **prostaglandin** $F_{2\alpha}$ produced in the endometrial cells by the action of phospholipase A_2 on lipid cell membranes, forming arachidonic acid.
   d. Associated symptoms include backache, nausea, vomiting, diarrhea, headache, and fatigue.
   e. Therapy is aimed at reducing prostaglandin production. Agents such as **prostaglandin synthetase inhibitors** or **oral contraceptives** are useful.

2. Pelvic adhesions
   a. Etiology. Adhesion formation occurs after trauma to the visceral or parietal peritoneum through **operative procedures** (70% of cases), **endometriosis, or infection and inflammation.** Foreign body granulomas caused by talc, gauze, or suture material also result in the production of adhesions.
   b. Pathogenesis
      (1) In cases that involve ischemic damage to peritoneum, lysis of fibrin does not occur because of reduced fibrinolytic activity and fibrinous adhesions.
      (2) Mechanical components have been proposed as the underlying mechanism of pain sensation caused by adhesions. Patients experience pain via mechanical stimulation of visceral nociceptors because of mechanical stretching of internal organs.
   c. Diagnosis
      (1) Patients with adhesions may often have a history of previous pelvic surgery, but many have no past history that may supply a reason for the existence of adhesions. Physical examination of the patient may also be noncontributory. Approximately 25% patients with adhesions have no preoperative findings on physical examination, which suggests the presence of adhesions.
      (2) Laparoscopy. Laparoscopic visualization of the abdomen and pelvis is essential. Detectable pathologic findings are documented in approximately 60% of patients; in 25% of these patients, adhesions are the primary condition. Laparoscopic lysis of adhesions in patients with chronic pelvic pain results in improvement of symptomatology in 65 to 85% of cases. This improvement is maintained in approximately 75% of patients 6 to 12 months after surgery.

3. **Endometriosis** (see Chapter 30). Approximately 25 to 40% of patients who undergo laparoscopy for chronic pelvic pain have evidence of endometriosis. Endometriosis is the presence of endometrial glands and stroma at sites other than the uterine cavity.

4. **Adenomyosis,** a condition characterized by the presence of ectopic foci of endometrium within the myometrium, may also cause chronic pelvic pain and severe dysmenorrhea. In the past, adenomyosis was diagnosed in the pathology laboratory after surgical removal of the uterus. Today, magnetic resonance imaging is a useful modality.

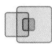

Study Questions for Chapter 29

Directions: *Each of the numbered items or incomplete statements in this section is followed by answers or by completions of the statement. Select the ONE lettered answer or completion that is BEST in each case.*

1. A 32-year-old woman, gravida 2, para 2 presents to your clinic reporting chronic abdominal and pelvic pain. The pain is intermittent, 6/10 intensity, worse when she lies on her left side, nonradiating, and occurs at different times throughout her menstrual cycle. Her past medical history is uneventful other than an appendectomy 4 years ago for a ruptured appendicitis. On physical examination of the abdomen in the supine position, you note a small linear scar in the right lower quadrant and active bowel sounds. The abdomen is diffusely tender to palpation, especially in the lower quadrants, and you do not palpate any masses. Her pelvic examination is unremarkable. The most likely diagnosis is

- **A** Torsion of ovarian cyst
- **B** Mittelschmerz
- **C** Adhesive disease
- **D** Psychogenic cause
- **E** Pelvic inflammatory disease

2. A 35-year-old gravida 4, para 3, SAB 1 who has a history of severe dysmenorrhea is seeing you for the first time. Six months ago, a laparoscopy, performed by another physician, showed no evidence of endometriosis or pelvic adhesions. She has essential hypertension and is taking a β-blocker. She has no known drug allergies. She has been happily married for 15 years and has regular but painful periods. Pelvic examination reveals an anteverted, anteflexed, slightly enlarged uterus that is fully mobile. There is no cul-de-sac nodularity. The next best step is

- **A** Blood tests (CBC, erythrocyte sedimentation rate)
- **B** Pelvic ultrasound
- **C** Magnetic resonance imaging (MRI)
- **D** Intravenous pyelogram (IVP)
- **E** Repeat laparoscopy

3. An 18-year-old nulligravid woman presents to your office because she has painful periods. She says she only has pain during the first 2 days of her periods, which are regular. The pain is always midline and 2 cm below the level of the umbilicus. She says Motrin helps ease the pain. She has no other medical or surgical history. Her pain is transmitted via

- **A** Sympathetic fibers to T10
- **B** Sympathetic fibers to T11
- **C** Parasympathetic fibers to S1
- **D** Parasympathetic fibers to L1
- **E** Pudendal nerve to S2–S4

4. A 33-year-old woman, gravida 5, para 4, TAB 1 presents to the clinic with left lower quadrant pain for 2 days. She describes the pain as intermittent initially but now constant, 7/10 intensity, nonradiating, and not associated with any other symptoms. Her last menstrual period was 2 months ago. She had a tubal ligation 3 years ago and a cholecystectomy 7 years ago. Her physical examination is as follows: T = 98.5, BP = 118/76, P = 89, R = 18. Abdominal examination reveals a scar on the right upper quadrant and a small scar within the umbilicus and right lower quadrant, present bowel sounds, slight tenderness to palpation in left lower quadrant, but no rebound tenderness and no guarding. Her pelvic examination reveals a uterus of normal size, shape, and contour, and no adnexal masses are appreciated. What is the next best step in management?

[A] Laparoscopy
[B] Laparotomy
[C] Antibiotics
[D] Naproxen
[E] Serum β-hCG

5. A 25-year-old woman, gravida 4, para 3, SAB 1 presents to your clinic for the first time reporting pelvic pain. She has had this pain for the last 10 years and has seen several physicians. She describes the pain as continuous and dull (4/10 intensity) with intermittent exacerbations (10/10). The pain occasionally radiates to her lower back and down her thighs. Nothing she takes or does seems to help her. The pain is not related to her menstrual cycle, which occurs only a few times a year. She has dyspareunia. She has a past medical history significant for asthma, peptic ulcer disease, and major depression. She has had a postpartum bilateral tubal ligation. She has had three hospitalizations within the last 10 years for suicide attempts. She also has a history of sexual abuse by a close family relative that occurred she was 13 years old. Currently, she is using an albuterol-metered dose inhaler, histamine receptor blocker, and an SSRI. On pelvic examination, the uterus cervix and uterus are midposition and normal in size and consistency, but there is diffuse pain in all areas of the pelvis, especially the right posterior cul-de-sac. The most likely cause of her pain is

[A] Endometriosis
[B] Uterine fibroids
[C] Mittelschmerz
[D] Pelvic adhesions
[E] Psychogenic cause

Answers and Explanations

1. The answer is C [IV B 2]. Due to her previous surgery and the fact that the appendix was ruptured, there is a high likelihood of adhesive disease inside the abdomen and pelvis. The fact that the pain is positional and not related to the menstrual cycle also suggests adhesions. There is no mention or ultrasound report of an ovarian cyst in the clinical scenario. Mittelschmerz is related to the menstrual cycle (occurs around time of ovulation). There is nothing in the scenario that suggests a psychogenic cause, although this should always be in the differential diagnosis. Pelvic inflammatory disease is unlikely given lack of evidence by pelvic or abdominal examination and lack of other associated findings, such as a fever or high WBC, or even an elevated erythrocyte sedimentation rate (ESR).

2. The answer is C [IV B 3]. A slightly enlarged uterus, symptoms of dysmenorrheal, and lack of pelvic pathology on laparoscopy suggest adenomyosis as the diagnosis. MRI is the best diagnostic test for this condition. Repeating the diagnostic laparoscopy is useful later if MRI is not diagnostic and the previous operative report was not descriptive or trustworthy. An IVP is not indicated given that pain from a kidney stone is remote for this clinical scenario. A pelvic ultrasound is less diagnostic than a laparoscopy, which has already been done. A CBC and erythrocyte sedimentation rate would not be helpful because pelvic inflammatory disease is low on the differential diagnosis.

3. The answer is B [II A 1]. Pain from dysmenorrhea is the result of contraction of the upper uterus caused by prostaglandin F2α and can be referred to the dermatome that is equivalent to where the pain signal ends up in the spinal cord. The uterus is innervated by the sympathetic fibers (not parasympathetic), which go to spinal cord segments T10, T11, T12, and L1. Because this patient's pain is slightly below the umbilicus (which is in the T10 dermatome), the pain signal reaches T11 and not T10. The pudendal nerve carries impulses from urogenitally derived structures, such as the bladder, rectum, perineum, and anus.

4. The answer is E [IV A 1]. The most important thing is to rule out pregnancy with a serum hCG level, especially because an ectopic pregnancy is a possibility given the patient's history of a tubal ligation. Simply giving an NSAID (naproxen) is not appropriate without ruling out acute causes. A laparoscopy or a laparotomy may be premature at this point given the stable vital signs and lack of other serum studies. Antibiotics are not appropriate because there is no mention of anything that may lead you to suspect pelvic inflammatory disease.

5. The answer is E [I A]. Given the patient's history of major depression, sexual abuse, suicide attempts, and long-standing pelvic pain, the most likely cause may be a manifestation of deep-rooted psychological difficulties. A team approach using a gynecologist, internist, psychiatrist, and a social worker would most benefit her. The pain is unrelated to her menses; therefore, you can rule out mittelschmerz and endometriosis. It is unlikely that a postpartum tubal ligation caused any or significant adhesions to account for her pelvic pain. There is no evidence of irregular uterine enlargement on pelvic examination.

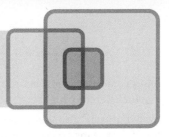

chapter 30

Endometriosis

SAMI I. JABARA AND RICHARD W. TURECK

I INTRODUCTION

A Definitions

1. Endometriosis is the **presence of functioning endometrial glands and stroma outside their usual location** within the uterine cavity. Significant pelvic adhesions with or without associated inflammatory cells or hemosiderin-laden macrophages often result.

2. Endometriosis is **primarily a pelvic disease** with implants in, or adhesions of, the ovaries, the fallopian tubes, uterosacral ligaments, rectosigmoid, bladder, and appendix. Less commonly, endometriosis can be found outside the pelvis, suggesting a metastatic spread.

3. This **generally benign disease** usually affects women in their reproductive years. However, there have been several case reports of endometrioid carcinoma developing within foci of endometriosis.

B Incidence.
The estimated incidence of endometriosis is 10 to15%. Recent data suggests that 30 to 40% of patients with infertility may have endometriosis. In addition, recent studies suggest existence of a hereditary tendency to initiate and propagate this disease; individuals in certain families tend to develop the more severe and recurrent forms of endometriosis.

II ETIOLOGY

A Causes

1. **Retrograde menstrual flow.** This theory postulates that the retrograde flow of menstrual debris through the fallopian tubes causes the endometrial cells to spread into the pelvis, form implants there, or serve as irritative foci, which stimulate coelomic metaplasia and differentiation of the peritoneal cells into endometrial-type tissue.
   a. **Clinical evidence.** Endometriosis is commonly found in dependent portions of the pelvis, most frequently on the ovaries, cul-de-sac, and uterosacral ligaments. Menstrual efflux from fallopian tubes has been observed during laparoscopy. In addition, patients with outflow obstruction (e.g., müllerian anomalies) have a significantly increased risk of endometriosis.
   b. **Experimental evidence.** Endometrial fragments from menstrual fluid can grow both in tissue culture and after injection beneath the skin of the abdominal wall.

2. **Hematogenous or lymphatic spread.** Endometriosis at sites distant from the pelvis may be caused by vascular or lymphatic transport of endometrial fragments. This could explain the presence of endometriosis at distant sites such as the brain and lungs.

3. **Metaplasia of the coelomic epithelium.** The transformation of coelomic epithelium results from some yet-unspecified stimuli, but it can occur early in puberty after a few menstrual cycles.

4. **Genetic and immunologic influences.** The relative risk of endometriosis is 7% in siblings, compared with 1% in control groups. An altered immunologic response may be involved in the pathogenesis of endometriosis.

B **Pain in endometriosis**

1. Lesions of the peritoneum can cause scarring and retraction of the peritoneum. They may also transmit pain through somatic afferent pain fibers.

2. Pain may result from elevated prostaglandins and histamines in endometriotic tissues and peritoneal fluids. In fact, levels of these compounds may be most elevated in patients with the earlier and more atypical forms of the disease. Liberal use of prostaglandin synthetase inhibitors may substantially help many women with endometriosis.

C **Infertility in minimal endometriosis.** Exactly how minimal endometriosis causes infertility is still under investigation.

1. Patients with endometriosis may have increased concentrations of macrophages in the ampullary portions of the fallopian tubes. Macrophages, chemotactically attracted to areas where endometriosis is present, may interfere with ovulation and corpus luteum formation and with fertilization through gamete phagocytosis. Factors produced by macrophages may interfere with sperm motility.

2. Prostaglandin $F_{2\alpha}$ increases the tone and amplitude of the cervical and uterine musculature and narrows the cervical os. It may increase the venous constriction of the uterus and the intensity of uterine contractions, therefore increasing the degree of dysmenorrhea. Prostaglandins also may interfere with placentation or implantation.

3. Interleukins are also secreted by the activated macrophages. Exposed embryos are less likely to progress to the eight-cell stage at 24 hours. Tumor necrosis factor and other cytokines may stimulate endometrial cell proliferation.

III SIGNS AND SYMPTOMS

A **Dysmenorrhea.** Secondary dysmenorrhea (menstrual pain secondary to an anatomic pelvic abnormality) is the most common symptom of endometriosis. The painful menses usually develop after years of relatively pain-free menses. With the increased use of laparoscopy, many adolescents with primary dysmenorrhea are being diagnosed with endometriosis.

B **Chronic pelvic pain.** Pelvic pain for more then 6 months (diffuse or localized in the pelvis) is considered chronic. However, many women with endometriosis are asymptomatic, and the degree of endometriosis often does not correlate with the existing amount of pain.

C **Dyspareunia.** Painful intercourse may be caused by:

1. Endometrial implants of the uterosacral ligaments

2. Endometriomas of the ovaries

3. Fixed retroversion of the uterus secondary to endometriosis and adhesions

D **Infertility.** Endometriosis has been demonstrated by laparoscopy in as many as 30 to 40% of women who are infertile.

1. Endometriosis may cause infertility when it interferes with tubal function and mobility, ovulation, steroidogenesis, and luteal function. Endometriosis may contribute to the **luteinized unruptured follicle syndrome,** in which the ovum is trapped in the follicle and not released with the luteinizing hormone (LH) surge.

2. Sufficient evidence supports the fact that minimal endometriosis is associated with infertility and that treating minimal endometriosis laparoscopically enhances fertility.

E **Associated symptoms**

1. **Urinary.** Urinary symptoms are common in patients with endometriosis; as many as one third of patients with endometriosis have urinary tract involvement. The highest frequency of such in-

volvement occurs in the bladder, followed in frequency by the lower ureter, upper ureter, and kidney. Symptoms range from intermittent dysuria, frequency, and urgency to complete ureteral obstruction. Gross or microscopic hematuria is present in many patients and frequently follows the menstrual cycle.

2. **Gastrointestinal.** Seven to thirty-five percent of all women with endometriosis have bowel involvement. Symptoms may vary from dyschezia (pain on defecation) and hematochezia (bloody bowel movements) to other symptoms of partial or complete bowel obstruction (e.g., abdominal bloating, intestinal cramps, nausea, and vomiting). Although severe cases of bowel involvement may be diagnosed by magnetic resonance imaging or computed tomography, the most practical method of diagnosis remains a radiographic evaluation of the bowel with barium contrast. Because endometriosis induces **severe inflammation** in the serosa, muscularis, and mucosa of the bowel, a **"tethering effect"** is often apparent on a barium enema or upper gastrointestinal series.

IV DIAGNOSIS

History and physical examination may be suggestive of endometriosis, but the only way to diagnose the condition is by visualization at surgery (usually laparoscopy) or by biopsy of implants.

A **History.**   The patient might have one or more of the characteristic symptoms (see III). A history of endometriosis in the patient's mother or sister is also important.

B **Pelvic examination.**   The pelvic examination in minimal endometriosis is usually normal.

1. **Nodularity and tenderness of the uterosacral ligaments** are characteristic findings on rectovaginal examination.

2. **Endometriomas** (ovarian cysts filled with old blood from endometriosis, forming **"chocolate cysts"**) are palpated as adnexal masses often fixed to the lateral pelvic walls or to the posterior cul-de-sac.

3. The uterus is often in a **fixed retroverted** position.

C **Laparoscopy and the classification of endometriosis**

a. **Appearance.** The classic endometriotic implant is characterized as brown or black pigmentation (**powder-burn lesion**) and fibrosis.

b. **Classification.** The extent of formation of classic lesions, ovarian involvement, and adhesive disease is classified by the American Society of Reproductive Medicine (formerly the Revised American Fertility Society). This classification system was originally developed to determine the efficacy of surgical therapy; however, it is somewhat inexact and may be very inaccurate in determining the activity and extent of disease.

c. **"Atypical" or "subtle" lesions.** Lesions ranging from **clear vesicular, white opacified, glandular excrescences, polypoid, or red hemorrhagic vesicles** have been increasingly apparent on laparoscopy and confirmed by biopsy to be endometriosis. Recent studies also suggest that these early implants may be the most metabolically active.

d. **Tissue damage.** Endometriosis may cause deep tissue damage, resulting in local scarring and reduplication of **peritoneum** and leading to **surface defects** or **Allen-Masters peritoneal defects.** Physicians should strongly suspect the possibility of endometriosis in all patients with demonstrated pelvic peritoneal defects at laparoscopy.

V TREATMENT

A **General considerations.**   Age of the patient, extent of disease, duration of the infertility, and severity of symptoms are important considerations. The patient's reproductive plans should also be taken into account.

1. Pregnancy tends to alleviate the symptoms of endometriosis.

2. CA-125 is increased in endometriosis. The CA-125 assay is a test for cell surface antigen found on coelomic epithelium, which includes the endometrium. This test is useful as a marker for response to treatment or recurrence but not as a diagnostic test because it **lacks specificity.**

B **Expectant treatment**

1. Expectant therapy may be appropriate in young women who have pelvic pain with apparent endometriosis on laparoscopy and no immediate interest in pregnancy. Goals are relief of the dysmenorrhea and prevention of further growth of endometriosis.
   a. **Oral contraceptive pills (OCPs).** Continuously administered OCPs are appropriate for mild disease because they reduce the amount of endometrial buildup and shedding, thereby preventing further growth of endometriosis.
   b. **Nonsteroidal anti-inflammatory drugs (NSAIDs).** The prostaglandin synthetase inhibitors are effective in controlling endometriosis-related dysmenorrhea. Women with endometriosis show increased concentrations of prostaglandins in the peritoneal fluid. When OCPs and NSAIDs are administered simultaneously, they have a synergistic effect.

2. Women with minimal disease and short-term infertility may be managed expectantly, but fertility may be an issue. Recent data has shown that conservative surgery (laparoscopic fulguration of endometriosis) is superior to expectant management in achieving fertility in the next year.

C **Medical therapy.** Ectopic endometrium responds to cyclic hormone secretion in a fashion similar to normal endometrium. **Hormonal suppression of menses constitutes the basis of medical therapy.**

1. **Gonadotropin-releasing hormone (GnRH) agonists.** These agents are the most commonly used method for medical treatment of endometriosis.
   a. **Mode of action.** GnRH is a decapeptide that controls the release of the anterior pituitary hormones (follicle-stimulating hormone and LH). GnRH has a very short half-life; it is rapidly destroyed by endopeptidases in the hypothalamus and pituitary gland. Normally, the release of GnRH is pulsatile. Chemical alterations of the amino acids at positions 6 and 10 produce synthetic derivatives of GnRH (GnRH analogs, GnRH agonists) that resist cleavage by endopeptidases but retain a high affinity for the pituitary GnRH receptor. If the gonadotrope is exposed to GnRH for a prolonged time, **downregulation** and **desensitization** occur, and gonadotropin secretion is suppressed.
   b. **Administration.** GnRH agonists may be administered intranasally, subcutaneously, or intramuscularly daily or as a depot injection every month or every 3 months.
   c. **Adverse effects**
      (1) Menopausal-type symptoms (e.g., hot flashes, decreased libido, vaginal dryness, and headaches) occur because of the hypoestrogenic state.
      (2) Prolonged use (more than 6 months) may result in significant bone loss, leading to osteoporosis. Using "**add-back therapy**" (estrogen and progestin) may minimize bone loss.
      (3) Flare-ups of endometriotic symptoms may occur in the first few weeks after treatment begins because of rapid elevations of steroid hormones. These symptoms typically abate. Recently, specific antagonists to GnRH have been developed.
   d. **Prognosis.** Amenorrhea and atrophic endometrial changes occur in most patients. Regression of endometriotic lesions occurs in 80% of cases, and symptomatic relief results in more then 50% of cases after 6 months of therapy. However, recurrence rates are 25 to 30% per year after therapy is discontinued.

2. **Danazol.** In the past, this synthetic 3-isoxazol derivative consistently improved symptoms of endometriosis. It has been now replaced by the GnRH agonists.

3. **OCPs**
   a. **Mode of action.** Continuously administered estrogen-progestin combination OCPs create a pseudopregnancy with amenorrhea. The pseudopregnancy causes decidualization, necro-

biosis, and resorption of the ectopic endometrium. This treatment is appropriate only in mild endometriosis that does not produce much distortion of the pelvic anatomy by adhesions or endometriomas.

   b. Dosage. The pills are given daily for 6 to 12 months. Addition of conjugated estrogens for short periods controls breakthrough bleeding.

   c. Prognosis. The recurrence rate is 15 to 25% in the following year, and the pregnancy rate is 25 to 50%.

D **Surgical therapy.** Medical therapy does not dissolve adhesions or eliminate endometriomas. Surgery is the treatment of choice in cases that present with considerable anatomic factors (e.g., adhesions and endometriomas). The success of surgery in relieving infertility is directly related to the severity of the endometriosis.

1. **Conservative surgery** involves the excision, fulguration, or laser vaporization of endometriotic tissue; the excision of ovarian endometriomas; and the resection of severely involved viscera, leaving the uterus and at least one ovary and fallopian tube intact. Studies have shown that gentle micromanipulation of the tissue, lysis of adhesions, and meticulous hemostasis improves fertility. **Reconstruction of all peritoneal surfaces** is essential. The raw areas in the pelvis can be covered with free peritoneal or omental graft to prevent adhesions.

2. **Radical surgery** involves a total hysterectomy and bilateral salpingo-oophorectomy.

   a. This approach is used in patients who do not desire future fertility or those whose endometriosis is so severe that it precludes any attempt at reconstruction. The rate of reoperation on women who have a hysterectomy without bilateral oophorectomy is high and varies from 15 to 40%.

   b. Estrogen replacement therapy is important in patients who undergo radical surgery to prevent osteoporosis and premature aging of the cardiovascular system. Estrogen replacement therapy carries only a small risk of inciting growth of residual endometriosis.

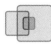

Study Questions for Chapter 30

DIRECTIONS: *Each of the numbered items or incomplete statements in this section is followed by answers or by completions of the statement. Select the ONE lettered answer or completion that is BEST in each case.*

1. A 34-year-old woman, gravida 0, has been trying to get pregnant for the last 3 years and has been unsuccessful. Her history is also significant for pelvic pain for several years and deep dyspareunia. On pelvic examination, you palpate a nodular, tender posterior fornix, a retroverted but normal-sized uterus, and a left adnexal mass. A recent pelvic ultrasound reveals a 6-cm right complex ovarian mass. Her CA-125 is elevated. What is the initial next step in management?

    [A] Expectant management
    [B] GnRH agonist
    [C] Diagnostic laparoscopy
    [D] Laparoscopy with cystectomy
    [E] Laparotomy with possible right oophorectomy

2. A 23-year-old woman, gravida 1, para 1, reports lower abdominal pain of 1 year's duration. She says that the pain is constant and dull and is worse around the time of her periods. She has no significant medical history and is taking birth control pills for contraception. You perform a laparoscopy and biopsy a lesion in the pelvic sidewall that looks like a clear vesicle. The pathology report is as follows: endometrial glands and stroma. What is the next best step in management?

    [A] Levonorgestrel and ethinyl estradiol
    [B] GnRH agonist
    [C] Conservative surgery
    [D] Total abdominal hysterectomy and bilateral salpingo-oophorectomy (TAH-BSO)
    [E] Danazol

3. A 25-year-old woman, gravida 3, para 3, who has been seen by a head and neck surgeon for the last 3 years because of cyclic nosebleeds is seeing you for an annual gynecologic examination. She tells you that she gets nosebleeds, only on the left side, every month, for two days after the start of her periods. She says that her nosebleeds stopped spontaneously during each pregnancy. Currently, she is married, sexually active, and not attempting pregnancy. The most likely cause of her epistaxis and the best management, respectively, is

    [A] Endometriosis by lymphatics and leuprolide
    [B] Endometriosis by blood vessels and oral contraception
    [C] Endometriosis by lymphatics and nasal electrocautery
    [D] Endometriosis by blood vessels and nasal electrocautery
    [E] Endometriosis by metaplasia and GnRH agonist

QUESTIONS 4–7

Match the statement below with the best word or words above. Each answer choice may be used once, more than once, or not at all.

    [A] Scarring and retraction
    [B] Prostaglandins
    [C] Allen-Masters lesions
    [D] Macrophages
    [E] Powder burn lesions

4. A 24-year-old woman with hematochezia during her menses

5. Patient with red hemorrhagic vesicles and white lesions who has a pelvic peritoneal defect on laparoscopy

6. May interfere with implantation of the embryo—one explanation for infertility in patients with endometriosis

7. Reason why naproxen may alleviate pain symptoms in a patient with endometriosis

Answers and Explanations

1. The answer is D [V D 1]. The most likely diagnosis here is an endometrioma of the right ovary. Because this patient has been attempting to get pregnant, conservative surgery to remove the endometrioma while preserving ovarian tissue and to fulgurate any endometriotic implants may improve her chances. Expectant management is not appropriate because she is infertile. Simple diagnostic laparoscopy without any treatment is also not appropriate. Medical therapy with a GnRH agonist may treat her symptoms, but it will not help her get pregnant. It is not necessary to perform a laparotomy and to remove what is most likely normal ovarian tissue.

2. The answer is B [V C 1]. The biopsy results show endometriosis; therefore, the best treatment at this point is a GnRH agonist. She is already on oral contraception (levonorgestrel and ethinyl estradiol) without any relief of her symptoms. Danazol is effective for endometriosis but, because of its many androgenic side effects, it is not preferred over leuprolide. Conservative surgery is not the next step, especially because she has no problem becoming pregnant. A TAH-BSO is too radical a procedure for this problem at this point in her life (she is young and still interested in childbearing).

3. The answer is B [II A 2]. Endometriosis at sites distant from the pelvis may be caused by vascular or lymphatic transport of endometrial fragments. The most likely explanation for endometriosis in the nose is vascular dissemination. Additionally, because this patient is interested in contraception, the best treatment for her would be oral contraceptive pills rather than leuprolide, which has side effects such as osteoporosis and premature menopausal symptoms. Cauterization of blood vessels in the nose is not the initial step in management of nosebleeds. Metaplasia does not account for distant site endometriosis.

4. A [II B 1 and III E 2] **5. C** [IV C d] **6. B** [II C 2] **7. B** [II B 1]. Endometriosis involving the bowel wall can cause scarring, retraction, and severe inflammation. A patient with endometriosis who has defects in the pelvic peritoneum because of local scarring has Allen-Master's defects. Infertility caused by minimal endometriosis may be related to macrophage response and prostaglandin F secretion. Prostaglandins may interfere with placentation and implantation. Naproxen is an NSAID and, as such, it is a prostaglandin synthetase or cyclooxygenase enzyme inhibitor.

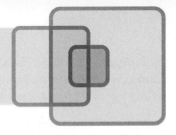

chapter 31

Ectopic Pregnancy
CLARISA GRACIA AND KURT BARNHART

I INTRODUCTION

An ectopic pregnancy is implantation of an embryo outside the uterus.

A Types
1. **Tubal (99%):** anywhere in the fallopian tube
   a. The most common site is the ampulla.
   b. Interstitial (cornual) pregnancies occur in the most proximal tubal segment, which runs through the uterine cornua. This type of ectopic pregnancy can grow to be quite large, and rupture may cause massive hemorrhage.
2. **Ovarian (0.5%):** on the ovary
3. **Abdominal (less than 0.1%):** in the abdomen, with possible adherence to the peritoneum, visceral surfaces, or omentum
4. **Cervical (0.1%):** in the cervix
5. **Heterotopic**
   a. Both intrauterine and ectopic pregnancies may occur concomitantly.
   b. This type of ectopic pregnancy is extremely rare (1 in 30,000 pregnancies).

B Prevalence. Ectopic pregnancies constitute 2% of all pregnancies. This proportion has increased over the past few decades.

C Significance. Ectopic pregnancy may lead to tubal rupture, massive intra-abdominal hemorrhage, and, ultimately, death. It also may result in tubal damage and has been associated with a poor reproductive outcome. It is the leading pregnancy-related cause of death in the first trimester.

II ETIOLOGY

A General considerations. The occurrence of ectopic pregnancy has been associated with abnormal function of the fallopian tubes. Normally, the tubes facilitate collection and transport of the oocyte and embryo into the uterus. The integrity of the fimbria, lumen, and ciliated mucosa appears to be important for transport. Conditions thought to prevent or retard migration of the fertilized ovum to the uterus predispose for ectopic pregnancy.

B Pelvic inflammatory disease (PID). The inflammation and scarring of intra- and extraluminal structures resulting from PID impair normal tubal function and foster implantation in the tube. Severe damage may lead to complete tubal blockage and infertility.

C Tubal surgery. Bilateral tubal ligation and tubal reanastomosis may lead to scarring and narrowing of the tube or false passage formation. Other pelvic and abdominal surgeries may also result in peritubal adhesions but have not been directly associated with ectopic pregnancy.

D **Artificial reproductive techniques.** Studies have documented increased risk of ectopic pregnancy with in vitro fertilization, gamete intrafallopian transfer, and superovulation, regardless of previous tubal damage. Retrograde embryo migration may be a possible mechanism.

E **Cigarette smoking.** Studies have shown that cigarette smoking causes tubal ciliary dysfunction. Smoking has been associated with ectopic pregnancy.

F **Intrauterine device (IUD).** Like any contraceptive method, the IUD protects against ectopic pregnancy. However, women who become pregnant with an IUD in place have a higher chance of having a tubal pregnancy than women without an IUD.

III SIGNS AND SYMPTOMS

A **Vaginal bleeding.** Light vaginal bleeding or spotting in the first trimester of pregnancy is the most common symptom of ectopic pregnancy. This bleeding usually begins 7 to 14 days after the missed menstrual period, and patients may interpret the bleeding as a menses.

B **Abdominal pain.** Unilateral pelvic pain is the second most common symptom. The pain may become severe and diffuse and may be associated with shoulder pain (caused by diaphragmatic irritation) if significant intra-abdominal hemorrhage exists.

C **Other symptoms.** Dizziness, fainting spells, and palpitations from hypotension resulting from intra-abdominal hemorrhage may occur.

D **Pregnancy status.** The standard urine pregnancy test is usually positive in the presence of an ectopic pregnancy. The serum pregnancy test, which is more sensitive, should be performed if the urine test is negative and clinical suspicion is high.

IV DIAGNOSIS

Because the symptoms of vaginal bleeding and pain in early pregnancy are not specific for ectopic pregnancy, these findings should not be used in isolation to diagnose this condition.

A **Physical examination.** In the presence of tubal rupture with intra-abdominal hemorrhage, patients may be hypotensive and tachycardic. In these cases, abdominal distention from hemoperitoneum and signs of an acute abdomen may be present with guarding, rebound, and cervical motion tenderness. In the absence of rupture, the physical examination may be completely normal. An unruptured ectopic pregnancy cannot be diagnosed by physical examination alone.

B **Differential diagnosis**

1. Adnexal torsion
2. Appendicitis
3. Spontaneous or threatened abortion
4. PID
5. Hemorrhagic corpus luteum
6. Endometriosis
7. Diverticulitis
8. Ovarian cyst

C **Diagnostic tests.** No single diagnostic test detects all ectopic pregnancies. A diagnostic strategy has been devised involving the use of several diagnostic modalities (Fig. 31-1).

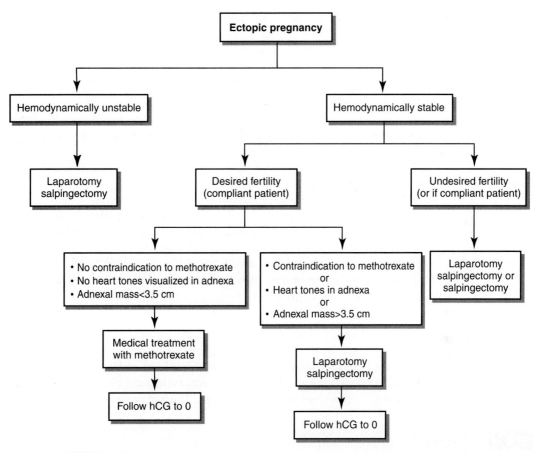

FIGURE 31-1 Treatment algorithm for ectopic pregnancy. hCG, human chorionic gonadotropin.

1. **Transvaginal ultrasound.** The first step in the evaluation of a suspected ectopic pregnancy is transvaginal ultrasound.
   a. It is difficult to diagnose an ectopic pregnancy by ultrasound alone. However, all viable intrauterine pregnancies can be visualized by transvaginal ultrasound at a gestational age greater than 5.5 weeks. Therefore, the **best way to diagnose** an ectopic pregnancy is to **rule out the presence of an intrauterine pregnancy** (heterotopic pregnancies are extremely rare).
   b. If an intrauterine pregnancy is detected on ultrasound, then ectopic pregnancy has essentially been excluded. If an ectopic pregnancy is visualized, then treatment may be pursued. If the ultrasound is nondiagnostic, then further evaluation is required.
2. **Human chorionic gonadotropin (hCG)**
   a. This hormone, which is produced by trophoblastic tissue, increases linearly in early pregnancy. hCG is used as a surrogate marker for gestational age because the exact gestational age at the time of presentation is often unknown.
   b. The **discriminatory zone** is defined as the quantitative hCG level above which all viable intrauterine pregnancies are visible by ultrasound. It is not the lowest hCG at which an intrauterine pregnancy can be visualized. The hCG level for transvaginal ultrasound, which varies by institution, is approximately 1500 to 2000 mIU/mL.
   c. If an intrauterine pregnancy is not identified by transvaginal ultrasound when the quantitative hCG level is higher than the discriminatory zone, then the gestation is, by definition, nonviable (either an abnormal intrauterine pregnancy or an ectopic pregnancy).

3. **Dilation and curettage (D&C).** When an intrauterine pregnancy is not identified by transvaginal ultrasound and the hCG level is greater than the discriminatory zone, a D&C may be performed to determine the location of the gestation. The absence of chorionic villi in the curettage specimen suggests the presence of an extrauterine, or ectopic, pregnancy.

4. **Serial hCG testing**
   a. If the quantitative hCG is below the discriminatory zone and the ultrasound is nondiagnostic, it is necessary to follow serial quantitative hCG levels to distinguish a viable intrauterine pregnancy from a nonviable gestation. Early in viable pregnancies, the **hCG concentration doubles approximately every 2 days** (minimum increase, 66%). If the hCG level increases above the discriminatory zone, a repeat ultrasound should be performed to confirm the presence of an intrauterine pregnancy.
   b. **hCG levels that fall or stabilize indicate nonviable pregnancies.**
      (1) When hCG levels decrease, they should be followed until the concentration of hCG is undetectable to confirm the diagnosis of a complete abortion. Ruptured ectopic pregnancies have occurred at very low hCG concentrations.
      (2) When hCG levels stabilize, a D&C should be performed to distinguish a nonviable intrauterine pregnancy from an ectopic pregnancy.

5. **Laparoscopy.** If the diagnosis is in doubt, laparoscopy may be performed to directly visualize the tubes and ovaries.

6. **Serum progesterone levels.** These measurements may be used as an adjunct to ultrasound and hCG. Progesterone levels less than 5 ng/mL are usually associated with nonviable pregnancies, and levels of 25 ng/mL or higher are usually associated with viable intrauterine pregnancies. However, these values are not absolute. Most patients evaluated for ectopic pregnancy have intermediate values, which are not helpful in diagnosis. The usefulness of progesterone is controversial.

V TREATMENT

A Surgical approaches

1. **Salpingectomy,** the removal of the fallopian tube containing the ectopic pregnancy, is the treatment of choice in the following situations:
   a. Future childbearing is not desired.
   b. The tube is severely damaged.
   c. Bleeding cannot be controlled.
   d. The ectopic pregnancy in that tube is recurrent.

2. **Linear salpingostomy,** the removal of the gestation through a linear incision in the fallopian tube, may be performed if future fertility is desired.
   a. This procedure is associated with a persistent ectopic pregnancy rate of 3 to 20%.
   b. Therefore, serial quantitative hCG values must be followed to ensure resolution.

3. **Operative laparoscopy** may be performed to confirm the diagnosis of ectopic pregnancy and to remove the abnormal gestation via salpingectomy or salpingostomy. This method is typically used in hemodynamically stable patients. Advantages of this technique over laparotomy include:
   a. Shorter hospital stay
   b. Faster postoperative recovery
   c. Better cosmetic result
   d. Potentially shorter operative time

4. **Laparotomy** is typically reserved for hemodynamically unstable patients who require emergent surgery for a ruptured ectopic pregnancy. This method may also be appropriate when laparoscopy is contraindicated or technically challenging because of extensive adhesive disease from prior surgery.

TABLE 31-1 Methotrexate Treatment in Ectopic Pregnancy		
Treatment Regimen	**Single Dose**	**Multidose**
Methotrexate	50 mg/m^2	1 mg/kg
Leucovorin	None	0.1 mg/kg every other day alternating with methotrexate
hCG monitoring	Days 0, 4, 7 Then weekly until level is undetectable	Every other day, then weekly until level is undetectable
Additional doses	Repeat dose if hCG does not decline 15% during days 4–7	Administer up to four doses if hCG does not decline 15% from previous value

hCG, human chorionic gonadotropin.

5. **Cornual resection** may be performed when an interstitial pregnancy occurs. The interstitial portion of the tube is removed via wedge resection into the uterine cornu.

6. **Oophorectomy** is indicated only when an ovarian ectopic pregnancy occurs and salvage of the affected ovary is not possible.

B **Medical approach.** Methotrexate, a chemotherapeutic agent, has been used successfully to treat small, unruptured ectopic pregnancies.

1. **Mechanism of action.** Methotrexate is a folic acid antagonist that interferes with DNA synthesis. Its action is principally directed at rapidly dividing cells, such as trophoblastic cells.

2. **Administration.** Methotrexate may be administered in a single intramuscular dose or in multiple doses with folic acid "rescue" (Table 31-1).

3. **Success rates** (73 to 94%). Decreased success has been noted with ectopic pregnancies of greater than 3.5 cm; with fetal cardiac activity; or with high hCG levels.

4. **Treatment failures.** Surgical management is usually necessary.

5. **Follow-up.** Serial hCG measurements must be observed after treatment to ensure resolution of the pregnancy.

6. **Complications** (approximately 5% of patients). Mild gastrointestinal symptoms such as nausea, vomiting, diarrhea, and stomatitis are typical. Potential life-threatening complications include pneumonitis, thrombocytopenia, neutropenia, elevated liver function tests, and renal failure.

7. **Contraindications.** Women who are breastfeeding or who have immunodeficiency, liver disease, renal disease, blood disorders, peptic ulcer disease, and active pulmonary disease should not receive methotrexate.

VI PROGNOSIS

A **Fertility.** Reported tubal patency after conservative therapy is approximately 70 to 80%. There appears to be no significant difference in tubal patency after salpingostomy in comparison to methotrexate. As many as 80% of women achieve pregnancy after an ectopic pregnancy, but only 33% deliver live infants. The best chance for future pregnancy in cases of tubal occlusion is in vitro fertilization.

B **Recurrence.** Of those women who achieve pregnancy after an ectopic pregnancy, as many as 27% will have another ectopic pregnancy. All patients should be told about the risk of recurrence risk and should notify a physician as soon as a menses has been missed to determine the location of the pregnancy.

Study Questions for Chapter 31

DIRECTIONS: Each of the numbered items or incomplete statements in this section is followed by answers or by completions of the statement. Select the ONE lettered answer or completion that is BEST in each case.

1. A 23-year-old gravida 2, para 1, ectopic 1 presents to your office because she missed her last period and has felt a sharp, intermittent pain on her left lower abdomen. She has no past medical history other than a left-sided ectopic pregnancy a few years ago, several years after vaginal delivery of her only son. Her in-office urine hCG is negative, so you order a serum β-hCG because of your high degree of suspicion. On physical examination, her BP = 110/74, P = 90, T = 97.8. She is obese, lacks peritoneal signs, and no masses are appreciated. A transvaginal ultrasound performed in your office reveals a 4.3-cm mass near the uterus-tubal junction. What is the next best step in management of this patient?

- A Laparoscopic salpingostomy
- B Laparoscopic salpingectomy
- C Methotrexate
- D Exploratory laparotomy
- E Repeat β-hCG in 2 days

2. A 23-year-old woman, gravida 3, para 1, SAB 1 presents to the emergency room reporting light vaginal bleeding and lower pelvic pain. Serum hCG is 3500 mIU/mL. She has a past medical history significant for diabetes mellitus and mild asthma. Her BP = 103/68, P = 88, T = 98.8. A 3-cm adnexal mass can be visualized on transvaginal ultrasound. The least invasive treatment of choice with the highest probability of future fertility is

- A Expectant management
- B Methotrexate
- C Laparoscopic salpingostomy
- D Laparoscopic salpingectomy
- E Laparotomy

3. A 36-year-old nulligravid woman is seeing you for her annual gynecologic care. She has a past medical history significant for pulmonary fibrosis. Within the past 3 years, all of the following are remarkable in her chart: bacterial vaginosis, candida, chronic endometritis, pyelonephritis, and three cycles of clomiphene therapy. She is a nonsmoker but does admit to drinking two to three alcoholic beverages every day. She has a family history significant for colon cancer in her maternal aunt. Which of the following places her at greatest risk for an ectopic pregnancy?

- A Age
- B Pulmonary fibrosis
- C Alcohol
- D Clomiphene
- E Chronic endometritis

4. A 21-year-old nulligravid woman, who had presented to the emergency room for spotting and abdominal pain yesterday but left against medical advice, is seeing you because she has not had a period for 7 weeks. You perform a transvaginal ultrasound, which shows an empty uterine cavity and no adnexal masses. Yesterday, her β-hCG was 4000 mIU/mL and today it is 4200 mIU/mL. The next best step in management of this patient is

- A Repeat β-hCG in 2 days
- B Laparoscopy

C Laparotomy
D Culdocentesis
E Dilatation and curettage

5. A 24-year-old gravida 2, para 1, ectopic 1 presents to your clinic for an annual pap smear. Before you end your interaction, you tell her that it is very important for her to give you a call or to come back to clinic if she misses her period. The reason for this advice is

A Given her history, she has a 33% chance of delivering a live infant
B Her fertility is in jeopardy if she delays diagnosis of a subsequent ectopic
C Her risk of a recurrent ectopic is approximately 20%
D Her risk of a recurrent ectopic is approximately 30%
E She is at increased risk for pelvic inflammatory disease

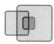

Answers and Explanations

1. The answer is D [V A 5 and I A 1 b]. The clinical scenario is that of an ectopic pregnancy in the interstitial portion of the left fallopian tube. Cornual pregnancies can grow quite large, and rupture may cause massive hemorrhage. The treatment of a corneal (interstitial) pregnancy is corneal resection. This requires a laparotomy. It is technically difficult to accomplish this via laparoscopy. Methotrexate is contraindicated in such a large ectopic pregnancy. Repeating hCG in 2 days is inappropriate because the tube can rupture at any time.

2. The answer is B [V B 7 and VI A]. This patient has an ectopic pregnancy that is amenable to treatment with methotrexate because she has no contraindications (mild asthma and diabetes mellitus are not contraindications). Although methotrexate and linear salpingostomy have comparable rates of tubal patency and fertility, methotrexate is the least invasive. Expectant management of a growing ectopic pregnancy is not appropriate given possibility of rupture and hemorrhage, which can be catastrophic. Salpingectomy is not preferred to salpingostomy in someone who desires future fertility. Laparotomy is not indicated in this patient, who is hemodynamically stable.

3. The answer is D [II D]. Clomiphene, human chorionic gonadotropin analogues, and follicle-stimulating hormone are all used by infertility doctors to induce superovulation (produce several follicles per cycle). All artificial reproductive technologies are risk factors for ectopic pregnancy. Only pelvic inflammatory disease is a risk factor for ectopic pregnancy, not chronic endometritis.

4. The answer is E [IV C 3]. When the quantitative hCG level is above the discriminatory zone (usually 1500 to 2000 mIU/mL depending on the ultrasound machine) and no pregnancy is visualized by transvaginal ultrasound, the pregnancy either is outside of the uterus or is an abnormal intrauterine pregnancy. To distinguish between the two, a uterine curettage should be performed. The presence of chorionic villi in the uterus indicates that the pregnancy was in the uterus and that the ectopic pregnancy does not exist. Repeating a quantitative hCG is not helpful because you already know the hCG is rising less than it should and there is no visualization of a sac in the uterus or the tube. Culdocentesis was performed in the past to confirm a ruptured ectopic pregnancy (because blood collects in the most dependent area, the cul-de-sac). Neither a laparoscopy nor a laparotomy is necessary yet because no mass has been visualized on ultrasound.

5. The answer is D [VI B]. Of those women who achieve pregnancy after an ectopic pregnancy, as many as 27% will have another ectopic pregnancy. All patients should be told about the risk of recurrence. The other answer choices are either false or not applicable to the question.

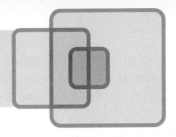

chapter 32

Uterine Leiomyomas

SAMI I. JABARA AND RICHARD W. TURECK

I · INTRODUCTION

Uterine leiomyomas, which are also known as myomas, fibroids, or fibromyomas, are proliferative, well-circumscribed, pseudoencapsulated, benign tumors composed of smooth muscle and fibrous connective tissue.

A Leiomyomas are the **most common uterine mass** and the most common neoplasm found in the female pelvis. They are present in 20 to 40% of women 35 years of age or older.

B They vary in diameter from 1 mm to more than 20 cm.

C Leiomyomas may be single but most often are multiple; 100 or more have been found in a single uterus.

II · ETIOLOGY

Leiomyomas are benign neoplasms consisting of a localized proliferation of smooth muscle cells and an accumulation of extracellular matrix. These smooth muscle tumors may be found in organs outside the uterus, including the fallopian tubes, vagina, round ligament, uterosacral ligaments, vulva, and gastrointestinal tract.

A **Cytogenetic studies** suggest that leiomyomas arise from a single neoplastic smooth muscle cell; in other words, they are **monoclonal** tumors resulting from somatic mutations. A variety of chromosomal abnormalities involving chromosomes 6, 7, 12, and 14 have been identified, suggesting a genetic role in the pathogenesis of these tumors. Disruption or dysregulation of the high mobility group genes on chromosome 12 appears to contribute to fibroid development.

B **Hormones** affect growth of leiomyomas but do not appear to be causal mechanisms. Evidence suggests that estrogen is a promoter of leiomyoma growth.

1. Leiomyomas are rarely found before puberty and stop growing after menopause.

2. New leiomyomas rarely appear after menopause.

3. Leiomyomas often grow rapidly during pregnancy.

4. Gonadotropin-releasing hormone (GnRH) agonists create a hypoestrogenic environment that results in a reduction of the size of leiomyomas. This effect is reversible on cessation of treatment.

C **Local and paracrine factors,** such as blood supply and proximity to other tumors, may account for variations in tumor volume and rate of growth. In addition, some peptide growth factors may play an etiologic role.

1. Epidermal growth factor (EGF) induces DNA synthesis in leiomyomas and myometrial cells.

2. Estrogen may exert its effect through EGF.

3. Recent studies in animals have shown that pirfenidone, an antifibrotic agent, suppresses leiomyoma growth via its potent inhibition of fibrogenic cytokines, including basic fibroblast growth factor, platelet-derived growth factor, transforming growth factor-β, and EGF.

III CLASSIFICATION AND PATHOLOGY

A **Classification of leiomyomas according to location.**   Three types of leiomyomas occur based on their location within or on the uterus.

1. **Intramural leiomyomas** are the most common variety, occurring within the walls of the uterus as isolated, encapsulated nodules of varying size. As these tumors grow, they can distort the uterine cavity or the external surface of the uterus. These tumors can also cause symmetric enlargement of the uterus when they occur singly.

2. **Submucous leiomyomas** are located beneath the endometrium and can grow into the uterine cavity. **Pedunculated leiomyomas** may protrude to or through the cervical os. These tumors are often associated with an abnormality of the overlying endometrium, resulting in abnormal bleeding. Anemia is a common problem.

3. **Subserous leiomyomas** are located just beneath the serosal surface and grow out toward the peritoneal cavity, causing bulging of the peritoneal surface of the uterus. These tumors may also develop a pedicle, become pedunculated, and reach a large size within the peritoneal cavity without producing symptoms. These potentially mobile tumors may present in such a manner that they need to be differentiated from solid adnexal lesions. When leiomyomas extend into the broad ligament, they are known as **intraligamentary leiomyomas**. Pedunculated leiomyomas may attach themselves to an adjacent structure such as the omentum, mesentery, or bowel; develop a secondary blood supply; and lose their connection with the uterus and primary blood supply. This situation occurs rarely, and the resulting structures are known as **parasitic leiomyomas**.

B **Pathology**

1. **Gross pathology.** Leiomyomas are **pseudoencapsulated** solid tumors, well demarcated from the surrounding myometrium. The **pseudocapsule** is not a true capsule and results from compression of fibrous and muscular tissue on the surface of the tumor. Because the vasculature is located on the periphery, the central part of the tumor is susceptible to degenerative changes. The tumors are smooth, solid, and usually pinkish-white, depending on the degree of vascularity. The surface typically has a trabeculate, fleshy, whorl-like appearance.

2. **Microscopic pathology.** Leiomyomas are composed of groups and bundles of smooth muscle fibers in a twisted, whorled fashion. Microscopically, these appear as smooth muscle cells in longitudinal or cross section intermixed with fibrous connective tissue. Vascular structures are few, and mitoses are rare.
   a. **Cellular leiomyomas** are tumors with mitotic counts of five to ten per 10 consecutive high-power fields that lack cytologic atypia.
   b. **Leiomyosarcomas** are a distinct clinical entity and in the past were diagnosed based on a **mitotic count** of ten mitotic figures per 10 high-power fields. Recently, the importance of other factors, such as **cellular atypia** and **coagulative necrosis** of tumor cells, has been recognized. These malignant tumors are found rarely in hysterectomy or myomectomy specimens.

C **Degenerative changes.**   A variety of degenerative changes may occur in leiomyomas that alter the gross and microscopic appearance of the tumors. Most of these changes have no clinical significance. Degenerative changes occur secondary to alterations in circulation (either arterial or venous), postmenopausal atrophy, or infection, or they may result from malignant transformation.

1. **Hyaline degeneration**, the most common type of degeneration, is present in almost all leiomyomas. It is caused by an overgrowth of the fibrous elements, which leads to a hyalinization of the fibrous tissue and, eventually, calcification.

2. **Cystic degeneration** may occasionally be a sequel of necrosis, but cystic cavities are usually a result of myxomatous change and liquefaction after hyaline degeneration.

3. **Necrosis** is commonly caused by impairment of the blood supply or severe infection. A specific kind of necrosis is the **red,** or **carneous,** degeneration, which occurs most frequently in pregnancy. The lesion has a dull, reddish hue and is believed to be caused by aseptic degeneration associated with local hemolysis.

4. **Mucoid degeneration** may occur when the arterial input is impaired, particularly in large tumors. Areas of hyalinization may convert to a mucoid or myxomatous type of degeneration; the lesion has a soft, gelatinous consistency. Further degeneration can lead to liquefaction and cystic degeneration.

5. **Infection** of a leiomyoma most commonly occurs with a pedunculated submucous leiomyoma that first becomes necrotic and then becomes infected.

6. **Calcification** of leiomyomas is a common finding in postmenopausal patients.

7. **Sarcomatous degeneration** occurs in less than 1% (0.13 to 0.29%) of leiomyomas. Whether this represents a true degenerative change or a spontaneous neoplasm is a subject of controversy. The presence of a leiomyosarcoma within the core of an apparently benign pseudoencapsulated leiomyoma suggests such a degenerative process. This type of sarcoma is usually of a spindle cell rather than a round cell type. The 5-year survival rate for patients with a leiomyosarcoma arising within a leiomyoma is much better than that for a true sarcoma of the uterus with extension of the sarcomatous tissue beyond the pseudocapsule of the leiomyoma.

IV   ASSOCIATED SYMPTOMS AND SIGNS

A Symptoms.   These vary greatly, depending on size, number, and location of the leiomyoma or leiomyomas. Most women with leiomyomas are asymptomatic; symptoms occur in 10 to 40% of patients.

1. **Abnormal uterine bleeding.** This is the most common symptom associated with uterine leiomyomas, occurring in as many as 30% of symptomatic women. The typical bleeding pattern is **menorrhagia,** or excessive bleeding at the time of menses (more than 80 mL). The increase in flow usually occurs gradually, but the bleeding may result in a profound anemia. The exact mechanisms of increased blood loss are unclear. Possible factors include necrosis of the surface endometrium overlying the submucous leiomyoma, a disturbance in the hemostatic contraction of normal muscle bundles when extensive intramural myomatous growth occurs, an increase in surface area of the endometrial cavity, or an alteration in endometrial microvasculature. In some cases, abnormal bleeding may be associated with anovulatory states. Frequently, leiomyomas are associated with polyps and endometrial hyperplasia, which may produce an abnormal bleeding pattern.

2. **Pain.** Uncomplicated uterine leiomyomas usually do not produce pain. Acute pain associated with fibroids is usually caused by either torsion of a pedunculated leiomyoma or infarction progressing to carneous degeneration within a leiomyoma. Pain is often crampy when a submucous leiomyoma within the endometrial cavity acts as a foreign body. Some patients with intramural leiomyomas experience the reappearance of dysmenorrhea after many years of pain-free menses.

3. **Pressure.** As leiomyomas enlarge, they may cause a feeling of pelvic heaviness or produce pressure symptoms on surrounding structures.
   a. **Urinary frequency** is a common symptom when a growing leiomyoma exerts pressure on the bladder.
   b. **Urinary retention,** a rare occurrence, can result when myomatous growth creates a fixed, retroverted uterus that pushes the cervix anteriorly under the symphysis pubis in the area of the posterior urethrovesicular angle.

c. Unilateral uretal obstruction can be caused by lateral extension or intraligamentous leiomyomas. A markedly enlarged uterus that extends above the pelvic brim may cause ureteral compression, hydroureter, and hydronephrosis.

d. Constipation and difficult defecation can be caused by large posterior leiomyomas.

e. Compression of pelvic vasculature by a markedly enlarged uterus may cause varicosities or edema of the lower extremities.

4. Reproductive disorders. Infertility secondary to leiomyomas is probably uncommon. Infertility may result when leiomyomas interfere with normal tubal transport or implantation of the fertilized ovum.

a. Large intramural leiomyomas located in the cornual regions may virtually close the interstitial portion of the tube.

b. Continuous bleeding in patients with submucous leiomyomas may impede implantation; the endometrium overlying the leiomyoma may be out of phase with the normal endometrium and thus provide a poor surface for implantation.

c. Increased incidences of abortion and premature labor occur in patients with submucous or intramural leiomyomas.

d. Less successful results with in vitro fertilization occur in patients who have large submucosal fibroids when compared to controls.

5. Pregnancy-related disorders. Uterine leiomyomas, found in 0.3 to 7.2% of pregnancies, are usually present before conception and may increase in size significantly during gestation.

a. Although women with leiomyomas have a higher **incidence of spontaneous abortion,** the tumors are an uncommon cause of abortion.

b. Red degeneration, or **torsion of a pedunculated fibroid,** may cause gradual or acute symptoms of pain and tenderness. These conditions must be distinguished from other causes of abdominal pain in pregnancy because treatment is conservative with symptomatic relief and observation. Surgical intervention is rarely, if ever, indicated.

c. Premature labor may be increased in women with leiomyomas.

d. In the third trimester, leiomyomas may be a factor in **malpresentation, mechanical obstruction,** or **uterine dystocia.** Large leiomyomas in the lower uterine segment may prevent descent of the presenting part. Intramural leiomyomas may interfere with effectual uterine contractions and normal labor.

e. Postpartum hemorrhage is more common in uterine leiomyomas.

B **Signs**

1. Physical examination. The diagnosis of uterine leiomyomas can be made with confidence in 95% of cases based on physical examination alone. Uterine size is defined as the equivalent gestational size as determined by abdominal and pelvic examination.

a. Abdominal examination. Uterine leiomyomas may be palpated as irregular, nodular tumors protruding against the anterior abdominal wall. Leiomyomas are usually firm on palpation; softness or tenderness suggests the presence of edema, sarcoma, pregnancy, or degenerative changes.

b. Pelvic examination. The most common finding is uterine enlargement. The shape of the uterus is usually asymmetric and irregular in outline. The uterus is usually freely movable unless residuals of an old pelvic inflammatory disease persist.

(1) In the case of **submucous leiomyomas,** the uterine enlargement is usually symmetric.

(2) Some **subserous leiomyomas** may be distinct from the main body of the uterus and may move freely, which often suggests the presence of adnexal or extrapelvic tumors.

(3) The **diagnosis of cervical leiomyomas or pedunculated submucous leiomyomas** may be made on examination if the tumor extends into the cervical canal. Occasionally, a submucous leiomyoma may be visible at the cervical os or at the introitus.

2. **Laboratory evaluation and diagnostic studies.** Additional diagnostic studies are based on individual presentation and physical examination. In asymptomatic patients with physical examinations consistent with leiomyomas, it is not necessary to obtain additional studies routinely.

   a. **Hemoglobin and hematocrit** is obtained in cases of excessive vaginal bleeding to assess the degree of loss and adequacy of replacement.

   b. **Coagulation profile** and **bleeding time** are ordered when the history is suggestive of a bleeding diathesis.

   c. **Endometrial biopsy** is performed in patients with abnormal uterine bleeding who are thought to be anovulatory or at increased risk for endometrial hyperplasia.

   d. **Ultrasonography** accurately assesses uterine dimension, leiomyoma location, interval growth, and adnexal anatomy.

      (1) Routine ultrasonography does not improve long-term outcome compared with clinical assessment alone. Pelvic ultrasound is appropriate in situations when clinical assessment is difficult or uncertain; when physical examination is suboptimal, as in cases of morbid obesity; or when adnexal pathology cannot be excluded on physical examination alone. Ultrasonography may be used to detect hydroureter and hydronephrosis in the patient with marked uterine enlargement.

      (2) **Sonohysterography** or intrauterine infusion of sterile saline at the time of ultrasound examination can identify the presence of pedunculated submucous leiomyomas and endometrial polyps.

   e. **Hysteroscopy** or **hysterosalpingography** may be used to evaluate the endometrial cavity in the workup of patients with uterine leiomyomas and infertility or repetitive pregnancy loss.

V   TREATMENT

Therapy for leiomyomas must be individualized and may be nonsurgical or surgical. Treatment decisions are based on symptoms, fertility status, uterine size, and rate of uterine growth.

A **Expectant management.**   In the absence of pain, abnormal bleeding, pressure, or large leiomyomas, observation with periodic examination is appropriate. This is especially true if the patient is nearing menopause, at which time the leiomyomas will atrophy as estrogen levels fall.

1. **Bimanual examinations** should be performed every 3 to 6 months to determine uterine size and the rate of tumor growth. After slow growth or stable uterine size has been confirmed, annual follow-up may then be appropriate. Rapid growth—a change of 6 pregnancy weeks in size or more in 12 months or less of observation—is an indication for surgical intervention. Follow-up with pelvic ultrasound should be performed if physical examination is inadequate because of obesity or if it is necessary to distinguish between a fibroid and an adnexal mass.

2. **Endometrial biopsy** may be indicated in patients with **increased bleeding.** Regular blood counts are warranted; iron deficiency anemia is common with menorrhagia, and oral iron may be required to replace losses associated with the uterine bleeding. Nonsteroidal anti-inflammatory drugs (NSAIDs) that inhibit prostaglandin synthesis, administered on a scheduled rather than as-needed basis, should be used to reduce menstrual blood flow. Low-dose oral contraceptives or progestin therapy may also reduce blood loss.

3. **NSAIDs** also treat pelvic discomfort or pressure.

B **GnRH agonists.**   Long-acting GnRH agonists suppress gonadotropin secretion and create a hypoestrogenic state similar to that observed after menopause. They are administered in the form of a subcutaneous implant or an intramuscular depot injection (every 4 weeks for 12 to 24 weeks).

1. Although individual response varies widely, a median reduction in uterine size of 50% has been observed. Maximum response is seen after 12 weeks of therapy, with no added advantage to 24

weeks of therapy. Decreased size is secondary to a decrease in blood flow and cell size; cell death and a decrease in cell number are not observed.

2. Leiomyomas rapidly regrow, returning to baseline size within 12 weeks after GnRH therapy is discontinued.

3. Use of GnRH agonist therapy is not recommended for longer than 24 weeks (6 months) because of the long-term effects of a hypoestrogenic state, most notably osteoporosis.

4. Long-term use of GnRH agonists with "add-back" hormone replacement therapy is another alternative. However, this regimen is costly and is still under investigation.

5. Because of potential side effects and expense, GnRH agonists are recommended for short-term use in selected cases only. For example:
   a. For large submucous leiomyomas to facilitate hysteroscopic resection
   b. For leiomyomas in symptomatic perimenopausal patients who wish to avoid surgery
   c. As presurgical treatment to decrease bleeding symptoms in patients with anemia who are taking iron

C **Surgery**

1. **Indications.** Surgical intervention is indicated when symptoms fail to respond to conservative management.
   a. **Excessive bleeding** that interferes with normal lifestyle or leads to anemia and **chronic pelvic pain or pressure**
   b. **Protrusion** of a pedunculated submucous leiomyoma through the cervix
   c. **Rapid growth** in a leiomyomatous uterus at any age. This finding warrants exploration because it may represent a leiomyosarcoma as opposed to a benign leiomyoma. Most often, leiomyosarcomas represent a distinct clinical entity rather than malignant degeneration within a leiomyoma. Because these malignancies occur primarily in women older than 40 years of age and their incidence increases with advancing age, any increase in uterine size in the postmenopausal woman warrants surgical exploration.
   d. **Repetitive pregnancy loss caused by leiomyomas** after other etiologies have been excluded
   e. **Infertility patients** with leiomyomas after evaluation and treatment of other causes. The location or size of the leiomyoma should indicate that it may be a cause of the infertility.
   f. **Arbitrary uterine size** (more than 12 pregnancy weeks) in asymptomatic patients. This criterion has traditionally been cited as an indication for surgery but has recently come under scrutiny. No controlled data indicates that the proposed benefits of surgery outweigh its risks. Expectant management of asymptomatic patients with uterine enlargement of greater than 12 pregnancy weeks' size with stable or slow growth is considered a reasonable treatment option. Surgical intervention is indicated if a patient is concerned about uterine size or is symptomatic.
   g. **Progressive hydronephrosis**, demonstrated by ultrasonography or intravenous pyelography, or **impaired renal function**.

2. **Surgical procedures.** The type of surgery to be performed depends on the age of the patient, the nature of the symptoms, the size and the location of the tumor, and the patient's desires about future fertility.
   a. **Myomectomy** involves the removal of single or multiple leiomyomas while preserving the uterus; this procedure is usually reserved for women who desire future pregnancy. Myomectomy is a reasonable approach in symptomatic women unresponsive to conservative treatment who desire uterine conservation. Eighty percent of patients report subjective improvement of symptoms, 15% of patients experience symptom recurrence, and 10% require additional treatment.
      (1) **Hysteroscopic resection** effectively treats submucous leiomyomas; 20% of women require additional treatment within 5 to 10 years.

(2) **Risks of abdominal myomectomy** include increased intraoperative blood loss, prolonged operative time, and increased postoperative hemorrhage compared to hysterectomy. These are offset by a decreased risk of infectious morbidity and ureteral injury.

(3) The **recurrence of leiomyomas after myomectomy** depends on race (higher in African Americans), patient age, and the completeness of the original myomectomy; 10-year recurrence rates of 5 to 30% have been reported.

(4) At the time of abdominal myomectomy, it may be necessary to open the uterine cavity to remove intramural or submucous leiomyomas completely. This is considered an indication for cesarean section in future pregnancies.

(5) **Term pregnancy rates after myomectomy** for infertility or repetitive pregnancy loss are 40%.

(6) Indications for **laparoscopic myomectomy** are the same as for abdominal myomectomy. Laparoscopic myomectomy may be associated with shorter recovery times, and uncertainty still exists over whether it is associated with less postoperative pelvic adhesions. Large, multiple, deep and lower posterior wall leiomyomas should be approached with caution; they are technically more challenging.

(7) **Laparoscopic myolysis** (using laser or coagulation current) and **cryomyolysis** (using a−180°C probe) of leiomyomas have resulted in a persistent decrease in the size of fibroids and appear quite promising.

b. Hysterectomy is the definitive treatment for uterine leiomyomas if the indications for surgery are present and if **childbearing is complete.**

(1) With hysterectomy, both the leiomyomas and any associated disease are removed permanently. There is no risk of recurrence.

(2) In patients with abnormal bleeding, other causes such as anovulatory states should be detected and treated before hysterectomy. Hysterectomy should not be performed on the assumption that the bleeding is caused solely by the leiomyomas. Biopsy of the endometrial cavity is essential before hysterectomy to rule out endometrial neoplasia. The absence of cervical malignancy must be ascertained before surgery.

(3) The patient's medical and psychological risks should be evaluated before surgical therapy.

(4) Ovaries need not be removed in women younger than 40 to 45 years of age. The patient must play an important part in the decision concerning oophorectomy at any age; little evidence supports the contention that the residual ovary after a hysterectomy is at greater risk for development of ovarian cancer. The long-term consequences of estrogen deprivation—osteoporosis and cardiovascular risk—and implications of estrogen replacement therapy should be addressed thoroughly before surgery.

c. Uterine artery embolization. Recently, this procedure has emerged as an alternative to traditional surgery. In uterine artery embolization, an interventional radiologist injects the desired previously mapped artery with embolic material, such as gel-foam pledgets or metal coils. This action occludes the vessel feeding the leiomyoma, depriving the tumor of its vascular supply and causing shrinking or necrosis and death of the leiomyoma.

(1) Recent studies have shown that uterine artery embolization is relatively safe. It results in a 60% reduction in size of fibroids and control menorrhagia in more than 90% of cases.

(2) Typical candidates are women with symptomatic fibroids who are approaching menopause, no longer desire fertility, have a large uterus, have multiple health risks for surgery, and have uncontrollable menorrhagia. Some of the risks associated with uterine artery embolization are fever, pain, infection, premature ovarian failure, possible need for hysterectomy, and pulmonary embolism.

Study Questions for Chapter 32

DIRECTIONS: Each of the numbered items or incomplete statements in this section is followed by answers or by completions of the statement. Select the ONE lettered answer or completion that is BEST in each case.

1. A 25-year-old woman, gravida 4, para 4, with a history of leiomyomas presents to the emergency department reporting pelvic pressure. She denies cardiac, renal, or hepatic symptoms. A pelvic ultrasound shows a 10-cm left uterine-adnexal mass that has the echogenicity of a fibroid. Pressure from the fibroid may also cause

- A Leg ulcers
- B Peau' de orange
- C Superficial thrombophlebitis
- D Deep venous thrombosis
- E Varicose veins

2. A 30-year-old woman, gravida 2, para 2 presents to you for her annual gynecologic visit. Currently, she has no symptoms. You perform a pap smear and a pelvic examination that reveals an enlarged, nontender, irregular uterus and no adnexal mass or tenderness. There are no vulvar or vaginal lesions. The most likely type of fibroid is a(n)

- A Anterior intramural fibroid (5-cm size)
- B Submucosal pedunculated fibroid (2-cm size)
- C Subserosal pedunculated fibroid (7-cm size)
- D Posterior intramural fibroid (5-cm size)
- E Intramural fibroid with a submucous component (5-cm size)

3. A 22-year-old woman, gravida 2, para 1 at 20 weeks of gestation presents to the emergency department reporting acute onset lower abdominal pain. She has a history of fibroids and an unknown abdominal surgery. Her vital signs are as follows: T = 99.2, BP = 105/68, P = 110, R = 28. There is a linear, 4-cm scar in the right lower quadrant, bowel sounds are present, and the abdomen is nontender except for spot tenderness in the midline, between the umbilicus and the symphysis pubis. There is no rebound tenderness or guarding. There is no costovertebral angle tenderness. Her fundus is 28 cm above the symphysis pubis. Her white blood cells are elevated, urinalysis is normal, and her liver function tests are within normal range. The most likely diagnosis is

- A Leiomyomatous degeneration (carneous type)
- B Leiomyomatous degeneration (myxomatous type)
- C Cystitis
- D Preeclampsia
- E Appendicitis

4. A 27-year-old woman, gravida 2, para 1 at 30 weeks of gestation presents to the clinic for a routine prenatal visit. Her pregnancy has been unremarkable thus far. "Serosal fibroids" are listed under her "problem list." Her fundus measures 37 cm from the symphysis pubis. In discussing possible complications of a fibroid uterus during pregnancy, you mention that she is at highest risk for

- A Preterm premature rupture of membranes (PROM)
- B Placenta previa
- C Pregnancy-induced hypertension (PIH)
- D Breech presentation
- E Placental abruption

5. A 49-year-old woman, gravida 3, para 2, SAB 1 who has a known myomatous uterus presents to you because of heavy bleeding during her periods and occasional spotting in between her periods. Her menses occur every 5 to 6 weeks and last 6 to 10 days. They are associated with painful cramps. She has no chronic medical problems. The next best step in management of this patient is

- [A] GnRH agonist for 3 months
- [B] GnRH agonist for 6 months and add-back hormones for last 3 months
- [C] Hysterectomy
- [D] Endometrial biopsy
- [E] Transvaginal ultrasound

Answers and Explanations

1. The answer is E [IV A 3 e]. Compression of pelvic vasculature by a markedly enlarged uterus may cause varicosities or edema (swelling) of the lower extremities. Peau' de orange is a skin edema that occurs in breast cancer. Leg ulcers are common in patients with a history of advanced diabetes or peripheral vascular disease. Superficial thrombophlebitis may result from stasis of blood in this patient, but it is not as common as vein varicosities. Deep venous thrombosis is not associated with leiomyomas.

2. The answer is C [III A 3]. Subserosal pedunculated fibroids are usually asymptomatic. A larger fibroid does not necessarily cause more symptoms unless it is in a critical location. An anterior large intramural fibroid may cause urinary symptoms because of pressure on the bladder. A large posterior intramural fibroid may cause bowel symptoms (constipation) because of pressure on the rectal area. A submucous fibroid or any intramural fibroid with a submucous component may cause bleeding (because of either local endometrial hyperplasia or a fragile endometrium overlying the fibroid area). The latter can also cause reproductive symptoms by interfering with implantation. A large intracavitary fibroid can even act as an intrauterine device (IUD).

3. The answer is A [III C 3]. A patient with a history of fibroids with this question's described physical examination findings during pregnancy most likely has carneous degeneration of her fibroids, which is quite painful. The RLQ scar and history of abdominal surgery suggest an appendectomy; therefore, appendicitis is not a possibility. Her BP and urinalysis (UA) are normal; therefore, preeclampsia is unlikely. Bladder infection is also unlikely given the lack of urinary symptoms and a normal urinalysis. The most common type of fibroid degeneration in pregnancy is carneous, not myxomatous.

4. The answer is D [IV A 5 d]. In the third trimester, leiomyomas may be a factor in malpresentation (breech), mechanical obstruction, and uterine dystocia. PIH and PROM are not related to fibroids (but premature labor is related). Placenta previa and abruption are unlikely with fibroids, especially when they are predominantly in the subserosal location.

5. The answer is D [V A 2 and V B 2]. You cannot assume that abnormal bleeding in a 49-year-old woman is caused by the leiomyomas simply because she has a myomatous uterus. At this age, the risk of endometrial disease, such as polyps, hyperplasia, and carcinoma, is significant and must be ruled out. Endometrial sampling is indicated before considering other therapy. Hysterectomy is the definitive treatment for fibroids and is a therapeutic option for someone who is finished with childbearing and who has inadequate relief with medical management (leuprolide). This option can be contemplated in this case only after endometrial neoplasia is ruled out. A transvaginal ultrasound is unnecessary because you already know that the patient has a fibroid uterus.

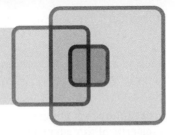

chapter **33**

Intimate Partner Violence and Sexual Assault

JANICE B. ASHER

I   **RELATIONSHIP VIOLENCE**

A **Introduction.** Relationship violence is the maintenance of power by one intimate partner, usually male, to control another intimate partner, usually female. The **National Center for Injury Prevention and Control (NCIPC)** of the **Centers for Disease Control and Prevention (CDC)** uses the broad term **intimate partner violence (IPV)** to refer to "actual or threatened physical or sexual violence or psychological and emotional abuse directed to a spouse, ex-spouse, current or former boyfriend or girlfriend, or current or former dating partner." Partners can be of the same sex.

1. **Frequency.** At the outset, episodes of violence may occur infrequently. Subsequently, they tend to occur more often.

2. **Severity.** Episodes of violence may begin as simple verbal or emotional assaults intended to intimidate and isolate the victim and may then escalate to the intentional infliction of brutal physical injuries.

3. **Role of the physician.** Relationship violence is a major public health concern. Physicians are frequently the only professionals with whom victims of relationship violence come in contact. Physicians have both the opportunity and the responsibility to address domestic violence with all of their female patients.

B **Epidemiology**

1. The CDC reports that 1.5 million women and 834,700 men are raped or physically abused by an intimate partner each year.

2. Overall, the lifetime incidence of relationship violence toward women is greater than 25%. More women present for medical care because of battering than the total number who present because of stranger rape, automobile accidents, and mugging.

3. Unfortunately, health care providers usually do not identify abused women, and their abuse-related symptoms are unrecognized. This is true even in cases of acute trauma. In one study, only 13% of women presenting to the emergency department for abuse-related injuries were asked about relationship violence.

C **Medical evaluation**

1. **Assessment.** Appropriate assessment of relationship violence is much more likely to save time and expense. The time needed to evaluate and treat abuse-related symptoms that are initially unrecognized may be considerable. Moreover, violence assessment is, in itself, a powerful intervention. By routinely asking questions about IPV, physicians are sending important messages:

that IPV is common, that it is an area of medical concern, and that the victim of violence can discuss the issue with a physician.

2. Screening

  a. Physicians should practice routine screening of all their female patients for relationship violence because the vast majority of women in abusive relationships do not spontaneously disclose that they are being abused. The primary reason that women give for not mentioning abuse is fear of retaliation by their partners who learn about the disclosure. Women also cite fear of police involvement and feelings of shame and embarrassment.

  b. Relationship violence occurs in **all racial, ethnic, religious, and socioeconomic groups,** and screening for those who fit a certain "profile" may exclude identification of some victims. Studies have shown the value of universal screening to increase the detection rate. The rate is much greater if the physician performs the screening and does not use a self-assessment tool, such as a questionnaire in an office waiting room.

  c. It is better to inquire about specific behaviors than to use general terms, because the term "abuse" means different things to different people. Recommended screening questions include:

   (1) Are you in a relationship in which you have been hit or physically threatened?

   (2) Are you in a relationship in which you have been forced to have sex?

   (3) Are you afraid of a current or ex-partner?

3. Clinical picture. More than 50% of abused women present with such somatic complaints as headache, abdominal pain, pelvic pain, fatigue, shortness of breath, gastrointestinal disturbances, sleep disorders, and other chronic conditions in addition to their physical injuries.

D Physician response

1. After obtaining the victim's history regarding the nature and severity of the abuse, it is important to communicate concern for the patient's safety in a nonjudgmental and compassionate way.

2. An understandable but **dangerous reaction by the physician** is to urge a patient to leave a violent relationship immediately. Abundant data indicate that abused women are most likely to be seriously injured or killed by their partners when they attempt to leave them. It is dangerous for victims to attempt to leave a relationship before they have **formulated well-developed safety and exit plan.**

3. A physician should focus on safety measures for patients and their children. Such measures include developing emergency exit plans, making copies of important documents, and keeping money in a place to which partners do not have access.

E Documentation. It is necessary to document patient statements regarding abuse and physical findings associated with battering as part of ensuring patient safety. Such documentation may eventually be useful in a court of law, particularly if custody issues arise. To protect the patient's confidentiality with regard to the abusive partner, documentation of abuse should not appear on the billing diagnosis if the patient's partner will receive insurance information.

1. Document the abuse in the patient's own words. For example, "Patient states, 'My husband, John Smith, hit me with his fists,'" is preferable to "history of trauma." Documentation should include the name of the perpetrator and nature of the weapon used. For description of injuries, dated photographs are ideal, but body maps or written descriptions are also acceptable.

2. Whenever possible, **document whether injuries appear recent or old.**

F Follow-up. Once a victim is identified, it is important that a physician refer the patient to a relationship violence expert, who may be a hospital-based or community-based social worker, a colleague who is knowledgeable about relationship violence, a local domestic violence advocacy organization, or the **National Domestic Violence Hotline** (1-800-799-SAFE).

II   VIOLENCE IN PREGNANCY

A **Introduction.**   Violence in pregnancy presents a unique challenge in that there are two victims: mother and fetus. Pregnancy offers physicians a tremendous opportunity for screening and intervention because of the

1. Increased availability of medical attention

2. Desire of pregnant women to ensure a healthy outcome for their infants

B **Epidemiology**

1. The leading cause of maternal mortality in pregnancy is homicide, and the most likely perpetrator is the woman's partner. More pregnant women die because of relationship violence than of any medical complication of pregnancy. The estimated incidence of relationship violence in pregnancy is 4 to 20%.

2. **Adolescents are overrepresented** among abused pregnant women. As many as 29% of pregnant adolescents experience abuse, including sexual abuse and assault.

3. The single **greatest risk factor** for relationship violence during pregnancy is a **history of violence within the year prior to the pregnancy**. In violent relationships, unintended pregnancy may in itself represent a manifestation of abuse; abused women may not be able to affect sexual activity or contraceptive use. Similarly, because abused women cannot necessarily practice "safe" sex, they are also at increased risk for sexually transmitted infections (STDs) during pregnancy.

4. Several studies have concluded that **violence during the postpartum period is even more common** than during pregnancy. In one study, 90% of women who were battered during pregnancy were abused by their partners within 3 months of delivery.

C **Obstetric complications associated with violence.**   Pregnant women in abusive relationships may have limited access to medical care, medications, or even food, which may have medical consequences. Several studies have found that abused pregnant women entered prenatal care significantly later than nonabused pregnant women; restricted access to medical care may explain this result.

1. An increased incidence of premature delivery, low birth weight, abdominal and vulvar trauma, cesarean section, and pyelonephritis may occur in women who suffer violence during pregnancy.

2. Abdominal trauma may cause injury to the mother but may also result in serious harm to the fetus, including fetal fractures, dermal scars, and even death.

III   SEXUAL ASSAULT

A **Introduction**

1. Sexual assault is a form of sexual activity that occurs without the consent of the victim and includes the use of force, implied force, or deception on the part of the assailant.

2. Sexual assault is an act that usually occurs in private.

3. Physicians play a crucial role in the 48 hours after an assault occurs; they must collect and document evidence properly for use by the police and the courts. Because only a small percentage of women receive emergency medical care or file a police report immediately after an assault, physicians must screen patients for a history of sexual assault to manage symptoms appropriately and to help patients receive aid for potentially devastating emotional sequelae.

4. **Rape** may be **broadly defined** as a form of sexual assault in which a bodily orifice is penetrated without consent by a genital organ or object wielded by another person. However, rape may be defined in different ways in various states and countries. For example, some jurisdictions include male rape whereas others (including the FBI) do not.

B Epidemiology. Sexual assault is the fastest growing crime in the United States. Of the approximately 1 million sexual assaults that occur each year, two thirds of incidents are not reported to the police, and two thirds of these acts are committed by a perpetrator known to the victim. Approximately 25% of females have been victims of sexual assault prior to 18 years of age.

C Medical evaluation. The physical examination has two purposes: **to evaluate injuries and to collect evidence.**

1. Photographs of external gynecologic injuries should be taken using a 35-mm camera, if possible. Smaller, less obvious contusions, abrasions, and tears are better captured through colposcopic imaging.

2. Only trained health care professionals should undertake evidence collection after sexual assault. Improperly collected and poorly handled evidence may negatively affect a victim's criminal case.
   a. If evidence is collected at the clinic site, it is of utmost importance that a chain of custody be established. All evidence must be collected securely, labeled, and sealed, and the physician responsible must know the location of the collected evidence or "rape kit" at all times.
   b. If an appropriately trained clinician is unavailable, or in the absence of an emergency department protocol, referrals to an established sexual assault center, which are designated in most large cities, should be made.

D Documentation. Medical documentation is an important forensic component in the management of a victim of a violent crime. Because medical documents are considered legal documents, the degree to which the physician accurately describes the care rendered may greatly affect a victim's legal case. The likelihood of rape charges and a resulting conviction are directly related to documentation of injuries.

E STD evaluation and prophylaxis. The estimated incidence of STDs resulting from rape is 3.6 to 30%.

1. Specimens from appropriate sites should be obtained to check for **gonorrhea** (*Neisseria gonorrhoeae*) and **chlamydia** (*Chlamydia trachomatis*).

2. Visible vesicles or ulcers may be cultured for **herpes.**

3. A wet mount of vaginal secretions can be examined for **trichomonas** (as well as for sperm). The absence of sperm does not mean that rape has not occurred. The act of rape is one of forced sexual contact, not necessarily ejaculation.

4. The patient needs to be advised that seroconversion for **syphilis** and **hepatitis B** takes 6 weeks. All patients who have not received the hepatitis B vaccine should be offered vaccination. **HIV** testing may also be performed at 6 weeks but should be repeated at 3 and 6 months.

F Pregnancy evaluation and prophylaxis

1. All female rape victims should undergo baseline pregnancy testing and be offered emergency contraception (often referred to as "the morning-after pill"). Emergency contraception reduces the risk of pregnancy when used within 72 hours after intercourse. Progesterone-only emergency contraception, which has recently become available, is more efficacious and has fewer side effects than estrogen–progesterone preparations.

2. The only absolute contraindication to emergency contraception is current pregnancy. Physicians may safely offer emergency contraception to women who would not ordinarily be considered good candidates for oral contraception because of concurrent medical problems. Most of the approximately 22,000 pregnancies per year in the United States that result from rape could be prevented if all women who had been raped received emergency contraception within 72 hours of the assault.

G Follow-up

1. In addition to collaborating with the local police, physicians should also offer to refer victims of rape to local victim advocacy agencies, including domestic violence and rape advocacy resources. When available and appropriate, victims' advocates should be present during the initial assault history and during the evidence collection procedure. The additional support offered by these specially trained advocates assists victims during the initial aftermath of the assault and during the longer recovery period.

2. **Psychological sequelae of rape** may be evident as long as 15 years after the assault. These sequelae include some or all of the features of **posttraumatic stress disorder**, which is chiefly characterized by four symptoms:
   a. Involuntary reexperiencing of the traumatic event through thoughts, nightmares, or flashbacks
   b. Avoidance of activities, including those that were previously pleasurable
   c. Avoidance of circumstances in which the rape occurred
   d. A state of increased psychomotor arousal, which may be associated with sleep disturbances and panic attacks

IV   ACQUAINTANCE RAPE AND DATING VIOLENCE

A Introduction. Adolescents and young adults are more likely to be victims of sexual assault than women in all other age groups. The prevalence of date rape ranges from 13 to 27% among college women and 20 to 68% among the general adolescent population. In one study, 41% of the women who had been raped stated that they were virgins at the time of the assault.

B Epidemiology. Rape statistics are difficult to obtain because of overall underreporting of sexual assault; it is not surprising that data about the incidence of acquaintance rape is limited.

1. **Association with drugs and alcohol**
   a. As many as 73% of assailants and 55% of victims have used alcohol or drugs immediately before the episode of sexual assault. Alcohol is a disinhibitor, but in itself, it does not cause violence.
   b. Drugs besides alcohol are rapidly gaining prominence in sexual assaults. These include flunitrazepam (Rohypnol), a fast-acting benzodiazepine; ketamine; and gamma-hydroxybutyrate and its congeners.
      (1) These drugs are added to the intended victim's drink without her knowledge or consent. In addition to causing disinhibition, one of the effects of such drugs is anterograde amnesia, which makes it difficult to obtain a history of the event.
      (2) Use of these drugs, which may cause symptoms similar to those of alcohol, should be suspected. Certain protocols exist in many emergency departments for urine or blood sample collection to test for the presence of such drugs. In the absence of protocols, the drug manufacturers can be contacted.

2. **Social and cultural factors.** Many cultural stereotypes and values support the notion that date rape simply does not exist or that, if it does, it is justifiable under a variety of circumstances.
   a. The perpetrator (and for that matter the victim) may have grown up in a family, peer group, or culture in which sexual aggression is part of the definition of manhood. Most perpetrators do not consider forceful or coercive sex in the context of a date to be rape.
   b. Many men, as well as women, believe that women are "supposed" to refuse sex and that men are "supposed" to pressure, coerce, or even force them.

C Medical evaluation

1. As with other types of rape, the approach to acquaintance rape should include identification and treatment of injuries; prevention of STDs and pregnancy; psychological assessment with appro-

priate referral for counseling; and, if the patient consents, collection of forensic evidence if the assault has occurred with 72 hours.

2. It is important for the physician to ascertain the victim's level of safety. As in other types of assault in which the victim knows the perpetrator, there may be a high risk of retaliation against the victim for seeking medical care. It is mandatory to review a safety plan with the victim prior to discharge.

D **Physician response.**   The importance of psychological support cannot be overemphasized. The victim is likely to feel traumatized and even ashamed.

1. A compassionate, nonjudgmental response is crucial in helping the victim of rape begin the process of psychological healing.

2. It is crucial to help the patient understand that while she needs to know how to ensure her personal safety as much as possible, she is in no way to blame for a sexual assault. That responsibility rests solely with the perpetrator.

3. It is important to stress to a patient that she can minimize the risk of being the victim of acquaintance rape by not drinking excessive alcohol or by not going to a secluded place with a date. That is by no means the same as saying that if she does not practice these risk-reduction behaviors, she is to blame for a rape. The responsibility for a crime always rests with the perpetrator.

E **Prevention.**   The possibility of dating violence, particularly in the context of drugs and alcohol, should be included in routine visits with adolescent patients. This discussion should also include information about STDs, emergency contraception, and long-term contraception. According to the Council on Child and Adolescent Health, such preventive counseling is particularly important at the precollege visit.

Study Questions for Chapter 33

DIRECTIONS: *Each of the numbered items or incomplete statements in this section is followed by answers or by completions of the statement. Select the ONE lettered answer or completion that is BEST in each case.*

1. A married, 26-year-old gravida 4, para 3 at 30 weeks of gestation presents to you for routine prenatal care. Her medical history is remarkable for active hepatitis B and moderate asthma. She had an appendectomy 4 years ago. She has no known drug allergies. All of her prenatal labs are in order. Upon measuring her fundus, you notice several bruises in the shape of a long cylindrical object on her shins and thighs. What is the best opening question to address relationship violence?

    A "When did your husband beat you?"
    B "Did your husband use a broom stick to beat you?"
    C "Are you afraid of your husband?"
    D "Is your husband physically abusing you with different objects around the house?"
    E "Is your relationship with your husband one which makes you want to hide from him?"

2. A 27-year-old gravida 3, para 2, SAB 1 has been beaten many times by her husband. She wants help, but she has not told anyone about what has been happening. The most likely reason that she has not told the physician is

    A She does not want to talk about the issue
    B She is afraid of breaking up her family
    C She knows that physicians are required to report domestic violence
    D She is afraid of retaliation by the partner, especially on the children
    E She has deep-rooted masochistic tendencies

3. A woman discloses to her physician that her husband beats her when he is drunk and that she is afraid of him. The physician's main role is to

    A Help the patient understand why she must leave the relationship immediately
    B Accept that this is a personal issue and not interfere
    C Report the abuse to the National Center for Injury Prevention and Control (NCIPC)
    D Involve a social worker
    E Focus on patient safety issues, such as exit plans and copies of important documents

4. Intimate partner violence significantly increases in incidence

    A After the first year of marriage
    B Shortly after the birth of an infant
    C After one partner retires
    D After a couples' children have left the home
    E In a household where one partner is a homemaker and the other the provider

Answers and Explanations

1. The answer is C [I C 2 c]. The best opening question is the one that is the most general but at the same time addresses the question of domestic violence. Answer choices A, B, and D are too specific and assume too much. Answer choice E is not bad but is not as broad and appropriate as C. All of the following would be good opening questions: (1) Are you afraid of a current or ex-partner? (2) Are you in a relationship in which you have been forced to have sex? (3) Are you in a relationship in which you have been hit or physically abused?

2. The answer is D [I C 2]. Women fear retaliation by the abusive partner if the partner finds out that she has disclosed the abuse. Abused women are more likely to disclose the abuse to their physicians than to anyone else—but only when asked. The most common reasons women give for staying in abusive relationships are fear of increased violence to themselves and their children if they leave and a lack of safe, affordable housing. A masochistic desire for pain and punishment is unusual. Only two states have mandated reporting laws related to the abuse of competent adults.

3. The answer is E [I D]. Urging a patient to leave a violent relationship immediately, before she has a well-developed safety plan, is fraught with danger for both herself and her children. Physicians should consider domestic violence and its consequences a medical issue of great importance. Details of the abuse should be documented, but the abuse should not be noted in the billing diagnosis if the abusive partner receives billing or insurance-related information. Passing off the patient, to NCIPC or a social worker, is not the primary role of the physician. Consultation with a social worker can be done after establishing a solid patient-physician relationship and after safety issues have been discussed.

4. The answer is B [II B 4]. The incidence of intimate partner violence is particularly high in the postpartum period. Other life events, such as marriage and retirement, are not associated with an increase in domestic violence. There is an increased incidence of violence when there is a short interpregnancy interval, not when children leave the home. In a homemaker-provider household there may be increased violence depending on the sex of the homemaker and provider, but this is not as significant as the increase in domestic violence in the postpartum period.

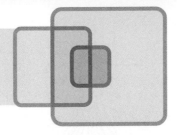

chapter 34

Disorders of the Pelvic Floor

CATHERINE S. BRADLEY

I INTRODUCTION

A Epidemiology

1. Urinary incontinence affects women five times more often than men.

2. From 10 to 25% of women 25 to 64 years of age and as many as 40% of women older than 65 years of age suffer from some form of urinary incontinence.

3. As many as 50% of all parous women have pelvic support defects, and 10 to 20% seek care for pelvic organ prolapse (POP).

4. In the United States, women have a lifetime risk of urinary incontinence or POP that requires surgical treatment of approximately 10%.

5. The true prevalence of fecal incontinence is unknown, but the disorder is estimated to affect as many as 10% of women older than 64 years of age.

6. Thirty percent of women with urinary incontinence also have fecal incontinence.

B Anatomy of the pelvic floor (Fig. 34-1)

1. The pelvic floor is made up of the **levator ani** and coccygeus muscles. The levator ani has several parts, including the puborectalis and pubococcygeus (also referred to as the pubovisceral muscle) and iliococcygeus muscles.
   a. These muscles, which create a hammock-like sling between the pubis and coccyx, are attached laterally along the pelvic sidewalls.
   b. The levator ani muscle is tonically contracted, providing a firm shelf posteriorly to support the pelvic contents and aiding with urinary and fecal continence.

2. **Endopelvic fascia** is a loose network of connective tissue, small vessels, lymphatics, and nerves, which surrounds and supports the pelvic organs and the vagina.

C Innervation of the pelvic floor and its functions

1. The levator ani is innervated by sacral nerve roots (S2–S4). This muscle group is tonically stimulated to contract, providing constant support to the pelvic organs.

2. Bladder filling and voiding functions are controlled by closely coordinated autonomic and somatic pathways.
   a. **Autonomic nervous system**
      (1) **Sympathetic** (thoracolumbar) nerves promote urine storage by **relaxing the bladder (detrusor) muscle** and contracting smooth muscle in the bladder neck and urethra. These nerves are inhibited during voiding.
      (2) **Parasympathetic** (sacral) nerves cause the detrusor muscle to contract. They are stimulated during micturition.
   b. The **somatic nervous system** controls the striated external urethral sphincter and levator ani muscle through the pudendal nerve and the sacral nerve roots (S2–S4). Inhibition of these nerves causes relaxation of the bladder outlet and pelvic floor, which must occur during voiding.

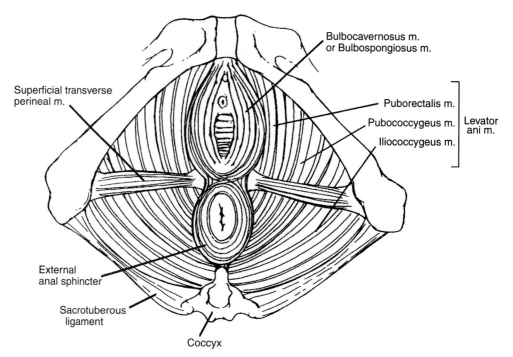

FIGURE 34-1 Levator ani muscles from below. The levator ani has several parts, including the pubovisceral and iliococcygeus muscles. m., muscle.

    c. The **central nervous system (CNS)** provides voluntary control and modification of micturition and defecation reflexes.

II   PELVIC ORGAN PROLAPSE (POP) (also called pelvic relaxation)

Such prolapse or protrusion of pelvic structures into the vaginal canal results from weakening or damage to pelvic support structures.

A   Risk factors

    1. Vaginal childbirth may damage or weaken pelvic support structures.

    2. Obesity, chronic cough, and chronic constipation may cause increased intra-abdominal pressures, increasing the risk of POP.

    3. Increasing age is associated with an increased risk of POP.

    4. A genetic predisposition for POP may exist in some women.

B   Terminology

    1. Cystocele is protrusion of the bladder behind the anterior vaginal wall.

    2. Uterine prolapse is descent of the uterus into the lower part of the vagina or through the vaginal opening.

    3. Vaginal vault prolapse is descent of the vaginal apex after hysterectomy.

    4. Enterocele is protrusion of small bowel behind the upper vaginal wall into the vaginal canal.

    5. Rectocele is protrusion of the rectum behind the posterior vaginal wall.

C   Symptoms.   Mild forms of POP are often asymptomatic. Advanced forms of POP may cause difficulty with urination or defecation. Associated symptoms may include:

    1. Bulge of tissue protruding through the vaginal opening

TABLE 34-1   The Halfway Grading System for Pelvic Organ Prolapse. Descent of the Most Dependent Portion of the Prolapse is Graded during Maximal Straining

Grade	Level of Prolapse
1	No prolapse
2	Descent halfway to the hymen
3	Descent to the hymen
4	Descent halfway past the hymen
5	Maximum possible descent for each site

2. Pelvic or vaginal **pressure**, especially after prolonged standing

3. Dyspareunia

D Evaluation

1. Prolapse is diagnosed on **pelvic examination**, performed in the lithotomy and standing positions.

2. The severity of prolapse may be classified according to systems that describe the location and severity of POP.
   a. Halfway system (Table 34-1)
   b. Pelvic Organ Prolapse Quantification (POP-Q)

E Treatment.   Asymptomatic POP does not require treatment.

1. **Pelvic floor muscle (Kegel) exercises** may improve symptoms caused by mild forms of prolapse.

2. **Pessaries** are devices placed in the vagina that support prolapse.

3. **Surgery** for POP aims to relieve symptoms and to restore normal anatomic relationships. The surgical procedure and approach (abdominal or vaginal) is tailored to the particular type of POP present.
   a. **Hysterectomy** for uterine prolapse
   b. **Anterior repair, paravaginal repair** for cystocele
   c. **Posterior repair** for rectocele
   d. **Enterocele repair**
   e. **Vaginal vault suspension**

III URINARY INCONTINENCE

A Types

1. **Stress urinary incontinence (SUI)** is the loss of urine that occurs with increased abdominal pressure, such as coughing or straining. SUI is the result of an **anatomic defect of the urethrovesical junction** or **urethra**. It most commonly occurs following pelvic floor muscle and nerve damage that resulted from childbearing.
   a. **Urethral hypermobility** is the most common form and is usually surgically correctable with the anatomic restoration of the urethrovesical junction.
   b. **Intrinsic urethral sphincteric deficiency** is less common and is caused by a weakened urethral sphincter.

2. **Urge incontinence** is defined by the symptom of urine loss that occurs when the patient experiences urgency, or a strong desire to void. This type of incontinence is often accompanied by

symptoms of urinary frequency, urgency, and nocturia. Urge incontinence includes the following subtypes:

    a. Detrusor overactivity (DO) (previously called detrusor instability), or overactive bladder, is caused by involuntary detrusor contractions. Its cause is usually unknown.

    b. Neurogenic DO is involuntary detrusor contractions associated with a neurologic disorder (e.g., stroke, spinal cord injury, or multiple sclerosis). It is a common cause of incontinence in elderly and institutionalized women.

3. Overflow incontinence occurs because of underactivity of the detrusor muscle. The bladder does not empty completely, and urine leakage occurs with stress or continuously.

4. Extraurethral sources of urine include genitourinary fistulas, which may be congenital or follow pelvic surgery or radiation. These typically cause continuous leaking of urine.

B **Evaluation**

1. A **detailed history** is essential and should include:

    a. Urinary symptoms, including the presence of voiding frequency, nocturia, urgency, precipitating events, and frequency of loss. A voiding diary allows the patient to document voiding frequency and incontinence episodes during a specific period.

    b. Previous urologic surgery

    c. Obstetric history, including parity, birth weights, mode of delivery

    d. CNS or spinal cord disorders

    e. Use of medications, including diuretics, antihypertensives, caffeine, alcohol, anticholinergics, decongestants, nicotine, and psychotropics

    f. Presence of other medical disorders (e.g., hypertension or hematuria)

2. Physical examination may detect:

    a. Exacerbating conditions, such as chronic obstructive pulmonary disease, obesity, or intra-abdominal mass

    b. Hypermobility of the urethra

    c. POP

    d. Neurologic disorders

3. Diagnostic tests

    a. A midstream urine specimen is collected for **urinalysis** or **culture and sensitivity**. Infection may aggravate urinary incontinence.

    b. Postvoid residual urine volume should be measured (by ultrasound or catheterization) after the patient has voided. Typically, the postvoid residual urine volume is less than 50 to 100 mL.

    c. The **Q-tip test** is an indirect measure of the urethral axis. A Q-tip is inserted into the urethra with the patient in the lithotomy position. If the Q-tip moves more than 30° from the horizontal with straining, **urethral hypermobility** is present.

    d. Urodynamic testing, including a cystometrogram and voiding studies, may be useful for demonstrating the type of incontinence present. These tests measure pressures within the bladder and abdomen during bladder filling and emptying.

3. Cystoscopy is performed in some patients to examine the bladder and urethral mucosa for abnormalities such as diverticula or neoplasms.

C **Treatment.** Therapy depends on the underlying diagnosis.

1. Treatment of exacerbating factors such as excess weight, chronic cough, or constipation may improve SUI.

2. Pelvic muscle rehabilitation may be helpful for both SUI and DO.

    a. Kegel exercises

    b. Vaginal cones

    c. Biofeedback

    d. Electrical stimulation

3. **Pessaries,** other intravaginal devices, and urethral plugs and inserts are useful conservative therapies for SUI.

4. **Drug therapy** is the mainstay of treatment for DO but is of limited value in treating SUI.
   a. **Antispasmodic agents** (oxybutynin and tolterodine) are highly effective and are the most commonly prescribed treatments for DO. However, they cause side effects, such as dry mouth and constipation, in about 25% of patients.
   b. **α-Adrenergic stimulating agents** (e.g., pseudoephedrine, imipramine) increase smooth muscle contraction in the urethral sphincter and may decrease SUI symptoms.
   c. **Estrogens** (systemic or vaginal) improve irritative bladder symptoms such as urgency and dysuria in postmenopausal women but do not significantly improve urinary leakage.

5. **Surgery** is extremely effective in the treatment of SUI. It is rarely helpful for DO and is generally reserved only for intractable cases.
   a. **Injection of bulking agents** around the urethra is a minimally invasive procedure to treat SUI resulting from intrinsic urethral sphincteric deficiency. Collagen, the bulking agent currently used most commonly, provides a temporary (3 to 12 months) cure or improvement rates as high as 70%.
   b. **Retropubic urethropexy** elevates the urethra and bladder neck by fixing the paraurethral connective tissues to the pubis. The most common type of retropubic operation performed is the **Burch** procedure, which suspends the vaginal fascia lateral to the urethra to the iliopectineal line (Cooper ligament). Burch procedures are most successful in patients who have SUI associated with urethral hypermobility, resulting in long-term cure rates of 75 to 90%. Postoperative complications are uncommon but may include urinary retention and new DO.
   c. **Transvaginal needle procedures** stabilize the bladder neck by anchoring vaginal tissue to the rectus fascia or symphysis pubis. These procedures have lower long-term cure rates than retropubic operations and suburethral slings.
   d. **Suburethral sling procedures,** which place various biologic and synthetic materials under the urethra, appear to effect treatment by partially obstructing the urethra during times of increased intra-abdominal pressure. Sling procedures differ according to the type of material and the sling fixation points used; however, they all have high cure rates (80 to 90%). Sling procedures are more effective than retropubic operations in patients with **intrinsic urethral sphincteric deficiency.** Complications of sling procedures may include infection and ulceration (especially with the use of synthetic grafts) and **urinary retention.**

IV   FECAL INCONTINENCE

The involuntary loss of stool or gas is a socially embarrassing disorder. Symptoms of fecal incontinence are often not reported to physicians.

A Pathophysiology

1. Fecal continence depends on stool consistency and volume, colonic transit time, rectal compliance, and innervation and function of the anal sphincter and pelvic floor.

2. Gastrointestinal and neurologic disorders may result in fecal incontinence.

3. Obstetric injuries to the pelvic floor, as well as denervation injuries related to childbirth or chronic straining, are the most common cause of fecal incontinence in women.

B **Symptoms**

1. Fecal urgency

2. Incontinence of flatus

3. Incontinence of stool

C **Evaluation.**   A detailed history and examination, including a vaginal and rectal examination, are essential. Useful tests for determining the etiology of fecal incontinence may include anal ultrasound, anal manometry, and pelvic floor nerve conductance studies.

D **Treatment.**   Therapy may include behavioral modification, pharmacologic agents, biofeedback, and surgery.

Study Questions for Chapter 34

DIRECTIONS: Each of the numbered items or incomplete statements in this section is followed by answers or by completions of the statement. Select the ONE lettered answer or completion that is BEST in each case.

1. A 60-year-old gravida 5, para 4, SAB 1 has been treated with vaginal estrogen therapy, various pelvic muscle rehabilitation therapies, and pessaries for symptoms of pelvic prolapse without incontinence for the two years. She desires definitive therapy. She has no past medical history other than hypertension for which she takes hydrochlorothiazide. All of her children were delivered vaginally. On pelvic examination, vaginal mucosa is pink and moist. The anterior vaginal wall prolapses up to the hymenal ring on Valsalva. When the anterior vagina is supported with half of the speculum, the uterus and cervix prolapse past the hymenal ring as well. There is no stress incontinence when the urethrovesical junction is supported and the cystocele reduced. The uterus is normal in size, contour, and consistency. The sacral neurologic examination is unremarkable. A urine culture is sent. The next best step in management of this patient is

- A Electrical stimulation of pelvic musculature
- B Abdominal hysterectomy and anterior repair
- C Vaginal hysterectomy and anterior repair
- D Vaginal hysterectomy, anterior repair, and suburethral sling
- E Burch retropubic urethropexy and anterior repair

2. A 32-year-old gravida 3, para 3 just delivered a viable female infant weighing 4000 g via cesarean section for nonreassuring fetal heart rate pattern. She received intrathecal (spinal) anesthetic and narcotic for pain relief during the procedure. Her Foley catheter is left in place for several hours after the cesarean section. This will prevent

- A Stress incontinence
- B Urge incontinence
- C Overflow incontinence
- D Bypass incontinence
- E Postoperative urinary tract infection

3. A 56-year-old gravida 2, para 2, who reports leaking urine when she coughs and exercises, is diagnosed with genuine stress urinary incontinence. A regimen of Kegel exercises does not improve her symptoms, and she desires more definitive treatment. Her doctor recommends laparoscopic retropubic urethropexy. When discussing the risks and benefits of the laparoscopic Burch procedure, the doctor should mention

- A Low short-term cure rates
- B 60% long-term cure rates
- C Risk of urinary retention
- D Alternative of drug therapy
- E Risk of graft infection and ulceration

4. A 67-year-old gravida 3, para 3 presents to your office reporting incontinence. She tells you that she voids almost 40 times during the day and has several episodes of nocturia. She says she feels like voiding 2 to 3 times an hour and that when she makes it to the bathroom, only small amounts of urine are voided. Her past medical history is remarkable for mild asthma for which she takes albuterol. Her previous gynecologist also placed her on estrogen patch, estrogen vaginal cream, and intravaginal progesterone tablets. She had a cholecystectomy 20 years ago and she is allergic to penicillin. Her BP = 130/80 mmHg, P = 80 bpm, height = 5 foot 4 inches, weight = 230 lbs. On physical examination you notice pink, moist vaginal epithelium with mild cystocele and well-supported proximal urethra. The next best step in management of this patient is

- [A] Urinalysis
- [B] Tolterodine
- [C] Pseudoephedrine
- [D] Pessary
- [E] Suburethral sling

5. A 55-year-old Caucasian woman, gravida 3, para 3 who delivered all of her children by scheduled cesarean sections (prior to initiation of labor) has mild pelvic organ prolapse. She had her last period 3 years ago and since that time has been on estrogen patches and progesterone vaginal tablets for treatment of hot flushes and vaginal dryness. She has no chronic medical problems but is on antibiotic therapy for acute bronchitis. Her family history is significant for osteoporosis diagnosed at an earlier age than average in her mother, two sisters, and grandmother. The strongest risk factor for pelvic relaxation in this patient is

- [A] Parity
- [B] Age
- [C] Hormone status
- [D] Genetic
- [E] Cough

Answers and Explanations

1. The answer is C [II E 3]. The patient has uterine prolapse and cystocele, and conservative treatment (pelvic muscle rehab, pessary, and estrogen) has failed. Therefore, the next best treatment is surgical. Cystocele can be cured with anterior repair. Uterine prolapse can be cured with a hysterectomy. Because the anterior repair is performed vaginally, it makes sense to do the hysterectomy vaginally as well (if there are no contraindications) so as to have only once incision site and faster recovery. A suburethral sling is unnecessary for this patient because, in the clinical scenario, "there is no stress incontinence when the urethrovesical junction is supported and the cystocele reduced." Electrical stimulation is a form of pelvic muscle rehabilitation that has been tried and failed.

2. The answer is C [III A 3]. Intrathecal anesthetic and narcotics blocks nerve impulses to and from the bladder. When the bladder becomes distended with urine, the afferent impulses cannot be transmitted, and therefore the bladder detrusor muscle is underactive. This results in overdistension of the bladder and overflow incontinence. The risk of urinary tract infection is increased with placement of a Foley catheter.

3. The answer is C [III C 4,5]. The laparoscopic Burch has similar cure rates as the nonlaparoscopic Burch. The short- and long-term cure rates are very high (about 90%). The main complication of a retropubic urethropexy is the small risk of urinary retention, which depends on how tight paraurethral tissue is approximated to Cooper's ligament. This can be measured subjectively by the size of dimple produced on the upper lateral fornices of the vagina. Only urge incontinence is effectively treated with drug therapy. Graft infection and ulceration is a risk of suburethral sling procedures.

4. The answer is A [III B 3a]. Although the clinical scenario is almost definitely urge incontinence, you must rule out urinary tract infection (UTI) because it may mimic symptoms of urgency. Once UTI is ruled out, you may begin therapy with tolterodine or oxybutynin. Pessary and suburethral slings are not as useful for detrusor overactivity as they are for stress incontinence.

5. The answer is D [II A]. The cause of pelvic organ prolapse (POP) is multifactorial. Genetics determine the subtype and density of collagen and connective tissue that a person inherits. Parity is not a risk factor in this patient because she has not had any vaginal deliveries and all of her cesarean sections were performed prior to initiation of labor. Nonchronic coughing (as in acute bronchitis) is not a risk factor for POP. This patient is only 55 years old; therefore, her age is not as large a determinant of her pelvic relaxation as in a woman who is 85 years old. This patient has been on hormone replacement since menopause; therefore, the tissues derived from the urogenital sinus have been stimulated adequately and continuously with estrogen.

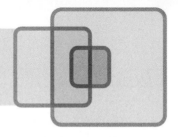

chapter 35

The Infertile Couple

MOLINA B. DAYAL AND STEVEN SONDHEIMER

I INTRODUCTION

A **Definition.** Infertility is defined as 1 year of unprotected intercourse without conception. This definition is not strict; many couples may seek medical attention before 1 year has passed.

1. **Fecundability**, or the monthly probability of pregnancy, is about 20% among fertile couples. The cumulative probability of pregnancy after 1 year approaches 85%.

2. **Primary infertility** refers to couples who have never established a pregnancy.

3. **Secondary infertility** refers to couples who have conceived previously (including miscarriages) but are currently unable to establish a subsequent pregnancy.

B **Incidence.** Approximately 15% of couples are infertile, using the criteria of at least 1 year of unprotected coitus.

C **Factors involved in fertility**

1. Spermatogenesis (male factor)

2. Ovulation (ovulatory factor)

3. Endometrial cavity size and shape (uterine factor)

4. Oviductal patency (tubal or pelvic factor)

5. Implantation (embryo quality, endometrial receptivity, and unexplained factors)

D **Causes of infertility**

1. Ovulatory dysfunction: 15%

2. Pelvic factors (endometriosis, tubal occlusion, adhesions): 35%

3. Male factor: 35%

4. Unexplained: 10%

5. Other (cervical factor): 5%

6. Multiple causes: 20 to 40%

II AGING AND FERTILITY

A **Female age** alone affects the ability to conceive and to carry a pregnancy. Spontaneous loss rates are higher in older women. Infertility increases with increasing age of the female partner. Age-related fertility rates for women in three age groups are as follows:

1. 25 to 29 years: 9%

2. 30 to 34 years: 15%

3. 35 to 39 years: 22%

B **Ovarian reserve** can be evaluated using either a follicle-stimulating hormone (FSH) level on menstrual cycle day 3 or a clomiphene challenge test.

1. An **elevated FSH** level at any time is correlated with fewer available oocytes and decreased oocyte quality. An FSH level greater than or equal to 25 IU/l (or 44 years of age or older) on menstrual cycle day 3 is associated with a chance of pregnancy close to zero with infertility treatment. Lower cutoff values have been reported (as low as less than 10 mIU/mL) because of different FSH assay reference ranges. A single elevated day 3 FSH value suggests a poor prognosis even when values in subsequent cycles are normal.

2. The **clomiphene citrate challenge test** is a **bioassay to FSH response** that reflects ovarian follicular capability. An FSH level on menstrual cycle day 10 is compared with a baseline FSH level on menstrual cycle day 3. An FSH response greater than or equal to the threshold level for the laboratory is associated with a significant prospect of failure to achieve a pregnancy, regardless of age.

3. For patients with extremely elevated day 3 FSH levels or clomiphene citrate challenge results, adoption or in vitro fertilization with donor oocytes should be recommended.

C **Paternal age** greater than 40 years is associated with a 20% greater chance of birth defects in the offspring. The capacity to fertilize is maintained.

III OVERALL TREATMENT GOALS

A Seek out and correct causes of infertility.

B Provide accurate information and dispel misinformation.

C Provide emotional support.

D Provide options for treatment and alternatives when treatment is not successful.

IV OVULATORY DYSFUNCTION

Inability of the ovaries to release ova on a cyclic basis accounts for approximately 40% of female infertility.

A **Etiology.**   **Anovulation** (lack of ovulation) or **oligo-ovulation** (occasional ovulation) may result from:

1. Androgen excess (polycystic ovary syndrome)
2. Hypothalamic causes (malnutrition, extreme weight loss, or excessive exercise)
3. Elevated prolactin levels (from medications or pituitary tumors)
4. Decreased ovarian reserve
5. Thyroid dysfunction

B **Diagnosis.**   Evaluation involves determining if ovulation occurs cyclically.

1. With **basal body temperature monitoring** (degrees Fahrenheit), the patient takes her temperature before getting out of bed in the morning.
   a. A **biphasic pattern** is seen with ovulation secondary to the thermogenic effects of progesterone secretion.
   b. Basal temperatures become elevated by 0.5 to 1.0° immediately after ovulation.
   c. At the end of a month-long cycle, the temperature in the first 10 to 14 days should be lower than in the last 10 to 14 days.

d. If this pattern is present, it can be assumed that the patient is ovulating because of increased progesterone levels.

2. A **serum progesterone level** greater than 10 nmol/L at midpoint of the luteal phase (approximately day 21 of the cycle) suggests ovulation.

3. An **endometrial biopsy** demonstrating a secretory pattern during the late luteal phase of the cycle (approximately cycle day 24) also suggests ovulation. Basal body temperature charts and luteal phase progesterone levels may be used in place of the endometrial biopsy during a general infertility evaluation.

4. **Urinary luteinizing hormone (LH) predictor kits** may also be used to detect a rise in LH immediately prior to ovulation. Patients begin testing their urine on cycle day 10 and continue testing until they detect a change in color on the indicator stick. It can be assumed that ovulation will occur within the following 24 to 36 hours.

5. Thyroid-stimulating hormone (TSH), prolactin, total testosterone, and FSH should be assessed if no evidence of ovulation is detected.

C Treatment

1. **Correction of underlying endocrine disorders**, such as thyroid disease and hyperprolactinemia, lead to spontaneous ovulation in many patients.

2. **Induction of ovulation**
   a. Clomiphene citrate is the **most commonly prescribed fertility drug;** it is most successful in women with normal estrogen levels. It is well suited for practitioners and patients because of its oral administration, ease of use, and minimal monitoring.
   (1) The usual starting dose in anovulatory women is 50 mg daily for 5 days early in the follicular phase (usually cycle days 5 to 9). Intercourse can be timed by using a urinary LH predictor kit or by triggering egg release with an injection of human chorionic gonadotrophin (hCG) when a follicle greater than 18 mm in diameter is noted on pelvic ultrasound.
   (2) If no measurable response to 50 mg of clomiphene occurs, the dose can be increased by 50 mg in subsequent cycles to a maximum of 150 mg.
   b. Injectable gonadotropins are administered by subcutaneous injection. Monitoring is more complex in that serial estradiol and pelvic ultrasounds are performed to assess patient response. Ovulation is triggered by administration of hCG after both estradiol levels and follicular size suggest follicular maturity.

V PELVIC FACTOR

This type of infertility involves a wide range of conditions and accounts for approximately **40% of female infertility.**

A Tubal factor.
The fallopian tube is responsible for efficient transfer of gametes and transport of the dividing embryo to the uterine cavity. It provides an environment in which capacitation of spermatozoa, fertilization, and early development of the embryo take place. Tubal disease or blockage can impair the ability to conceive.

1. **Diagnosis.** Evaluation involves determining if tubal occlusion exists.
   a. Hysterosalpingography is a radiologic study that provides visualization of the **internal lumen and patency** of the fallopian tube using a radiopaque contrast dye. This method neither allows for visualization of the external surface of the tubes nor provides external assessment of pelvic adhesions or anatomic relationships within the pelvis. A hysterosalpingogram is usually obtained before performing a laparoscopy because it is less costly and less invasive.
   b. Laparoscopy allows direct visualization of the external surface of the fallopian tube to identify abnormalities in structure or location and to detect peritubal or pelvic adhesions.

Laparoscopy does not provide any information on tubal patency unless a dye (usually indigo carmine) is injected through the cervix and is allowed to spill into the pelvic cavity under direct visualization.

2. **Treatment. In vitro fertilization (IVF)** is most successful, but treatment may also be achieved surgically.
    a. Tubal anastomosis for reversal of sterilization
    b. Salpingoplasty for occluded distal or proximal fallopian tubes
    c. Lysis of peritubal adhesions
    d. IVF and embryo transfer (ET) when fallopian tubes are absent or damaged

B **Endometriosis** (see Chapter 30) is a common gynecologic disorder estimated to affect 71% of women with pelvic pain alone and nearly 85% of women with both infertility and pelvic pain. Despite the association of endometriosis and infertility, there is **inconclusive evidence that endometriosis is a direct cause of infertility**, unless there is anatomic distortion of the pelvis secondary to endometriotic lesions or adhesions.

1. **Diagnosis. Laparoscopy with histologic confirmation by biopsy** is definitive. Laparoscopy also allows direct visualization of the pelvic cavity and its contents.

2. **Treatment. Expectant management** may be effective. Only one prospective randomized study comparing surgical ablation of minimal and mild endometriosis with expectant management has demonstrated a higher pregnancy rate in the surgically treated group. No difference in pregnancy rates is noted with more severe stages of endometriosis. For this group of patients, IVF is beneficial.

C **Uterine factor.** The uterus is responsible for providing an environment suitable for sperm transport, development of the embryo prior to implantation, and carriage of the pregnancy. Uterine factors thought to play an important role in infertility include **myomas** (fibroids), **polyps, synechiae** (scar tissue from prior uterine procedures), **infection**, and congenital **anatomic anomalies**. Myomas, polyps, synechiae, and anatomic abnormalities **are associated more with pregnancy loss than infertility**.

1. **Diagnosis.** Evaluation involves hysterosalpingography, hysteroscopy, magnetic resonance imaging (MRI), sonohysterography, endometrial biopsy, and (sometimes) laparoscopy.
    a. **Hysterosalpingography** allows visualization of the internal contour of the uterine cavity by injection of a radiopaque contrast medium under fluoroscopic radiography through the cervix. Aside from detecting tubal pathology, this **technique detects synechiae, congenital anatomic anomalies,** and **fibroids** if they distort the uterine cavity.
    b. If an abnormality is detected on the hysterosalpingogram, a **hysteroscopy** can be performed for confirmation of the abnormality and further evaluation of the uterus. Hysteroscopy allows for direct internal inspection of the uterine cavity. Many abnormalities, including **synechiae, fibroids, polyps, and uterine septae can be surgically corrected** at the time of hysteroscopy.
    c. If a congenital uterine anomaly is suspected after hysterosalpingography, a **pelvic MRI** may be helpful in assessing the external and internal contours of the uterus. This technique also allows inspection of the urinary tract given a high rate of associated anomalies. **Laparoscopy** is a more invasive method of obtaining information about the external contour of the uterus.
    d. **Sonohysterography** is another technique used to assess the uterine cavity. A sonohysterogram is performed by placing a small balloon-tipped cannula into the uterus via the cervix and infusing the cavity with sterile saline. A vaginal ultrasound is performed simultaneously. Small polyps and fibroids impinging on the uterine cavity can be detected by this method. However, this method **does not allow assessment of the external surface of the uterus**.
    e. An **endometrial culture or sampling by biopsy** can help identify uterine infection.

VI MALE FACTOR INFERTILITY

Abnormalities in semen volume, sperm count, or motility can significantly affect a couple's ability to conceive. The following tests can be used to evaluate infertility secondary to male factor:

A A **semen analysis** should be the initial test obtained on all males in couples seeking treatment. The sample is generally collected after 2 to 5 days of abstinence. The World Health Organization standards are as follows:

1. Volume: more than 2.0 mL
2. Count: more than 20 million sperm/mL
3. Motility: more than 50% with forward progression
4. Morphology: more than 35% with normal, oval heads, and a single tail
5. White blood cells: less than 1 million/mL

B The **postcoital test** checks receptivity of the cervical mucus and the ability of sperm to reach and survive in the mucus. Cervical mucus is examined microscopically between 2 and 12 hours after coitus at midcycle for number of sperm per high power field and percentage and quality of motility.

1. A **satisfactory test** is one in which the mucus exhibits a ferning pattern (secondary to high estrogen levels) and can be stretched to greater than or equal to 5 cm, and where greater than 5 motile spermatozoa are seen per high power field.
2. An **unsatisfactory test** may result from azoospermia (no spermatozoa in the ejaculate), poor inherent sperm motility, improper coital technique, or a small ejaculate volume. The overall validity of the postcoital test is questionable given its lack of standardization and predictive value. The postcoital test is useful in confirming that intercourse did in fact take place.

C **Semen is extremely antigenic** and is normally isolated from the immune system by the blood–testes barrier. If this barrier is broken (via trauma or surgery), **sperm antibodies** can form. Occasionally, these sperm antibodies may be responsible for impaired fertility. To date, the clinical significance of sperm antibodies remains unclear.

D Tests of **fertilizing capacity of spermatozoa** have been devised to assess the ability of sperm to fertilize an ovum. Note that these tests are of **unclear prognostic value** and are not used often because of **lack of standardization**. A practical use for these tests might be to identify abnormalities of sperm not evident in studies of such parameters as count and morphology (i.e., semen analysis).

1. The **zona-free hamster ovum penetration test** evaluates the ability of sperm to penetrate a hamster ovum without a zona present. The patient's sperm is compared with a known, fertile sperm sample.
2. The **human zona binding assay** tests the ability of sperm to attach to the zona. The ratio of the number of patient sperm attached to the zona is compared with the number of a known, fertile control.

E Treatment

1. **Medical therapies** include **correction of underlying hormonal disorders** (e.g., thyroid disorders, prolactin excess, and dietary disturbances) and **donor insemination** for severe oligospermia (few sperm) or azoospermia (no sperm). Intrauterine insemination (IUI) may also be performed as part of routine treatment of patients undergoing ovulation induction to improve pregnancy rates.
2. **Surgical therapies** involve vasectomy reversal, varicocele repair, IVF, percutaneous epididymal sperm aspiration (only in IVF), or testicular biopsy (only in IVF).

VII CERVICAL FACTOR

The cervix is the first major barrier encountered by sperm after arrival in the female reproductive tract. Spermatozoa migrate rapidly through the endocervical canal and have been demonstrated to be in the fallopian tube as early as 5 minutes after deposition at the cervix.

A **Abnormalities in the cervix or the cervical mucus** may interfere with sperm migration. Previous cervical surgery (e.g., conization or electrocautery for cervical dysplasia) may lead to mucous depletion.

B The **postcoital test,** as previously described (see VI B), may evaluate for cervical factor infertility. Intrauterine insemination bypasses the cervix and can therefore be used as a treatment modality for cervical factor infertility.

VIII UNEXPLAINED INFERTILITY

This diagnosis refers to couples in whom no identifiable cause of infertility can be found, and it accounts for approximately 10% of infertility. Superovulation with either clomiphene citrate or injectable gonadotropins is usually attempted before considering assisted reproductive technology (IVF). The pregnancy rate per cycle for unexplained infertility couples and IUI alone is 2.7%; this increases to 6.1% if injectable gonadotropins are used and to 15% with both injectable gonadotropins and IUI.

IX ASSISTED REPRODUCTIVE TECHNOLOGY

A In **IVF and ET,** oocytes are surgically retrieved directly from maturing ovarian follicles after ovarian stimulation with injectable gonadotropins and pituitary suppression with gonadotropin-releasing hormone agonists and antagonists. Oocytes are usually retrieved **transvaginally.** These oocytes are then placed in a dish with sperm where fertilization is allowed to take place in vitro. After fertilization and embryo division (to the 8- to 10-cell or blastocyst stage), the embryo is transferred back into the uterus.

B In **intracytoplasmic sperm injection,** a micromanipulation technique, a sperm is injected directly into the cytoplasm of the oocyte to enhance fertilization. This method is often used for **male factor infertility.** Pregnancy rates are independent of any semen analysis parameter because sperm are directly injected into ova by an embryologist.

C In **gamete intrafallopian transfer (GIFT),** oocytes are retrieved from ovaries as previously mentioned (see IX A). The oocyte and spermatozoa are not placed into a dish for fertilization but are placed together within the distal fallopian tube, allowing for natural fertilization. This procedure normally requires a **laparoscopic approach.** Another procedure that involves the same principles as GIFT is **zygote intrafallopian transfer (ZIFT),** except that a zygote (present after fertilization in vitro) is replaced into the fallopian tube for further development. This also requires a **laparoscopic approach.** Both GIFT and ZIFT are seldom used and have been replaced by IVF and ET.

Study Questions for Chapter 35

DIRECTIONS: Match each clinical scenario with the most likely location for the cause of infertility. Each answer may be used once, more than once, or not at all.

QUESTIONS 1–6

- A Ovary
- B Fallopian tubes
- C Uterus
- D Cervix
- E Immune system

1. A 25-year-old woman, gravida 2, para 2 has been trying to get pregnant for the last 2 years. She has no medical problems. She had surgery for a ruptured appendix 5 years ago. Her periods are regular and last 3 to 4 days. She denies smoking, drinking alcohol, or using drugs. Her husband is 28 years old, is healthy, and has a normal sperm count.

2. A 29-year-old gravida 4, para 1, SAB 4 presents to you because she has not been able to bear children. Although she becomes pregnant, she is not able to carry the pregnancy past 14 weeks. Her bimanual examination reveals an irregularly enlarged uterus (14-week size). Her husband is 34 years old and is healthy as far as his wife knows (he is not in the office for evaluation).

3. A 32-year-old gravida 2, para 0, SAB 2 presents to you because she has lost two pregnancies in the second trimester. She says that both times she did not have any labor contractions or pain prior to passing a liveborn infant that died shortly afterward.

4. A 30-year-old gravida 1, para 1 presents to you because she and her husband have been trying to have a second child for the last 3 years. She has mild asthma for which she takes albuterol. She has a history of abnormal pap smears and three loop electro-excision procedures (LEEP). Her husband is 31 years old, is healthy, and has a normal sperm count.

5. A 27-year-old woman, gravida 2, para 2 presents to you because she has not been able to get pregnant after reversal of her husband's vasectomy. She has no medical problems.

6. A 22-year-old nulligravid woman and her husband have been trying to get pregnant for the last 18 months. She has no know medical problems and has never had any surgery. She says her periods are irregular. She gets about four to five periods per year. She is 5 feet 2 inches tall and weighs 210 lbs. On review of systems, she reports hair growth on her abdomen and chin.

DIRECTIONS: Each of the numbered items or incomplete statements in this section is followed by answers or by completions of the statement. Select the ONE lettered answer or completion that is BEST in each case.

7. Among 100 healthy, fertile couples, approximately how many will become pregnant within 1 month if they have regular intercourse?

- A 15
- B 20

C 35
D 45
E 85

8. A 26-year-old nulligravid and her 26-year-old husband are seeing you because they have not been able to get pregnant for the last 3 years. The woman has regular periods every 30 days that last 4 days. Both of them have no medical problems or past surgical history. Both deny smoking, caffeine use, herbal remedy use, alcohol abuse, or drug use. The husband's sperm analysis reveals a volume of 2.5 mL, total count 20×10^6 sperm/mL, 30% forward progression, 30% normal morphology, and 200,000 WBC/mL. The next best step in management of this couple is

A Semen wash, intrauterine insemination (IUI), and clomiphene citrate
B In vitro fertilization and embryo transfer (IVF-ET)
C Intracytoplasmic sperm injection (ICSI)
D Gamete intrafallopian transfer (GIFT)
E Egg retrieval, in vitro fertilization, and intrafallopian transfer

Answers and Explanations

1. B [V A 2 c] **2. C** [V C] **3. D** [VII A] **4. D** [VII A] **5. E** [VI C] **6. A** [IV A 1]. In question 1, the woman has had surgery for a ruptured appendicitis. When an intra-abdominal infection is present (from either a ruptured viscus or pelvic inflammatory disease), there is a risk of adhesion formation, including adhesion of the fallopian tubes to other structures. This prevents proper egg retrieval and transport by the tube, which can be confirmed by hysterosalpingography or laparoscopy. In question 2, this patient most likely has submucosal fibroids in her uterus that are contributing to her miscarriages. This can be confirmed by hysterosalpingography or, better yet, hysteroscopy. In question 3, painless dilation of the cervix with second-trimester loss suggests cervical incompetence. Her history, serial cervical length measurements, and easy passage of a dilator through the cervix can suggest this diagnosis. The treatment is cervical cerclage. In question 4, this patient has had three previous surgical procedures (LEEP) on her cervix, which may not be able to perform its functions (e.g., no cervical mucus production). After reversal of a vasectomy, the normal blood–testes barrier (which isolates the sperm from the immune system) may have been breached, and thus sperm antibodies can enter the testes. In question 6, this patient's signs and symptoms suggest polycystic ovarian syndrome. These patients are oligo-ovulatory.

7. The answer is B [I A 1]. The monthly probability of pregnancy is 20% among fertile couples.

8. The answer is C [VI A and IX B]. In this clinical scenario, it appears that the wife is ovulatory and has no reason for having tubal or uterine abnormalities. The husband, however, has abnormal sperm parameters. Although the volume, sperm count (low normal value), and white blood cell count satisfy the WHO criteria, the percent normal morphology and percent forward progression are low. ICSI is a micromanipulation technique in which sperm is injected directly into the cytoplasm of the oocyte to enhance fertilization. This method is often used for male factor infertility (as in this case). Pregnancy rates are independent of any semen analysis parameters. The other answer choices (IVF, GIFT, and ZIFT [answer E]) all involve placing the egg near sperm and allowing fertilization to occur in a Petri dish (IVF, ZIFT) or the fallopian tube (GIFT). Theoretically, for fertilization to occur, normal sperm parameters are necessary, which are lacking in this patient's husband. Because the woman is ovulatory (regular cycles every month), she does not need clomiphene. Furthermore, sperm washing with IUI concentrates the sperm that bypasses the cervix by placing the sperm inside the uterus. This technique may wash out sperm antibodies, but it does nothing for abnormal sperm motility or morphology.

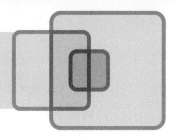

chapter 36

Menopause

ANN STEINER

DEFINITIONS

A **Menopause**

1. Menopause is the period in which a **permanent cessation of menses occurs because of loss of ovarian activity.** The cessation of menses reflects the reduction of ovarian estrogen production to **levels insufficient to produce proliferation of the endometrial lining.**

2. Menses usually cease between **50 and 52 years of age;** the median age of menopause is 51.3 years, with a range of 48 to 55 years.

3. **Premature menopause** is defined as the permanent cessation of menses occurring before 40 years of age.

B **Perimenopause**

1. The **perimenopause** refers to the period just before and after the menopause, usually ranging from 45 to 55 years of age.

2. The **transition** is a term used to describe the years leading up to and preceding the menopause.
   a. This period is marked by menstrual cycle irregularity, reflecting a gradual decline in and fluctuation of ovarian function.
   b. The median age of onset of menstrual irregularity is 47.5 years; the transition lasts an average of 4 years. Ten percent of women abruptly stop menstruating without preceding cycle irregularity.

C **Climacteric**

1. **Climacteric** is a broad term encompassing the transitional years, the menopause, and the postmenopausal years.

2. This period reflects the decline and loss of ovarian function and the long-term consequences of reduced estrogen levels.

II **PHYSIOLOGY OF THE PERIMENOPAUSE**

A **Ovarian function.** A period of waxing and waning ovarian function occurs before the menopause. It is a time of fluctuation in hormone production and reduced fecundability.

1. The **number of remaining follicles is reduced** and those remaining are less sensitive to gonadotropin stimulation. Follicular function varies not only from one individual to another but also from cycle to cycle within the same individual. As follicular maturation declines, ovulation becomes less frequent as the menopause approaches.

2. Although fertility rates are markedly reduced, **conception** can occur during this time of fluctuating ovarian activity.

B Endocrinology

1. **Inhibin** production by the ovary depends on the number of existing ovarian oocytes and therefore is reduced. Inhibin exerts a negative feedback on the secretion of follicle-stimulating hormone (FSH) by the pituitary.

2. An increase in **FSH** levels results from the decreased circulating levels of inhibin and the loss of negative feedback. This is the earliest evidence of a change in ovarian function. Elevated FSH levels can be seen with both normal and abnormal cycles.

3. **Luteinizing hormone (LH)** secretion escapes the negative feedback of inhibin, and LH levels are not affected by the loss of inhibin production. LH levels rise much later in the transition than FSH levels; sustained elevations may not be seen until after the menopause.

4. **Estradiol** levels fluctuate but remain within the wide range of normal until follicular development ceases altogether.

5. **Progesterone** levels fluctuate depending on the presence and adequacy of ovulation and are frequently low during the transition.

6. **Androgen** levels steadily decline during the transition period.

C Menstrual cycles.
Changes in the menstrual cycle reflect changes in ovarian function and circulating levels of ovarian steroids and pituitary gonadotropins.

1. **Changes in menstrual cycle regularity** occur as a woman progresses through her forties. Cycle length is determined by the length of the follicular phase. It is variable and may be normal, shortened, or prolonged.

2. **Shortening of cycle length** occurs early in the transition and is associated with ovulatory cycles, a shortened follicular phase, and elevated FSH levels.

3. **Anovulatory cycles** and **prolonged cycles** become more frequent as the menopause approaches, resulting in dysfunctional uterine bleeding (DUB) and oligomenorrhea.

III PHYSIOLOGY OF THE MENOPAUSE

A Ovarian function.
Follicular reserve is depleted and is manifested by a permanent cessation in menses.

1. **Few follicular units remain in the postmenopausal ovary,** and those present are no longer capable of a normal response despite stimulation by markedly elevated gonadotropins.
   a. **FSH receptors** are absent on a cellular level.
   b. **Estradiol** production by the ovary depends on FSH stimulation and is negligible in the postmenopausal ovary.
   c. **Estrone,** a less potent estrogen, is also produced in negligible amounts by the postmenopausal ovary.

2. **Ovarian stromal tissue** continues to produce androgenic steroid hormones for several years after the menopause.
   a. Although there is a lack of FSH receptors, ovarian stromal cells possess LH receptors and respond with the production of **ovarian androgens** (e.g., androstenedione, testosterone, and dehydroepiandrosterone [DHEA]).
   b. **Androstenedione** and **DHEA** production continues but at a decreased rate. **Testosterone** production remains stable or may be slightly increased.

3. When menses have been absent for 1 year, conception is no longer an issue.

B Endocrinology

1. **FSH levels** are elevated 10 to 20 times above premenopausal levels, reaching a plateau 1 to 3 years after the menopause, after which there is a gradual decline. This reflects loss of the negative feed-

back effects of both inhibin and estradiol. FSH levels never return to the premenopausal range, even with estrogen replacement therapy, reflecting the influence of inhibin.

2. **LH levels** rise two- to threefold after the menopause, reaching a plateau in 1 to 3 years, after which there is a gradual decline. This reflects the loss of the negative feedback effect of estradiol. LH levels never reach those of FSH because of the shorter circulating half-life of LH (30 minutes as opposed to 4 hours).

3. Although **ovarian estrogen production** is negligible after the menopause, there is individual variation in circulating estrogen levels because of peripheral conversion of androgenic precursors to estrone. Estrone, a less potent estrogen, is the principal estrogen after the menopause.
   a. **Androgens,** which serve as precursors for estrogen, continue to be produced by the postmenopausal ovary and the adrenal gland.
   b. **Aromatase enzymes** that convert androgens to estrone primarily (and estradiol to a lesser degree) are present in peripheral tissues but are **predominantly present in adipose tissue.**
   c. Estrogen levels vary with the degree of adiposity; **obesity** can lead to a state of relative estrogen excess.

4. **Peripheral testosterone levels** are decreased despite sustained or increased production rates by the ovary. Circulating testosterone levels are the net result of androstenedione and testosterone production by the adrenal gland and the ovary.
   a. Testosterone and androstenedione production by the adrenal gland does not decrease for several years after the menopause.
   b. Testosterone production by the ovaries does not decrease for several years after the menopause.
   c. Androstenedione production by the ovary is markedly reduced after the menopause and accounts for the fall in circulating testosterone levels characteristic of this time.

5. **DHEA levels** are reduced after the menopause. However, DHEA sulfate levels, which reflect adrenal gland activity, are unchanged.

C Menstrual cycles

1. Menopause is a retrospective diagnosis and is said to have occurred when there is the **absence of menses for 12 months in a woman older than 45 years of age.**

2. The reduced level of estrogen is no longer sufficient to induce endometrial proliferative changes capable of producing menstruation.

D Premature menopause or premature ovarian failure is the cessation of menses in a woman **younger than 40 years of age** (see Chapter 20).

1. The frequency of premature ovarian failure is 0.3%. This is the diagnosis in 5 to 10% of women with secondary amenorrhea (hypergonadotropic amenorrhea).

2. Most women with premature menopause undergo premature oocyte atresia and follicular depletion. This results from one of three mechanisms:
   a. Decreased initial germ cell number at birth
   b. Accelerated oocyte atresia after birth
   c. Postnatal germ cell destruction

3. A small number of affected women have abundant remaining follicles and elevated gonadotropins, suggesting a blockade of gonadotropin stimulation or biologically inactive gonadotropins.

4. Etiologies of premature ovarian failure and hypergonadotropic amenorrhea are diverse and fall under one of the following categories:
   a. Genetic and cytogenetic abnormalities
   b. Enzymatic defects

    c. Physical insults
    d. Autoimmune disturbances
    e. Abnormal gonadotropin structure or function
    f. Idiopathic

IV CLINICAL MANIFESTATIONS OF THE PERIMENOPAUSE

A **Manifestations of estrogen excess** During the perimenopause, some women present with evidence of estrogen excess rather than deficiency.

1. **DUB** is abnormal uterine bleeding that is excessive in amount, duration, and frequency secondary to prolonged exposure of the uterine lining to estrogen stimulation unopposed by progesterone.
   a. Anovulatory cycles, common to the perimenopausal transition, result in unopposed estrogen stimulation of the endometrial lining and result in DUB, which occurs with increased frequency in perimenopausal women.
   b. Increased endogenous estrogen can also be caused by increased peripheral conversion of androgen precursors to estrone and estradiol. This is most frequently seen in obese perimenopausal women.
   c. Less commonly, pathologic conditions are associated with increased estrogen production (ovarian tumors) or decreased metabolic clearance of estrogen (hepatic or renal disease), leading to elevated circulating estrogen levels.

2. **Endometrial neoplasia**
   a. Prolonged unopposed estrogen stimulation of the endometrial lining may lead to endometrial pathology, which manifests as **abnormal uterine bleeding.**
   b. Abnormal uterine bleeding that occurs in a woman older than 40 years of age, or in a younger woman because of prolonged anovulatory cycles, must be evaluated with sampling of the endometrium to rule out organic disease. **Endometrial biopsy** is usually sufficient; **dilation and curettage (D&C)** is performed when biopsy results are inconclusive.
   c. **Simple hyperplasia** has a low risk of progression to endometrial carcinoma and can be treated medically.
   d. **Complex hyperplasia without atypia** is a more advanced type of hyperplasia, with a 3% risk of progressing to endometrial carcinoma. Complex hyperplasia may also be treated medically, including posttreatment biopsy.
   e. **Complex hyperplasia with atypia** is associated with an increased risk of an associated carcinoma. Further evaluation with hysteroscopy and D&C is warranted before treatment to rule this out. Because of an approximately 25% risk of progression to endometrial carcinoma, hysterectomy is the treatment of choice for this condition.
   f. **Carcinoma of the endometrium** should be suspected in all women older than 35 years of age who present with abnormal bleeding. As much as 10% of postmenopausal bleeding is secondary to a carcinoma.

B **Manifestations of hormonal fluctuation**

1. **Menstrual cycle changes.** Some change in the character of the menstrual cycle is the most common manifestation of the perimenopause.
   a. **Menorrhagia** is increased blood flow (**more than 80 mL**) at the time of menses. Cycles are **regular** and ovulatory. Increased flow may result from a relative reduction in progesterone levels.
   b. **Metrorrhagia** is menses at **irregular intervals** with normal or reduced volume or flow. Shortening of cycle length is a common change reported early in the transition. Cycle length remains longer than 21 days but is typically shorter than cycles experienced during the reproductive years. Cycles are ovulatory with a shortened follicular phase.

c. Midcycle spotting. With a drop in estradiol levels just before ovulation, midcycle estrogen withdrawal bleeding may occur.

d. Oligomenorrhea. As the menopause approaches, missed periods are common, and cycle length increases until a permanent cessation of menses occurs.

2. **Other symptoms.** Many women who are still menstruating experience a variety of symptoms traditionally attributed to the menopause. These symptoms are thought to result from the fluctuation of hormone levels that occurs from cycle to cycle.

    a. Hot flushes or flashes. Many women experience hot flushes before the menopause. Frequently, occurrence of these symptoms is not consistent from cycle to cycle.

    b. Headaches. Premenstrual migraines may appear or worsen during this time.

    c. Premenstrual psychological symptoms. Some women report the onset or worsening of premenstrual symptoms, such as depression, anxiety, and irritability, during the transitional years.

    d. Sleep disturbances. Interrupted sleep, with or without hot flushes, is often reported by women during these years.

C Treatment

1. **Progesterone supplementation.** Periodic administration of a progestin is used to treat conditions associated with estrogen excess.

    a. Dysfunctional uterine bleeding can be treated with intermittent progestin therapy (medroxyprogesterone acetate), which provides estrogen antagonism and allows for the orderly sloughing of the endometrium. This prevents uncontrolled uterine bleeding and the development of endometrial hyperplasia.

        (1) Medroxyprogesterone acetate, 10 to 30 mg for 10 to 14 days each month, is administered for 3 to 6 months. Therapy may be continued for the long term until there is a lack of withdrawal bleeding. No further bleeding signifies a reduction of estrogen levels to the menopausal range.

        (2) Norethindrone acetate can be substituted for women who do not tolerate medroxyprogesterone acetate.

    b. Simple and complex hyperplasia may be treated effectively with progestin supplementation. Treatment with medroxyprogesterone acetate as described for DUB is prescribed. Follow-up biopsy is performed after 3 months of treatment to verify resolution of the hyperplasia.

    c. Complex hyperplasia with atypia may be treated with high-dose progestin if surgical therapy is not an option, after the presence of carcinoma has been excluded. Follow-up biopsy after 3 months of treatment is mandatory to verify resolution.

        (1) Medroxyprogesterone acetate, 30 mg, is given daily for 3 months.

        (2) Megestrol, 20 to 60 mg, is given daily for 3 months.

2. **Oral contraceptives** are an attractive alternative in women older than 40 years of age who are normotensive nonsmokers.

    a. Low-dose oral contraceptives (less than 35 μg) are effective treatment for abnormal bleeding associated with the perimenopause.

    b. Oral contraceptives often provide relief of other symptoms, such as vasomotor symptoms. Oral contraceptives are also an effective method of contraception for women older than 40 years, and they carry no increased risk in nonsmokers.

    c. Because **oral contraceptives** contain **five to seven times the estrogen equivalent of postmenopausal hormone replacement therapy**, it is desirable to change therapy with the onset of menopause. FSH levels are obtained annually after 45 years of age on day 5 to 7 of the menstrual cycle. Oral contraceptives are stopped when the serum FSH level is consistently greater than 30 IU/l.

3. **Hormone replacement therapy** refers to the combined use of estrogen and progestogen. **Estrogen replacement therapy** refers to the use of estrogen without a progestogen (see section VI for more details).
   a. **Estrogen replacement therapy** may be used to treat perimenopausal symptoms in women with oligomenorrhea before permanent cessation of menses.
   b. **Natural progesterone or synthetic progestin** is added sequentially or continuously to provide endometrial protection to women who have their uterus. These are called progestogens.

4. **Nonsteroidal anti-inflammatory drugs (NSAIDs)** effectively reduce menstrual blood flow by 40 to 60% in women with ovulatory cycles. NSAIDs may be useful in the treatment of menstrual migraines.

V   CLINICAL MANIFESTATIONS OF MENOPAUSE

A **Target organ response to decreased estrogen.**   Estrogen-responsive tissues are present throughout the body. Chronic reduction of estrogen results in the following manifestations:

1. **Urogenital atrophy.** The vagina, urethra, bladder, and pelvic floor are estrogen-responsive tissues. Decreased estrogen levels after the menopause result in a generalized atrophy of these structures.
   a. There is a reduction in the height of **vaginal epithelium** and decreased vascular flow. The vaginal epithelium becomes pale, thin, and dry. Maturation of the vaginal epithelium is estrogen dependent. After the menopause, there is a shift (regression) in the maturation index, with a preponderance of immature cell types (basal and parabasal) over mature cell types (intermediate and superficial). There is a shift of the vaginal pH from acidic to alkaline.
   b. The vaginal walls lose elasticity and compliance; the **vagina becomes smaller,** and the size of the upper vagina diminishes.
   c. The **labia minora** have a pale, dry appearance, and there is a reduction of the fat content of the **labia majora.**
   d. The **pelvic tissues and ligaments** that support the uterus and the vagina **lose their tone,** predisposing to disorders of pelvic relaxation.
   e. The **epithelium of the urethra and bladder** mucosa becomes atrophic; there is a loss of urethral and bladder wall elasticity and compliance.

2. **Uterine changes**
   a. The **endometrial tissue becomes sparse,** with an atrophic appearance.
   b. The **myometrium atrophies,** and the **uterine corpus decreases in size.** There is a reversal of the corpus–cervical length ratio compared with the reproductive years.
   c. The **squamocolumnar junction** relocates high in the endocervical canal; the cervical os frequently becomes stenotic.
   d. **Fibroids,** if present, reduce in size but do not disappear.

3. **Breast changes**
   a. Progressive fatty replacement with atrophy of active glandular units
   b. Regression of fibrocystic changes

4. **Skin changes.** Skin collagen content and skin thickness decrease proportionately with time after the menopause.

5. **Bone changes.** Bone loss is accelerated for the first 5 to 7 years after the menopause associated with decreased estrogen levels.
   a. The greatest effect is seen in **trabecular bone,** particularly in the spine.
   b. Excessive loss predisposes to the development of **osteoporosis** and increased fracture risk.

6. **Hair changes.** As estrogen decreases, circulating androgens increase and the chance of developing increased facial hair and androgenic alopecia increases.

7. **Brain changes.** Estrogen receptors are located throughout the brain. Reduced estrogen levels may affect cognitive function and moods after the menopause, although the precise contribution has not been fully defined.

8. **Cardiovascular changes.** The incidence of cardiovascular disease increases after the age of 50 years in women coincident with the age of menopause. Cardiovascular disease is the cause of the largest number of deaths of menopausal women.

B **Symptoms related to estrogen reduction.** Symptoms are the manifestation of target organ response to declining estrogen levels.

1. **Vasomotor instability**
   a. **Hot flushes or flashes** are the most common symptom related to the menopause and occur in 75 to 85% of perimenopausal women.
      (1) Flushes appear to be more frequent and severe at night or during times of stress. They also can be precipitated by foods and beverages that are hot or spicy or contain methylxanthines; they can be precipitated by alcohol as well.
      (2) The vasomotor instability lasts for **1 to 2 years** in most women but may last for as long as 5 years or more in up to one third of symptomatic women.
   b. Hot flushes are the result of **inappropriate stimulation of the body's heat-releasing mechanisms** by the thermoregulatory centers in the hypothalamus. Although the core body temperature is normal, the body is stimulated to lose heat. The onset of the flushes initially depends on a reduction of previously established estrogen levels. Flushes do not occur in hypoestrogenic states, such as gonadal dysgenesis.
   c. Flushes are characterized by **progressive vasodilation of the skin over the head, neck, and chest,** accompanied by reddening of the skin, a feeling of intense body heat, and perspiration. Palpitations or tachycardia may accompany the flush. The flush may last a few seconds to several minutes and recur with variable frequency.
   d. Treatment
      (1) **Hormone replacement or estrogen replacement** reduces or eliminates hot flushes.
      (2) **Progestins, clonidine, methyldopa, vitamin E, and herbal remedies** are used to treat hot flushes in women in whom estrogen is contraindicated. Relief is not as complete as that seen with estrogen therapy.
      (3) **Venlafaxine,** an inhibitor of serotonin and norepinephrine reuptake, given in low doses has been effective in reducing or eliminating vasomotor instability in 60% of symptomatic women.

2. **Altered menstrual function.** Oligomenorrhea is followed by amenorrhea. If vaginal bleeding occurs after 6 months of amenorrhea, endometrial disease (e.g., polyps, hyperplasia, or neoplasia) must be ruled out.

3. **Vaginal atrophy**
   a. **Dyspareunia** (painful intercourse). This common symptom is related to the menopause.
      (1) Changes in the vaginal epithelium and vaginal vasculature lead to decreased lubrication during sexual activity. Decreased compliance and elasticity of the vaginal wall contribute to vaginal stenosis.
      (2) Continued sexual activity into the menopause is associated with increased vaginal blood flow and fewer problems with sexual function compared with women who are less frequently sexually active.
   b. **Atrophic vaginitis**
      (1) The postmenopausal vagina becomes more susceptible to pathogenic and nonpathogenic organisms.
      (2) Atrophy of the vaginal mucosa and changes in pH predispose to vaginitis, which presents with symptoms of discharge, pruritus, odor, and irritation.
   c. **Treatment.** Symptoms related to vaginal atrophy respond to estrogen therapy.

4. **Urinary tract symptoms.** Changes in the mucosal lining of the urethra and bladder may lead to symptoms of dysuria, nocturia, urinary frequency, urgency, and urge incontinence.
    a. **Urinary conditions. Urinary stress incontinence** may progressively worsen after the menopause because of urethral changes and a loss of pelvic support. There is an increased incidence of **bacteriuria** in the postmenopausal woman compared with women in the premenopausal age group.
    b. **Treatment.** Vaginal, urethral, and bladder symptoms improve with estrogen therapy.

5. **Osteoporosis.** This systemic skeletal disease is characterized by **low bone mass** and **microarchitectural deterioration of bone structure,** both of which result in fragile bones that are at an increased risk for fracture. Osteoporosis may be a primary disease state or may be secondary to other diseases that affect calcium and bone metabolism.
    a. **Epidemiology and etiology**
        (1) Peak bone mass is reached in the late twenties for trabecular bone and the early thirties for cortical bone. Thereafter, there is a gradual loss of bone with aging. **Bone loss is accelerated for the first 5 to 7 years after the menopause** as a direct result of declining estrogen levels. Osteoporosis is more common in women than in men because of lower peak bone mass and higher rates of bone loss.
        (2) **Risk factors** other than age and gender include inadequate calcium intake; sedentary lifestyle; smoking; alcohol use; premature menopause; genetic predisposition; white and Asian race; chronic glucocorticoid use; and hyperthyroidism, including excessive thyroid replacement.
        (3) Osteoporosis has reached epidemic proportions in the United States; an estimated 1.3 million fractures occur annually.
            (a) Approximately 25% of white American women older than 60 years of age who are not treated with estrogen replacement have spinal compression fractures.
            (b) Approximately 32% of white American women older than 75 years of age suffer hip fractures; there is an excess mortality rate of 10 to 30% at 1 year after fracture. Thirty percent of survivors no longer live independently.
        (4) Osteoporosis results when **bone resorption outweighs bone formation.** Trabecular bone is at greater risk than cortical bone because it is more metabolically active and structurally more porous. The bones most commonly affected by fracture are the vertebrae, distal radius, hip, and humerus; however, all bones are at risk.
    b. **Diagnosis.** Osteoporosis is diagnosed late in the disease, when fractures typical of the disease occur (e.g., spinal compression fractures [dowager hump]).
    c. **Imaging modalities** can be used to detect bone loss and bones at risk for fracture earlier in the disease.
        (1) **Single-photon absorptiometry,** used very seldom today, was the first modality used to measure bone density at the wrist.
        (2) **Dual-photon absorptiometry** also is used very seldom today because of the use of a radionuclide source and inability to differentiate cortical and trabecular bone.
        (3) **Dual-energy x-ray absorptiometry** is the most popular technique used today to measure bone density. An x-ray tube has replaced the radionuclide source, and independent measurements can be made at the hip, spine, and other bone sites.
        (4) **Quantitative computed tomography** gives the most precise measurement of bone density at specific sites. However, its use has been limited by expense and higher radiation doses.
    d. **Prevention of osteoporosis** is the key to management (see VI A 2). Exercise, adequate calcium intake, and estrogen replacement after the menopause play key roles in prevention. The higher a woman's bone mineral density at the onset of menopause, the more bone she will have to lose to be at risk for osteoporotic fractures.

6. The **menopausal syndrome.** This term has been used to cover several symptoms, such as fatigue, headache, nervousness, loss of libido, insomnia, depression, irritability, palpitations, and joint and muscle pain.
   a. Progressive improvement of some of these symptoms occurs with hormone replacement.
   b. Addition of low doses of androgen in addition to hormone or estrogen replacement may enhance the therapeutic response.
   c. The etiology of these symptoms may be multifactorial. Underlying medical illness should be considered in the differential diagnosis.

VI ESTROGEN REPLACEMENT THERAPY

A **Benefits and indications.** Currently, the best reason to use hormone or estrogen replacement in the menopause is related to quality of life issues. If a woman feels better using these medications, the risks (see VI B) may be justified.

1. **Treatment of menopausal symptoms**
   a. **Hormone or estrogen replacement** usually **eliminates or significantly reduces hot flushes** and night sweats. Progestins alone are less effective than conjugated estrogen, estrone, or estradiol, but they may provide relief in women who have contraindications to estrogen use.
   b. Estrogen replacement can be used for relief of symptoms associated with **urogenital atrophy.**
      (1) **Atrophic vaginitis** and resulting **dyspareunia** may be treated with vaginal and oral estrogens. Long-term use is required for this purpose, and complete response may take 3 or 4 months. Estrogen replacement therapy restores vaginal elasticity, vasculature, and tone. Nonhormonal vaginal lubricating agents maybe useful as well.
      (2) **Urinary symptoms,** especially **urgency, may** improve with systemic or topical estrogen use.
   c. **Affective symptoms**—depression, insomnia, irritability, and loss of concentration—may improve with estrogen therapy, especially if these symptoms begin with the onset of menopause.
      (1) Other causes should be considered when little or no response is seen with estrogen replacement.
      (2) Addition of low-dose testosterone may achieve a better therapeutic response.
   d. **Decreased libido** may respond to hormone replacement or estrogen replacement. Addition of low-dose testosterone may achieve a better therapeutic response than estrogen alone.
      (1) Libido may improve after treatment for dyspareunia.
      (2) Often, other underlying factors, such as psychosocial issues and fatigue, affect sexual desire in addition to the hormonal changes associated with the menopausal state.
   e. **Vaginal relaxation** usually is not responsive to estrogen therapy alone.

2. **Prevention and treatment of osteoporosis**
   a. **Prevention** involves hormone or estrogen replacement after the menopause. Estrogen acts through an **antiresorptive effect.** Although estrogen is not approved for the treatment of osteoporosis, it does appear to decrease the fracture risk in women with osteoporosis.
      (1) Accelerated bone loss that occurs after the menopause can be prevented with early estrogen replacement therapy. Transdermal and oral preparations effectively reduce bone loss. Hormone or estrogen replacement is associated with a 50% reduction in fracture risk.
      (2) **Adequate calcium intake** must also be ensured through diet or supplementation; 1000 to 1500 mg of elemental calcium plus vitamin D is required daily, depending on how much estrogen is given.
      (3) A regular program of weight-bearing **exercise** is necessary to stimulate bone formation and to ensure maintenance of muscle tone.
   b. **Other antiresorptive agents** used to treat osteoporosis include calcitonin, bisphosphonates, and selective estrogen receptor modulators, such as raloxifene.

3. **Effects on Alzheimer dementia and cognitive function** are not clear at this time. Studies have shown that estrogen replacement therapy given for 1 year **does not** slow cognitive decline in women with mild to moderate Alzheimer dementia. Hormone replacement therapy may have enhanced cognitive effects in women with menopausal symptoms.

B **Risks and contraindications**

1. **Absolute contraindications.** The use of estrogen replacement therapy is contraindicated in women with conditions that could potentially worsen with estrogen exposure or conditions that affect the metabolism and clearance of estrogen.
    a. **Medical conditions related to estrogen exposure**
        (1) Recent vascular thrombosis
        (2) Neuro-ophthalmologic vascular disease
        (3) Recent history of endometrial carcinoma
        (4) History of breast cancer (except in certain circumstances)
        (5) Undiagnosed vaginal bleeding
    b. **Conditions related to estrogen metabolism**
        (1) Acute hepatic disease
        (2) Chronically impaired liver function

2. **Relative contraindications.** The following conditions may worsen with estrogen exposure and therefore are relative contraindications to replacement. However, with adjustments in dosage or route of administration, hormone replacement therapy is used safely and successfully on an individual basis.
    a. Seizure disorders
    b. High serum triglycerides
    c. Current gallbladder disease
    d. Migraine headaches

3. **Endometrial cancer.** Estrogen therapy increases the risk of endometrial hyperplasia and carcinoma when used without progestin.
    a. The **risk of endometrial cancer** and hyperplasia is raised 2- to 20-fold depending on the duration of exposure and dose of estrogen. Risk is duration- and dose-dependent.
    b. **Addition of a progestogen** for at least 12 days per month reduces that risk to less than 1 to 2%. There is actually a decreased relative risk of endometrial cancer in women who are on combined estrogen and progestin replacement therapy.
    c. Hormone replacement therapy may be considered in women who have been successfully treated for stage I endometrial carcinoma.

4. **Cardiovascular disease.** The estrogen–progestin arm of the **Women's Health Initiative**, a large prospective randomized primary prevention trial of postmenopausal hormones, was closed 3 years prematurely, in the spring of 2002, because of unexpected adverse outcomes. There was an increased risk of heart attack, stroke, and thromboembolism in women who took hormone replacement therapy. The effect of estrogen replacement therapy is still being evaluated. It was recommended that hormone replacement therapy **not be given for prevention of cardiovascular disease.** Other studies have demonstrated additional clinical benefits and risks.
    a. Estrogen may have potentially **beneficial effects on cardiovascular disease**, such as favorable lipid effects, reduced lipoprotein a, inhibition of oxidation of low-density lipoprotein, improved endothelial vascular function, and reversal of postmenopausal increases in fibrinogen and plasma-activator inhibitor type 1.
    b. Potentially **detrimental estrogen effects** may include increased triglycerides, activation of coagulation, and increased levels of C-reactive protein.

5. **Breast cancer.** The controversy surrounding the risk of breast cancer in women who use estrogen replacement therapy continues. Fear of breast cancer is one of the most common reasons

women choose not to use estrogen after the menopause. The Women's Health Initiative showed a significantly **increased risk of invasive breast cancer in women who used conjugated estrogen and medroxyprogesterone.**

6. **Uterine bleeding.** The return of periods is another common reason women avoid estrogen replacement therapy after the menopause.

   a. **Progestin** is added to estrogen therapy to prevent endometrial hyperplasia and carcinoma. This results in withdrawal bleeding when progestin is given sequentially, or breakthrough bleeding when progestin is given continuously.

      (1) Progestin given sequentially on a monthly basis (see VI C 3 a) results in regular withdrawal bleeding. The duration and flow usually decrease with time and may cease altogether.

      (2) Progestin given continuously does not induce cyclic bleeding but is associated with irregular spotting and bleeding, particularly during the first year.

      (3) Progestin is also associated with other side effects that are often poorly tolerated, including depression, irritability, mastalgia, and bloating.

   b. Abnormal bleeding that occurs during hormone replacement therapy must be evaluated with **endometrial sampling** to rule out endometrial disease. Bleeding that continues after sampling and appropriate management should be evaluated with **hysteroscopy** or **sonohysterography.**

C Current standard regimens

1. **Unopposed estrogen.** Estrogen is given unopposed and on a daily basis. This is the treatment of choice in **women who have undergone hysterectomy.** This regimen can be used in women who cannot tolerate side effects related to progestational agents, provided there is adequate surveillance of the endometrial lining. **Endometrial biopsy on an annual basis** is recommended.

2. **Cyclic combined therapy.** Estrogen is given on days 1 to 25 of the month, and the progestogen is given for the last 12 days of the cycle (days 14 to 25). This regimen is rarely used because women may become symptomatic on hormone-free days.

3. **Sequential combined therapy.** Estrogen is administered every day, and progestogen is administered for 12 to 14 days every month. Scheduled bleeding should occur on completion of the progestogen.

4. **Continuous combined therapy**

   a. Estrogen and progestogen are administered daily. There are **advantages** to maintaining a constant hormonal environment.

      (1) There is no scheduled withdrawal bleeding or resumption of menstrual-like bleeding; this was the initial reason this therapy was introduced.

      (2) Symptoms that worsen with hormonal fluctuations, including mood disturbances, migraines, and cyclic mastalgia, are improved.

      (3) The regimen is easy for patients to remember.

   b. The **disadvantage** to this regimen is the occurrence of irregular spotting and bleeding in up to 40% of women during the first year. This becomes a source of concern for the patient and physician and is an indication for biopsy.

5. **Periodic or quarterly progestogen**

   a. Progestogen is administered for 14 days once every 3 months to reduce the number of withdrawal bleeds and progestin side effects. The quarterly progestin schedule is usually used in association with daily, low-dose estrogen.

   b. Withdrawal bleeding may be heavy when it does occur.

   c. Long-term endometrial protection has not been documented.

6. **Local applications**

   a. **Topical estrogen** is used intravaginally to treat symptoms of **urogenital atrophy** and **dyspareunia.** Estrogen-containing creams, tablets, and synthetic rings are available for this use.

Peak systemic absorption is in the first few days of initial use. Once the vaginal mucosa becomes cornified, there is minimal systemic absorption of estrogen.

    b. Progestin intrauterine devices are being used as a way to provide endometrial protection and avoid the side effects of systemic progestin.

D **Current agents**

1. **Estrogens.** Estrogens, for the purpose of replacement, are administered orally or transdermally. The current trend is to give the lowest dose of estrogen necessary to relieve menopausal symptoms and to continue estrogen only as long as is necessary for relief of symptoms. Evaluation of need may require periodic alteration or cessation of dosing.

    a. Conjugated estrogens are the preparation that has been used for the longest time for hormone replacement. The most commonly used dose is 0.625 mg administered according to the various schedules discussed (see VI C). Low-dose therapy is 0.3 mg.

    b. Estrone sulfate is administered in dosages of 0.625 to 1.25 mg according to one of the regimens discussed (see VI C).

    c. Estradiol can be administered orally or transdermally.

      (1) Oral dosing is 0.5 to 2 mg (the lowest is the most popular).

      (2) Patches are available for use at doses of 0.025 to 0.1 mg. Patches are changed once or twice a week, depending on the particular brand.

      (3) A combination estrogen–progestin patch is available.

2. **Progestogens.** Progestogens are administered according to the regimens described for the purpose of prevention of endometrial hyperplasia and endometrial carcinoma (see VI C).

    a. The most commonly used agent is **medroxyprogesterone acetate.** Starting doses depend on the regimen used.

      (1) 5 mg for 12 days monthly for sequential therapy

      (2) 5 mg for 14 days for 3-month (quarterly) therapy

      (3) 2.5 or 5 mg for continuous regimens

    b. Other progestins are used, including **norethindrone acetate.** Doses vary according to regimen.

    c. Natural oral micronized progesterone is also used in 100- or 200-mg doses. Compared with the synthetic progestogens, there may be fewer associated side effects, such as breast tenderness.

VII **RECOMMENDATIONS FOR CARE OF THE MENOPAUSAL WOMAN**

A **Health risk assessment and physical examination**

1. Identification of risk factors for cardiovascular disease and cancer in medical, social, family, lifestyle history

2. Annual determination of height, weight, and blood pressure

3. Annual physical examination, including breast and pelvic examination

B **Age–risk appropriate screenings.** Screening tests are performed to detect risk factors and early disease in asymptomatic patients.

1. Cholesterol screening according to age and prior values

2. Fasting blood sugar screening according to risk and age

3. Mammography every 1 to 2 years from 40 to 50 years of age, annually after 50 years of age, and in women taking hormone replacement therapy

4. Pap smear every 1 to 3 years depending on age, risk, and previous results

5. Bone density screening for osteoporosis beginning at age 65 years, earlier in women with risk factors for fractures or in women whose decision to begin treatment would be influenced by screening results

6. Routine screening for colon cancer beginning in low-risk women at age 50 years. This includes yearly fecal occult blood testing plus flexible sigmoidoscopy every 5 years, colonoscopy every 10 years, or double-contrast barium enema every 5 to 10 years.

C **Healthy lifestyle promotion**

1. Smoking cessation and alcohol limitation
2. Nutritional assessment and recommendations about fat, cholesterol, calcium, and caloric intake
3. Exercise recommendations
4. Identification of physical abuse and substance abuse
5. Screening for symptoms of depression
6. Counseling about prevention of falls

D **Menopause management**

1. Hormone replacement therapy counseling if indicated
2. Nonhormonal management of symptoms
3. Problem-related evaluation and management

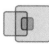

Study Questions for Chapter 36

DIRECTIONS: *Each of the numbered items or incomplete statements in this section is followed by answers or by completions of the statement. Select the ONE lettered answer or completion that is BEST in each case.*

1. A 61-year-old Asian woman just underwent a dual-energy x-ray absorptiometry (DEXA) scan, which placed her T-score three standard deviations below the mean. She has no known medical problems. She is 5 foot 3 inches tall and weighs 92 lbs. She denies using alcohol and she is an ex-smoker (she smoked half a pack per day for 13 years). She stopped having periods at age 52. She was never on hormone replacement therapy. She does not report experiencing vaginal dryness or hot flushes. The most effective next step in management of this patient is

- A Estrogen
- B Progestin
- C Vitamin D and calcium
- D Alendronate
- E Swimming

2. A 52-year-old woman, gravida 2, para 2 presents to your clinic reporting insomnia, hot flashes, and an anxious mood. According to her DEXA scan, she has severe osteopenia. Her last menstrual period was 2 years ago. She has no medical problems other than migraines. She is Caucasian, 5 feet 7 inches tall, and weighs 110 pounds. She is a smoker and drinks 1 to 2 glasses of wine with dinner. The most important reason to begin hormone replacement therapy (HRT) is to

- A Decrease risk of coronary artery disease
- B Decrease risk of Alzheimer's disease
- C Decrease risk of osteoporosis
- D Treat vaginal dryness and dyspareunia
- E Make her feel better

3. A 54-year-old woman presents to you because her hot flashes and night sweats are interfering with her daytime activities and her sleep. Her last menstrual period was 16 months ago. Her past medical history is remarkable for gallstones, which are symptomatic when she strays away from her low-fat diet. She denies smoking or drinking alcohol. Her family history is remarkable for breast cancer in her maternal aunt. The next best step in the management of this patient is

- A Oral medroxyprogesterone acetate
- B Transdermal estrogen replacement with progestin
- C Methyldopa
- D Oral micronized progesterone
- E Soy products, ginseng, and dong quai

4. A 19-year-old woman who is was born with wide-set nipples and a webbed neck was diagnosed with Turner syndrome (X0) by karyotype. This patient has only had a few, light periods since age 16 years. Patients with Turner syndrome undergo premature menopause because of accelerated follicle depletion. Patients with Turner syndrome _____ hot flashes because _____.

- A report; estrogen withdrawal during perimenopause
- B report; stimulation of heat-releasing mechanisms in the hypothalamus
- C do not report; they never had estrogen sensitization of brain tissues
- D do not report; centers in the hypothalamus are defective
- E do not report; their thermoregulatory centers are insensitive to estrogen

5. A 54-year-old woman wants treatment for her hot flushes. She says she is educated and has read about all of the risks and benefits of hormone replacement therapy. She tells you that her previous physician put her on a regimen that caused irregular spotting (which was not bothersome to her.) However, the regimen also caused irritability, depression, mastalgia, bloating, and weight gain. The best treatment option for this patient is

(Note: HRT = hormone replacement therapy [estrogen + progestin], ERT = estrogen replacement therapy, EMB = endometrial biopsy)

A ERT
B ERT + annual EMB
C HRT (cyclic combined)
D HRT (continuous combined)
E HRT (sequential combined) + annual EMB

Answers and Explanations

1. The answer is D [VI A 2]. The bisphosphonates (e.g., alendronate) are effective in both decreasing the rate of bone loss in women with normal or low bone density and reducing the risk of fracture in women with osteoporosis (as in this woman). Although retrospective studies suggest that estrogen may also reduce the incidence of fracture in women with osteoporosis, the hormone is not currently approved for this use. Progestogens do not have a consistent effect on bone loss and are currently not approved to treat osteoporosis. Swimming is not a weight-bearing exercise (as opposed to walking) and has minimal effect on prevention of bone loss. Calcium and vitamin D are both essential in patients at risk for and those who have osteoporosis. However, the most successful therapy in a patient with this degree of osteoporosis requires use of bisphosphonates (T-score three standard deviations [SD] below the mean; the T-score [measured in standard deviations] compares the bone density of a patient to that of a young healthy woman). Most experts consider SD of 2.5 or more below the mean as the definition of osteoporosis.

2. The answer is E [VI A 1 and B 4]. Currently, the best reason to use estrogen in menopause is to treat vasomotor (which she has) and urogenital symptoms (which she does not have). It may also have other benefits, such as its effect on cognitive function and depression. As of 2004, there is no evidence that estrogen is useful in decreasing heart disease or Alzheimer's disease. The efficacy of estrogen treatment for osteoporosis is established, but the risks may outweigh the benefits in this patient. Osteoporosis is effectively treated with bisphosphonates. This patient is not reporting vaginal dryness or dyspareunia.

3. The answer is B [VI D 1 and V B 1 d 2]. This patient is experiencing severe hot flashes that are affecting her quality of life, and she therefore needs effective therapy. Hormone replacement therapy (HRT), either in the form of oral estrogen and progestogen, transdermal estrogen and progestogen, or some other form that achieves significant systemic blood levels of estrogen, effectively treats vasomotor activity (hot flashes). Progestins alone, clonidine, methyldopa, vitamin E, and herbal remedies have been used in women with hot flashes who have absolute contraindications to estrogen use (this woman has a relative contraindication). These treatments are not as effective as estrogen. Testimonials and case reports have shown that herbal remedies may improve hot flashes and vaginal dryness. Soy products, ginseng, and don quai contain phytoestrogens (such as genistein and equol), which have not been shown (in placebo-controlled trials) to effectively treat menopausal hot flushes. Further scientific evidence is needed before physicians can prescribe alternatives to traditional estrogen therapy as their first choice.

4. The answer is C [V B 1 b]. Hot flashes are the result of inappropriate stimulation of the body's heat-releasing mechanisms by the thermoregulatory centers in the hypothalamus. The onset of flushes initially depends on a reduction of previously established estrogen levels. Most patients with Turner syndrome do not have high enough estrogen levels to sensitize the thermoregulatory centers because they are hypoestrogenic. Therefore, withdrawal of estrogen (during menopause) in a hypoestrogenic person does not result in hot flashes.

5. The answer is B [VI C 1]. This patient wants effective treatment for her hot flashes. Both HRT (any regimen) and ERT are effective treatments of hot flashes. Because this patient is unable to tolerate the side effects related to progestational agents (e.g., bloating, depression, irritability, mastalgia, and weight gain), she is not a candidate for any type of HRT. Therefore, ERT is the treatment of choice. The problem with ERT is that the unopposed estrogen causes endometrial hyperplasia and can lead to endometrial carcinoma. Therefore, it this treatment option is chosen, you must provide adequate surveillance of the endometrial lining with yearly EMBs.

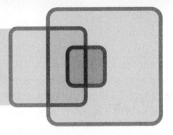

chapter 37

Pelvic Malignancies

CHRISTINA BANDERA

I CERVICAL CANCER

Cervical cancer is the most preventable gynecologic cancer because of the Pap smear. George Papanicolaou developed a method of identifying abnormal cells in exfoliative cytology in the 1920s and published his work in the 1940s. Pap smear screening is now an integral part of health care in the United States. In developing countries, where Pap smears are not routinely performed, cervical cancer remains the most common cause of cancer death in women.

A Epidemiology and etiology

1. **Frequency peaks** between 45 and 60 years of age

2. **Increased incidence** is related to:
   a. First intercourse at a young age
   b. Marriage or conception at a young age
   c. Multiple sexual partners
   d. Cigarette smoking. Byproducts of cigarette smoke are concentrated in cervical mucus and have been associated with a depletion of the cells of Langerhans, which are macrophages that assist in cell-mediated immunity.
   e. High-risk sexual partners (e.g., those whose previous sexual partners developed precancerous or cancerous conditions of the cervix)
   f. Immunosuppression (e.g., from HIV infection)

3. **Infectious associations**
   a. **Human papilloma virus (HPV)**, a double-stranded DNA virus, appears to be involved in the pathogenesis of cervical cancer. Incorporation of the E6 and E7 open reading frames into the cervical cell genome is associated with progression to invasive disease.
      (1) HPV is detected in more than 90% of cervical cancers. It is also detected in precancerous dysplastic lesions.
      (2) Certain HPV subtypes (16, 18, 31, 33, and 45) are commonly associated with high-grade neoplasms and cervical cancer.
   b. **Herpes simplex virus-2 (HSV-2)**. HSV-2 DNA and messenger RNA sequences have been found in cervical cancer cells and may increase the likelihood of HPV infection.

B Preinvasive cervical disease

1. **Pap smear screening.** The **cervical transformation zone (TZ)** is the site of most **squamous preinvasive and invasive neoplasms**. The TZ undergoes a transformation from mucus-secreting glandular cells to non–mucus-secreting squamous cells in a normal process called **metaplasia** (change in growth). **Active metaplasia** is most susceptible to infection by HPV.
   a. **Types of Pap smears**
      (1) A **traditional Pap smear** is performed using a wooden spatula to wipe cells from the surface of the cervix and a brush to wipe cells from the endocervical canal. The cells are smeared onto a slide that is fixed and stained for cytologic evaluation.

403

    (2) A **liquid cytology** method (e.g., Thin Prep, AutoCyte) is commonly used to create a Pap smear that is easier to evaluate. The specimen is collected by wiping cells from the cervix and endocervix. The cells are then suspended in liquid, which is processed to remove blood, mucus, and debris. The remaining concentrated suspension of cells is used to create a stained slide for evaluation. The specimens collected in this fashion can also be used to identify HPV subtypes, providing information that may help assess risk in a patient with a progressing lesion.

  b. Efficacy of cytologic screening programs

    (1) **Invasive carcinoma of the cervix** is usually preceded by a spectrum of **preinvasive disease**, which can be detected cytologically (e.g., with the Pap smear). Detection and simple local treatments of preinvasive cervical disease can prevent invasive cancer.

    (2) **Regular cervical cancer screening programs** have demonstrated a significant decrease in mortality from cervical cancer. Unscreened populations can have as high as a 10-fold or greater increase in mortality from cervical cancer.

  c. Frequency of cervical cytologic screening

    (1) Screening should be initiated at the onset of sexual activity or age 18 years.

    (2) Women with high-risk factors (see I A 2) should be screened annually.

    (3) Women with low-risk factors and three consecutive negative annual Pap smears can be screened less frequently at the discretion of the physician.

  d. Evaluation of the abnormal Pap smear. The **Bethesda System** uses descriptive terms that correlate with histology. This analysis includes:

    (1) A statement regarding the adequacy of the sample

    (2) A general categorization statement (optional)

    (3) A descriptive diagnosis regarding benign or reactive changes, low- or high-grade intraepithelial cell abnormalities, glandular cell abnormalities, or the presence of malignant cells

2. Further diagnosis with colposcopy. The Pap smear carries a false-negative rate of 15 to 40% for invasive cancers, and colposcopy provides a more definitive diagnosis. This technique involves using magnification to inspect the TZ after applying a 3 to 5% acetic acid solution. Biopsies are performed of abnormal-appearing epithelium. Colposcopically directed biopsies carry an accuracy of 85 to 95%. **Endocervical curettage** is performed in conjunction with colposcopy to rule out dysplasia within the canal that is not visualized.

3. Treatment. Therapeutic recommendations are based on colposcopic biopsy.

  a. Low-grade lesions can be treated surgically or followed conservatively. Although there is a 60% incidence of regression, there is a 15% incidence of progression to a high-grade abnormality.

  b. Destruction or excision of the TZ may be performed using the following methods:

    (1) **Cold knife conization** is the gold standard because a pathologic specimen with clean margins is obtained. This procedure is performed in the operating room using a scalpel. It is recommended in the following circumstances:

      (a) Significant dysplastic lesions with either a nonvisualized component or a positive endocervical canal curettage

      (b) High-grade lesions that do not correlate with colposcopic findings

      (c) Premalignant or malignant glandular cell abnormalities

    (2) **Loop excision** is commonly called a loop electrosurgical excision procedure (LEEP) or large loop excision of transformation zone (LLETZ). This procedure is easily performed in the office with local anesthesia. A hot metal loop is used to excise a wedge of cervical tissue. Disadvantages include a cautery artifact at the margin of the specimen and a limited biopsy size because of lack of general anesthesia or size of the metal loop.

    (3) **Cryotherapy** involves freezing the cervix in the office. It has the disadvantages of yielding no tissue for pathologic evaluation and potential scarring.

    (4) **Laser vaporization** or **laser conization** is also performed at some centers.

    c. Cure rates for preinvasive disease after one treatment range from 85 to 95%. Repeat treatment of the adequately evaluated persistent lesion results in a cure rate of 95%.

    d. The risk of premalignant lesions persisting or recurring is 5 to 15%. Of these lesions, 85% are detected within 2 years of the initial treatment. **Follow-up** should include:

        (1) Cytologic evaluation every 3 to 6 months for the first year posttreatment

        (2) Repeat colposcopic evaluation for persistent or recurrent abnormalities

        (3) Hysterectomy for patients who have persistent severe lesions despite repeated conservative local destructive techniques

C **Microinvasive carcinoma of the cervix** Much controversy surrounds the exact definition of "early" invasive cancer of the cervix. A commonly adopted definition in the United States is a depth of invasion less than or equal to 3 mm, lesion width of less than or equal to 7 mm, and no evidence of lymphatic or vascular space involvement.

    1. Diagnosis can be made only by means of a thoroughly examined cone biopsy specimen.

    2. The **incidence of pelvic lymph node metastases** is less than 4%.

    3. The treatment of choice is **total abdominal hysterectomy**, although cervical conization with negative margins may be used in women who wish to preserve fertility.

    4. The **cure rate** is 95%.

D **Invasive carcinoma of the cervix**

    1. Symptoms

        a. Postcoital or irregular bleeding is the most common symptom.

        b. Malodorous, bloody discharge; sciatica; leg edema; and deep pelvic pain are seen in advanced disease.

    2. Histology. Squamous carcinomas (80%) and adenocarcinoma (15%) account for most invasive cervical cancer. There appears to be no difference in survival rates between women with these two groups of cancer when the lesions are matched for grade, size, and stage. Rare tumors of the cervix include small cell carcinomas, sarcomas, and lymphomas.

    3. Staging (Table 37-1). Staging is **clinical** and does not change after surgery. Assessment for staging is based on cervical biopsies, physical examination, radiologic imaging of the kidneys and ureters to identify hydronephrosis caused by tumor extension, proctoscopy, cystoscopy, and chest radiography.

    4. Treatment. Therapeutic measures are governed by the patient's age and general health and by the clinical stage of the cancer. Primary modalities include surgery and radiotherapy. Chemotherapy is commonly used as a radiation sensitizer.

        a. Surgery. This modality may be considered for patients with stage I or IIA disease. Typically, a **radical hysterectomy** with para-aortic and pelvic lymphadenectomy is performed. This procedure involves en bloc removal of the uterus, cervix, upper third of the vagina, parametrium, and uterosacral and uterovesical ligaments. In addition, the lymphatic nodes of the lower para-aortic, common iliac, and pelvic regions are removed en bloc.

            (1) Comparable cure rates between surgery and radiotherapy are the rule in the treatment of early-stage disease. The best treatment of very bulky cervical cancers, which appear to be limited to the cervix, is still debated, but will usually be multimodal.

            (2) The **ovaries may be preserved with** surgical treatment, allowing for continued hormonal function in premenopausal women.

            (3) Five-year survival rates with surgery alone range from 75 to 100% for stage IA and IIA patients, depending on operative findings. Postoperative radiation with or without chemotherapy may improve survival in some cases.

        b. Radiotherapy. This treatment modality may be used for **all stages of cervical cancer,** either for curative or palliative intent. A series of randomized trials in the 1990s solidified the role of

---

TABLE 37-1   Staging System for Cervical Cancer

Stage I: Carcinoma is confined to cervix
  Stage IA: Microscopic tumors ≤5 mm deep or ≤7 mm wide
      Stage IA1: Invasion ≤3 mm in depth and ≤7 mm in width
      Stage IA2: Invasion >3 mm and ≤5 mm in depth, and ≤7 mm in width
  Stage IB: All other cases of stage I

Stage II: Carcinoma extends beyond cervix but not onto pelvic sidewall. Cancer extends into vagina but not lower third.
  Stage IIA: No obvious parametrial involvement
  Stage IIB: Obvious parametrial involvement

Stage III: Carcinoma extends to pelvic sidewall. On rectal examination, there is no cancer-free space between tumor and pelvic sidewall. Tumor extends to lower third of vagina. All cases of hydronephrosis and nonfunctioning kidney should be included in stage III diagnoses unless another cause for these conditions can be found.
  Stage IIIA: Tumor extends to lower third of vagina, with no extension to pelvic sidewall
  Stage IIIB: Extension onto pelvic sidewall, hydronephrosis, or nonfunctioning kidney

Stage IV: Carcinoma extends beyond true pelvis or clinically involves mucosa of bladder or rectum
  Stage IVA: Spread to mucosa of bladder or rectum
  Stage IVB: Spread beyond true pelvis

---

chemotherapy as an effective radiation **sensitizer.** Currently, chemotherapy, usually weekly intravenous cisplatin, is **included in most situations in which radiation therapy is used.**

   (1) Primary treatment usually involves **external beam radiotherapy (EBRT)** to the pelvis followed by intracavitary treatment or **brachytherapy.**
   (2) EBRT may be extended to include the para-aortic lymph nodes if they are involved or are at high risk for occult involvement.
   (3) Radiotherapy may be administered **after radical hysterectomy** for high-risk patients, including those with positive surgical margins, lymph–vascular space involvement, and disease within lymph nodes.
   (4) **Five-year survival rates with radiotherapy alone** are comparable for survival with surgery alone for stages IA and IIA disease.
   (5) For advanced-stage disease localized to the pelvis, five-year survival varies from 50 to 80%. For metastatic disease out of the pelvis, survival is less than 15%.

5. Follow-up. Approximately 35% of patients with invasive cervical cancer are estimated to have persistent or recurrent disease. Most of these (85%) have a recurrence of disease within 3 years of the initial treatment.
   a. Frequent checkups are mandatory in the first 3 years. Evaluations include pelvic examinations, careful palpation of nodal groups, Pap smears, and radiologic imaging.
   b. Suspicious signs and symptoms include a persistent cervical or vaginal mass, unilateral leg edema, hydronephrosis, pelvic or sciatic pain, vaginal discharge, and palpable supraclavicular or groin nodes.

6. Treatment of recurrent disease. Treatment depends on whether recurrent disease is confined to the pelvis or is distant.
   a. Pelvic confined
      (1) Of **patients treated primarily with surgery,** 25% are saved after recurrence of the disease with pelvic radiotherapy.
      (2) In **patients treated primarily by radiotherapy** and in whom extensive presurgical and intraoperative evaluations reveal no evidence of metastatic tumor, partial or total **pelvic exenteration** (e.g., en bloc removal of the uterus, cervix, vagina, parametrium, bladder,

and rectum) is appropriate. This surgery often involves colostomy, urinary diversion, and vaginal reconstruction. It can be curative in up to 70% of cases.

    b. Distant recurrence. These patients are usually treated with chemotherapy. Cures are exceedingly rare, and response rates are variable and of limited duration. Radiotherapy can be used for the palliation of painful metastases.

II   ENDOMETRIAL CANCER

This disease is the most common gynecologic malignancy and the most curable.

A Epidemiology

1. **Incidence.** Endometrial cancer will eventually affect 2 to 3% of women in the United States.
2. **Risk factors.** Increased risk of endometrial cancer has been associated with factors related to prolonged or increased estrogen exposure without the controlling effects of adequate progestin or progesterone. Conditions associated with excess estrogen include:
   - **a. Early menarche**
   - **b. Late menopause**
   - **c. Obesity** resulting in increased conversion of androstenedione to estrone in fat cells
   - **d. Chronic anovulation or polycystic ovarian disease,** which is associated with conversion of adrenal or ovarian androstenedione (an androgenic precursor to estrogens) in the peripheral adipose tissue to estrone (a weak estrogen). As a result, ovulation and the subsequent production of progesterone, a potent "antiestrogenic" hormone, ceases. Unabated stimulation of the endometrium by estrone leads to endometrial hyperplasia (a premalignant lesion) and endometrial carcinoma.
   - **e. Exogenous unopposed estrogen.** A significant correlation exists between use of exogenous oral estrogen and endometrial cancer when estrogen therapy is administered without the protective effects of a progestin.
   - **f. Tamoxifen.** This agent acts as an antiestrogen in the breast but stimulates the endometrium similarly to estrogen, resulting in an increased risk of endometrial cancer (relative risk of 7). The therapeutic benefit in appropriately selected women with breast cancer outweighs this risk.
   - **g. Estrogen-secreting tumors.** Granulosa and theca cell ovarian tumors produce active estrogen and have been associated with a 25% incidence of a concurrent endometrial carcinoma.
   - **h. Other factors.** A history of breast and ovarian cancers is associated with an increased risk of a concomitant endometrial carcinoma. In addition, a history of hypertension and diabetes mellitus is associated with an increased risk of endometrial carcinoma, although these factors may be related to obesity.
3. The **Lynch II syndrome,** also called **hereditary nonpolyposis colorectal cancer syndrome,** is an autosomal dominant inherited predisposition to developing cancer. Endometrial cancer is the second most common cancer in women of Lynch II families. It is recommended that affected women consider prophylactic hysterectomy when childbearing is complete.
4. Factors associated with **decreased risk** are smoking, high parity, and use of oral contraceptives. Endometrial cancer that occurs in the absence of estrogenic risk factors is rare and often has a worse prognosis with more aggressive cell types and early metastases.

B Endometrial hyperplasia, which may be a precursor to endometrial carcinoma

1. **Types of endometrial hyperplasia** are classified based on the extent of endometrial gland crowding and on cellular atypia.
   - **a. Simple hyperplasia** without atypia is associated with a 1% risk of progression to cancer. For simple hyperplasia with atypia, the risk is 8%.
   - **b. Complex hyperplasia** without atypia is associated with a 3% risk of progression to cancer. For complex hyperplasia **with atypia, the risk is 29%.**

2. The **diagnosis of endometrial hyperplasia** must be established with adequate sampling of the endometrium in any woman with abnormal bleeding who is older than 35 years of age.

3. Treatment of endometrial hyperplasia
   a. **Young women desiring fertility** may be treated with 3 to 6 months of progestin therapy, followed by a repeat endometrial sampling.
   b. Proper sampling of the endometrium of **perimenopausal and postmenopausal women** with dilation and curettage (D&C) to ensure proper diagnosis is essential.
      (1) For hyperplasia without atypia, initial treatment is **conservative**: 3 to 6 months of progestin therapy followed by a repeat endometrial sampling.
      (2) **Hysterectomy** is recommended for women with complex atypical hyperplasia and for women with persistent hyperplasia after treatment with a progestational agent.

C Endometrial carcinoma

1. **Symptoms.** The most common symptom of endometrial carcinoma is irregular menses or postmenopausal bleeding. Any woman older than 35 years of age with heavy menses or bleeding throughout the month should have an endometrial biopsy.

2. **Age.** The median age for endometrial cancer is 61 years. The largest number of patients is between 50 and 59 years of age.

3. **Histology.** The **principal histologic subtype** of endometrial carcinoma is **endometrioid adenocarcinoma** (75 to 85%). The remaining subtypes include mucinous, papillary serous, clear cell, and squamous carcinoma. **Papillary serous and clear cell** subtypes are associated with a lower survival rate. Histologic differentiation correlates with depth of myometrial penetration, pelvic and periaortic lymphatic metastases, and overall 5-year survival.

4. **Staging** is based on surgical findings (Table 37-2).

5. Diagnosis and staging evaluation
   a. **D&C.** This procedure is the definitive method of diagnosis. However, an **office biopsy** may yield a diagnosis without the additional need for a D&C.

TABLE 37-2 Staging System for Endometrial Carcinoma

Stage I: Confined to uterus
  Stage IA: Tumor limited to endometrium
  Stage IB: Tumor invades less than one-half of the myometrium
  Stage IC: Tumor invades more than one-half of the myometrium

Stage II: Involvement of cervix
  Stage IIA: Endocervical glandular involvement
  Stage IIB: Cervical stromal invasion

Stage III
  Stage IIIA: Tumor invades serosa or adnexa, or positive peritoneal cytology
  Stage IIIB: Vaginal metastases
  Stage IIIC: Metastases to pelvic or paraaortic nodes

Stage IV: Mucosal involvement of bladder or rectum or extension beyond true pelvis
  Stage IVA: Tumor invades bladder or bowel mucosa
  Stage IVB: Distant metastases, including inguinal lymph nodes

For all stages, the degree of differentiation is noted. G1, G2, G3.

   b. Preoperative workup should include a chest radiograph. A computed tomography (CT) scan or other imaging studies of the abdomen and pelvis is optional.

6. **Treatment.** A surgical staging evaluation includes total abdominal hysterectomy, bilateral salpingo-oophorectomy, peritoneal cytology (e.g., washings of the pelvis and abdomen), and omentectomy. **Intraoperative evaluation** of the depth of uterine invasion may be performed by a pathologist. Sampling of **nodes from the pelvic and para-aortic regions** is recommended for patients with poorly differentiated cancer, tumor invasion through more than half of the uterine wall, or cervical extension of tumor. Some experts recommend sampling the lymph nodes in all cases because of the uncertainty associated with intraoperative frozen section.

   a. **Low-risk patients** comprise those with **stage IA, grade 1 or 2 carcinomas.** This group of tumors has few poor prognostic features. Surgery (total abdominal hysterectomy and bilateral salpingo-oophorectomy) alone is usually considered adequate treatment. Disease-free survival rate is 96%.

   b. **Intermediate-risk patients** are those with **grade 3 tumors; stage IB, IC, IIA, IIB; and positive peritoneal cytology with less than one-third myometrial invasion** and **no other extrauterine spread.** These patients may be offered pelvic irradiation, vaginal cuff irradiation, or hormonal therapy.

   c. **High-risk patients** include those with **adnexal spread, node metastases, outer one-third myometrial invasion,** or **grade 3 tumors with any invasion.** Adjuvant radiotherapy may be beneficial.

   d. **Stage IV carcinomas.** Treatment in these patients must be individualized. In most instances, treatment programs involve surgery with adjuvant radiation therapy, chemotherapy, or hormonal therapy.

   e. **Recurrent disease.** Treatment for recurrent disease must be individualized, depending on the extent and site of recurrence, hormone receptor status, and the patient's health. Treatment programs may include exenterative procedures, radiotherapy, chemotherapy, and hormonal therapy.

III ▪ EPITHELIAL OVARIAN CANCER

This is cancer arising from the epithelial surface of the ovary. Epithelial ovarian cancer accounts for 90% of ovarian cancers. It is the most difficult gynecologic cancer to diagnose because symptoms are nonspecific. The remaining 10% of ovarian cancers, classified as "nonepithelial ovarian cancers," arise from the ovarian germ cells, or sex cord and stromal cells; for a detailed description, see IV.

A Epidemiology

1. **Incidence.** The incidence begins to increase in the fifth decade and continues to increase until the eighth decade. Ovarian cancer is the **leading cause of death attributable to gynecologic cancers in the United States.** Approximately 1 in 70 women (1.7%) will contract ovarian cancer.

2. **Risk factors**

   a. **Family history** of ovarian cancer is the strongest risk factor for the disease; however, **most ovarian cancer is not familial.**
      (1) The risk is 4 to 5% if one relative is affected.
      (2) The risk is 7% if two relatives are affected.

   b. **Mutations in autosomal-dominant tumor suppressor genes, BRCA1 and BRCA2,** which are located on chromosomes 17 and 13, respectively, are identified in 5 to 10% of patients with ovarian cancer.
      (1) These genes account for most cases of familial breast ovarian cancer and confer an increased risk of ovarian cancer. The penetrance of the genes is variable but may confer a risk of 20 to 50%.

(2) Approximately 2% of Ashkenazi Jews are carriers of mutations in one of these genes. **Familial breast ovarian cancer syndrome** should be suspected if multiple family members have breast and ovarian cancer, if the age of onset of cancers is early, if multiple primary sites of cancer are noted in one patient, or if male breast cancer occurs in the family (likely BRCA2 mutation).

c. Low parity and infertility are risk factors associated with excess ovulation, which, in turn, may be an irritant to the ovary, increasing the propensity for cancer development.

3. Use of **oral contraceptives** is correlated with a **decreased risk** of ovarian cancer. Whether this is a marker for fertility rather than an independent protective factor is unclear.

4. **Preventive measures** include **prophylactic oophorectomy,** which should be offered to high-risk patients. These patients still have a 2% risk of developing primary peritoneal carcinoma, a cancer that is histologically identical to ovarian carcinoma but arises from the epithelial surfaces of the abdomen and pelvis. Older women having pelvic surgery should consider prophylactic oophorectomy even if they are not considered high risk.

B **Diagnosis**

1. Ovarian cancer usually produces **nonspecific symptoms** until the disease is advanced. In more than 70% of cases, the ovarian disease has spread beyond the pelvis before the diagnosis is made.
   a. Abdominal distention caused by ascites is often the presenting complaint.
   b. Lower abdominal pain, a pelvic mass, and weight loss are additional features.

2. **Early diagnosis of ovarian cancer** is rare, but it may be identified on bimanual pelvic examination or using radiologic imaging studies.

3. There is **no reliable screening test.**
   a. Although **CA-125 levels** are elevated above the normal range in more than 85% of patients with advanced ovarian cancer, these levels should not be used for screening purposes because of the high number of false-negative and false-positive results. This is especially true in early disease when screening would be of most benefit.
   b. Pelvic ultrasound is helpful in characterizing the size and architecture of the adnexal mass. Approximately 95% of ovarian cancers are larger than 5 cm. Multicystic and solid components and free fluid in the cul-de-sac are ultrasonic features suggestive of ovarian carcinoma. Ultrasound screening combined with CA-125 testing has not been shown to improve early detection rates, even in high-risk patients.
   c. For lack of better strategy for screening, many physicians offer annual or biannual testing with **CA-125 and ultrasound to patients with a family history of ovarian cancer.**

4. **Abdominopelvic CT scan, barium enema,** and **chest radiography** are helpful in the evaluation of disease in women suspected of having ovarian cancer.

C **Staging.** Surgical findings are used to stage ovarian cancer (Table 37-3). More than 70% of patients have stage III disease at the time of diagnosis.

D **Predominant histologic types**

1. **Serous** tumors account for 40% of ovarian carcinoma.
2. **Mucinous** tumors account for 10% of ovarian carcinoma.
3. **Endometrioid tumors** account for 10% of ovarian carcinoma.
4. **Clear-cell carcinoma,** which is more common in Asia, accounts for 6% of ovarian carcinoma. These cancers appear to be more resistant to chemotherapy than serous, mucinous, and endometrioid ovarian carcinomas.
5. **Small-cell ovarian cancers** are rare and have a poor prognosis.
6. **Borderline ovarian tumors (also called "ovarian carcinoma of low malignant potential")** account for 15% of epithelial malignancies. This distinct type of ovarian carcinoma has the potential

TABLE 37-3   Staging System for Ovarian Cancer

Stage I: Limited to ovaries
Stage IA: Limited to one ovary; no ascites containing malignant cells; no tumor on external surface of ovary; capsule intact
Stage IB: Limited to both ovaries; no ascites containing malignant cells; no tumor on external surface of ovary; capsule intact
Stage IC: Tumor either stage IA or IB but with ascites containing malignant cells, tumor on surface of one or both ovaries, or rupture of tumor capsule

Stage II: Involvement of one or both ovaries with pelvic extension
Stage IIA: Extension or metastases to uterus or tubes or both
Stage IIB: Extension to other pelvic tissues
Stage IIC: Tumor either stage IIA or IIB but with ascites containing malignant cells, tumor on surface of one or both ovaries, or rupture of tumor capsule

Stage III: Involvement of one or both ovaries with peritoneal metastases outside pelvis or superficial liver metastases or retroperitoneal nodes containing cancer
Stage IIIA: Tumor limited to pelvis with negative nodes but microscopic seeding of peritoneum
Stage IIIB: Peritoneal implants ≤2 cm in diameter with negative nodes
Stage IIIC: Implants >2 cm in diameter or positive retroperitoneal or inguinal nodes

Stage IV: Involvement of one or both ovaries with distant metastases; this can include positive pleural effusion and intrahepatic metastases

to metastasize but not to invade tissues. The cell type may be papillary serous or mucinous. With surgical debulking, most of these cancers are curable. The average age at diagnosis is 48 years. Patients with these tumors have higher survival rates, and most are diagnosed in stage I.

E **Clinical course of ovarian carcinoma**

1. The **initial spread** of ovarian carcinoma is to adjacent peritoneal surfaces, omentum, and retroperitoneal lymph nodes.

2. **Extra-abdominal and intrahepatic metastases** occur late in the disease and only in a small percentage of cases.

3. **Bowel obstruction** occurs as a terminal event and results from massive serosal involvement.

F **Treatment.**   A combination of surgery and chemotherapy is necessary.

1. **Goals of surgery** are to determine the extent of the disease through **staging** and to remove or **debulk** as much tumor as possible. Surgery may include the following:
   a. Exploratory laparotomy through a vertical abdominal incision, allowing a thorough evaluation of the upper abdomen
   b. Peritoneal washings from the pelvis and upper abdomen
   c. Inspection of all peritoneal and diaphragmatic surfaces
   d. Excision of pelvic and para-aortic lymph nodes
   e. Omentectomy
   f. Debulking tumor with the goal of leaving behind as little residual disease as possible

2. **Ovarian cancer is extremely sensitive to chemotherapy.** However, this cancer has a tendency to recur.
   a. **Paclitaxel** and **carboplatin** are currently the standard treatment for all patients with ovarian cancer who have a tumor of stage IB or greater. Patients with stage IA grade 1 or 2 cancers may forgo chemotherapy.

b. Side effects of paclitaxel include neuropathy, alopecia, myelosuppression, neuropathy, hypersensitivity reaction, and bradycardia.

c. Side effects of carboplatin include nausea and vomiting, myelosuppression, and constipation.

G **Recurrent ovarian cancer.** Retreatment involves surgery, paclitaxel, and carboplatin, or second-line treatment agents. With time, ovarian cancer develops chemotherapy resistance. Because advanced ovarian cancer usually recurs and 5-year survival in stage III disease is only 20%, patients should be encouraged to enroll in clinical trials using novel treatments.

IV NONEPITHELIAL OVARIAN CANCER

This form of ovarian cancer arises from the germ cells and sex cord stromal cells of the ovary. These rare cancers account for less than 10% of ovarian tumors. Staging is the same as for epithelial ovarian cancer (see Table 37-3). Treatment consists of surgical staging or debulking, occasionally followed by chemotherapy as detailed for each cancer subtype.

A **Germ cell tumors.** Benign germ cell tumors, called "dermoids," account for 25 to 30% of ovarian neoplasms. Malignant germ cell tumors are believed to arise from primitive germ cells in the ovary. These cancers represent 5% of all ovarian malignancies but account for more than two thirds of all malignant ovarian neoplasms in women younger than 20 years of age. When disease is limited to one ovary, it is appropriate to **leave the uterus and other ovary in place,** as long as a complete staging, including pelvic and para-aortic lymph node dissection, is performed.

1. **Dysgerminomas.** Histologically, the undifferentiated germ cells present as sheets of uniform polyhedral cells. There is a characteristic lymphocytic infiltrate within delicate fibrous septa. Other characteristics of dysgerminomas include the following:
   a. They are the **most common malignant germ cell tumor,** accounting for approximately 40% of this type of tumor.
   b. Ninety percent of dysgerminomas are found in women younger than 30 years of age.
   c. The propensity for lymphatic invasion is great.
   d. Syncytiotrophoblasts in the tumor occasionally secrete detectable amounts of human chorionic gonadotropin (hCG).
   e. Bilateral tumors occur in more than 20% of cases; 50% of these are macroscopic.
   f. Tumors are exquisitely sensitive to chemotherapy, and the cure rate approaches 95%.

2. **Immature teratomas.** Histologically, a mixture of differentiated fetal tissue representing three germinal layers is present. Usually the immature element is **neural tissue.** Immature teratomas are further characterized by the following:
   a. They account for 20% of all germ cell tumors.
   b. Tumors are rarely bilateral, although 10% of patients have a benign dermoid in the contralateral ovary.
   c. Prognosis is excellent. Adjuvant chemotherapy is recommended for most patients. Patients with low-grade, stage I disease may be followed with surgery alone.

3. **Endodermal sinus tumors or yolk sac tumors.** The classic histologic finding is the **Schiller-Duval body,** a central vessel lined with columnar cells. Endodermal sinus tumors are further characterized by the following:
   a. They account for 20% of all germ cell tumors.
   b. The **median age of patients** with endodermal sinus tumors is 19 years.
   c. Tumors are rarely bilateral.
   d. Alpha-fetoprotein (AFP) is detectable in the serum of most patients and acts as a tumor marker.
   e. All patients should receive postoperative chemotherapy.
   f. In patients with complete surgical excision of tumor prior to chemotherapy, survival is 96%. Survival with incomplete resection is 55%.

4. **Embryonal carcinomas.** The histologic appearance of undifferentiated embryonal tissue consists of solid sheets of anaplastic cells with abundant clear cytoplasm, hyperchromatic nuclei, and numerous mitotic figures. Embryonal carcinoma is further characterized by the following:

   a. This rare cancer occurs in young females; the **median age of patients** with embryonal carcinoma is 15 years.

   b. Tumors elaborate both AFP and hCG. These trophic hormones may be responsible for precocious puberty in prepubertal girls.

   c. Most often, tumors are unilateral with explosive growth tendencies, leading to large tumor masses and acute abdominal pain. Tumors are rarely bilateral.

   d. Surgery and chemotherapy result in cures for approximately one third of patients.

5. **Nongestational choriocarcinomas.** These primary tumors must be distinguished from metastatic disease to the ovary from gestational choriocarcinomas. The histologic appearance is that of atypical to highly anaplastic cytotrophoblastic and syncytiotrophoblastic elements. These tumors are further characterized by the following:

   a. This rare cancer usually occurs in women of reproductive age.

   b. Tumors are rarely bilateral.

   c. hCG is detectable in the serum of most patients and acts as a tumor marker.

   d. Tumors can present as a pelvic mass and precocious puberty in prepubertal girls.

   e. Treatment with surgery and chemotherapy results in 80% survival.

6. **Polyembryonal cancer.** This cancer has the histologic appearance of embryoid bodies in various states of development. This tumor is further characterized by the following:

   a. This rare cancer usually occurs in women of early reproductive age.

   b. Tumors are rarely bilateral.

   c. hCG and AFP are often detectable in the serum of patients and act as a tumor marker.

7. **Mixed germ cell tumors.** Approximately 10% of germ cell tumors are comprised of two or more subtypes of cancer. Treatment and prognosis are based on the most severe element.

B **Sex cord stromal neoplasms.** The sex cord cells are granulosa cells and the male homolog, the Sertoli cells. Stromal cells include theca cells, Leydig cells, and fibroblasts. Tumors arising from these cells often produce estrogens and androgens. Granulosa cells, Sertoli cells, and theca cells are usually estrogenic. Leydig cells and specific steroid cells are usually androgenic.

1. **Juvenile granulosa cell tumors** that occur in premenarchal women induce abnormal bleeding and breast development. Early-stage disease is curable with surgery, but the prognosis for disease spread beyond the ovary is poor.

2. **Adult granulosa cell tumors** have the following characteristics:

   a. They are bilateral in less than 5% of cases.

   b. Tumors vary in size from microscopic to tumors that fill the abdomen.

   c. Tumors are characterized histologically by **Call-Exner bodies** (e.g., rosettes or follicles of granulosa cells, often with a central clearing).

   d. Ninety percent of cases present as stage I disease and are usually curable. More advanced stage disease is prone to recurrence, often many years after initial treatment.

3. **Sertoli-Leydig cell tumors or arrhenoblastoma** are rare tumors of mesenchymal origin.

   a. Their usual endocrine activity is androgenic.

   b. Defeminization is the classic feature of the androgen-secreting tumors, including breast and uterine atrophy, which is followed by masculinization, including hirsutism, acne, receding hairline, clitorimegaly, and deepening of the voice. Prognosis is based on the extent of differentiation.

C **Gonadoblastomas.** These tumors are composed of **germ cells and stromal cells**. They occur in **dysgenic ovaries** commonly present in individuals with a Y chromosome because of a mosaic genotype (46X/46,XY) or testicular feminization (46,XY with androgen insensitivity). Both ovaries are usually affected, and it is recommended that these individuals undergo prophylactic bilateral oophorectomy. **Dysgerminomas** or occasionally other germ cell malignancies occur in 50% of patients with gonadoblastomas.

V VAGINAL CANCER

A **Squamous cell carcinomas.** These cancers are usually located in the upper half of the vagina. They are the most common histologic type.

1. Symptoms
   a. The most common symptom is **vaginal discharge,** which is often bloody.
   b. Because of the **elasticity of the posterior vaginal fornix,** tumors may be large before they are symptomatic.

2. **Age.** This rare, malignant cancer occurs in women between 35 and 70 years of age.

3. **Lymphatic spread.** The upper vagina is drained by the common iliac and hypogastric (internal iliac) nodes, whereas the lower vagina is drained by the regional lymph nodes of the femoral triangle.

4. **Staging** (Table 37-4)

5. **Treatment.** Treatment is primarily by radiotherapy. Large carcinomas of the vault or vaginal walls are treated initially with external radiation; this shrinks the neoplasm so that local radiation therapy will be more effective. Occasionally, vaginal cancer is amenable to primary surgical excision or to excision with a radical hysterectomy and upper vaginectomy.

6. Five-year survival rates
   a. **Stage I:** 80 to 90%
   b. **Stage II:** 60%
   c. **Stage III:** 40%
   d. **Stage IV:** 0%

B **Diethylstilbestrol (DES)-related adenocarcinoma (clear cell carcinoma)**   DES was used in the 1940s through the early 1970s in high-risk pregnancies (e.g., diabetes, habitual abortion, and threatened abortion) to prevent miscarriage. In all documented cases of genital tract abnormalities, maternal DES use began before the 18th week of pregnancy.

1. Age
   a. The mean age for development of clear cell adenocarcinoma of the vagina is 19 years for patients with a history of DES exposure.
   b. The risk for development of these carcinomas through the age of 24 years in DES-exposed women has been calculated to be between 0.14 and 1.4/1000.

TABLE 37-4   Staging System for Vaginal Cancer
Stage I: Limited to vaginal mucosa
Stage II: Involvement of subvaginal tissue but no extension onto pelvic sidewall
Stage III: Extension onto pelvic sidewall
Stage IV: Extension beyond true pelvis or involvement of mucosa of bladder or rectum

2. **Characteristics of clear cell carcinoma**
    a. Approximately 40% of the cancers occur in the cervix, and the other 60% occur primarily in the upper half of the vagina.
    b. The **incidence of lymph node metastases** is high—about 16% in stage I and 30% or more in stage II.

3. **Treatment**
    a. If the cancer is confined to the cervix and the upper vagina, radical hysterectomy and upper vaginectomy with pelvic lymphadenectomy and ovarian preservation are recommended.
    b. Advanced tumors and lesions involving the lower vagina are treated more appropriately by radiation, which should include treatment of the pelvic nodes and parametrial tissues.

4. **Prognosis. Five-year survival rates** are better than those for the squamous tumors of the cervix and upper vagina, probably because of earlier detection.

VI VULVAR CARCINOMA

A Epidemiology. Factors associated with vulvar carcinoma include the following:

1. A history of vulvar condylomata or granulomatous venereal disease

2. A history of vulvar Paget disease

3. A history of vulvar carcinoma in situ

4. A history of cervical or vaginal cancer

5. More than 50% of the patients are between the ages of 60 and 79 years. Fewer than 15% are younger than 40 years of age.

B Etiology. Little is known about causal factors in vulvar carcinoma. Recently, HPV types 16 and 18 have been detected in squamous cancer of the vulva.

C Symptoms. Recognition of a lesion is often accompanied by a delay in diagnosis because of either self-treatment by the patient or lack of recognition by the treating physician. Vulvar cancer usually presents with:

1. A history of chronic **vulvar irritation** or soreness

2. A **visible lesion on the labia,** which is often painful or pruritic

D Histology. Squamous carcinoma comprises 90% of these tumors. The remaining 10% consist of malignant melanoma, basal cell carcinoma, and sarcoma. The Bartholin gland may give rise to vulvar adenocarcinoma.

E Patterns of spread

1. **Local expansion** involves the contiguous structures of the urethra, vagina, perineum, anus, rectum, and pubic bone.

2. **Lymphatic spread** follows the lymphatic drainage pattern of the vulva, which includes superficial inguinal nodes, deep femoral groups, and pelvic nodes.

3. **Hematogenous spread** occurs in the advanced or recurrent cases.

F Diagnosis. Incisional or excisional biopsy of the suspect lesion under local or general anesthesia confirms the diagnosis.

G Pretreatment evaluation. Clinical assessment of tumor size (T), nodes (N), and metastases (M) and surgical staging are appropriate (Table 37-5).

TABLE 37-5   Clinical Assessment and Staging System for Vulvar Carcinoma

ASSESSMENT

Tumor size (T)
T1: Tumor ≤2 cm in size that is confined to vulva
T2: Tumor >2 cm in size that is confined to vulva
T3: Tumor of any size that spreads to urethra, vagina, perineum, or anus
T4: Tumor of any size that infiltrates bladder and rectal mucosa or is fixed to bone

Node (N)
N0: No regional nodes palpable
N1: Unilateral regional lymph node metastases
N2: Bilateral regional lymph node metastases

Metastases (M)
M0: No metastases
M1: Distant metastases, including pelvic nodes

STAGING

Stage I: T1 N0 M0
Stage II: T2 N0 M0
Stage III: T3 N0 M0, T3 N1 M0, T1 N1 M0, T2 N1 M0
Stage IVA: T1 N2 M0; T2 N2 M0; T3 N2 M0; or T4, any N, M0
Stage IVB: any T, any N, M1

H **Treatment.**   Surgical treatment is individualized.

1. **T1 lesions (tumor 2 cm or smaller in size)**
   a. Radical local excision of the lesion with a 1-cm margin laterally and a depth down to the inferior fascia is indicated when:
      (1) Biopsy of the tumor reveals a depth of invasion of less than 1 mm
      (2) Tumor is unifocal
      (3) Remaining vulva is normal
   b. No groin dissection is necessary.

2. **T2 and early T3 tumors without suspect inguinal nodes**
   a. Radical vulvectomy may be partial or total, depending on the size and location of the lesion.
   b. Bilateral inguinal and femoral lymphadenectomy may be warranted. Ipsilateral inguinal and femoral lymphadenectomy may be considered when the lesion is well lateralized.

3. **Tumors with disease in inguinal nodes** are treated with lymphadenectomy. If there are more than two histologically positive nodes, external beam radiation is administered to the groin and pelvis.

4. **Advanced disease.** Individualized treatment may include surgery, radiation, and chemotherapy. Pelvic radiotherapy is recommended for patients with involved nodes. Survival is poor.

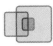

Study Questions for Chapter 37

DIRECTIONS: *Match the statement below with the best system above. Each answer may be used once, more than once, or not at all.*

QUESTIONS 1–2

[A] Brain
[B] Ureter
[C] Liver
[D] Intestine
[E] Spleen

1. Advanced cervical cancer can affect this structure by extension and pressure effects.

2. Advanced ovarian cancer often affects this structure by spread and encroachment.

DIRECTIONS: *Each of the numbered items or incomplete statements in this section is followed by answers or by completions of the statement. Select the ONE lettered answer or completion that is BEST in each case.*

QUESTIONS 3–4

A 48-year-old woman, gravida 2, para 1, SAB 1 reports bleeding after intercourse. Speculum examination reveals a lesion on the cervix that involves the upper vagina. Bimanual examination does not reveal parametrial thickening.

3. Given the above information and assuming the rest of her work-up is normal, she has stage _____ cervical cancer.

[A] IA2
[B] IIA
[C] IIB
[D] IIIA
[E] IIIB

4. After performing an intravenous pyelogram, it is discovered that her left kidney has hydronephrosis. There is no history of kidney disease in this patient. Cystoscopy, sigmoidoscopy, and chest radiograph are all unremarkable. The final stage of her cervical cancer is

[A] IIA
[B] IIB
[C] IIIA
[D] IIIB
[E] IV

5. A 42-year-old woman, gravida 1, para 1 presents to you because she wants to decrease her risk of ovarian cancer via a prophylactic oophorectomy. She has no chronic medical problems. Her gynecologic history is remarkable for first sexual intercourse at age 15 years, four sexual partners in her entire life, and breastfeeding of her only child. Her pap smear has shown exposure to human papilloma virus (HPV). She is currently taking birth control pills. She smokes one pack per week (for the last 10 years)

and has an occasional drink with her husband. Her family history is remarkable for breast cancer in her mother and ovarian cancer in her maternal aunt. The most significant risk factor for developing ovarian cancer is her

- [A] Family history
- [B] HPV
- [C] Low parity
- [D] Birth control pills
- [E] Smoking

6. A 43-year-old woman, gravida 1, para 0, SAB 1 has undergone colposcopy for evaluation of a high-grade lesion found on Pap smear. The squamocolumnar junction was visible in its entirety, and the endocervical curettage was normal. A directed biopsy of the cervix revealed a 1-mm focus of invasion. The next best step in management is

- [A] Endometrial biopsy (EMB)
- [B] Cryotherapy of cervix (Cryo)
- [C] Cold knife conization of cervix (CKC)
- [D] Simple hysterectomy and bilateral salpingo-oophorectomy (TAH-BSO)
- [E] Radical hysterectomy (Rad Hyst)

QUESTIONS 7–11

DIRECTIONS: Match the statement below with the histology above. Each answer may be used once, more than once, or not at all.

- [A] Squamous
- [B] Serous
- [C] Mucinous
- [D] Endometrioid
- [E] Clear
- [F] Small
- [G] Papillary serous
- [H] Dysgerminoma
- [I] Teratoma
- [J] Endodermal sinus
- [K] Choriocarcinoma
- [L] Sertoli-Leydig
- [M] Gonadoblastoma
- [N] Melanoma

7. Most common histology for cervical cancer

8. Subtype of endometrial cancer with very poor prognosis; is also type of borderline ovarian tumor

9. Most common malignant germ cell tumor

10. Uncommon, aggressive vulvar cancer that is known as the most common cancer to metastasize to the placenta

11. Most common endometrial cancer

Answers and Explanations

1. B [Table 37-1] **2. D** [Table 37-3, III E 3]. Cervical cancer extends laterally toward the pelvic sidewall and can encroach on the ureter resulting in hydronephrosis (Stage IIIB). However, ovarian cancer spreads out over the peritoneal surface and implants on the peritoneum and intestinal wall. This can eventually lead to bowel obstruction.

3. The answer is B [Table 37-1]. Carcinoma that extends beyond the cervix but not onto the pelvic sidewall is considered stage II. If there is also no parametrial involvement, then it is a IIA.

4. The answer is D [Table 37-1 and I D 3]. Staging for cervical cancer is entirely clinical (cervical biopsies, physical examination, imaging of kidneys, sigmoidoscopy, cystoscopy, and chest radiograph) rather than surgical (as for the rest of the gynecologic cancers).

5. The answer is A [III A 2, 3]. The family history of ovarian cancer is the strongest risk factor for developing ovarian cancer, especially if it is a first-degree relative. The familial breast ovarian cancer syndrome that is usually associated with an autosomal dominant mutation in the BRCA1 and BRCA2 genes should be suspected when multiple breast and ovarian cancers occur in one family. Mutations in these genes account for 5 to 10% of all cases of ovarian cancer. Oral contraception is associated with a decreased risk of ovarian cancer. HPV is associated with cervical, not ovarian, cancer. Low parity is a risk factor for ovarian cancer but is not the strongest risk factor here. Smoking is associated with many types of cancers but does not have a large relative risk in ovarian cancer.

6. The answer is C [I C 1]. The diagnosis of microinvasive cervical cancer can be made only by thorough examination of a cone biopsy specimen. If the diagnosis of microinvasion is confirmed, further treatment may involve a simple hysterectomy only. An endometrial biopsy is not necessary for further evaluation of HGSIL (high-grade cervical lesion). Cryotherapy is not a good option because it may not completely destroy the microinvasive lesion (therefore no cure) and it does not provide a pathologic specimen for further evaluation of the lesion. In this patient, a TAH-BSO is not the best initial step here because this patient has no children and is still of childbearing age. A radical hysterectomy is too radical of a procedure for a microinvasive lesion. It is not without complications (e.g., urinary retention).

7. A [I D 2] **8. G** [II C 3 and III D 6] **9. H** [IV A 1] **10. N** [VI D] **11. D** [II C 3]. The most common histologic type of cervical cancer is squamous cell carcinoma (80%), followed by adenocarcinoma (15%). Papillary serous subtypes of endometrial carcinoma are associated with increased aggressiveness and low survival. However, papillary serous carcinoma of the ovary is a borderline ovarian tumor that can be treated with surgical debulking. Most of these cancers are curable. Dysgerminomas are the most common malignant germ cell tumors. Ninety percent are found in women younger than 30 years of age. These tumors are exquisitely sensitive to chemotherapy. The most common histology for vulvar carcinoma is squamous cell carcinoma (90%). Melanomas are uncommon vulvar cancers, but they are aggressive and tend to metastasize to distant locations (such as placenta and brain). The principal histologic subtype of endometrial carcinoma is endometrioid adenocarcinoma (75 to 85%).

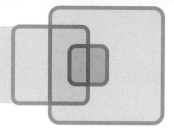

chapter 38

Medicolegal Considerations in Obstetrics and Gynecology

WILLIAM W. BECK, JR.

I · INTRODUCTION

Law defines modes of behavior among the members of a society and the groups within a society, such that conflicting interests may be resolved in a civilized fashion. Medicine is one such group. In medicine, the law permeates, defining and regulating the relationship between the physician and patient, the physician and hospital, and the physician and society. Moreover, legal issues dealing with access to medical care and consumer demands regarding health care are dominant in public policy discussions. Obstetrics and gynecology is at the cutting edge of these matters because the field involves the most critical aspects of life: conception, reproduction, and abortion. Thus, it is important for the student of medicine to understand, in a preliminary fashion, the legal issues that involve the practice of obstetrics and gynecology.

II · MALPRACTICE

A **Definition.** Malpractice is **professional misconduct** whereby a physician departs from the standards of reasonable physicians, through either a lack of skill or a lack of knowledge in carrying out professional duties.

B **Elements of negligence**

1. **Duty.** A physician has a particular duty or obligation to the patient. A **physician–patient relationship** exists when a patient comes to a physician, who agrees to undertake her care in a fiduciary manner. It is a form of **implied contract.** In this relationship, a physician must act:
   a. In accordance with standards established or accepted by a reasonable fraction of the profession practicing in a given area
   b. As a reasonable physician, taking reasonable care of a patient and not taking unreasonable risks

2. **Breach of duty.** A physician who fails to act on a specific occasion in accordance with professional norms has departed from the standard of care and has committed a breach of the duty owed to the patient. This breach must be substantiated by the testimony of an expert.

3. **Causation.** The breach of duty owed must be the proximate cause of a patient's injury for a malpractice action to exist.

4. **Damages.** Actual loss, injury, or damage must have occurred, although pain and suffering is a common report.

C **Recovery.** The patient or plaintiff must prove that it is more probable than not that the elements of negligence are satisfied (**preponderance of evidence**) to recover compensation for the damage incurred.

III PRECONCEPTION ISSUES

A constitutional right of privacy protects an individual's procreative choice from government intrusion. The **right to use contraception** was the earliest right to reproductive freedom (*Griswold v Connecticut*, 1965).

A Oral contraceptives

1. Most lawsuits regarding oral contraceptives are **product liability** cases against the manufacturer.
   a. The general rule is that a manufacturer must provide patients with a written warning of all untoward side effects.
   b. A physician must inform patients of the possible side effects and explain the alternative methods of contraception. All of these discussions must be documented.
2. A physician has a duty to:
   a. Perform a thorough physical examination
   b. Perform relevant laboratory examinations
   c. Warn patients of possible adverse side effects
   d. Closely monitor patients in whom side effects develop

B Intrauterine devices (IUDs) have been the center of legal and medical controversy surrounding contraceptives ever since the Dalkon Shield was recalled in 1974.

1. All IUDs, except for Mirena (hormone-containing device) and the ParaGard (a copper-containing device), have been withdrawn by the manufacturers because of litigation costs. Most lawsuits have been product liability cases, with claims that the IUD has caused:
   a. Uterine and pelvic infections
   b. Infertility
   c. Uterine perforation
   d. Ectopic pregnancy
2. A physician has a duty to:
   a. Inform patients of the risks involved with IUD insertion and use
   b. Explain alternative methods of contraception and their risks
   c. Perform a physical examination
   d. Perform a Papanicolaou (Pap) test and cervical cultures
   e. Examine patients in 3 months after insertion of an IUD and yearly thereafter

C Sterilization. This surgical procedure is undertaken for the express purpose of eliminating reproductive capacity.

1. Voluntary sterilization
   a. **Public hospitals** cannot refuse to perform sterilization procedures because it would abridge a woman's reproductive right of privacy.
   b. **Private physicians and hospitals** may, however, decline to perform this procedure on moral grounds.
   c. **Federal funding regulations** require that a Department of Health and Human Services consent form be signed 30 to 180 days before surgery. Consent cannot be obtained if the patient is:
      (1) Younger than 21 years of age
      (2) In labor
      (3) Under the influence of alcohol or drugs
      (4) Mentally incompetent
      (5) Having an abortion. Federal regulation is such that tubal ligation and abortion cannot be performed at the same time because the federal government will not fund abortion.

   d. A physician has a duty to inform patients that:
     (1) The operation will result in sterility.
     (2) The procedure is permanent.
     (3) There are alternative forms of contraception.
     (4) There is no guarantee of sterility; pregnancy occurs at a rate of 15 to 20/1000 cases over 10 years, with ectopic pregnancy being the main concern.

  2. Involuntary sterilization. Some states authorize involuntary sterilization of genetically retarded wards of the state. However, it is generally required that the patients:
   a. Have permanent medical conditions
   b. Have adequate sexual capacity
   c. Have a high probability of transmitting a genetic disease
   d. Be unable to care for children
   e. Be unable to use alternative methods of contraception

IV. GENETIC COUNSELING

Five percent of all newborns are born with a congenital disorder.

A. Routine genetic screening
  1. Legislation requires **phenylketonuria** and **hypothyroid** testing in newborns.
  2. Testing for **cystic fibrosis** should be discussed and offered at the prenatal visit.
  3. There are centers for voluntary **screening of sickle cell disease, homocystinuria, galactosemia,** and **maple syrup urine disease.**
  4. Prenatal **maternal serum α-fetoprotein (MSAFP)** or **multiple marker** (MSAFP, human chorionic gonadotropin, and estradiol) testing to determine the risk of neural tube defects and Down syndrome is routinely recommended for all women, including those younger than 35 years of age.

B. Particular genetic problems of which a physician must be aware include the following:
  1. Teratogens
   a. Rubella
   b. Phenytoin
   c. Alcohol
   d. Tobacco
   e. Illicit drugs (e.g., cocaine)
  2. Autosomal dominant disorders
   a. Neurofibromatosis
   b. Hereditary familial polyposis
  3. Autosomal recessive disorders
   a. Cystic fibrosis
   b. Infantile polycystic kidney disease
   c. Congenital deafness
   d. Tay-Sachs disease
   e. Thalassemia
  4. X-linked disorders
   a. Duchenne muscular dystrophy
   b. Hemophilia

C. Referral to a genetic counselor is appropriate for pregnant women if there is:
  1. A genetic or congenital abnormality in a family member
  2. A family history of a genetic problem

   3. Abnormal development in a previous child

   4. Mental retardation in a previous child

   5. Maternal age 35 years or older

   6. Specific ethnic background suggestive of a genetic abnormality (e.g., Tay-Sachs disease in Ashkenazi Jews, among others)

   7. Exposure to drugs or teratogens

   8. A history of three or more spontaneous abortions

D **Amniocentesis** must be offered to pregnant women if there is:

   1. Maternal age 35 years or older

   2. A history of multiple miscarriages

   3. A family history of genetic disease

   4. An abnormal MSAFP

V TERMINATION OF PREGNANCY

A **Right of privacy.** A woman's right to abortion falls within a right of privacy interpreted by the United States Supreme Court to exist within the Constitution. This right was upheld in *Roe v Wade*, 1973.

B **Trimester model**

   1. During the first trimester, the decision to abort is a decision that is strictly between a woman and her physician.

   2. During the second trimester, the state may impose regulations reasonably related to a woman's health.

   3. After the second trimester or after the fetus is viable, the state may regulate abortion, except when necessary to preserve a woman's health.

C **State restrictions.** Since 1973, the time of the abortion decision, states have formulated many laws to limit a woman's access to abortion. For example, in *Planned Parenthood v Casey*, 1992, the United States Supreme Court upheld a **Pennsylvania** statute.

   1. Restrictions on elective abortion imposed by the statute
      a. Physicians are required to discuss the nature, risks, and alternatives to abortion, as well as the gestational age of the fetus.
      b. A 24-hour waiting period is required between the time this information is given and the time the abortion is performed.
      c. Either parental consent or, alternatively, judicial bypass if parental consent is denied, is required for a minor.

   2. The Supreme Court struck down the provision of the statute that required spousal notification.

VI NEW REPRODUCTIVE TECHNOLOGIES

New techniques have created a change in society's concept of the family. Examples include artificial insemination by husband or donor; in vitro fertilization and embryo transfer (IVF/ET); and other assisted reproductive techniques, including gamete intrafallopian transfer, zygote intrafallopian transfer, and intracellular spermatozoa injection, donor oocytes, and embryo and oocyte freezing. A child may be born with as many as five parents: a genetic father, a social father, a genetic mother, a gestational mother, and a social mother. These technologies create legal issues of linkage, inheritance, legitimacy, adultery, confidentiality, the legal status of residual embryos, the particular "parental" responsibilities for a child's diseases and defects, and the legal status and rights of each "parent."

A **Artificial insemination**

1. **Definition.** Inoculation of a husband's semen (artificial insemination by husband [AIH]) or a donor's semen (artificial insemination by donor [AID]) into the female genital tract is called artificial insemination.

2. **Consent of the husband.** When the husband of a child's mother consents to AID, the husband obtains the same legal right and obligations as a natural parent, including:
   a. The duty to support the child
   b. The right to visitation in case of divorce

3. **Right to privacy.** Given the United States Supreme Court's recognition of a right to privacy, when a single woman requests AID, a public institution providing these services cannot abridge this woman's right to privacy and, thus, would logically have to provide this service; however, a private practitioner could choose not to provide this service.

4. **A physician has a duty to explain** that there is:
   a. No guarantee of pregnancy
   b. A possibility of birth defects that may be attributable to unknown recessive genes of the donor
   c. Little chance of sexually transmitted disease (STD) transmission because of screening and the quarantined freeze preservation of semen

5. **Liability** may arise when:
   a. A physician has not adequately screened a donor for genetic defects or STDs, including HIV.
   b. A husband's consent has not been obtained.

B **In vitro fertilization (IVF)**

1. **Definition.** In IVF, sperm and ova are obtained and incubated outside the body, and then the blastocyst is implanted into a uterus.

2. **Legal concepts**
   a. When a husband provides sperm, and a wife provides an ovum, traditional family principles apply. This is similar to AIH.
   b. When a donor provides sperm and a wife provides an ovum, legal concepts of AID and adoption apply.
   c. When the ovum comes from a female donor and is fertilized and then transferred into another woman's uterus, the legal relationships that arise are complex and not clearly formulated. The essential question is whether genetic material, a contractual relationship, or carrying and giving birth determine the claim of motherhood.

C **Surrogate motherhood**

1. **Definition.** When a wife is incapable of bearing a child, a couple enters into a contract with another woman (a surrogate mother), who agrees to be artificially inseminated with the husband's semen, to carry and bear a child, and to relinquish her rights to the child. In exchange, she receives payment for medical care, lost wages, clothing, and hospitalization.

2. **Arguments against surrogate motherhood**
   a. It undermines the traditional family model.
   b. It threatens the institution of marriage.
   c. It cheapens and destroys maternal bonding.
   d. It treats children as commodities.
   e. It exploits poor women as vehicles to fulfill the dreams of the rich.

3. **Problems arising in the surrogate contract**
   a. Surrogate mothers develop maternal feelings toward their infants and refuse to give them to the husband and his wife.

b. Surrogate mothers decide not to honor the contract and terminate the pregnancy.

c. Surrogate mothers expose the fetus to teratogens or addicting drugs.

d. The infant is defective, and the contractive couple decides not to accept it.

e. There is a multiple gestation.

D **Embryo freezing**

1. **Definition.** Embryo freezing entails the freezing of unused fertilized ova for future implantation.

2. **Problems**

a. Concerns have been raised as to the propriety of eugenic considerations and commercialism.

b. The disposition of unused embryos has been deemed unethical by some critics.

c. If the parents die, the rights and obligations of frozen embryos have yet to be decided.

VII BIRTH-RELATED SUITS

A **Wrongful conception**

1. **Definition.** Conception is deemed wrongful if it arises after:

a. Failed sterilization

b. Ineffective prescription of contraception

c. Failure to diagnose pregnancy in a timely fashion

d. Unsuccessful abortion

2. **Liability** arises secondary to a physician's negligence, resulting in the birth of an unplanned child. Negligence is based on:

a. Improper performance of a sterilization procedure or an abortion

b. Failure to ascertain the success of the procedure

c. Failure to inform the woman about the possibility of procedural failures

B **Wrongful birth and wrongful life**

1. **Wrongful birth** is an action brought by parents of a child, alleging that a child with a congenital defect was born because of negligent genetic counseling. Thus, a physician has failed to:

a. Recognize a genetic problem

b. Recognize a condition that places a fetus at risk for a genetic problem

c. Inform the mother of the ability to detect genetic problems and to offer termination

2. **Wrongful life** is an action similar to wrongful birth. However, the **child brings suit against the physician,** alleging that no life at all would have been preferable to life with a congenital defect.

VIII BIRTH INJURY

A **Definition.** A birth injury results when an obstetrician's neglect results in injury to a child (e.g., birth trauma, brain damage, or neurologic damage).

B **Negligence** may arise from a failure to:

1. Monitor fetal heart rate adequately

2. Assess the degree of risk of a pregnancy

3. Perform expedient delivery, resulting in perinatal asphyxia that leads to brain damage

4. Monitor a pregnancy adequately

5. Use obstetric forceps properly

6. Recognize possible macrosomia and the potential for shoulder dystocia and resulting Erb palsy

C Brain damage. Current studies indicate that it is impossible to isolate a single cause of brain dysfunction. The National Institutes of Health has stated that:

1. **Mental retardation is multifactorial,** resulting from a combination of genetic, biochemical, viral, and developmental factors, and is not necessarily related to birth trauma.

2. **Severe mental retardation and epilepsy** are possibly associated with birth asphyxia but only when accompanied by cerebral palsy, which is associated with birth asphyxia, prematurity, and intrauterine growth retardation.

IX INFORMED CONSENT

A General definition. "Every human being of adult years and sound mind has a right to determine what shall be done with his own body" (*Schloendorff v Society of New York Hospital*, 1914).

B Negligence theory of consent. To sue successfully under this theory, the patient or plaintiff must show that:

1. A physician was under a duty to disclose an adequate amount of material information.

2. A physician disclosed an inadequate amount of material information.

3. The patient agreed to therapy based on this inadequate information.

4. The patient was harmed.

5. If the significant information had been given, the suggested therapy would have been refused.

C Disclosure rules establish the appropriate standard of care in obtaining informed consent. States differ as to which standard is applicable.

1. **Majority rule.** A physician needs to disclose only information that a reasonable physician would disclose and need not disclose information that would not customarily be disclosed. This rule operates from the physician's point of view.

2. **Minority rule.** A physician needs to disclose only information that a reasonable patient in similar circumstances would wish to know to make a reasonable decision.

D General guidelines in obtaining informed consent

1. A physician must obtain a patient's informed consent before treating her.

2. A physician must provide information concerning the probable benefits, risks, and nature of the suggested diagnostic or therapeutic interventions.

3. A physician must provide an explanation of reasonable alternatives to the recommended intervention and the consequences of no intervention.

4. Information must be:
   a. What a reasonable practitioner would reveal under similar circumstances
   b. What a reasonable patient would consider significant under similar circumstances

E Exceptions to informed consent include the following:

1. If a risk is not reasonably foreseeable, it need not be disclosed.

2. Disclosure may be partial if full disclosure would be detrimental to a patient's best interest.

3. If the danger is commonly known, it can be assumed that the patient knows of the danger.

4. The patient may request not to be told of risks.

5. If the risk concerns improperly performing an appropriate procedure, it need not be disclosed.

6. In an emergency, where delay would result in death or serious injury and where a patient is unable to reflect and give an informed decision, informed consent is not required.

7. If a patient is declared either generally or specifically incompetent, informed consent cannot legitimately be obtained.

F **Procedure for obtaining informed consent.**   Informed consent is a process by which a physician imparts information to a patient who, by virtue of this information, may intelligently decide whether to submit to and participate in the physician's proposed intervention. Thus, the physician must do the following:

1. Discuss the need for the intervention.

2. Discuss the intervention honestly and explain it in layman's terms along with the reason for its necessity.

3. Explain the risks inherent in the procedure.

4. Explain alternatives and the probable result of no intervention.

5. Allow the patient to ask questions.

6. Document the conversation, listing the major risks and alternatives presented.

7. Explain that it is the patient's right to know a reasonable amount about the proposed intervention and that this right is being forfeited if she refuses to discuss the intervention. Document this discussion.

8. Inform the patient about the risks and the recovery time.

9. Refrain from altering records.

10. Personally obtain the consent, not relegating this duty to a nurse or staff member.

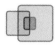

Study Questions for Chapter 38

DIRECTIONS: *Each of the numbered items or incomplete statements in this section is followed by answers or by completions of the statement. Select the ONE lettered answer or completion that is BEST in each case.*

1. It is important for a physician to _____ when counseling a couple who wishes artificial insemination.

A Explain that divorce absolves the husband from child support
B Explain that there is no guarantee of pregnancy if protocol is followed
C Explain that, with screening, birth defects are not possible
D Explain that transmission of STDs is very likely
E Explain that a divorce excludes the husband from access to the child

2. An obstetrician is called at home by a woman who is in labor. Although she has never been to see the obstetrician for a prenatal visit, she would like him to deliver her infant. The obstetrician refuses to attend to her because he is in the middle of dinner. She subsequently delivers a healthy infant at home. If this woman sues the physician for negligence, which of the following would be his best defense?

A Labor is not a disease, so it was not necessary to attend to this pregnant woman
B Because the woman did not come for prenatal visits, she is not entitled to a physician
C Because the woman gave birth to a healthy infant, no harm was done
D The physician never accepted the woman as his patient
E The patient was contributorily negligent in not calling the physician long in advance of active labor

3. A gynecologist has a long-standing relationship with a patient. The woman becomes pregnant but does not inform her gynecologist of her pregnancy and is not scheduled to see him until the next annual visit. One Saturday she calls to report nausea and vomiting but is unable to reach her physician, who is on vacation and has left no other physician to take care of his patients. Three months later the patient goes into preterm labor and delivers a premature infant. The infant ultimately dies 1 month later. In a lawsuit, which of the following statements is the physician's best defense?

A No physician-patient relationship existed
B The physician did not breach any duty owed to the patient
C The premature delivery and fetal death was unrelated to the physician's time on vacation
D A premature infant is not a viable human being
E The woman has not suffered any injuries

4. A 34-year-old gravida 1, para 1 delivers a boy with Tay-Sachs disease. Eight years later, she and her husband obtain the services of a lawyer and sue the physician, alleging that he was remiss in genetic counseling, and because of this, a child with an irreversible neurologic disease had to be brought into the world. The best term to describe this lawsuit is

A Wrongful birth
B Wrongful conception
C Wrongful life
D Medical malpractice
E Wrongful counseling

5. A 21-year-old gravida 7, para 4, SAB 2 at 8 weeks of gestation is on her way to the operating room for an elective termination. She has been married for 7 years, has four healthy children, and is finished with childbearing. She has no medical problems except for mild lung fibrosis. Her family history is

remarkable for mental retardation in a first-degree relative who has Fragile X syndrome. She has already signed a consent form to have a laparoscopic tubal ligation after the dilation and curettage. The most compelling reason to abstain from performing the tubal ligation is

- A Her age
- B Her family history
- C Her impending abortion
- D She has received mind-altering medications
- E She is on her way to the operating room

6. Because of new reproductive technologies, a child may be born with as many as ___ parents. (What is the maximum number of "parents," genetic and/or social a child can have?)

- A 2
- B 4
- C 5
- D 6
- E 7

Answers and Explanations

1. The answer is B [VI A 2, 4, 5]. The couple who wishes artificial insemination by donor (AID) must be told of the risks of acquiring birth defects due to unknown recessive genes of the donor. There is no guarantee of pregnancy. Even though there is little risk of sexually transmitted disease because of screening and quarantined freeze preservation of semen, there is no guarantee against that transmission. It is essential that the husband give his consent because, in doing so, he is accepting all responsibility for the child born through the donor insemination process. In addition to that responsibility, in case of divorce, the husband maintains his right to visitation and is responsible for child support.

2. The answer is D [II B 1–4]. For a physician to be sued for negligence, the plaintiff must clear four hurdles. These are (1) that a duty existed; (2) that the duty was breached; (3) that, because of the breach of duty, harm was directly caused; and (4) real damage occurred. In this case, no physician-patient relationship existed because the physician refused to help a person who was not his patient. Although it might be argued that it would have been morally correct for the physician to attend to this woman, the law does not recognize a duty to rescue. A physician–patient relationship must be entered into voluntarily and cannot be coerced on either part.

3. The answer is C [II B 1–4]. Although the physician was negligent in not having another physician cover for him while he was on vacation, his negligence did not proximately cause his patient's ultimate injury. Any relationship between the physician's negligence of not being present and the patient's premature delivery 3 months later is too remote to establish causation. Because a premature infant was born and lived for 1 month, it is a human being and a legal entity that can maintain a lawsuit. Also, the mother can maintain a lawsuit apart from her infant.

4. The answer is A [VII B 1]. Wrongful birth actions are brought by the parents of a child with a congenital defect, alleging that a physician was remiss in genetic counseling, and because of this, a defective child was allowed to be born. In general, these cases have been successful, especially in cases where testing would have been easy, such as in prenatal testing for Tay-Sachs disease. Wrongful life actions that are brought by a child, alleging that no life would have been better than life with congenital defects, have generally been unsuccessful. Compensation prior to these injuries, however, may be granted on negligence theory. In cases involving wrongful conception (namely, parents seeking compensation for a normal child resulting from a failed sterilization), willingness to compensate has been low. In cases in which the resulting child was abnormal, medical expenses for the care of the infant have been granted. Important to the determination of wrongful conception is documentation of whether the mother was informed of the possibility of failure of the sterilization procedure. There is no such term as "wrongful counseling." Medical malpractice is an umbrella term, and it does not specifically describe this clinical scenario.

5. The answer is C [III C 1 c]. Federal regulations require that consent for sterilization cannot be obtained if the patient is under 21 years, in labor, under the influence of alcohol or drugs, mentally incompetent, or having an abortion (dilation and curettage or dilatation and evacuation). Federal regulation is such that a tubal ligation and abortion cannot be performed at the same time.

6. The answer is C [VI]. A child may be born with as many as five parents—a genetic father (sperm donor), a social father (person who raises the child), a genetic mother (egg donor), a social mother (person who raises the child), and a gestational mother (the person whose uterus carries the child to term).

Cases Studies

Hormone Replacement Therapy

A 53-year-old woman comes to her physician for a routine gynecologic examination. Once in the office, she starts to cry and asks how she knows when she is through menopause and how long it will take. She explains that her life is not the same anymore and that it must be due to "the change." She has not been to the gynecologist for several years. Her friends and family encouraged her to come today to get help.

QUESTIONS

■ *What is the definition of menopause?*

■ *When does menopause normally occur?*

DISCUSSION

Menopause is the point in time marked by the permanent cessation of menses. The diagnosis of menopause is made retrospectively. Menopause is defined as the absence of a menstrual period for 6 to 12 months in a woman 45 years of age or older. The cessation of menses reflects a decline in ovarian function. The average age of menopause is 51.4 years, with a normal age range of 48 to 55 years. Perimenopause is the period of time just before and after the permanent cessation of menses. The few years preceding menopause, characterized by a fluctuation of ovarian function, are referred to as the transition. The average length of transition is 4 years. This patient could be anywhere along the spectrum of declining or reduced ovarian function. How a woman experiences menopause is related to the hormonal changes characteristic of this time as well as other factors, such as psychosocial issues, the presence of medical illness, and general physical condition.

> The patient states that her last period was about 14 months ago but that she really has not been herself for the last 2 years. During this time, she has been experiencing what she thinks are hot flashes that have been getting progressively worse. They seem to occur most often at night, and she does not remember when she last had a full night's sleep. Before this she usually adjusted quite well to changes in her life. Now, she cannot seem to cope. She is grateful that her husband is very patient with her; after years of a rewarding sexual relationship, she has very little interest or enjoyment in their sex life.

QUESTIONS

■ *What are the characteristic symptoms of menopause?*

■ *What is the endocrinology, physiology, and clinical course of hot flushes?*

■ *What vaginal changes are characteristic of menopause?*

■ *How does menopause affect sexual function?*

DISCUSSION

The most common symptom of the menopausal period is the hot flush. Seventy-five to eighty-five percent of women experience hot flushes to some degree; they are the most common reason women seek treatment during menopause. Many women notice the onset of hot flushes before the permanent cessation of menses. Hot flushes may occur during the transition, most typically during periods of amenorrhea when circulating estradiol levels are reduced. Hot flushes occur in response to a reduction of estradiol levels from previously established levels. Women with hypogonadism secondary to gonadal dysgenesis who have always had low estrogen levels do not experience hot flushes. It has been noted that there is a surge of luteinizing hormone (LH) just before the onset of the hot flush. However, it is unlikely that the LH surge plays a causative role because women with hypopituitarism and no LH surge still experience hot flushes. Hot flushes are caused by an inappropriate stimulation of the heat-losing mechanism in the thermoregulatory center of the hypothalamus. Core body temperature has been measured and noted to be normal when the body is stimulated to lose heat to reduce core temperature. There is a corresponding decrease in core body temperature after the hot flush occurs. A prodromal aura usually signals that the hot flush is going to occur, followed by a increasing sense of warmth progressing from the waist and over the chest, neck, and face. This sense of warmth is accompanied by peripheral vasodilation with a flushing of the skin, perspiration, and, at times, heart palpitations. Hot flushes last from seconds to minutes and may be repetitive. They tend to occur more frequently at night and may be a source of significant sleep disturbances. Chronic sleep deprivation can result in fatigue, depression, anxiety, and an overall decreased sense of well-being. Hot flushes tend to decrease in frequency with time, although they may persist for more than 3 to 5 years in up to 33% of women. The pattern of symptoms seen in this patient is typical of the menopause experience. Insomnia and depression are symptoms of the menopausal period that may occur independently of hot flushes. However, the mood disturbances experienced by this woman may be secondary to the disruption in her life from hot flushes.

Dyspareunia (painful intercourse) is another common symptom experienced after menopause. The vagina is an estrogen-sensitive organ. When circulating estradiol levels decline after menopause, the vaginal epithelium atrophies, the vagina loses elasticity and compliance, and lubrication decreases. As discomfort with intercourse increases, enjoyment and interest decline. Women also report decreased libido during the perimenopause and beyond, unrelated to dyspareunia. The etiology of waning interest in sexual activity is usually multifactorial, with a complex interplay of hormonal, psychological, and social factors. Some women experience a new enjoyment of sexual activity after the menopause with children moving away and no risk of pregnancy.

> The role of estrogen replacement therapy for relief of menopausal symptoms is discussed with the patient. She is eager to experience relief of her symptoms but is concerned because she has read that a risk of breast cancer is associated with estrogen replacement therapy. Further history shows the patient has no history of breast biopsy or problems, and a negative family history for breast, ovarian, and colon cancers. She has not had a mammogram and does not do breast self-examination regularly. She has four children; she had her first when she was 23 years of age. She has no known medical problems and is not taking any medications. She does not take vitamins or calcium supplements. The patient works as a secretary, and she does not exercise regularly; she neither smokes nor drinks alcohol. She gets one serving per day of dairy products, does not pay attention to fat in her diet, and drinks four to five cups of coffee per day. The patient's father died from a heart attack at age 62; he had his first heart attack at age 47. Her mother is alive and well at age 78. The patient has never had her cholesterol measured.

QUESTIONS

- *What are the benefits of estrogen replacement therapy?*
- *What are the risks of estrogen replacement therapy?*
- *What are the contraindications of estrogen replacement therapy?*

DISCUSSION

Estrogen is approved for use after menopause to treat menopausal symptoms and to prevent and treat postmenopausal osteoporosis. Estrogen, compared with placebo, has consistently reduced the severity, frequency, and intensity of hot flushes. With improvement in hot flush frequency, an improvement in sleep and mood is also noted. Estrogen replacement also effectively relieves symptoms related to urogenital atrophy. After 3 to 4 months of use, women experience an increase in vaginal lubrication, decreased discomfort with intercourse, and an improvement in symptoms of urinary urgency and frequency. Estrogen replacement alone is often insufficient to improve decreased libido. If a lack of desire is related to vaginal discomfort, marked improvement is often noted with replacement therapy. Adding androgens, in a low dose, to the hormone replacement therapy regimen may provide further improvement in the level of sexual desire.

Osteoporosis is a systemic skeletal disease characterized by a decrease in bone mass with microarchitectural distortion associated with increased fragility of bone and susceptibility to fracture. The sites most frequently involved with fracture include the vertebrae, hip, and wrist, although all bones are at risk. Risk factors for osteoporosis include advanced age, female gender, white or Asian race, tobacco use, alcohol use, inadequate calcium intake, sedentary lifestyle, high protein diet, and excessive caffeine use. Medications associated with an increased risk of osteoporosis include chronic corticosteroid use and excessive thyroid replacement. Peak bone mass is reached for both trabecular and cortical bone by age 30. Thereafter, there is continuous age-related bone loss. For the first 5 to 7 years after menopause, the rate of bone loss accelerates secondary to reduced circulating estradiol levels. Estrogen replacement therapy prevents the accelerated bone loss associated with menopause and effectively reduces the risk of fracture by up to 50%. Effective protection requires at least 3 to 5 years of estrogen use; bone loss occurs after cessation of therapy. Other measures, such as adequate calcium intake and exercise, are important in the prevention and treatment of osteoporosis.

In the past, women had been routinely prescribed hormone replacement therapy for heart disease and osteoporosis prevention based on observational data. Recently, a large study showed an increase in the risk of coronary heart disease with the use of estrogen and progestin in healthy postmenopausal women. The Women's Health Initiative discontinued one of the trials early because the rate of nonfatal coronary events increased, as did the number strokes and venous thromboembolism events. A separate study, the HERS trial, showed that hormone replacement therapy did not reduce coronary events in women with established heart disease. Despite the improved lipid profiles seen with estrogen, these recent studies support the lack of a role for estrogen-progestin in the primary or secondary prevention of coronary disease in postmenopausal women.

Other benefits attributed to estrogen use after menopause include a maintenance of skin thickness, treatment of androgenic alopecia, and increased sense of well-being. Preliminary evidence suggests that estrogen use may be associated with slowing the progression of memory loss associated with Alzheimer's dementia. Ongoing research will further define this proposed benefit.

Unopposed estrogen replacement therapy in a woman who has not undergone hysterectomy is associated with an increased risk of endometrial hyperplasia and carcinoma. Risk increases with increasing dose and duration of use. Adding a progestin at currently recommended doses and duration to the replacement regimen effectively decreases the risk to less than 1%. Adding progestin also enhances the protective effect estrogen exerts on bone.

Long-term progestin use is associated with a reduction in colorectal cancers and in increase in invasive breast cancers. Of note, short-term use of estrogen-progestin therapy, defined as less than 5 years' duration, is not associated with an increased risk of breast cancer.

Women who are not candidates for hormone replacement therapy are those with conditions that could be worsened by hormone use or conditions that would impair the metabolism of estrogen, leading to unpredictable circulating estrogen levels. These risk factors are a history of one or more of the following: breast cancer, endometrial cancer (except stage I disease), recent thromboembolic disease, hormone-related thromboembolic disease, and acute or chronic hepatic disease. Other conditions are relative contraindications in that they are not life-threatening but could be worsened with hormone use. These conditions include the presence of a seizure disorder, history of migraine headaches, cholelithiasis, and hypertriglyceridemia. Adjustment of the regimen or route of administration often allows safe, effective use of hormones in women with these conditions.

Hormone replacement therapy in postmenopausal women needs to be tailored to the risks and benefits' profile of each individual patient. The patient in this case will benefit from hormone replacement therapy for symptom management. Her history does not contain any absolute or relative contraindications to therapy. With her menopausal symptoms and risk of osteoporosis, a short course may be considered.

> Physical examination reveals the patient to be normotensive and of average weight. Breast examination is normal, and breast self-examination was taught. Pelvic examination showed atrophic vaginal changes, a normal-sized uterus, and adnexae that were not palpable. Rectal examination was negative for masses and occult heme. A pap smear was obtained; mammography was ordered; and cholesterol and high-density lipoprotein (HDL) tests were ordered. Colorectal cancer screening with sigmoidoscopy was discussed.

QUESTIONS

▪ *What are the components of routine health maintenance that are important to include in the clinical encounter with a menopausal patient?*

▪ *How should hormone replacement therapy be prescribed and how should the patient be counseled?*

▪ *What follow-up should be recommended?*

▪ *When would an endometrial biopsy be recommended?*

DISCUSSION

Frequently, the only encounter the postmenopausal woman has with the health care system is for gynecologic care. It is of utmost importance to take full advantage of this opportunity to provide counseling on healthy lifestyle recommendations and obtain appropriate screenings according to the patient's age and risk profile. Blood pressure, weight, and height should be obtained on an annual basis. Breast self-examination should be reviewed and recommended to be done monthly. Clinical breast examination should be done annually; mammography should be obtained annually after the age of 50. Before age 50, mammographic screening should be obtained every 1 to 2 years beginning at age 40. A normal mammogram should be documented before initiation of hormone replacement therapy. A pelvic examination is recommended on an annual basis. A pap smear should be obtained annually; longer screening intervals can be used in the low-risk patient with a history of normal pap smears. After age 50, cholesterol screening should be obtained every 2 to 3 years, if normal, and more frequently if abnormal. Before age 50, levels should be obtained every 5 years. Smoking cessation should be initiated when indicated. Recommendations about adequate calcium intake should be made, including a total of 1,000 mg for the woman receiving hormone replacement therapy and 1,500 mg when not receiving hormone replacement therapy. This total is the sum of both dietary and supplemental intake. Counseling regarding daily physical activity and an aerobic exercise program should be provided. Screening for colorectal cancer includes annual rectal examination and guaiac testing. Sigmoidoscopy in the patient of average risk and colonoscopy in the high-risk patient are recommended at intervals (1 to 5 years) according to risk and previous findings. The role of routine bone density measurements to detect osteoporosis has yet to be defined. Bone density measurements are obtained in the postmenopausal woman when the results would impact therapy; when the woman has asymptomatic hyperparathyroidism; and when the woman has a history of chronic corticosteroid use.

Estrogen replacement therapy should be prescribed for symptom relief and osteoporosis prevention. Progestin is added either sequentially (10 to 14 days/month) or continuously to provide endometrial protection. Prescribing progestin sequentially has the disadvantage of inducing menstrual-like bleeding on a monthly basis. Continuous progestin therapy avoids regular cyclic bleeding but is associated with a higher incidence of irregular bleeding that is unpredictable in terms of amount, frequency, and duration. The lowest recommended dose of estrogen should be the starting point; this varies with the type of estrogen prescribed. Increasing the dose of estrogen may be necessary to obtain maximum symptom relief; this should be done for the shortest duration possible. A patch can be prescribed for those women who prefer this route of administration; in women in whom there is an advantage to bypassing the first-pass hepatic effect; or in women in whom consistent bioavailability is critical. Avoiding the first-pass effect on the liver may be advantageous in women who have cholelithiasis, women taking anticonvulsant medication, and women with a history of thromboembolic disease. Consistent bioavailability may be a factor in women who have depressive symptoms and hormone-related migraine headaches; avoiding fluctuations in serum estrogen levels may enhance the response to hormone therapy. Women with skin sensitivities may not tolerate patch therapy.

Adequate counseling about the risk, benefits, and expected side effects of hormone replacement therapy is a critical component of the menopausal encounter. Compliance with hormone replacement therapy continues to be a significant problem. Only 10 to 25% of appropriate candidates opt to initiate hormone replacement. Only 30% of these women continue therapy after 1 year. The patient should be warned that breast fullness, tenderness, or enlargement is not unusual, initially, and that it usually subsides with continued use. Initial water retention and weight gain may occur. Substantial weight gain has not been demonstrated to be secondary to hormone therapy. Woman who wear contact lenses may experience an intolerance for previously comfortable lenses secondary to fluid retention and change in corneal shape. If the patient is placed on a sequential regimen, she should be informed that normal bleeding occurs on completion of the progestin component. Bleeding that occurs at any other time is considered abnormal. Bleeding may be similar in amount to previous menses; lighter bleeding or no bleeding is an acceptable pattern as well. Patients often equate the presence of withdrawal bleeding with adequate endometrial protection. The woman needs to be assured that endometrial shedding is not essential to obtain endometrial protection. If a woman is started on continuous combined therapy, she should be warned about the likely occurrence of irregular bleeding. There is no normal expected bleeding pattern with this regimen. What is important to define is what is abnormal. Heavy, persistent, or frequent bleeding should be considered abnormal. The patient should be instructed to call the physician if she experiences abnormal bleeding or symptoms that are new, persistent, and bothersome. After initiation of therapy, the patient should return in 3 months to review her response to therapy and any voice any questions or concerns. Once the patient's response to therapy has stabilized, she can return to routine, annual follow-up.

Routine endometrial biopsies are not necessary before the initiation of hormone replacement therapy but should be obtained in women who experience postmenopausal bleeding and in women who experience abnormal bleeding while taking hormone replacement therapy. On a sequential regimen, abnormal bleeding is any bleeding that occurs at a time other than with progestin withdrawal. On a continuous regimen, bleeding that is persistent, heavy, or prolonged is considered abnormal.

CASE 2

Secondary Amenorrhea

A 28-year-old woman presents to her physician's office with amenorrhea of 6 months' duration. Her medical history includes a spontaneous vaginal delivery 1 year ago. This delivery was followed by postpartum endometritis and bleeding, which necessitated a dilation and curettage and a blood transfusion. The patient nursed her infant for 4 months and stopped because of lack of milk. She had two spontaneous light bleeds 6 weeks apart before becoming amenorrheic. She states that she always had irregular cycles and actually took 1 year to become pregnant. She has lost 50 lb. since her pregnancy.

QUESTIONS
▪ *What is the differential diagnosis of secondary amenorrhea?*
▪ *Do the events before or after the pregnancy help to narrow the diagnosis?*

DISCUSSION
This is a clinical picture of secondary amenorrhea with a significant differential diagnosis. With the history alone, the etiology of the amenorrhea could be pregnancy or could be secondary to hypothalamic, pituitary, ovarian, or endometrial dysfunction. In this case, the secondary amenorrhea could be hy-

pothalamic due to stress or the significant weight loss. Normally a 50-lb. weight loss might explain the amenorrhea; however, the patient may have lost the weight in an effort to reestablish her prepregnancy weight. Either a pituitary adenoma with increased levels of prolactin or Sheehan's picture (hypoactive thyroid, adrenal, and ovarian function because of decreased stimulating hormones) secondary to post-partum bleeding, hypotension, and pituitary necrosis could cause the amenorrhea. The ovary might be the cause because of either an ovarian tumor or polycystic ovaries (irregular menses and relative infer-tility) or premature failure. The tumor and the premature failure are rare possibilities. Finally, the en-dometrium could be replaced by scar tissue (Ascherman's syndrome) secondary to the postpartum endometritis and curettage.

> Physical examination shows no significant abnormalities. Breast examination is normal without any galactorrhea. Pelvic examination shows a normal sized, firm uterus with no apparent adnexal masses. The result of a urine pregnancy test is negative. A 5-day course of oral progesterone pro-duces no withdrawal bleeding within 10 days.

QUESTIONS

- *What is the significance of the absence of withdrawal bleeding?*
- *Does the absence of withdrawal bleeding eliminate any of the compartments in the etiology?*

DISCUSSION

The negative pregnancy test result rules out pregnancy. The absence of a progesterone withdrawal flow means either that the endometrium is unresponsive to hormonal stimulation (synechiae), that the ovary cannot produce estrogen (premature failure), or that the ovary is inadequately stimulated because of low gonadotropins (pituitary or hypothalamic causes). This clinical test does not, therefore, elimi-nate any of the compartments as possible causes of the amenorrhea.

> The patient is given sequential estrogen and progesterone and has a withdrawal flow within 3 days. Her thyroid function studies and cortisol levels are within normal limits. There is no eleva-tion of her prolactin level.

QUESTIONS

- *What does the bleeding following sequential estrogen/progesterone therapy indicate?*
- *Why are the normal values of the pituitary target glands important?*

DISCUSSION

The withdrawal bleeding following sequential estrogen/progesterone therapy establishes the fact that the endometrium can respond if properly stimulated. This finding rules out intrauterine synechiae and polycystic ovaries. With polycystic ovarian disease and its estrogenic state, the endometrium would have been proliferative and would have bled with the initial progesterone challenge. The normal thy-roid function tests and cortisol levels effectively rule out Sheehan's syndrome, a panhypopituitary state with low levels of all pituitary hormones. The normal prolactin level rules out a prolactin-secreting mi-croadenoma that could be the cause of the amenorrhea secondary to suppression of follicle-stimulating hormone (FSH) and luteinizing hormone (LH). What is not yet ruled out is either premature ovarian failure or hypothalamic amenorrhea (hypogonadotropic hypogonadism).

> The final and definitive test in this clinical picture is a gonadotropin assay (FSH and LH) assay; both levels are reported back as very low.

QUESTION

- *How do the FSH and LH levels differentiate between premature ovarian failure and hypothalamic amen-orrhea?*

DISCUSSION

The low level of gonadotropins indicates that the etiology of the amenorrhea is most likely hypothala-mic in nature. The fact that the thyroid and adrenal glands are functioning normally eliminates the possibility of a nonresponsive pituitary. The gonadotropins would have been high in premature ovarian failure because of the lack of ovarian estrogen and the lack of consequent negative feedback on the hypothalamus. Thus, the cause of this postpartum patient's secondary amenorrhea is hypothalamic in nature, possibly due to the large amount of weight loss, but most probably due to the stress of new motherhood; this condition was foreshadowed by her inability to nurse because of a decreased milk supply.

Female Urinary Incontinence

A 46-year-old woman, gravida 4, para 4, presents to her physician's office with complaints of urinary incontinence.

QUESTION

▪ *What are the causes of urinary incontinence in women?*

DISCUSSION

There are three general categories of female urinary incontinence. Genuine stress urinary incontinence (GSUI) is the most common and is generally caused by an anatomic defect of the posterior urethrovesical angle. GSUI usually is a result of pelvic floor muscle damage from childbearing.

Urge incontinence associated with detrusor instability (DI) is another common cause of female urinary incontinence. DI is defined by the onset of spontaneous detrusor contractions with bladder filling; it may also be caused by neurologic disease.

Mixed incontinence includes both stress and urge components in the cause of urine loss.

QUESTION

▪ *What questions might the physician ask this patient to further evaluate her urinary incontinence?*

DISCUSSION

In evaluating a patient with urinary incontinence, it is essential to obtain a voiding diary. In the diary the patient should document the times and amounts that she voids, the times that she is incontinent, and the precipitating events.

The patient should also complete a thorough urologic questionnaire, which should inquire about how often she voids during the day and night, the amounts of urine voided or leaked, the presence of an urgency to void, whether she has a history of urinary infections or stones, and when her incontinence began. It should also include questions regarding what medications she takes and what precipitates her urine loss.

> The patient tells the physician that she typically loses urine with coughing or sneezing and that she sometimes doesn't make it to the bathroom in time. She noticed that these symptoms began after the birth of her second child, improved for a time, but have since worsened. She has to wear a diaper, which becomes soaked from leaking urine. Her diary shows that she drinks a cup of coffee and a glass of orange juice in the morning and a glass of iced tea at lunch. She doesn't drink any liquids after dinner for fear that she may have to get up during the night. She usually gets up to void once during the night. Her voiding diary demonstrates more episodes of leakage in the mornings than at any other time of day. She presently takes hydrochlorothiazide and verapamil for her hypertension.

QUESTIONS

▪ *What kind of incontinence might this patient have?*
▪ *What part of her history could be exacerbating her incontinence?*
▪ *What might be done to improve her symptoms?*

DISCUSSION

Because she first reported symptoms after childbirth, and because her urine loss typically occurs with an increase in abdominal pressure (i.e., with coughing or sneezing), the patient most likely has stress incontinence. However, a patient's history does not always correlate with the type of urinary incontinence. This diagnosis should be confirmed with the demonstration of urine loss with the Valsalva maneuver, accompanied by a descent of the posterior urethrovesical angle. Detrusor instability should also be excluded cystometrically.

Coffee and tea can irritate the bladder mucosa and can exacerbate incontinence. The patient should be advised to avoid caffeine and tea intake. Her use of hydrochlorothiazide, a diuretic, and verapamil, a calcium channel blocker, also may be exacerbating her incontinence; she might be switched to an alternative medication with fewer effects on the bladder. The patient should also be instructed on how to perform Kegel exercises, which strengthen the pubococcygeus muscles and can improve incontinence symptoms in up to 75% of individuals.

QUESTION

- *What elements of the physical examination are important to obtain?*

DISCUSSION

The physical examination is necessary to exclude a neoplasia, diverticulum or fistula, and pelvic mass. The examination should assess the patient's hormonal status; check for the presence of a cystocele, rectocele, and uterine prolapse; and evaluate for pelvic floor muscle tone. A neurologic examination of the perineum and lower extremities should also be performed to exclude neuromuscular disorders such as multiple sclerosis.

The patient's physical examination demonstrates a moderate uterine prolapse and a moderate cystocele and rectocele. The result of her neurologic examination is normal.

QUESTION

- *What other evaluation can be performed to confirm the diagnosis?*

Once a presumptive diagnosis of stress incontinence has been established, office cystometrics can be performed to confirm the diagnosis and to exclude detrusor instability or mixed incontinence as the cause of urine loss. The office evaluation should include a post-void residual test, which should be less than 100 ml; this catheterized sample should be sent for culture and sensitivities to exclude urinary tract infection. Simple cystometrics can be performed by filling the bladder through a catheter, noting the patient's first sensation to void, and when she senses a maximally full bladder. If the patient develops spontaneous bladder contractions with bladder filling, this is indicative of detrusor instability, and not stress incontinence. If leakage of urine can be demonstrated with a full bladder with straining, this is indicative of stress incontinence. In the presence of both, further studies must be performed to evaluate for mixed incontinence or other causes.

CASE 4

Hypertension in Pregnancy

A 33-year-old African-American primigravid woman presents for prenatal care at 10 weeks' gestation by her last menstrual period. Her blood pressure taken in the office is 150/100.

QUESTIONS

- *How common is hypertension in pregnancy?*
- *What is the most likely diagnosis?*

DISCUSSION

Hypertensive disease occurs in 8% to 11% of all pregnancies. It is second only to embolism as a cause of maternal mortality. Hypertension during pregnancy is divided into pregnancy-induced hypertension

(PIH) and chronic hypertension. PIH usually occurs in the second half of pregnancy. Hypertension that occurs before 20 weeks' gestation, even in the absence of a history of hypertension, is defined as chronic hypertension. The one exception is patients with gestational trophoblastic disease, who may develop PIH before 20 weeks' gestation. The most likely diagnosis in this patient is chronic hypertension, but gestational trophoblastic disease should be excluded by ultrasonography.

> Further questioning provides a history of essential hypertension since age 25. The patient reports that she is currently taking enalapril for control of her blood pressure. The remainder of her history is noncontributory, and a routine gynecologic examination is remarkable only for a 10-week–sized uterus.

QUESTIONS

▪ *Should the patient's medication be continued?*

▪ *How else should she be evaluated?*

DISCUSSION

Enalapril and other angiotensin-converting enzyme (ACE) inhibitors should not be continued in pregnancy. Their use beyond the first trimester has been associated with fetal hypocalvaria, renal failure, oligohydramnios, and fetal and neonatal death. If the patient's blood pressure is persistently 150/100, she should be treated to prevent maternal morbidity. The antihypertensive of choice in pregnancy is alpha-methyldopa. Further evaluation of this moderately hypertensive woman should include a complete physical examination including cardiac and funduscopic evaluation. Laboratory evaluation should include a complete blood count, urinalysis, serum creatinine, 24-hour urine test for protein and creatinine clearance, and serum electrolytes. An electrocardiogram, a chest radiograph for cardiac contour, and an ophthalmologic evaluation should also be considered. An ultrasound should be performed to confirm the patient's dates and exclude a hydatidiform mole.

The patient should be seen every 2 weeks, and serial sonography for fetal growth is indicated. Once the patient is in the third trimester, fetal surveillance is indicated. The clinician should be alert to signs and symptoms of placental abruption and superimposed PIH, which are common in pregnant women with chronic hypertension.

> The patient's physical examination and laboratory evaluation are normal. Her pregnancy remains uncomplicated until 35 weeks' gestation, when she calls the physician's office with a complaint of a headache.

QUESTIONS

▪ *What should the physician be concerned about?*

▪ *What should the physician do next?*

DISCUSSION

The patient should be instructed to come in immediately for evaluation. Symptoms such as headache, visual changes, and epigastric pain may indicate PIH in any pregnant patient. Patients with chronic hypertension are especially at risk for superimposed PIH and preeclampsia.

> The patient is seen on the labor floor, and her blood pressure is persistently 180/120. Urine protein is noted to be +2. The patient complains of a persistent headache that is not relieved by Tylenol. Physical examination is unremarkable, and her cervix is noted to be 1 cm dilated and 90% effaced with the fetal vertex at −1 station. Fetal monitor demonstrates irregular contractions and fetal heart rate in the 140's and reactive.

QUESTIONS

▪ *What is the physician's diagnosis now?*

▪ *What laboratory studies are indicated?*

▪ *How should the patient be managed?*

DISCUSSION

Based on the patient's blood pressure and symptoms, the patient meets criteria for the diagnosis of su-perimposed severe PIH. Laboratory evaluation should include a complete blood count to look for hemoconcentration and thrombocytopenia, a serum creatinine and uric acid test to identify renal dys-function, and liver function tests to identify a transaminitis. If the platelet count is abnormal, or if the patient has clinical signs of abruption, complete coagulation studies should be ordered. Because the di-agnosis of severe PIH has been made, the indicated treatment is delivery of the fetus to prevent both ma-ternal and fetal morbidity and mortality. Vaginal delivery is preferred, and with a favorable cervix in-travenous oxytocin may be given. The patient should also receive parenteral magnesium sulfate for seizure prophylaxis.

CASE 5

Menopause

A 51-year-old woman presents to her physician's office complaining of mood swings, vaginal dryness, and hot flashes for the past several months. She had a total abdominal hysterectomy 4 years ago sec-ondary to uterine myomas.

QUESTIONS

☐ *What are the potential causes of this patient's complaints?*

☐ *What laboratory values would help confirm the diagnosis?*

DISCUSSION

Given the patient's age and symptoms, she is most likely going through menopause. It must be con-sidered that, as women age, their risk for thyroid disease increases. The most common complaints that will bring a menopausal woman to her physician are hot flashes, irregular menses, vaginal dryness, mood swings, and sleep disturbances. This patient has undergone a hysterectomy so has not experi-enced irregular menses. Most women will begin to experience menstrual irregularities as the first sign of impending menopause. The irregularities are quite similar to the menstrual irregularities experi-enced by adolescents. The cessation of menses defines menopause. When a woman has had her uterus removed, the physician relies on symptoms to make the diagnosis. Serum levels of follicle-stimulating hormone and luteinizing hormone increase due to the loss of negative feedback from estrogen and in-hibin from the ovary. In this situation, these values help confirm the diagnosis of menopause. A mat-uration index from the vaginal mucosa may be obtained to determine if the vaginal symptoms are caused by atrophy.

> On further questioning, the physician discovers that the patient's mother died from a pulmonary embolus after surgical pinning of a fractured hip.

QUESTION

☐ *How will this information impact patient management?*

DISCUSSION

This patient's mother may have suffered a fractured hip secondary to osteoporosis. A family history of osteoporosis is the strongest risk factor for the development of osteoporosis. This patient should be ad-vised of her increased risk of osteoporosis and instructed as to how she can decrease her risk and keep her bones healthy. The health cost of osteoporosis is great. Over 10 billion dollars are spent every year caring for men and women who have osteoporosis. For elderly patients who suffer a hip fracture, the rate of morbidity is high. The mortality rate approaches 25% for women who have a hip fracture. The most common cause of death for women undergoing hip replacement or pinning of a fracture is pul-monary embolus. These elderly patients commonly have multiple medical problems complicating their recovery.

The physician discusses the use of estrogen replacement therapy, calcium supplementation, weight-bearing exercise, and the avoidance of smoking and alcohol to decrease the patient's risk of osteoporosis. The patient refuses estrogen replacement therapy because she is afraid of increasing her risk of breast cancer.

QUESTION

▪ *What other therapy should the physician offer this patient?*

DISCUSSION

If the patient has already developed osteoporosis, she can be treated with alendronate sodium (Fosamax). This is a new class of drugs that inhibits osteoclastic resorption of bone. It is approved for use in menopausal women who have documented osteoporosis. This diagnosis can be made by demonstrating osteoporosis on a dual-energy x-ray absorptiometry (DEXA) bone scan. Adequate calcium supplementation is mandatory with this therapy. The patient should be advised to continue weight bearing exercise and the avoidance of alcohol and smoking.

Before leaving the physician's office, the patient asks the physician to recommend an internist for her. The physician gives the patient the name of an internist, explaining to her that all the routine primary care screenings will be forwarded.

QUESTION

▪ *What other studies should be ordered before the completion of the visit?*

DISCUSSION

This patient needs a screening blood pressure measurement, urinalysis, weight measurement, and a screening cholesterol test. Total cholesterol and high-density lipoprotein are satisfactory. In addition, the patient should have a rectal examination with stool guiaic. After the age of 50, all men and women should have screening sigmoidoscopies performed every 3 to 5 years. Starting at age 65 all women should be screened for thyroid disease with a thyroid-stimulating hormone. The patient should be reminded about the need for yearly pap smears and mammograms.

The patient returns 2 months later stating that she and her husband have not been able to have intercourse due to severe pain. She is distressed by this and would like to resume a normal sex life.

QUESTIONS

▪ *What should the physician tell this patient?*
▪ *What are the patient's options?*

DISCUSSION

Vaginal dryness is a common complaint in menopausal women. This dryness is due to a decrease or lack of secretions. The pain with intercourse is due to the lack of lubricant as well as vaginal atrophy from estrogen deprivation. Most patients will have significant relief from the use of a lubricant with intercourse. Patients must be advised that continued sexual activity is necessary or the pain with intercourse will worsen. A maturation index can be helpful to confirm vaginal atrophy. A careful examination to diagnose vaginitis is mandatory. For those patients with severe atrophy who do not respond to lubricant, a trial of oral or local premarin therapy is indicated. Although there is systemic absorption of premarin cream applied to the vagina, the levels are much lower than with oral therapy.

This patient was willing to try the local premarin and had complete resolution of her symptoms. The patient returned 1 year later for her annual examination and was doing quite well. She has had a normal sex life with her husband, and the hot flashes have tapered. The only complaint that she has is mild bone pain in her back.

QUESTION

▪ *What could the physician recommend for this patient?*

DISCUSSION

Bone pain is common in menopausal women. These symptoms commonly abate with estrogen replacement therapy. The patient should be informed of this and should have a DEXA bone scan to check for osteoporosis. If osteoporosis is diagnosed, the physician should suggest that the patient begin estrogen replacement therapy. Because she has had a hysterectomy, the patient can take just estrogen daily.

Abnormal Papanicolaou (Pap) Test

A 28-year-old woman (G_1P_{0010}) presents to her gynecologist for a yearly examination. She has no complaints and no history of medical problems or prior surgery. She is interested in birth control and would like to take oral contraceptive pills.

QUESTIONS

- *What elements of the patient's history are important in addition to her medical history?*
- *What aspects of routine health maintenance are part of a yearly gynecologic visit?*

DISCUSSION

It is important to learn about the patient's prior pregnancies and their outcomes, her menstrual history, history of sexually transmitted diseases (STDs), and any past abnormal pap tests. Social history is also significant. Discussion of smoking, alcohol and drug use, and sexual orientation and sexual history is also appropriate.

At a yearly gynecologic visit, the physician should perform a complete physical examination, including a breast and pelvic examination. A pelvic examination should include both visual examination of the female genitalia using a bivalve speculum and a bimanual examination to palpate the cervix, uterus, and adnexa. A pap test should be performed, and tests for STDs may also be necessary, particularly for chlamydia, which is often asymptomatic. The patient should be instructed in breast self-examination.

> The patient reports that she had her first period at 12 years of age. Her menses are regular; they occur every 4 weeks and last for 5 days. Occasionally, she has mild cramps. She estimates that she has had about 10 to 12 sexual partners. Her only pregnancy ended in an elective termination 12 years ago. She states that she has never had gonorrhea or chlamydia, but a few years ago she did receive treatment for genital warts. She thinks she may have once had an abnormal pap smear, but she is not sure about the details of the abnormality and never returned to the clinic. The patient is unmarried and works as a sales clerk. She smokes one to two packs of cigarettes per day, consumes alcohol occasionally, and denies drug use.
>
> Pelvic examination is unremarkable. A pap test is performed, and cultures for gonorrhea and chlamydia are obtained.

QUESTIONS

- *When should screening for cervical cancer take place?*

DISCUSSION

Screening for cervical cancer has decreased both the incidence of the disease and the associated mortality rate. In 2002, the American Cancer Society issued new recommendations for cervical cancer screening, which were endorsed by both the Gynecologic Cancer Foundation and the Society of Gynecologic Oncologists. Screening should begin about 3 years after the onset of vaginal intercourse, but no later than age 21 years. Traditional pap smears should be obtained yearly, but liquid-based pap tests may be performed every two years. For women older than age 30 with three prior consecutive normal pap tests, the screening interval may be extended to one test every 2 to 3 years. Women over the age of 70 who have had at least three normal pap tests and no abnormal tests in the previous 10 years may choose to stop testing after discussion with their physician. Also, screening is not necessary in women who have undergone hysterectomy with cervical removal unless the surgery was done as treatment for cervical cancer or cervical dysplasia. Women who are chronically immunosuppressed, such as those with HIV infection or organ transplants, should continue getting pap tests at the usual interval.

Although the new recommendations state that women over the age of 70 may consider discontinuing routine cervical cancer screening under certain circumstances, a misperception exists that pap tests are unnecessary in postmenopausal and elderly women. Approximately 11 million women in the United States older than 65 years of age have not had cervical cancer screening in the past year. Unfortunately, about 25% of all cervical cancers and 41% of all cervical cancer deaths occur in this age group. Pap testing remains important throughout a woman's life.

After the physician and patient discuss use of contraceptives and prevention of STDs, the patient is given a prescription for oral contraceptive pills. The physician strongly recommends that the patient stop smoking, particularly because of the increased risk of deep venous thrombosis in smokers who take oral contraceptives. The physician tells the patient that the office will call with her test results and reminds her to return next year for a yearly examination.

One week later, the physician receives the test results. The gonorrhea and chlamydia cultures are negative, but the pap test shows a low-grade squamous intraepithelial lesion (LGSIL), changes associated with human papilloma virus (HPV), and cervical intraepithelial neoplasia grade I (CIN I).

QUESTIONS
- *What is the significance of LGSIL?*
- *What is the relationship between HPV infection and cervical dysplasia?*
- *What are the risk factors for cervical dysplasia in this patient?*
- *What is colposcopy?*
- *What follow-up is appropriate in this case?*

DISCUSSION
To standardize the reporting of Pap test results, the Bethesda System was introduced in the late 1980s. The term "low-grade squamous intraepithelial lesion," or LGSIL, includes the cytologic changes caused by HPV and mild dysplasia (CIN I). The term "high-grade squamous intraepithelial lesion," or HGSIL, includes moderate (CIN II) and severe dysplasia (CIN III), as well as carcinoma in situ. Another common Bethesda System diagnosis uses the term "atypical squamous cells of undetermined significance," which denotes an abnormality that exceeds the usual changes of an inflammatory process but is not severe enough to qualify as dysplasia.

Most, but not all, dysplastic lesions of the cervix are associated with HPV infection, although most women who are infected with HPV never develop cervical dysplasia. HPV also causes genital condyloma, but infected women may have no symptoms. More than 70 different serotypes of HPV have been identified. Types 16 and 18 have been associated with cervical cancer, and types 6 and 11 have been associated with cervical dysplasia and genital warts. Host integration of the E6 and E7 HPV genes can cause immortalization of human genital epithelial cells and may contribute to the development of carcinoma.

Risk factors for cervical dysplasia and cervical cancer include early age at first intercourse, large number of sexual partners, multiparity, and a history of STDs. Other important risk factors include smoking, lower socioeconomic status, and exposure to diethylstilbestrol in utero. Many of these risk factors are likely to be related to the risk of exposure to HPV, a sexually transmitted virus that is widely present in the general population. Depending on the population tested and the technique used, 9 to 38% of women are positive for HPV. In some high-risk populations, the prevalence may be as high as 50%. This patient's risk factors include an early age at first intercourse, multiple sexual partners, a history of genital warts (which indicates exposure to HPV), and tobacco use.

It is important for patients with LGSIL to be observed closely. One option is to perform repeat pap testing every 4 to 6 months for 2 years until three consecutive negative results are obtained. At that point, yearly testing may be resumed. If LGSIL continues, colposcopy with directed biopsy is indicated. A second option is to perform colposcopy directly.

Colposcopy, an office procedure, involves examination of the cervix under a stereoscopic, binocular, low-magnification microscope. The colposcope is used to view the cervix while a dilute acetic acid solution is applied. The acetic acid causes abnormal areas of the cervix to turn white. These areas are referred to as "acetowhite epithelium." The practitioner must take care to examine the entire squamocolumnar junction and transformation zone (area of squamous epithelium that replaced the original glandular columnar epithelium via a normal metaplastic process) because these areas are the most common sites for dysplastic lesions. Condylomas and low- and high-grade dysplastic lesions have a characteristic appearance that can include acetowhite changes, abnormal blood vessels, mosaicism, and punctation. The practitioner identifies abnormalities and biopsies the most atypical areas for histologic analysis. Endocervical curettage (ECC) is used to sample the endocervical canal.

Once LGSIL has been confirmed histologically, there are several treatment options. The most common option is to continue with frequent pap tests every 4 to 6 months for 2 years. Local excision or ablation may be warranted in patients with persistent lesions. Electrocautery, cryotherapy, and laser ablation may all be performed in the office or as outpatient surgery.

> The physician calls the patient and recommends that she schedule an appointment for colposcopy in the next 1 or 2 months. However, she does not return for a follow-up visit. She comes to the office 8 years later reporting vaginal spotting after sexual intercourse that has persisted for the last 5 months. She has no new medical problems and has continued to smoke one to two packs of cigarettes per day. Since her last visit to your office, she has not had a gynecologic examination.
>
> Pelvic examination reveals a friable cervix without gross lesions. The uterus and adnexa are otherwise of normal size and contour. A pap test shows a high-grade squamous intraepithelial lesion (HGSIL) and changes associated with HPV.
>
> The patient, who is frightened by the bleeding, keeps her appointment for colposcopy. The entire transformation zone and squamocolumnar junction is well visualized. A suspicious area with abnormal vessels and mosaicism is seen on the cervix at the 3 o'clock position. Biopsies of this area confirm severe dysplasia (CIN III). ECC is negative.

QUESTIONS

- ☐ *What is the pathophysiology of cervical dysplasia and cervical cancer?*
- ☐ *What is the next step in evaluation and treatment?*

DISCUSSION

CIN I and II lesions are similar in terms of their natural history. More advanced CIN III lesions are more likely to persist and progress to invasive cancer. Although CIN I progresses to cancer in only 1% of patients, studies have shown that approximately 30% of patients who allow their severe dysplasia to remain untreated eventually develop invasive cancer over 10 years of follow-up. No method reliably predicts which lesions will develop into more advanced dysplasia or to invasive cancer and which will simply persist or regress. In addition, no dependable procedure exists to determine how rapidly the progression to a more serious lesion may occur.

Typically, patients with severe dysplasia are counseled to undergo cone biopsy of the cervix. This is preferable in many cases because ablative therapies, such as cryotherapy and laser ablation, do not provide a tissue sample for histologic diagnosis. In addition to providing therapeutic removal of the dysplastic cells, cone biopsy may be diagnostic. It may be performed to help clarify a diagnosis and to preclude invasive cancer in the following situations: inadequate colposcopic examination (incomplete visualization of the transformation zone or abnormal lesions), high-grade dysplasia on endocervical curettage, adenocarcinoma in situ, significant discrepancy between findings on pap smear and biopsy, or possible invasive carcinoma on colposcopy (even if biopsies show only carcinoma in situ).

Conization of the cervix removes a cone-shaped piece of tissue from the cervix. The biopsy can be performed by applying a cold knife cone technique (using a scalpel) as an outpatient surgical procedure under anesthesia or as a loop electrocautery excision procedure (or LEEP) in the office under local anesthesia.

Although cold knife cone biopsy is an extremely safe procedure, it does have some risks. The most common side effect is bleeding, which may occur in less than 10% of patients. Physicians usually take precautions by injecting the cervix with a local anesthetic mixed with epinephrine, which causes vasoconstriction in the cervix, and by applying Monsel's solution to the cervix after achieving hemostasis with electrocautery to further coagulate bleeding. Infection occurs less commonly, and patients are advised to avoid sexual intercourse, tampons, and douching for several weeks after the biopsy to promote healing. Infertility is rarely associated with cone biopsy. Cervical stenosis occurs when scarring after the procedure causes an abnormal narrowing in the opening of the cervix. This may block the entry of sperm into the uterus or change the normal mucous secretions of the cervix, making the environment inhospitable to sperm. Cervical deformity and possible second-trimester miscarriage through premature cervical dilation is another rare risk of the cone biopsy. This effect is usually associated only with removal of large portions of tissue during the biopsy. Most women do not have problems with either becoming pregnant or carrying a pregnancy to term after a cone biopsy.

> The patient undergoes cold knife cone biopsy. Histologic examination confirms the presence of a CIN III lesion and involvement of the endocervical glands. The margins of the specimen are free of dysplasia.

QUESTION

▪ *What is the appropriate follow-up?*

DISCUSSION

The patient has been adequately treated for her CIN III lesion. However, she still requires frequent pap tests to ensure that a lesion does not recur. She should undergo pap tests every 4 to 6 months for the next 2 years. After a cone biopsy, the physician must pay careful attention that the endocervix is adequately sampled by the pap test. Stenosis and scarring may make sampling of the area difficult; however, given the extent of the lesion and the involvement of endocervical glands on the cone biopsy specimen, routine cytologic examination is important. If ap tests cannot adequately sample the endocervix, ECC may be required.

CASE 7

Postmenopausal Bleeding

A 58-year-old woman presents to her gynecologist reporting a 2-month history of vaginal spotting.

QUESTIONS

▪ *What is the differential diagnosis of postmenopausal vaginal bleeding?*
▪ *What details of the history and physical examination would be helpful?*

DISCUSSION

Postmenopausal bleeding should never be ignored. In most women, the bleeding is benign, but in approximately 15% of cases, the bleeding results from endometrial cancer. The most common cause of postmenopausal bleeding is atrophy of the endometrium or vagina. Other causes include exogenous estrogen use, endometrial or cervical polyps, and endometrial hyperplasia, as well as cervical cancer, estrogen-producing ovarian tumors, urethral caruncle, and genital trauma.

The astute physician should ask about the quality, quantity, and timing of bleeding. A general medical, surgical, and gynecologic history may identity risk factors for endometrial hyperplasia and carcinoma. It is important to know what medications the patient is taking because use of exogenous estrogen may cause as much as 30% of postmenopausal bleeding. Physical examination, including pelvic examination, is necessary to exclude obvious causes such as trauma, urethral caruncle, cervical polyp or cancer, and ovarian masses that may produce estrogen. Atrophy of the genital tract is also usually apparent on pelvic examination.

The patient reports that the bleeding is light and intermittent; she wears a sanitary pad occasionally. She has diabetes mellitus type 1 and hypertension, for which she takes insulin and hydrochlorothiazide, respectively. She has had no prior surgery. She has never been pregnant. Until she was 53 years of age, her periods occurred normally every month. She does not have hot flashes and does not use hormone replacement therapy or dietary supplements. She denies any history of abnormal Papanicolaou (pap) smears or sexually transmitted disease. She is a widow and works as an executive secretary. She does not smoke and denies illicit drug use but has one or two drinks per week.

On physical examination, the patient is 5 foot 3 inches tall and weighs 254 lbs. She is moderately obese with no palpable abdominal masses. On pelvic examination, her vulva is free of lesions, and her vagina shows only scant old blood in the vault. The cervix appears small but otherwise normal. Because of her habitus, the uterus and adnexa are not palpable.

QUESTIONS

▪ *What is the next step in the workup of this patient?*
▪ *What are the risk factors for endometrial cancer?*

DISCUSSION

Endometrial biopsy is used to exclude endometrial cancer and hyperplasia in cases of abnormal vaginal bleeding. This rule is true applies to both pre- and postmenopausal patients because, although the median age at diagnosis of endometrial cancer is 61 years, 20 to 25% of cases are diagnosed before menopause, and 5% are diagnosed before 40 years of age. In most patients, endometrial biopsy may be performed in the office with minimum discomfort. Outpatient techniques for endometrial sampling are about 90% accurate for the diagnosis of carcinoma. Dilation and curettage may be necessary in the following situations: cervical stenosis is present, the office procedure is nondiagnostic, bleeding persists after a negative office procedure, or a patient cannot comfortably tolerate the procedure without anesthesia.

Some physicians may use pelvic ultrasound as a diagnostic tool. Ultrasound may be necessary to exclude a hormonally active ovarian tumor but is more commonly used in this instance to examine the thickness of the endometrial stripe. No cases of cancer have been reported in patients with an endometrial stripe thickness of 4 mm or less, but there is no consensus on the histologic diagnosis for a given endometrial stripe thickness. The cost-effectiveness of ultrasound has not been established for the evaluation of vaginal bleeding; therefore, the preferred first step remains the office endometrial biopsy.

Most risk factors for endometrial cancer involve increased exposure to estrogen. One of the most obvious sources of estrogen exposure is iatrogenic. Women who take unopposed estrogen replacement therapy are at high risk for the development of endometrial hyperplasia and carcinoma; these women should undergo yearly endometrial biopsy to screen for abnormalities, even in the absence of symptoms. Tamoxifen, frequently used to treat breast cancer, has proestrogenic effects on the endometrium and may also predispose patients to endometrial cancer.

Normal physiologic variations, such as obesity, nulliparity, and late menopause, also increase endogenous estrogen exposure. Obesity increases the body's exposure to estrogen through increased peripheral production of estrogens by body fat and through decreased levels of both circulating progesterone and sex hormone–binding proteins. Endometrial cancer is three times more likely in individuals who are 20 to 50 pounds overweight when compared to those of a normal weight, and the cancer is ten times more likely in individuals who are more than 50 pounds overweight. In nulliparous women, the risk is two times greater than that of women with one child, and three times greater than that of women with five or more children. Late menopause (beginning later than 52 years of age) is associated with a greater than twofold risk.

Medical conditions commonly associated with endometrial cancer are hypertension and diabetes. Prior oral contraceptive use and cigarette smoking appear to have a protective effect against the development of endometrial cancer.

The physician performs an endometrial biopsy in the office. Because the uterus and adnexa are not palpable, a pelvic ultrasound is ordered. The patient is instructed to make an appointment 2 weeks from now to discuss the test results.

At her next appointment, the physician reviews the results of the endometrial biopsy, which shows complex hyperplasia without atypia. The ultrasound reveals normal-appearing ovaries and a small uterus with an endometrial stripe of 12 mm.

QUESTIONS

▣ *What is the significance of complex hyperplasia?*

▣ *What are the treatment options?*

DISCUSSION

Endometrial hyperplasia is classified based on glandular architecture as simple (regular) or complex (irregular with back-to-back crowding). Cytologic atypia may be present or absent. Of patients with simple hyperplasia without atypia on biopsy, only about 1% progress to, or already have, concomitant carcinoma. The rate or progression of concomitant carcinoma for patients with complex hyperplasia without atypia is about 3%. These forms of hyperplasia often regress with progesterone therapy.

Treatment of hyperplasia without atypia depends on patient age, reproductive desire, and symptoms. For perimenopausal patients, progesterone therapy, with biopsy in 3 to 6 months, may be appropriate. For women interested in future childbearing, oral contraceptive pills for 3 months and then repeat biopsy to monitor regression of the lesion may be sufficient. Oral contraceptives may be continued in patients who do not wish to have children immediately. Cyclic progesterone withdrawal may be used instead of oral contraceptives in anovulatory patients. For patients who experience heavy bleeding or who have a suspected estrogen-secreting ovarian neoplasm, hysterectomy with bilateral salpingo-oophorectomy may be warranted.

Because the patient's symptoms are minor and she is reluctant to undergo major surgery, the physician and patient agree on a course of progesterone therapy. The patient is given a schedule for intramuscular injection of medroxyprogesterone acetate with a follow-up endometrial biopsy 4 months from now. The repeat biopsy reveals complex hyperplasia with atypia.

QUESTIONS

▣ *What is the significance of atypical hyperplasia?*

▣ *What are the treatment options for this patient?*

DISCUSSION

Cytologic atypia is characterized by nuclear enlargement, irregularity, and hyperchromasia. These lesions rarely respond to progesterone therapy and have a greater tendency to progress to carcinoma. For patients with simple atypical hyperplasia, 8% either may possess a coexisting focus of carcinoma or will eventually progress to cancer. For patients with complex atypical hyperplasia, this value increases to as high as 29%.

Because of the high risk of carcinoma, the treatment of choice for this postmenopausal patient with complex atypical hyperplasia is hysterectomy with bilateral salpingo-oophorectomy. This treatment is appropriate for all patients except those who have serious concomitant medical problems that present unacceptable surgical risks. In such cases, high-dose progesterone therapy may be attempted. Younger patients, or those who wish to be able to bear children, may be treated with a trial of hormonal therapy and followed closely with endometrial biopsy to monitor success of treatment.

CASE 8

Pelvic Pain

A **38-year-old woman** ($G_{4}P_{3013}$) presents to the emergency room with right lower abdominal pain that has been increasing in intensity over the past 4 days. The pain has been accompanied by nausea but no vomiting. The patient states that her last menstrual period was 6 to 7 weeks ago and that she had some spotting on the previous day. Her menstrual cycles are irregular, ranging from 30 to 50 days, and she has an intrauterine device (IUD) in place for birth control.

QUESTIONS

- ▫ *What are some of the possible causes of this patient's pain?*
- ▫ *What are some of the nongynecologic causes of right lower quadrant pain?*

DISCUSSION

This patient's history suggests a wide range of possible causes for pelvic pain. A benign or malignant ovarian mass could cause pain, either because of expanding size or torsion of the cyst or tumor. Although the patient has had very irregular and sometimes long menstrual cycles, she could have ovulated and become pregnant even with an intrauterine device (IUD) in place. With an IUD, there is an increased possibility of ectopic pregnancy. However, the patient also could have an intrauterine pregnancy with a corpus luteum cyst that has either ruptured or twisted. Pelvic infection inside or outside the uterus must be considered, again because of the presence of the IUD. Unilateral tuboovarian abscess also can be associated with IUD use. Gastrointestinal conditions such as appendicitis or a passing kidney stone also are possible sources of right lower quadrant pain. Although this patient has no history of myoma uteri, a degenerating myoma also can cause intense pelvic pain.

> Physical examination in the emergency room reveals a temperature of 99.8°F, blood pressure of 140/80, and a normal examination with the exception of the abdomen and pelvis. The abdomen is soft, with active bowel sounds, and there is guarding without rebound in the right lower quadrant. Pelvic examination shows a parous cervix with clear, watery mucus and no visible IUD strings. The uterus is anterior, slightly enlarged, and nontender. A tender, 3-cm × 4-cm mass is anterolateral to the uterus on the right, seemingly very close to the uterus.

QUESTIONS

- ▫ *What additional information has been gained from the physical examination of this patient?*
- ▫ *What laboratory studies should be ordered at this time?*

DISCUSSION

The physical examination certainly adds important information to the history, making some diagnoses less likely than others. The temperature of 99.8°F is slightly higher than normal but not in the range expected in the setting of an acute appendicitis; it also makes generalized pelvic infection unlikely. The cervical mucus is clear, not purulent, which further suggests that infection is not a problem. Additionally, the uterus itself is not tender and there is no tenderness of the left side.

The history of IUD placement combined with the absence of IUD strings on pelvic examination could be significant. Despite the absence of significant temperature elevation, a chronic right-sided tuboovarian abscess could exist (again, recall that unilateral tuboovarian abscess can be associated with IUD use). Or, the IUD could have perforated the uterus (no strings were seen), moved into the peritoneal cavity, and established an abscess involving the fallopian tube, ovary, or bowel. The slight temperature elevation, the presence of the IUD, the possible late menses, the tender mass, and slight bleeding could represent a right tubal pregnancy or, possibly, an intrauterine pregnancy with a bleeding or ruptured corpus luteum. The tender right adnexal mass could represent a degenerating myoma or an ovarian cyst or tumor undergoing torsion. A temperature of 99.8°F would be consistent with either of these conditions.

> After 2 hours in the emergency room, the patient's condition has not changed. By this time, some laboratory values are available. The hemoglobin is 12.1 g/dl, and the white cell count is 11,000 with a slight shift to the left. Urinalysis shows no bacteria, white cells, or red cells. The serum human chorionic gonadotropin (hCG) test is negative.

QUESTIONS

▢ *How have these laboratory results helped to narrow the differential diagnosis?*

▢ *What diagnostic studies should be obtained at this point?*

DISCUSSION

The early laboratory results for this patient help to narrow the differential diagnosis. The negative serum hCG rules out pregnancy (intrauterine or ectopic). In retrospect, the clear, watery mucus now makes sense: If the patient had ovulated, or if she was pregnant, progesterone would be in the system, changing the cervical mucus to a viscous, cloudy fluid. The absence of significant findings on urinalysis effectively rules out urinary tract infection as well as a kidney stone passing through the ureter.

Several diagnostic possibilities still exist, however. The slightly elevated white cell count with the slight shift to the left could be compatible with a chronic right tuboovarian abscess in association with the IUD, a twisted right ovarian mass, or a degenerating myoma. In thinking about the ovarian possibilities, either a functional cyst or a neoplastic process under torsion could simulate the clinical situation as presented. A cystic teratoma (dermoid cyst) of the ovary would be high on the list because of the anterolateral position.

At this point it is important for the clinician to get some idea of the nature of the mass because of differences in management plans. A tuboovarian abscess would initially be treated with hospitalization and intravenous antibiotics. A degenerating myoma would be treated with analgesics. An ovarian mass undergoing torsion is a clinical emergency that would be treated with exploratory laparotomy and, most likely, salpingo-oophorectomy.

Ultrasound examination of the pelvis is performed while the patient still is in the emergency room. The examination shows a 3-cm × 4-cm complex mass with solid and cystic elements. The right ovary cannot be identified. The IUD is seen within the cavity of the uterus.

QUESTIONS

▢ *How has the ultrasound examination helped to narrow the differential?*

▢ *What would be the next step in evaluating this patient?*

DISCUSSION

Unfortunately, the ultrasound findings are not very helpful in narrowing the diagnostic possibilities in this case, as they could represent any of the remaining diagnoses. The complex solid and cystic mass could be a tuboovarian abscess, a degenerating myoma with cystic areas, a cystic teratoma, an endometrioma, or a benign or malignant ovarian tumor. The endometrioma probably could be ruled out because of the patient's multigravid state; endometriosis commonly is associated with infertility. At this point, an ovarian mass that is twisted or in torsion should be placed at the top of the list, with the degenerating myoma next. A unilateral tuboovarian abscess still is a possibility, but the nontender uterus, the minimally elevated temperature and white cell count, and the clear cervical mucus all make this diagnosis less likely than the other two conditions.

Because of the need to make a diagnosis, it is important to directly observe this patient's pelvis. Approximately 6 hours after she appeared in the emergency room, she is taken to the operating room and laparoscopy is performed. Examination shows no sign of infection in the pelvis, no pathology associated with either ovary, and no evidence of either a tuboovarian abscess or cyst of the right tube and ovary. However, the uterus is distorted by a 3-cm × 4-cm sessile myoma in the right corneal aspect. The myoma is closely attached to the uterus but is not a part of the uterine wall, and it appears to be slightly darker than the rest of the uterine fundus.

QUESTION

▢ *What kind of follow-up is advisable for this patient?*

DISCUSSION

Having considered the various clinical possibilities and having used the available diagnostic tools (i.e., laboratory, ultrasound, and laparoscopic evaluation), a final diagnosis is made. In this patient, the pelvic pain was caused by a degenerating myoma and should be self-limited with bed rest and analgesia. If the problem is recurrent, it would be appropriate to consider a myomectomy in the future. A degenerating myoma is an unusual cause for pelvic pain and is not an emergency. Conversely, the most important conditions to rule out in any woman with one-sided pelvic pain and a palpable mass are ectopic pregnancy and torsion of an adnexal mass—conditions that are emergencies and demand immediate attention.

Unexplained Vaginal Bleeding

A 38-year-old woman presents to the emergency room complaining of heavy vaginal bleeding that has persisted for 1 week. She feels weak and dizzy. The patient states that her last menstrual period was 10 weeks ago. She was last seen by her gynecologist 2 years ago.

QUESTIONS

▪ *What are potential causes of this patient's bleeding?*

▪ *What further history should be obtained?*

DISCUSSION

Abnormal vaginal bleeding is one of the most common gynecologic complaints, whether in the office, over the phone, or in the emergency room. This patient has symptoms of acute blood loss (i.e., weakness, dizziness), which could be secondary to the presumed uterine bleeding. A large number of conditions might cause this type of bleeding, but a complication of pregnancy must be high on the list of diagnostic possibilities for any woman of reproductive age. The patient's last menstrual period was 10 weeks ago, which means she could be pregnant.

Endometrial neoplasia or dysfunctional bleeding secondary to anovulation or some endogenous source of estrogen (i.e., a granulosa cell tumor) also is a likely cause of the bleeding. In addition, uterine myomas with submucous myomas can cause prolonged, heavy bleeding. Hematologic disorders such as leukemia and idiopathic thrombocytopenia (ITP) are rare but distinct possibilities; however, if ITP were the cause, it would be more likely to manifest at about the time of menarche. Endometritis and endometrial polyps also can be associated with heavy vaginal bleeding.

> On further questioning, the patient states that, for as long as she can remember, she has had irregular cycles ranging from 30 to 90 days. She had a pregnancy 10 years ago, which ended in spontaneous abortion. She has engaged in unprotected intercourse since her last menstrual period. The patient gives no history of easy bruising or abnormal bleeding from her gums or from cuts. She says that she thinks her uterus may be enlarged.

QUESTION

▪ *What is the significance of the patient's pattern of menstrual cycles?*

DISCUSSION

The additional history does not help to narrow the diagnosis much, but it does suggest anovulatory or unopposed estrogen bleeding as a good possibility. Any woman with the varied menstrual cycle lengths described by this patient is not ovulating regularly and may not be ovulating at all. However, because she has been pregnant once, a complication of pregnancy still is a possibility. With anovulatory cycles or hormonally active tumors, prolonged heavy bleeding is the result of unopposed estrogen continuously stimulating the endometrium. This condition can lead to a hyperplastic, sometimes atypical, and occasionally neoplastic endometrium. It is doubtful that cervical cancer is the cause of bleeding in this patient, since she was seen by a gynecologist 2 years previously, at which time it is appropriate to assume that a Pap smear was taken. Bleeding from endometrial polyps, endometritis, or submucous myomas still must be considered possibilities, especially with a history of an enlarged uterus. A bleeding diathesis cannot be ruled out from the history alone.

> Physical examination of the patient shows a well-nourished, well-developed female in mild distress, with no evidence of bruising and no petechiae. Her vital signs show a pulse of 90 and a blood pressure of 110/65 prone and a pulse of 110 and pressure of 90/45 standing. Abdominal examination shows a firm, irregular suprapelvic mass, just palpable above the symphysis. Pelvic examination reveals a firm, smooth cervix that appears slightly open, with a steady stream of blood coming through the os. The uterus is firm, irregular, and the size of a 12-week gestation, with presumed lateral and fundal myomas; it is not possible to palpate the adnexa accurately due to the enlarged uterus. A urine pregnancy test is negative, and the complete blood count shows a hemoglobin of 5.6 g/dl, a white cell count of 9600 with a normal differential, and a normal platelet count. Prothrombin time (PT) and partial thromboplastin time (PTT) are normal.

QUESTIONS

▪ *Which diagnoses are less likely based on the physical examination finding?*

▪ *Which diagnostic studies should be performed now?*

▪ *What would be the initial therapy for this patient?*

DISCUSSION

The physical examination and few laboratory findings help to direct the clinician's thinking about this case. The low hemoglobin level certainly indicates significant blood loss and explains the patient's weakness and dizziness. ITP, leukemia, and other hematologic problems are excluded by the laboratory findings. The negative pregnancy test is not absolute, but a pregnancy advanced enough to give this kind of clinical picture certainly should show up on a urine test. Pathologic conditions of the endometrium (i.e., endometritis, hyperplasia, carcinoma, polyps, or submucous myomas) cannot be diagnosed by a physical examination without sampling the endometrium. The combination of myomas and unopposed estrogen bleeding is a likely possibility, because a woman can bleed significantly from either of these causes without the other. An ovarian tumor still is a possibility, because the enlarged, irregular uterus prevented an accurate examination of the ovaries. At this point, it is important to stop the bleeding and make a diagnosis.

> Based on the suspicion that unopposed estrogen is partly responsible for the bleeding and with the need to stop the bleeding as quickly as possible, the emergency room physician decides on a course of intravenous (IV) estrogen. However, realizing the need to sample the endometrium before any hormone manipulation, the physician first performs an endometrial biopsy, sampling all four quadrants of the uterus. After completing the biopsy and beginning an IV infusion of 25 mg of conjugated estrogen (estrone), the physician sends the patient for pelvic ultrasound. The ultrasound report notes an enlarged uterus with multiple subserous myomas, an endometrial cavity with markedly thickened endometrium, and a left ovary that is 4 cm × 4 cm × 5 cm and solid.

QUESTIONS

▪ *What is learned from the ultrasound report?*

▪ *What are some of the causes of unopposed estrogen secretion?*

DISCUSSION

Now the pieces of the diagnostic puzzle are falling into place. The pelvic ultrasound is very helpful because it demonstrates an ovarian mass and subserous myomas. Because of the position of the myomas, they should not be contributing to the bleeding; on the other hand, submucous myomas could have been responsible for the whole clinical picture. The thickened endometrium probably is the result of prolonged unopposed estrogen stimulation. Without the biopsy report, endometrial pathology cannot be ruled out, although endometritis seems unlikely at this point. The finding of an ovarian mass suggests a cause for the unopposed estrogen secretion, the endometrial thickening, and the abnormal bleeding. A granulosa cell tumor secreting estrogen could be responsible for all of these clinical features.

The patient is admitted to the hospital with an order to infuse 25 mg of conjugated estrogen every 4 hours. By the third dose, the bleeding has stopped and the patient is started on a daily dose of progestin. The same day, the endometrial biopsy report shows adenomatous endometrial hyperplasia. The patient is discharged on 3 weeks of progestin and daily iron, with a plan to readmit her in 4 to 6 weeks (when her blood count is normal) for exploratory laparotomy and excision of the presumed estrogen-secreting ovarian tumor.

QUESTIONS

☐ *Why is estrogen used as the initial treatment for this patient?*

☐ *What is the physiologic mechanism of this patient's bleeding?*

DISCUSSION

Although the cause of this patient's bleeding and adenomatous hyperplasia is unopposed estrogen secretion from an estrogen-secreting tumor, high doses of IV estrogen are needed to stabilize the endometrium. The bleeding is caused by irregular breakdown and shedding of the hyperplastic endometrium. Estrogen has its primary effect on the vascular element of the endometrium, supporting the small vessels and healing the areas of endometrial degeneration. Once the bleeding stops, progestin must be added to stabilize the endometrium and to allow an orderly sloughing after 3 to 4 weeks. The hyperplasia is solely the result of the unopposed estrogen and would be reversed by either ongoing, intermittent progestin administration (i.e., for 12 days each month) or by removal of the estrogen source. In this case, the latter is indicated because the source is an ovarian tumor that may be malignant.

Comprehensive Examination

QUESTIONS

1. This morning, a 21-year-old woman, gravida 2, para 2 delivered a female neonate weighing 3950 g with APGAR scores of 9 and 9 at 1 and 5 minutes, respectively. She has no medical problems and her pregnancy was without complications. She delivered via spontaneous vaginal delivery at term and incurred a second-degree laceration, which was repaired. Her predelivery hemoglobin was 12.8. Today her physical examination is unremarkable: her vital signs are T = 97.9, BP = 105/78, P = 90, R = 18, and she has minimal lochia (changing three soaked pads in a 24-hour period). Her labs are as follows: hemoglobin = 12, hepatitis B surface antigen nonreactive (HBsAG negative), Venereal Disease Research Laboratory (VDRL) nonreactive, blood type O Rh +/antibody −, and gonococcus and chlamydia culture negative. She is not interested in any form of contraception. She is breastfeeding successfully. What is the next step in management?

- **A** Consult lactation nurse
- **B** Prescribe FeSO4
- **C** Obtain rubella antibody titers
- **D** Administer RhoGAM
- **E** Discharge from hospital

2. A 22-year-old woman, gravida 1, para 0 at 36 weeks of gestation presents to the labor and delivery department reporting severe back pain. She describes the pain as constant lower back pain, 7 of 10 in intensity, and without radiation to any other area of the body. Resting improves her pain, whereas bending and standing for prolonged periods seem to aggravate her pain. She denies past medical history or any trauma. She is allergic to sulfa drugs. Her vital signs are as follows: T = 98.8, P = 100, BP = 104/68, R = 20. Her physical examination is unremarkable except for tenderness in her back and in the midline and para-lumbar regions from L3 to sacral spine. There is no costovertebral angle tenderness. Her cervix is closed. Fetal heart rate is 135 bpm and reactive and there are no uterine contractions. Urine dipstick of a clean-catch midstream urine specimen reveals the following: RBC 0, nitrite 0, leukocyte esterase 0, ketones 0, protein 1+. What is the initial step in management?

- **A** Urinalysis and urine culture
- **B** Magnetic resonance imaging (MRI) of spine
- **C** Pain reliever containing codeine
- **D** Ibuprofen
- **E** Rest and massage

3. A 19-year-old primigravid woman at 20 weeks of gestation presents to the emergency department because of severe headache and loss of sensation throughout the right side of her body. She has a history of two seizures within the last 3 years, which allegedly occurred without any explanation. Today, her vital signs are as follows: T = 99.1, BP = 195/110, R = 24, P = 124. Her pupils are fully dilated and react equally to light. Her nasal septum is nondeviated, pale, and eroded. Her heart is tachycardic with 2/6 systolic murmur heard best at the right sternal border. She does not allow you to examine her extremities. She has no known drug allergies. She denies use of nicotine but admits to past heroine use. She also admits to using cocaine in the past. Given her history, her baby may be at risk for

- **A** Cystic kidney
- **B** Duodenal atresia
- **C** Deafness
- **D** Hepatitis
- **E** Chorioretinitis

4. A 57-year-old woman underwent a total abdominal hysterectomy, bilateral salpingo-oophorectomy and staging procedures for ovarian cancer. She was NPO for 8 hours prior to her surgery. Her preoperative hemoglobin was 11.7 and the estimated blood loss during the 4-hour operation was approximately 300 mL. Today is postoperative day # 1. The patient's pain is well controlled on patient controlled analgesia (PCA) with continuous basal low dose. She has not passed flatus yet and has not had anything to eat or drink. She has a Foley catheter, a subcutaneous drain, and an intraperitoneal drain in place. She is receiving Lactated Ringer's solution (LR) at maintenance rate. Her 24-hour total input/output values are as follows: 8200 mL/7600 mL (urine output was 120 mL/hr). Her vital signs are T = 98.7 BP = 128/82, P = 86, R = 12. Her physical examination is unremarkable. Her abdominal examination is significant for decreased bowel sounds and is soft. Her incision is nontender, clean, dry, and intact with staples in place. Her hemoglobin today is 10.6 and her electrolytes are within normal range. What is the next step in management?

- A Transfuse 2 units of packed red blood cells
- B Increase her intravenous fluids
- C Discontinue Foley catheter
- D Initiate bilateral lower extremity sequential compression devices

5. A 39-year old woman, gravida 3, para 3 presents to your office reporting "sexual dysfunction." She denies any medical problems but has a history of total abdominal hysterectomy and bilateral salpingo-oophorectomy performed a year ago for benign ovarian and uterine pathology. She has no known allergies and only drinks alcohol a few times per year. She says she is frustrated with herself because she lacks the desire to have sex with her husband even though everything is fine between the two of them. She tells you that her husband always initiates sex, but once they have begun to have intercourse she becomes excited and is able to achieve orgasm. She denies marital or relationship problems. She denies history of sexual abuse. She denies change in sleep patterns, appetite, loss of concentration, or loss of interest in previously pleasurable activities. Which of the following would most likely help this patient?

- A Superphysiologic androgen treatment
- B Sildenafil citrate (Viagra)
- C Water-based lubricant
- D Fluoxetine

6. A 23-year-old woman, gravida 1, para 0 at 15 weeks of gestation is seeing you for routine prenatal care. She has an extensive past medical history. She is purified protein derivative (PPD) positive and is on cyclosporine therapy to prevent kidney transplantation rejection. She is hepatitis B surface antigen positive. She has recently undergone breast augmentation (two sizes up). She has a strong family history of lactose intolerance that causes excessive flatulence and abdominal pain. What in her history is an absolute contraindication to breastfeeding her infant?

- A HBsAg+
- B Breast augmentation
- C Cyclosporin
- D PPD+
- E Lactose intolerance

7. A 25-year-old woman, gravida 2, para 0 at 7 weeks of gestation presents to you because of painful urination. She has a stinging sensation immediately after she urinates but not during urination. Her temperature is 97.6° and her physical examination reveals multiple painful vesicles and raw areas on the inner labia minora and inferior to the urethra. You perform a culture of the lesions to confirm your suspicion. The next best step in management of this condition during pregnancy is

- A Cesarean section for active lesions
- B Valacyclovir therapy now and suppression during pregnancy
- C Artificial rupture of membranes early in labor
- D Do nothing

8. A 24-year-old primigravid woman (12 weeks of gestation) who is a competitive downhill skier is seeing you for routine prenatal care and counseling about participation in sports during pregnancy. She is 5 feet 10 inches tall and weighed 130 lbs prior to becoming pregnant. She wants to remain active during her pregnancy. Of the listed activities below, which is the safest for this woman during pregnancy?

- A Soccer
- B Scuba diving
- C Basketball
- D Horseback riding
- E Tennis

9. A 22-year-old East Asian woman, who immigrated less than a year ago, presents to the emergency department reporting lower abdominal pain, dysmenorrhea, and menorrhagia. She has had no surgeries in the past but had an unknown lung disease that was treated in her country 2 years ago. Her vital signs are as follows: BP = 128/74, P = 88, T = 100.5, R = 16. On physical examination, her lungs are clear to auscultation, abdomen is nonobese, bowel sound is positive, and her abdomen is tender to palpation, especially in the lower quadrants. There is no rebound tenderness or abdominal distension. Pelvic examination reveals bilateral tender, firm adnexal masses, thickening and tenderness of uterosacral ligaments and broad ligaments, and uterine tenderness. Speculum examination reveals a tender but smooth, normal- appearing cervix with blood at external os; no discharge is noted. A pap smear is performed, and chlamydia and gonorrhea cultures are sent. An endometrial biopsy is performed to culture bacteria, if any. Significant labs are as follows: hemoglobin = 9 g/dL, ESR = 105 mm/hr, and β-hCG is negative. Given these facts, the best diagnosis is

- A *Actinomyces israelii*
- B *Mycobacterium tuberculosis*
- C *Neisseria gonorrhea*
- D Colorectal carcinoma
- E Ovarian carcinoma

10. A 24-year-old woman, gravida 4, para 2, SAB 1 at 26 weeks of gestation is seeing you for a routine prenatal visit. She has a history of one previous cesarean section with low transverse uterine incision (confirmed by operative report), which was performed at 37 weeks of gestation for multiple gestation (twins). She has had a successful vaginal delivery of a 3600-g female neonate after the cesarean section. During this pregnancy, she had fetal ultrasounds performed for various reasons at 13, 18, and 24 weeks of gestation, which, when plotted on singleton fetal growth curves, estimate the weight of the fetus at 4400 g at 40 weeks of gestation. The patient is interested in being induced with prostaglandin agents before 40 weeks when she is considered "term." She has a past medical history of hypertension and a surgical history significant for myomectomy (without entering into the uterine cavity, as per the operative report). The two facts in her history that increase her likelihood of successful VBAC (vaginal birth after cesarean section) are _____ and _____.

- A Current fetal weight and indication for previous cesarean section
- B Past surgical history and indication for previous cesarean section
- C History of successful VBAC and indication for previous cesarean section
- D History of successful VBAC and past surgical history
- E Desire for prostaglandin induction and number of previous low transverse cesarean sections

11. A 70-year-old patient with end-stage ovarian cancer and documented bowel obstruction has undergone several unsuccessful cycles of commonly recommended chemotherapy. The patient is advised by her gynecologic oncologist to receive a cycle of an experimental chemotherapy agent to try to reduce the size of her cancer implants. She refuses treatment and says she would rather die sooner and in peace at her home that receive more therapy in the hospital. Which ethical principle best describes this situation in which the physician does not influence the patient to take the drug because it is experimental and allows her to go home with narcotics for pain relief?

A Beneficence
B Nonmaleficence
C Justice
D Paternalism

12. A 25-year-old woman, gravida 1, para 0 at 22 weeks of gestation presents to you because she is suddenly concerned about the well-being of her baby. She says she had a severe flu during her first trimester which lasted 4 days and disappeared. She did not think anything of it then but she is now concerned after talking with her friends. You perform a complete ultrasound evaluation of the fetus and discover ascites, hydrops, ventriculomegaly, calcification of the lateral borders of the lateral ventricles, and liver calcifications. Based on the appearance of the fetus, what test would you perform?

A Amniocentesis with PCR and culture for cytomegalovirus (CMV)
B Amniocentesis with PCR for parvovirus B19
C Amniocentesis with PCR and culture for varicella zoster (VZV)
D Amniocentesis with PCR for toxoplasmosis
E Cervical and vulvar culture for herpes simplex (HSV)

13. Mrs. Hendersen lives in California and has five daughters (Molly and Mary are twins):

Molly is 15 years old and is currently serving on active duty with the U.S. Navy
Megan is 14 years old, living at home, and divorced
Mary is 15 years old, lives in an apartment on her own, and manages her own financial affairs
Mandy is 16 years old, pregnant, and wants to have bunion surgery during pregnancy because it is 100% covered by her insurance
Melinda is 12, lives at home, and has contracted Chlamydia infection
For this *hypothetical scenario*, which daughter would require parental consent for medical treatment in the state of California?

A Molly
B Megan
C Mary
D Mandy
E Melinda

14. A 25-year-old woman, gravida 2, para 1, ectopic 1 presents to the emergency department reporting sharp right lower quadrant pain. Her last menstrual period was 33 days ago (her periods are usually regular and occur every 28 days). She denies vaginal bleeding or sexual intercourse within the last 3 weeks. Her vital signs are as follows: T = 97.9, BP = 105/67, P = 100, R = 16. On abdominal examination she is nondistended but has voluntary guarding and is moderately tender to palpation. She denies having a past medical history except for treatment of an ectopic pregnancy with methotrexate 2 years ago. Her serum β-hCG is positive. Transvaginal ultrasound examination reveals no sac in the uterus, a 3.2 cm by 3.3 cm right complex adnexal mass, and fluid in the cul-de-sac. The best diagnosis is

A Corpus luteal cyst
B Luteoma of pregnancy
C Theca lutein cyst
D Appendicitis

15. In women, low levels of androgens are responsible for hair growth in the axillae, lower pubic triangle, forearms, and legs, and it may play a role in libido. Most circulating testosterone (not androgen) in premenopausal women comes from the

A Adrenal gland
B Fat cells
C Muscle

    [D] Ovaries
    [E] Skin

16. A 28-year-old woman, gravida 1, para 0 at 12 weeks of gestation is seeing you for routine prenatal care. She tells you she loves to eat seafood, especially fish. You advise her to limit her overall fish eating to once a week, to limit consumption of predatory fishes, and to avoid eating raw fish or sushi that may be of questionable quality. This advice was given to prevent an adverse outcome from

    [A] *Schistosoma japonicum*
    [B] *Wuchereria bancrofti*
    [C] *Ascaris lumbricoides*
    [D] Lead
    [E] Mercury

17. A 26-year-old woman, gravida 5, para 1, SAB 3 at 8 weeks of gestation by her last menstrual period presents to your office for prenatal care. She has a history of microinvasive cervical cancer that was treated with cold knife conization. Ever since the procedure, she has been unable to carry a baby to term. She miscarries and is unaware that it is occurring because her cervix dilates without any pain. What is the best management of this patient?

    [A] Daily transvaginal ultrasound with cervical length measurement
    [B] Placement of cerclage at 14 weeks and removal at 38 weeks or earlier
    [C] Placement of cerclage at 17 weeks and removal at 39 weeks or earlier
    [D] Bedrest and Foley catheter
    [E] Magnesium sulfate

18. The main difference between leuprolide (a GnRH receptor agonist) and gonadotropin releasing hormone (GnRH) is

    [A] GnRH causes a larger release of gonadotropins than leuprolide
    [B] GnRH has a longer half-life than leuprolide
    [C] Leuprolide is more resistant to endopeptidases than GnRH
    [D] GnRH causes down-regulation faster than GnRH
    [E] Leuprolide has ten times the potency of GnRH

19. A 5-year-old girl is brought in to see you because her mother believes she is menstruating. The mother tells you that her little girl's underpants always have had spots of blood. The mother lives with her boyfriend and her two daughters. Her other daughter is 4 years old and does not have similar complaints. You examine the girl under anesthesia and do not see any bruising or tearing in the vaginal or perineal area. Using a nasal speculum, you view inside the vagina and discover a large, grapelike mass in the anterior wall of the upper vagina. The mass bleeds easily upon contact with a cotton swab. The best management is

    [A] Child protective services
    [B] Leuprolide
    [C] Chemotherapy
    [D] Podophyllin resin
    [E] Estrogen cream

20. Gonadotropin releasing hormone (GnRH) is produced in the

    [A] Hypothalamus, arcuate nucleus
    [B] Hypothalamus, median eminence
    [C] Hypothalamus, paraventricular nucleus
    [D] Cerebral cortex
    [E] Anterior pituitary

21. A 22-year-old woman, gravida 1, para 1 at 9 weeks of gestation presents to you for her first prenatal visit. She has type 2 diabetes mellitus and has had an average fasting blood glucose of 230 mg/dL for the last 3 months. When she obtains an ultrasound to evaluate fetal anatomy, the most characteristic finding would be

   A A hole between the right and left atrium
   B Lack of the S1, S2, S3 spinal cord segments
   C Large fetus
   D Lack of lung development

22. A 29-year-old woman, gravida 3, para 2 at 27 weeks of gestation failed both the 1-hour glucose screening and the standard 3-hour glucose tolerance test. She was unable to keep her fasting glucose less than 95 mg/dL and her 2-hour postprandial glucose less than 120 mg/dL. She was placed on a self-administering insulin regimen. She is is at risk for

   A Delivering a fetus with ventricular septal defect
   B Delivering a fetus with encephalocele
   C Delivering a fetus with pulmonary hypoplasia
   D Persistent glucosuria during pregnancy
   E Cerebrovascular accident (CVA)

23. A 25-year-old woman, gravida 1, para 0 at 18 weeks of gestation is seeing you for her routine prenatal visit. Several years prior to her pregnancy she was diagnosed with an endocrine disorder because her thyroid-simulating hormone (TSH) was increased and her free T_4 was below normal range. She also has a history of mild hypertension. This patient is at risk for

   A Abnormal fetal scalp development
   B Large fetus
   C Delivering a fetus with a higher than average IQ
   D Separation of the placenta from the uterus
   E Maternal kidney infections

24. A 29-year-old gravida 3, para 0, SAB 2 at 26 weeks of gestation presents to you for severe bilateral leg pains. She has sickle cell anemia and has had similar episodes in the past that have been treated symptomatically. She is asymptomatic and afebrile, other than a productive cough of 1 week's duration on review of systems. Her prenatals labs are up to date. Her fundus measures 25 cm. Her legs are tender to touch. You do not notice redness, swelling, or calf cords. You admit her to the hospital, place her on oxygen by mask, and give her intravenous fluid and scheduled intravenous meperidine injections for pain. Which of the following is essential during this hospitalization?

   A Transfusion
   B Sputum culture
   C Folic acid
   D Pneumococcal vaccine
   E Stool for ovum and parasites

25. A 24-year-old woman, gravida 1, para 1 just delivered a viable male infant weighing 3900 g with APGAR scores of 9 and 9 at 1 and 5 minutes, respectively. After delivery of her infant, the woman's uterus was atonic and she incurred a second-degree laceration. Total estimated blood loss was 480 mL. During the immediate postpartum period there will be a(n)

   A Increase in heart rate
   B Decrease in blood volume
   C Increase in cardiac output
   D Increase in leg edema
   E Increase in tidal volume

26. A 25-year-old woman, gravida 1, para 0 at 25 weeks of gestation by her last menstrual period is seeing you for a routine prenatal visit. Her fundus measures 21 cm so you decide to obtain an ultrasound. The following are remarkable on sonogram: amniotic fluid index of 3.4 cm, enlarged cerebral ventricles, and hydropic placenta. The most likely karyotype of this fetus is

- [A] 69,XXX
- [B] 47,XXY
- [C] 47,XYY
- [D] 45,X
- [E] 45,X/46,XY

27. A 25-year-old gravida 4, para 0, SAB 4 presents to you for evaluation of recurrent miscarriages. The entire workup is normal except for her karyotype of 45,XY,t(13q14q), which is a robertsonian fusion translocation. A reasonable approach to management of this patient is

- [A] Reassurance
- [B] Donor insemination
- [C] Amniocentesis and selective termination
- [D] IVF-ET
- [E] Intracytoplasmic sperm injection (ICSI) and embryo transfer (ET)

28. A 68-year-old gravida 3, para 3 who has her last menstrual period 18 years ago presents to you reporting vulvar pruritus. Her medical history is significant for type 2 diabetes and hypertension. She had an appendectomy and a cholecystectomy a long time ago. Upon examination, the vulva appears shiny, pale, and white around the labia majora. It also blends smoothly into the labia minora. You perform a biopsy (the results are shown in the following figure).

The next best step in management of this patient is

- [A] Estrogen cream
- [B] Steroid cream

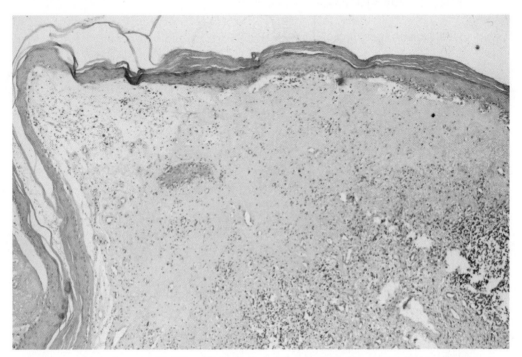

Question 28 figure. Courtesy of Jeff Cao, MD (Loma Linda University Medical Center, Department of Pathology)

C Testosterone cream
D Laser ablation
E Simple vulvectomy

29. Select the answer choice that best answers the following three questions:
(1) The most common type of suture utilized in gynecologic surgery is ___.
(2) The above suture loses 50% of its tensile strength by ____ week(s).
(3) The braided type of the above suture has the advantage of ____ .

A (1) absorbable (2) 4 weeks (3) pliability
B (1) nonabsorbable (2) does not lose its strength (3) tensile strength
C (1) absorbable (2) 3 weeks (3) tensile strength
D (1) absorbable (2) 8 weeks (3) resists harboring organisms
E (1) absorbable (2) 1 week (3) flexibility

Directions: For each of the following processes, list the best reason why a woman could experience unexpected vaginal bleeding. Each answer choice may be used once, more than once, or not at all.

QUESTIONS 30–33
A Progesterone withdrawal bleeding
B Progesterone breakthrough bleeding
C Estrogen withdrawal bleeding
D Estrogen breakthrough bleeding

30. Depot medroxyprogesterone acetate

31. Removal of corpus luteum

32. Spotting after low dose estrogen therapy

33. Bilateral salpingo-oophorectomy (BSO)

A 26-year-old nulligravid woman presents to your office reporting white nipple discharge. Upon further questioning, she tells you that she has irregular periods. In fact, she has only had five periods this year. Her serum prolactin level is elevated (90 ng/mL) and her TSH is within normal limits. Magnetic resonance imaging shows a microadenoma in the pituitary gland.

QUESTIONS 34–35

34. If she is interested in becoming pregnant, the best next step is`
A Bromocriptine
B External radiation therapy
C Thyroid hormone
D Medroxyprogesterone acetate
E Clomiphene citrate

35. If she is not bothered by her symptoms of oligomenorrhea and galactorrhea, the next best step in management is
A Observation
B Cytology of nipple discharge
C Medroxyprogesterone acetate

D Bromocriptine
E Vitamin D

36. A 20-year-old gravida 1, para 1 undergoes an operation for a unilateral adnexal mass with a normal contralateral ovary. Microscopic image of a section through the mass is depicted below:

The best way to manage this condition is

A Unilateral oophorectomy
B Bilateral oophorectomy
C Bilateral salpingo-oophorectomy
D Total abdominal hysterectomy and bilateral oophorectomy
E Chemotherapy

37. A 63-year-old woman with a left, 9-cm adnexal mass and an elevated CA-125 is found to have papillary serous carcinoma with spread to the omentum, bowel, and the diaphragm. A total abdominal hysterectomy and a bilateral salpingo-oophorectomy, omentectomy, and debulking of the tumor to less than 1cm residual disease are performed. The current treatment regimen with the *least toxicity* (least number of side effects) for advanced ovarian cancer is

A Cyclophosphamide and doxorubicin
B Cisplatin (Platinol) and paclitaxel (Taxol)
C Carboplatin (Paraplatin) and paclitaxel (Taxol)
D Methotrexate, actinomycin D, and folic acid
E Vincristine, actinomycin D, and cyclophosphamide

38. Radiation is used as primary or adjuvant therapy in management of some cancers. The most radiosensitive noncancerous tissue is the

A Liver
B Rectum

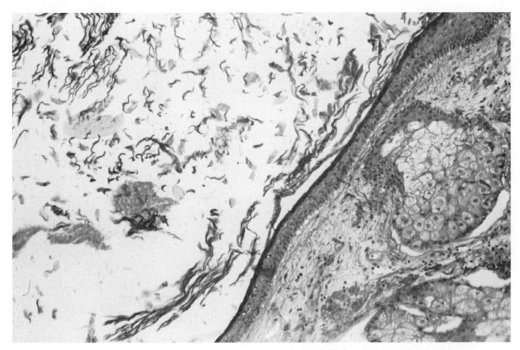

Question 36 figure. Courtesy of Jeff Cao, MD (Loma Linda University Medical Center, Department of Pathology)

C Cervix
D Bladder
E Ovary

Directions: In the evaluation of an infertility patient, tests are performed at specific times during the 28-day menstrual cycle. Match the test below with the best time to perform the test.

QUESTIONS 39–41

A Day 3 (early follicular)
B Day 8 (mid-follicular)
C Day 14 (ovulation)
D Day 21 (mid-luteal)
E Day 26 (late luteal)

39. **Hysterosalpingogram** to evaluate the uterine cavity and patency of fallopian tubes

40. **FSH levels** to evaluate ovarian follicular reserve

41. **Serum progesterone** to document ovulation

42. A 22-year-old gravida 2, para 0, SAB 2 presents to your office for a routine annual gynecologic visit. She tells you she has had two miscarriages, the first at 15 weeks and the second at 18 weeks of gestation. Her medical records indicate a right femoral vein thrombosis 4 years ago. She has also tested positive for VDRL, but her FTA-ABS test is negative. She had an appendectomy 7 years ago for a ruptured appendix. She does not smoke, drink alcohol, or use any illicit drugs. She has no known drug allergies. Her physical examination is unremarkable other than a single, 1-cm maculopapular rash on her right forearm. All of her serum chemistries and cell counts are within normal limits. The best diagnosis in this patient is

A Syphilis
B Antithrombin III deficiency
C Fitz-Hugh-Curtis syndrome
D Systemic lupus erythematosus
E Antiphospholipid syndrome

Directions: Match the statement below with the most appropriate vitamin or mineral above. Each answer may be used once, more than once, or not at all.

A Vitamin A   F Vitamin K
B Pyridoxine (B_6)   G Nicotinic acid
C Vitamin C   H Folic acid
D Vitamin D   I Iron
E Vitamin E   J Calcium

QUESTIONS 43–44

43. Immediately after vaginal delivery, a newborn is given _____.

44. A patient taking prophylactic medication for tuberculosis should also be taking _____.

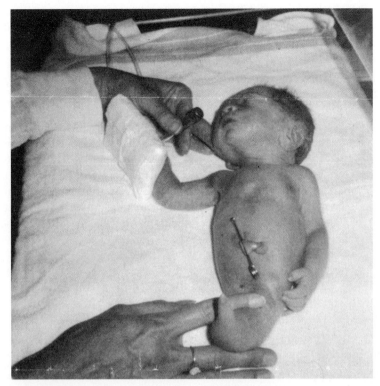

Question 45 figure. Reprinted with permission from Reece EA, Coustan DR, eds. Diabetes Mellitus in Pregnancy. 2nd Ed. New York: Churchill Livingstone, 1995;243.

45. The following photograph shows a baby born with a unique congenital anomaly. You conclude that _____ .

- [A] The infant has mesomelic dwarfism
- [B] The infant has osteogenesis imperfecta
- [C] The infant has pulmonary hypoplasia
- [D] The mother has an endocrinologic disorder
- [E] The mother has a hemoglobinopathy

46. A 24-year-old gravida 3, para 3 just delivered a male infant who weighs 3800 g and has low APGAR scores. The pregnancy was uncomplicated and the fetal monitoring strip was unremarkable. Time from complete cervical dilation to delivery of the infant was less than 1 hour, and the patient received local anesthetic and intravenous meperidine for pain control at completion of cervical dilation. The infant is lethargic and limp. The next best step in management of the infant is

- [A] Intravenous D_{10} in water
- [B] Naloxone
- [C] Intramuscular vitamin K
- [D] Intravenous calcium
- [E] Measurement of serum electrolytes

47. A 21-year-old gravida 1, para 0 at 40 weeks of gestation is in the second stage of labor. She has been pushing for almost 2 hours without an epidural in place. Examination reveals a cervix that is fully dilated and effaced. Fetal station is 0 according to location of fetal calvarium but is +2 in relation to the leading part of the fetal scalp. After delivery of the infant there is molding and edema of the fetal presenting part. The edema resolves in 3 days. There are no neurologic sequelae. The most likely diagnosis is

A Subdural hematoma
B Intraventricular hemorrhage
C Caput succedaneum
D Cephalohematoma

48. A 29-year-old gravida 1, para 0 at 30 weeks gestation presents to your office because she is concerned about her unborn baby's well-being. A relative from her native country just visited her recently and he frequently appeared to be coughing up bloody sputum. You perform a purified protein derivative (PPD) test on her by injecting a PPD intracutaneously and measuring a diameter of induration of 7 mm two to three days after placement. Her medical records indicate that her PPD was negative 2 years ago and that she is currently HIV negative. You are not sure what to do next so you perform a chest radiograph with abdominal shielding and the results are read as normal by the radiologist. The next best step in management of this patient is

A Repeat PPD testing postpartum
B Repeat chest radiograph postpartum
C Give isoniazid and vitamin B_6 postpartum
D Give isoniazid and vitamin B_6 now

49. Given the statements below, choose the answer choice that has the most number of true statements about breast conditions or disorders:

(1) Mammographically detected clusters of calcifications less than 2 mm in size require biopsy
(2) Dominant, well-circumscribed, smooth masses much larger than other masses require biopsy
(3) Fibrocystic disease is associated with elevated blood levels of luteinizing hormone
(4) A fat necrosis mass requires excisional biopsy to distinguish it from carcinoma
(5) Pathologic nipple discharge is usually intermittent, unilateral, and serous

A 1, 2, 3
B 1 & 3 only
C 1, 3, & 5
D 1, 2, & 4
E 1, 3, 4, & 5

50. A 24-year-old gravida 1, para 0 at 18 weeks of gestation is having a routine obstetrical ultrasound when the following is seen on cross-section of the head at the level of the cerebellum:

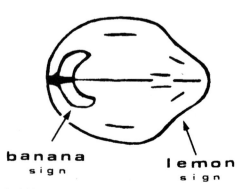

Question 50 figure. Modified from Nicolaides KH, Campbell S, Gabbe SG, Guidetti R. Ultrasound screening for spina bifida: Cranial and cerebellar signs. Lancet 1986;2:72.

The best diagnosis is

- [A] Encephalocele
- [B] Hydrocephalus
- [C] Spina bifida
- [D] Meningomyelocele
- [E] Holoprosencephaly

51. A 26-year-old nulligravid woman presents to you because she has been unable to become pregnant for the last 3 years. She has no known medical problems other than a history of chlamydia that was treated 7 years ago. She has never had any surgeries. She does not smoke or consume any alcohol or drugs. Her husband of 4 years has fathered a child with his previous partner and is in good medical condition. You see bilateral hydrosalpinges on hysterosalpingogram.

The next best step in the treatment of her infertility is

- [A] Clomiphene citrate and intrauterine insemination (IUI)
- [B] Recombinant follicle stimulating hormone and IUI
- [C] IVF-ET
- [D] Bilateral salpingectomy and IVF-ET
- [E] ICSI and ET

52. When performing an abdominal hysterectomy, one of the first steps after entering the peritoneal cavity and establishing good visualization is to clamp, transect, and suture ligate the round ligaments. This interrupts an artery that is a branch of [the] _____ artery. Furthermore, the round ligaments attach the uterus to the _____ .

- [A] Sampson's; labia majora
- [B] External iliac; labia majora
- [C] Internal iliac; labia minora
- [D] External iliac; labia minora
- [E] Ovarian; labia majora

Answers and Explanations

1. The answer is C. It is crucial to obtain a rubella antibody titer before discharging this patient from the hospital. If she does not have immunity to rubella and becomes pregnant in the future, her fetus is at risk for congenital rubella syndrome, which consists of neurologic (e.g., microcephaly), cardiovascular (e.g. patent ductus arteriosus), ocular (e.g., blindness), and inner ear (sensorineural deafness) abnormalities. Because she is breastfeeding successfully and this is not her first baby, she probably does not require help from a lactation nurse. This patient's postpartum hemoglobin is 12.0; therefore, she does not need additional iron, which can worsen constipation. RhoGAM would not benefit a patient who is Rh-positive and antibody-negative. Discharging from the hospital without first knowing her rubella immunity status is poor management.

2. The answer is E. Midline lower back pain is common late in pregnancy and less tolerable in a primigravid. It results from ligament and joint changes that occur during normal pregnancy. It is important to rule out a urinary tract infection (UTI) and pyelonephritis in any pregnant woman who reports back pain. Because this patient's urine dipstick is normal, she is afebrile, and lacks costovertebral angle tenderness, you can confidently rule out urinary tract infection. Therefore, a urine culture and antibiotics are not necessary. An MRI is not necessary at this point because her back pain can be explained by her pregnancy, lack of infection, and lack of history of any trauma. It is better to avoid ibuprofen during pregnancy for management of pain and inflammation because theoretically, it can cause closure of the fetal ductus arteriosus. It is prudent to avoid narcotics (codeine) for management of benign pain *initially* because not only can it produce tolerance, it can also exacerbate the constipation of pregnancy. It is probably more prudent to try acetaminophen alone before resorting to narcotics for this type of pain.

3. The answer is D. Although this patient denies drug abuse, this case scenario is that of a cocaine abuser or addict. The patient has just had a cerebral infarct (stroke), has a history of seizures, is severely hypertensive and mydriatic, and probably has an eroded nasal septum because she snorts cocaine. She may have needle tracks on her extremities and thus does not want you to examine them. Intravenous drug users are at risk for acquiring hepatitis B and C. Both can be vertically transmitted. Cocaine use is not associated with cystic kidney disease, deafness, or chorioretinitis. It is associated with intestinal atresia, but not of the duodenum.

4. The answer is D. In a patient who has not had excessive bladder manipulation or injury and who has adequate urine output, it is safe to discontinue the Foley catheter in the first postoperative day. She is not a candidate for blood transfusion. Her hemoglobin has decreased appropriately for the amount of blood she lost during surgery. She has stable vital signs and good urine output. There is no need to increase her intravenous fluid rate since her urine output is adequate and her input exceeds her output in a 24-hour period. Because a patient undergoing surgery is at risk for thromboembolic phenomena during and after surgery, it is wise to start bilateral lower extremity sequential compression devices (i.e., thromboguards) on the way to the operating room instead of initiating them after surgery.

5. The answer is A. In a young patient such as this who has undergone oophorectomy, androgen therapy (in the form of oral testosterone undecenoate, fluoxymesterone, methyltestosterone, or topical testosterone) is likely to help treat decreased libido. Estrogen supplementation is also helpful in treating decreased libido and in counteracting premature menopausal signs and symptoms, but it does not consistently increase libido as do supraphysiologic levels of androgens. Lubrication is useful during intercourse when there is insertional dyspareunia (painful sexual intercourse). There are no controlled studies on the effectiveness of sildenafil for treatment of decreased libido. The antidepressant fluoxetine, an SSRI, has been associated with sexual dysfunction.

6. The answer is C. The only absolute contraindication to breastfeeding is cyclosporine. Other medications that are contraindicated during breastfeeding are bromocriptine, cocaine, cyclophosphamide, doxorubicin, ergotamine, methotrexate, lithium, PCP, phenindione, and radioactive iodine. None of the hepatitis infections are absolute contraindications to breastfeeding. Breast augmentation and reduction are not contraindications, but treatment of breast cancer is a contraindication. PPD+ is not a contraindication, but active tuberculosis is a contraindication. Infant galactosemia, not a family history of lactose intolerance, is an absolute contraindication to breastfeeding.

7. The answer is B. Herpes simplex should be treated and suppressed during pregnancy using nucleoside analogues to decrease the frequency of cesarean section for active herpes, to reduce viral shedding and pain, and to heal lesions. None of the antiviral drugs in this class is approved for use during pregnancy by the FDA in 2003. Although acyclovir has more data demonstrating its safety, valacyclovir has better bioavailability (twice a day versus five times a day dosing for treatment), is class B (instead of acyclovir which is class C), and is now widely available. Artificial rupture of membrane (AROM) is the opposite of what you want to do when treating someone with a history of herpes simplex because rupture of membranes hastens spread of infection to the fetus.

8. The answer is E. Tennis would be safe to play as long as she is not too vigorous and takes care not to fall. Recreational activities that involve a high potential for contact (soccer and basketball) or increased risk of falling (horseback riding and downhill skiing) are not advisable during pregnancy. Scuba diving should also be avoided because the fetus is at increased risk for decompression sickness.

9. The answer is B. Pelvic tuberculosis is a rare disease. Facts in this scenario that, when combined, point to the diagnosis are as follows: (1) individual from an East Asian country recently immigrated to the United States (there is a high incidence of pulmonary tuberculosis in those regions); (2) low-grade fever: (3) history of lung disease (pulmonary tuberculosis); (4) bilateral adnexal masses and thickening around ligaments and uterus (frozen pelvis); (5) anemia; and (6) elevated ESR. Pelvic tuberculosis usually occurs when pulmonary tuberculosis spreads to the pelvis hematogenously. This can take a long time because this bacteria is very slow to divide. Possible procedures that may help elucidate the diagnosis would be to (1) culture the tissue sampled from the endometrial biopsy, which would reveal mycobacteria that can be stained by acid fast method; (2) perform a PPD, which would be positive; or (3) perform a chest radiograph, which would show old healed tuberculosis shadows. Pelvic tuberculosis should be treated with chemotherapy (four drugs: INH, ethambutol, rifampin, and pyrazinamide); surgery should be reserved for failures or progression of disease despite chemotherapy. Cancer (adnexal masses) and gonorrhea (tenderness, low-grade fever, and pelvic inflammatory type signs and symptoms) do not account for all of the facts in this clinical scenario. Actinomyces is a bacterium that is most likely associated with IUDs and causes classic draining sinuses with "sulfur granules."

10. The answer is C. The success rate of VBAC is quoted between 60 and 80%. Success is at the higher end if there is a history of one or more previous successful vaginal births after cesarean section and if the reason for the initial cesarean section was a non-recurring one (e.g., a non-recurring reason is fetal distress or breech whereas a recurring reason is failure to progress or labor dystocia). All of the other facts (such as macrosomia, previous uterine surgery, and prostaglandin agent induction) decrease the likelihood of vaginal delivery. In fact, use of prostaglandin agents to induce a VBAC is contraindicated because the uncontrollable uterine stimulation increases the risk of uterine rupture. Also, the number of previous cesarean sections also influences chances of successful VBAC. Currently, no data supports VBAC with a history of more than two previous low transverse cesarean sections.

11. The answer is B. Because the physician does not know the efficacy of the experimental drug and because he allows the patient to go home without undergoing any additional unproved and unnecessary drug therapies or procedures, he is displaying the ethical principle of nonmalfeasance (avoiding doing harm). He is also respecting the patient's autonomy by letting her go home without therapy, but the question is referring to the physician not insisting on a therapy because it is experimental. "Paternalism" is when a physician overrides a patient's autonomy because he or she knows what is best for the patient. Therefore, if the physician gave the chemotherapy despite the patient's wishes, that would be considered paternalism. "Beneficence" is when a physician prescribes a drug or therapy that has been proven to benefit the patient. Justice is the obligation to treat equally all those who are alike according to whatever criteria are selected.

12. The answer is A. Calcification of the lateral borders of the lateral ventricles (periventricular calcifications) is a specific sign for infection with cytomegalovirus. Intracranial calcification is also present with toxoplasmosis, but the pattern of calcification is diffuse rather than in the periventricular region. VZV can cause hydrops and hyperechogenicity in the liver but cannot cause intracranial calcifications. Parvovirus may manifest as hydrops fetalis on ultrasound. This patient has no history of genital lesions, thus you would not be suspecting HSV.

13. The answer is D. Molly does not need parental consent because she is on active military duty. Megan can consent for herself because she was previously married. Mary can sign for herself because she is older than 15 years, does not live at home, and manages her own financial affairs. Melinda does not need parental consent because she is at least 12 years old and has a contagious, communicable, infectious disease. Although Mary is pregnant, she will require parental consent because the care that she requires is not related to the prevention or treatment of pregnancy. Had Mary had placenta previa, she could consent because it is a condition related to pregnancy. Here are other conditions listed by the California Healthcare Association Consent Handbook as reasons parental consent would not be required: unmarried individual needing emergency care; individual emancipated by court at any age seeking an abortion, care for rape, or care for sexual assault; individual 12 years of age and older needing care for alcohol, drug abuse, or outpatient mental health treatment; and individual 17 years of older donating blood. A minor making an anatomic gift (e.g., kidney donation) would need written consent of a parent or guardian.

14. The answer is A. The clinical features described in this case scenario suggest a bleeding corpus luteal cyst during pregnancy. This patient probably has an early intrauterine pregnancy (that is not yet detectable by transvaginal ultrasound technology) along with a persistent corpus luteal cyst that is ruptured and hemorrhagic (which has caused the bleeding "fluid in the cul-de-sac"). Ectopic pregnancy would be the second best diagnosis but is less likely because of lack of vaginal bleeding. Note that vaginal bleeding associated with an ectopic pregnancy is caused by the pregnancy in the tube, which produces high levels of "pregnancy hormones," including estrogen, which causes growth of the endometrium. Theca lutein cysts result from extremely high β-hCG levels (as in a molar pregnancy) or from clomiphene therapy. These are usually *bilateral*, massive, and disappear spontaneously when the source of hCG is gone. Luteomas of pregnancy are massive, bilateral, *solid*, tumorlike growths that may occur during pregnancy and regress spontaneously. Luteomas can cause virilization of the mother and rarely of the fetus. Appendicitis is always in the differential of right lower quadrant pain, but it does not explain all of the findings in this clinical presentation.

15. The answer is E. In women, androgens come from the adrenal gland, ovary, and peripheral transformation of preandrogens. Most testosterone (more than 50%) comes from peripheral (skin and liver) conversion of preandrogens. The ovary and adrenal glands also produce some testosterone. The preandrogens are androstenedione, which is produced equally by the ovary and the adrenal gland, and dehydroepiandrosterone (DHEA), which is mostly derived from the adrenal gland. DHEA-sulfate (DHEA-S) is produced only by the adrenal gland. These hormones are here listed in order of potency (from least potent to most potent): DHEAS < DHEA < androstenedione < testosterone < DHT (2x testosterone).

16. The answer is E. Pregnant women are advised to avoid raw seafood and to limit overall cooked seafood (1) to prevent parasitic infections from Anisakis (intestinal nematode or roundworm), *Clonorchis sinensis* (trematode or fluke), *Paragonimus westermani* (trematode acquired from eating raw crab), *heterophyes heterophyes* (trematode), and *Diphyllobothrium latum* (cestode, the fish tapeworm) and bacterial infections from *Vibrio cholera* and *Vibrio parahaemolyticus;* and (2) because ingestion of mercury in fish causes neurodevelopmental problems in the developing fetus. Predatory fish like shark or whales are especially harmful because they eat other fish, which concentrates mercury in their bodies. *Schistosoma japonicum* infection is acquired through skin puncture, not ingestion. *Wuchereria bancrofti* is acquired from a mosquito bite. Acariasis is acquired from ingestion of eggs in soil contaminated with human feces. Lead ingestion and toxicity are acquired from old homes with peeling, lead-based paint, lead pottery, and lead bullets, and usually not from fish.

17. The answer is B. This clinical scenario is that of cervical incompetence caused by an acquired cause (conization). A cerclage is placed between weeks 12 to 16 and then removal at 38 weeks of gestation or earlier if labor begins. Transvaginal ultrasound to measure cervical length is a good idea but not on a daily basis. Bedrest, Trendelenburg positioning, and Foley catheter placement may have some use in patients with cervical dilation and a bulging amniotic membrane. Magnesium sulfate is used for preterm labor (which is a symptomatic phenomenon—regular uterine contractions). This patient has cervical incompetence.

18. The answer is C. Chemical alterations of the amino acids at positions 6 and 10 produce synthetic derivatives of GnRH (GnRH analogs or agonists) that are resistant to cleavage by endopeptidases (therefore a longer half-life, not potency) but retain a high affinity for the pituitary GnRH receptor.

19. The answer is C. Although the clinical scenario may lead you to think of child abuse (management—child protective services), condyloma acuminata (management—podophyllin resin), or precocious puberty (management—leuprolide), the actual evidence points to the diagnosis of sarcoma botryoides because of its appearance and occurrence in this particular age group. Sarcoma botryoides is the most common malignant vaginal tumor. This cancer usually extends locally and rarely metastasizes to a distant location. Primary treatment consists of surgical debulking and chemotherapy. Estrogen cream may be useful for prolapsed urethra or labial agglutination.

20. The answer is A. GnRH is a decapeptide produced by hypothalamic neurons, principally from the arcuate nucleus, and is transported along axons that terminate in the median eminence around capillaries of the primary portal plexus. It is then secreted into the portal circulation, which carries it to the anterior lobe of the pituitary gland.

21. The answer is B. Preexisting diabetes has many effects on pregnancy. The most characteristic of all is caudal regression (also known as sacral agenesis). Other congenital malformations, such as ventricular septal defect (VSD), situs inversus, anencephaly, and spina bifida also can occur in someone with preexisting diabetes who has poor glycemic control. However, none of these malformations are as characteristic of diabetic embryopathy as sacral agenesis. Macrosomia or growth retardation can occur in the fetus of a diabetic mother. Pulmonary hypoplasia is uncommon; however, slowing of lung maturation does occur and can lead to neonatal respiratory distress syndrome.

22. The answer is D. Patients with gestational diabetes mellitus (as opposed to preexisting diabetes mellitus) **are not** at risk for fetal anomalies (encephalocele, VSD, or pulmonary hypoplasia). CVAs can occur in patients with preeclampsia, not gestational diabetes.

23. The answer is D. Patients with hypothyroidism usually do not achieve pregnancy because they have reduced fertility. Those who become pregnant are at risk for spontaneous abortion, preeclampsia, abruptio placentae, stillbirth, and intrauterine growth restriction (not macrosomia). In addition, this patient has hypertension, which also puts her at increased risk for placental abruption. Infants of untreated women with significantly increased TSH levels may be at risk for decreased performance on IQ tests (an exact, average numerical decrease in IQ). Pyelonephritis is more common in patients with sickle cell trait. Abnormal fetal scalp development or aplasia cutis is a rare, reversible condition that may develop from treatment with methimazole for hyperthyroidism.

24. The answer is B. It is essential to screen and treat patients with sickle cell disease for infectious processes, especially if they are symptomatic, because infections can incite painful crisis and can lead to other serious conditions. Because this patient has a productive cough, it is a good idea to culture the sputum. Also, because these patients are at risk for urinary tract infections, you can also send a urinalysis and a urine culture. A stool culture for ova and parasites is useless because the patient does not have those symptoms. Daily folic acid and an up-to-date pneumococcal vaccine are important in a sickle cell patient. However, they are not the reason the patient has been hospitalized.

25. The answer is C. Although immediately after delivery there will be a drop in the cardiac output and blood pressure, during the *postpartum period* there is a 10 to 20% increase in blood volume resulting from absence of a uteroplacental circulation and shifting of fluids from the interstitium (third space) into the intravascular compartment. By definition, this patient has lost less than 500 mL of blood (the definition of postpartum hemorrhage).

26. The answer is A. Small for dates uterus, large placenta (as a result of villous hypertrophy), and the appearance of the fetus all suggest a partial molar pregnancy. Triploidy (69,XXX) is the most common karyotype.

27. The answer is C. A robertsonian fusion translocation, 45,XY, t(13q14q), means that chromosomes 1 through 12 and 15 through 22 are paired and that there is an X and a Y chromosome; however, one of the pair of chromosome 13 and one of chromosome 14 are translocated, forming one fused chromosome (i.e., there is one chromosome 13, one chromosome 14, and a long chromosome 13/14). Donor egg, not donor insemination, would be appropriate because of the abnormal maternal karyotype. Reassurance is not appropriate for someone who has had four spontaneous abortions. A 10% risk exists that this woman would give birth to an infant with trisomy 13. Therefore, identifying an abnormal fetus and selectively aborting it would be an option other than egg donation. Current federal guidelines and technology do not allow us to analyze the chromosomal make-up of an individual egg and sperm *prior* to using that egg or sperm for fertilization. Preimplantation genetic diagnosis (PGD), however, allows us to diagnose inheritable diseases and screen for aneuploidies by removing one cell from a *fertilized* egg that has divided several times (8-cell stage) prior to implantation inside the uterus (PGD is not an answer choice).

28. The answer is B. Histologic criteria for lichen sclerosus include a thin epithelium with a decreased number of cell layers and loss of the undulating rete ridges. Therefore, this micrograph is depicting lichen sclerosus, which is best treated with a high-potency steroid cream, such as clobetasol. Testosterone cream was advocated in the past but is not the treatment of choice after a recent placebo-controlled study showed its lack of efficacy in comparison to steroid creams. Estrogen cream is used for pediatric conditions, such as labial agglutination, or for atrophic vulvovaginitis in postmenopausal women. Laser ablation is good treatment option for vulvar dysplasia. Simple vulvectomy is the treatment for vulvar cancer.

29. The answer is C. The most common suture used in gynecologic surgery is polyglactin 910 (VICRYL or Polysorb), usually the braided type. This suture is absorbed by hydrolysis rather than by enzymatic processes (which occur in absorption of chromic or plain sutures). Polyglactin loses 25% of its strength in 2 weeks, loses 50% of its tensile strength in 3 weeks, and is completely absorbed by 9 to 10 weeks (2.5 months). The braided type of this suture has the advantage of increased tensile strength, pliability, and flexibility; however, it has the disadvantage of harboring organisms between its grooves and resistance as it passes through tissue, especially if it is not coated.

30. B; 31. A; 32. D; 33. C. Progesterone breakthrough bleeding occurs when there is a high ratio of progesterone relative to estrogen. Depot medroxyprogesterone acetate results in atrophy of the endometrium. Removal of the corpus luteum is similar to pharmacologic therapy with progesterone for several days and then discontinuing treatment. Progesterone withdrawal bleeding occurs only if the endometrium is stimulated to grow first by estrogen. Low doses of estrogen can lead to intermittent spotting caused by variable growth and response of the endometrium to the insufficient dose of estrogen. Estrogen withdrawal bleeding occurs upon discontinuation of estrogen, either through oophorectomy, radiation of the ovaries, or another method.

34. A; 35. C. The pituitary prolactinoma is causing this patient to have galactorrhea and oligomenorrhea. If this patient desires fertility or is bothered by her symptoms, the initial step in management is to start bromocriptine. Even if bromocriptine does not decrease her prolactin levels, it will help her to ovulate. However, if this patient is not bothered by these symptoms, then she can take a progestational agent 10 days a month to prevent endometrial hyperplasia. Remember, because she has periods, she must be producing estrogen; therefore, unopposed estrogen leads to endometrial hyperplasia.

36. The answer is A. The photomicrograph is that of a benign cystic teratoma or dermoid. These cysts have a wall of epidermis from which hair shafts may protrude. Teeth or simple calcifications may also be found within the wall of the cysts. Structures from other germ layers, such as cartilage, bone, and thyroid tissue, can be found inside as well. Microscopically, the cyst wall is composed of stratified squamous epithelium, which is the most common element to become malignant (only 1% of dermoids undergo malignant transformation). Dermoids should be removed intact, and a cystectomy (most desirable treatment) or a unilateral oophorectomy (in women of reproductive age who desire future fertility) should be performed if the involved ovary is salvageable and the contralateral ovary is free of disease. Although a cystectomy is preferred over an oophorectomy, it is not one of the answer choices. A bilateral oophorectomy is not necessary because there is no mention of bilateral involvement.

37. The answer is C. Advanced ovarian cancer is best treated with surgery (as described in the clinical scenario) in combination with chemotherapy. Currently, the treatment regimen with the best outcome is paclitaxel and a platinum agent (cisplatin or carboplatin). Because carboplatin is as effective as cisplatin and has less toxicity, it is the treatment of choice. Cyclophosphamide and doxorubicin have activity against ovarian cancer but are currently not first-line chemotherapy. Methotrexate, actinomycin D, and folic acid are used for gestational trophoblastic tumors. Vincristine, actinomycin D, and cyclophosphamide (VAC regimen) are used for ovarian germ cell tumors.

38. The answer is E. The approximate maximal amount of tolerated radiation for each tissue type is as follows: kidney, <2,000 rads; ovary, <2,500 rads; liver, <3,000 rads; rectum, <5,000 rads; bladder, <7,000 rads; and cervix/vagina, <20,000 rads. Cancer cells have greater sensitivity to radiation than normal tissue, and normal tissue has a greater ability to recover after radiation. To improve tolerance of normal tissue to radiation, the maximal tissue dose (i.e., 5,000 rads) is fractionalized (i.e., given in daily doses over a few weeks instead of all at once).

39. B 40. A 41. D The best time to perform a hysterosalpingogram to evaluate the contour of the uterine cavity and the architecture of the fallopian tubes is during the mid-follicular phase. At this time, the uterine lining is thin (because menstrual bleeding has already occurred) and ovulation has not yet occurred. Therefore, the chance of pregnancy is low. High FSH levels on day 3 of the menstrual cycle may indicate low follicular reserve and a low probability of achieving pregnancy with ovulation induction agents, such as clomiphene and recombinant FSH. An elevated serum progesterone level 7 days after the expected ovulation day is a sign that ovulation has occurred.

42. The answer is E. This patient meets three major criteria for antiphospholipid syndrome. She has a false-positive test for syphilis; she has a history of a thrombotic event (venous or arterial); and she has history of two unexplained second trimester losses. Ninety percent of patients with anti-phospholipid syndrome will also have a positive lupus anticoagulant *and* positive anti-cardiolipin antibodies (IgG or IgM). Other criteria include a connective tissue disease and autoimmune thrombocytopenia. Neither protein C deficiency nor antithrombin III deficiency can adequately explain this patient's entire medical history. This patient does not meet 4 of the 11 criteria needed to diagnosis systemic lupus erythematosus (SLE). These criteria are discoid rash, oral ulcer, photosensitivity, arthritis, malar rash, immunologic disorder, neurologic disorder, renal disorder, antinuclear antibody, serositis, and hematologic disorder (mnemonic: DOPAMIN RASH). SLE is usually not associated with thrombotic events or second-trimester losses. This patient does not have syphilis because her FTA-ABS is negative. Fitz-Hugh-Curtis syndrome is diagnosed in someone patients with a history of pelvic inflammatory disease in whom the infection has spread to the upper abdomen, forming "violin string" adhesions between the liver capsule and the diaphragm. It is a perihepatic inflammation originating from peritoneal or vascular spread of either *Neisseria gonorrhoeae* or *Chlamydia trachomatis*.

43. The answer is F. Newborns are deficient in vitamin K not only because they lack the bacterial intestinal flora that synthesize vitamin K, but also because they do not receive vitamin K from the mother due to lack of free vitamin K. Clotting factors II, VII, IX, and X depend on vitamin K for their synthesis. Therefore, vitamin K prevents hemorrhagic disease in the newborn.

44. A patient taking isoniazid should also take vitamin B_6. The two main side effects of isoniazid are drug-induced hepatitis (which increases as with older age) and peripheral neuropathy. Vitamin B_6 has been shown to be protective against peripheral neuropathy.

45. The answer is D. The photograph depicts caudal regression or sacral agenesis. Women who have pregestational diabetes mellitus with uncontrolled blood sugar levels are at risk for congenital malformations (such as congenital heart defects, neural tube malformations, etc.). Sirenomelia is a severe form of this unique congenital anomaly that occurs 200 times more in infants of mothers with diabetes mellitus. In dwarfism, you would see severely shortened bones (e.g., the radius and ulna) and not sirenomelia. In osteogenesis imperfecta, you may see fractures in utero (e.g., crumpling of the tibia and fibula) by ultrasound. Pulmonary hypoplasia would be diagnosed by ultrasound well before the baby's birth (it is diagnosed when gestational-age–dependent fetal thoracic circumference divided by the abdominal circumference is less than 80% [TC/AC <0.8]).

Pulmonary hypoplasia is unlikely when gestational-age–dependent fetal thoracic circumference divided by abdominal circumference exceeds 80% (TC/AC >0.8).

46. The answer is B. The cause of neonatal depression is maternal narcotic administration. Because labor was rapid, there was not sufficient time for metabolism of the narcotic and thus the narcotic crossed the placenta and depressed the neonate. The appropriate management steps include airway, breathing, and circulation, then naloxone (0.1 mg/kg intramuscularly, intravenously, or intratracheally).

47. The answer is C. Caput succedaneum, or "caput," is a soft tissue swelling of the scalp that involves the presenting portion of the head. There is occasional bruising, and the lesion always extends across suture lines. The edema also resolves in less than a week. However, a cephalohematoma is a hemorrhage underneath the periosteum of the skull (and thus does not extend across suture lines). This is also seen as swelling in the newborn. Cephalohematomas are more serious and may be associated with skull fractures; however, they usually resolve without any residual findings within a few weeks (less than 1 month). Subdural hematomas are serious and may result from trauma (such as shaken baby syndrome). They result from rupture of cortical veins and accumulation of blood between the dura layer and inner table of the skull. Subdural hematomas can be seen as slits on computed tomography scan. Intraventricular hemorrhages usually occur in preterm infants and lead to progressive hydrocephalus, bulging fontanelle, and neurologic signs.

48. The answer is D. A PPD induration (not erythema) of 5 mm or more is considered positive in patients with known or suspected HIB, close contacts with a person with active disease, or radiographic (adenopathy, multinodular upper lobe infiltrate, cavitation, upper lobe loss of volume, and old dense nodules in hilar area with or without fibrotic scars) or clinical evidence of tuberculosis. An induration of 10 mm or more is considered positive in anyone with chronic illness (diabetes mellitus, renal failure, hematologic disease, chronic alcoholic) and in intravenous drug users, health care workers, residents of health care institutions or prisons, certain immigrants and members of minority groups, immunosuppressed individuals, malnourished persons, and silicosis patients. Everyone else is considered PPD+ if the induration is 15 mm or more. In a patient who is PPD+, chest radiograph negative, and younger than 35 years of age who has converted within the last 2 years, the next best step is to begin antepartum isoniazid and vitamin B_6. If the same patient had converted beyond 2 years, then the best management would have been postpartum isoniazid and vitamin B_6. Collection of sputum samples is useful in someone who is PPD+, chest radiograph negative, and has respiratory symptoms. There is no need to repeat PPD or chest radiograph postpartum with the information in this clinical scenario.

49. The answer is D. Mammographically, calcifications that are less than 2 mm in size ("micro"); clustered along ducts; have more than five calcification per cm^2; or are dominant, well-circumscribed, smooth masses that are significantly larger than any other mass in either breast should be biopsied. Fibrocystic disease is associated with elevated blood levels of estrogen, not LH. Fat necrosis does require biopsy to distinguish it from carcinoma because it may feel and look like carcinoma on mammogram. Pathologic breast discharge is usually unilateral, spontaneous, and may be associated with a breast mass. It may be bloody, serous, or green-yellow. Only about 10% of pathologic nipple discharge is caused by breast cancer.

50. The answer is C. The "lemon sign" is a sensitive nonspinal marker for spina bifida. The "lemon" and "banana" (not seen here) signs are two sonographic signs of Arnold-Chiari malformation seen in spina bifida. The frontal bones of the skull are scalloped, giving a lemonlike configuration. When the cerebellum is seen, it is flattened and centrally curved, obliterating the posterior fossa and resulting in a bananalike appearance. Meningomyelocele is a subtype of spina bifida and cannot be diagnosed on a sonographic image of the skull. Holoprosencephaly results when there is failure of cleavage of the prosencephalon. In its most severe form, it gives rise to a single common ventricle, fused thalami, absent third ventricle, and olfactory bulbs. It is associated with varying degrees of facial malformations and is seen in trisomy 13. An encephalocele is a herniation of intracranial contents through a bony defect. Most commonly, they are occipital in location and midline. A posterior encephalocele with herniation of the cerebellum is termed the Chiari type III deformity, which is a major cause of hydrocephaly.

51. The answer is D. This patient has a history of chlamydia infection, which is usually asymptomatic and goes untreated for a period of time, and has evidence of bilateral hydrosalpinges on the hysterosalpingogram. A hydrosalpinx forms inside the fallopian tube after resolution of a bacterial infection (salpingitis) and results in an occluded, cystlike structure filled with clear fluid, which can drain into the uterine cavity. The hydrosalpinx prevents the blunted fimbriae of the fallopian tube from retrieving the oocyte immediately after ovulation. In the past, management of this condition was simply with IVF-ET or ICSI-ET. However, evidence shows that pregnancy rates are higher when the hydrosalpinges are removed and then IVF-ET is done because toxic substances inside the hydrosalpinges may flow into the uterine cavity, decreasing embryo implantation rates. It is not necessary to induce superovulation with clomiphene or R-FSH when the fallopian tube is unable to "pick up" the oocyte.

52. The answer is B. Suture ligation of the round ligament interrupts blood emerging from the external iliac artery to Sampson's artery (which is located within the round ligament). The round ligaments go through the inguinal canal and attach to the dermis of the labia majora.

Index

Page numbers in italics denote figures; those followed by a t denote tables; those followed by a Q denote questions; those followed by an E denote explanations.

Disseminated intravascular coagulopathy
(DIC), 101, 104, 172
Diuresis, postpartum, 27
Diuretics, 438
Diverticulitis, 330
DNA analysis, 62, 68
DNA hybridization techniques, 310
Domestic violence, 48, 49t, 361–363, 367Q,
368E
Donor insemination, 383
Dopamine agonists, 224
Doppler velocimetry, 198
Dose threshold, 77
Douching, 290
Down syndrome
amniocentesis for, 68
maternal age and, 62t
MSAFP for, 63
multiple marker screening for, 3, 39, 55,
58Q, 60E, 64, 70Q, 72E
Doxorubicin, 467E, 471E
Doxycycline
for chlamydia, 303, 304, 315Q, 317E
for gonorrhea, 303
for granuloma inguinale, 305
for lymphogranuloma venereum, 305
for pelvic inflammatory disease, 323,
327E
for syphilis, 307
Drospirenone, 275
Drug abuse (*see* Substance abuse)
Drugs
amenorrhea from, 223
androgenic, 261
category A, 42
category B, 42
category C, 42
category D, 42
category X, 42
congenital abnormalities from, 76–79
date-rape, 365
dysfunctional uterine bleeding and, 236
hirsutism from, 260
over-the-counter, 76
in pregnancy, 42, 53, 76–79
recreational, 78
violence and, 365
Dual-energy x-ray absorptiometry, 394,
400Q, 402E, 441, 442
Dual-photon absorptiometry, 394
Duchenne muscular dystrophy, 34, 68
Duct ectasia, 284
Ductal papilloma, 282
Ductus arteriosus, 13, 14, 163
Ductus venosus, 13, 14, 17Q, 19E
Due date (*see* Estimated date of delivery)
Duodenal atresia, 39
Dura, 146, 152Q, 153E
Duty, 420
Dwarfism, 472E
Dyschezia, 337

Dysfunctional uterine bleeding, 233–240,
241–242Q, 243E
in adolescents, 253
case study of, 450–452
diagnosis of, 236–238, 237t, 241Q, 243E,
450–452
estrogen breakthrough, 233, 234, 460Q,
471E
estrogen-progesterone withdrawal,
233–234
estrogen withdrawal, 236
etiology of, 234–235, 450–452
leiomyomas and, 353, 355, 359Q, 360E
in menopause, 390
in perimenopause, 388, 391
progesterone breakthrough, 236, 460Q,
471E
treatment of, 238–240, 241–242Q, 243E,
391, 452
Dysgenesis, gonadal, 222, 254, 432
Dysgerminomas, 247, 412, 414, 419E
Dysmenorrhea, 216, 218Q, 220E
in adolescents, 252–253
endometriosis and, 336, 338
pelvic pain from, 330, 332Q, 334E
primary vs. secondary, 330
Dyspareunia
endometriosis and, 336
estrogen replacement therapy for, 395
menopause and, 393, 432
pelvic inflammatory disease and, 318
pelvic organ prolapse and, 371
topical estrogens for, 397
Dysplasia
cervical, 443–445
vulvar, 470E
Dyspnea, 190
Dystocia, 130, 131, 137

Eating disorders, 253
EBRT (External beam radiotherapy), 406
Ebstein anomaly, 80
ECC (Endocervical curettage), 404, 444, 445
Echocardiography, 67, 72E, 181, 189, 199Q,
201E
Eclampsia, 51, 175
Ectoparasites, 313–314
Ectopic pregnancy, 343–347, 348–349Q,
350E
abdominal, 343
cervical, 343
combination oral contraceptives and, 274
corneal, 350E
diagnosis of, 64, 344–345, 450, 468E
etiology of, 343–344
hCG levels and, 2, 3, 10
heterotopic, 343
intrauterine devices and, 271, 448
ovarian, 343

pelvic inflammatory disease and, 60E,
318, 322, 343
pelvic pain from, 329
risk factors for, 8Q, 10E, 48, 60E, 347,
349Q, 350E
treatment of, 345, 346–347, 348–349Q,
350E
tubal, 343
Ectopic ureter with vaginal terminus, 247
EDD (*see* Estimated date of delivery)
Edema
fetal scalp, 463–464Q, 473E
in preeclampsia, 173
in pregnancy, 36, 145
pulmonary, 115Q, 117E
Edward syndrome, 39, 55, 64, 68
Eflornithine hydrochloride, 264
EGF (Epidermal growth factor), 351
Ehlers-Danlos syndrome, 62
Ejaculate, 41
Electrical stimulation
for urinary incontinence, 373
for uterine prolapse, 377E
Electrolysis, 264
Elliot forceps, 136
Embolism, pulmonary, 169, 192, 193
Embolization, uterine artery, 357
Embryo freezing, 425
Embryo implantation, 5
Embryo transfer, 381, 383, 465Q, 474E
Embryonal carcinomas, 247, 413
Emergency contraception, 276, 279Q, 280E,
364
Emollient creams, 30
Enalapril, 439
Encephalocele, 473E
Endocardial fibroelastosis, 85Q, 86E
Endocervical curettage (ECC), 404, 444, 445
Endocrine system, fetal, 1, 2, 6, 11–13,
15–16
Endocrinology of pregnancy, 1–7, 8–9Q,
10E
Endocytosis, 11, 18Q, 19E
Endodermal sinus tumors, 247, 412
Endometrial ablation, 240
Endometrial biopsy
for anovulation, 380
for dysfunctional uterine bleeding, 238,
241Q, 243E, 451–452
for infertility, 381
for leiomyomas, 355, 359Q, 360E
for postmenopausal bleeding, 446
Endometrial cancer, 407–409, 418Q, 419E
clear cell, 408
combination oral contraceptives and, 274
diagnosis of, 408–409, 446–447
dysfunctional uterine bleeding and, 243E,
450
endometriosis and, 335
epidemiology of, 407, 446

Menarche, 251
Mendelian abnormalities, 62
Meningoencephalitis, 80
Meningomyelocele, 70Q, 72E, 473E
Menometrorrhagia, 233, 253
Menopausal syndrome, 395
Menopause, 387–399, 400–401Q, 402E (*see also* Perimenopause)
  androgens and, 388, 389
  care for, 398–399, 434, 441–442
  case study of, 440–442
  estrogen replacement therapy for, 395–398, 400Q, 402E, 431–435
  late, 446
  leiomyomas and, 355, 440
  osteoporosis and, 392, 394, 400Q, 402E, 440–441
  physiology of, 388–390
  premature, 387, 389–390, 400Q, 402E
  signs and symptoms of, 392–394, 431–432
Menorrhagia, 390
Menstrual cycle, 211–217, *215*, 218–219Q, 220E
  body temperature and, *215*
  follicular phase, 211, 233
  hirsutism and, 260
  luteal phase, 211, 233
  menopause and, 389, 393
  natural family planning and, 277
  normal physiology, 221, 233–234
  oogenesis, *213*, 213–216
  perimenopause and, 388, 390
  varied, 450
Menstruation
  normal physiology, 216, 233–234
  postpartum, 27
  retrograde, 335
Mental retardation, 75, 79, 80, 81, 89, 426
Meperidine, 117E, 147
Mercury, 457Q, 469E
Metabolic acidosis, fetal, 118
Metabolism
  fetal, 12–13
  inborn errors of, 62
Metaplasia, 403
Metastasis (*see also* Lymph node metastasis)
  from cervical cancer, 407
  from ovarian cancer, 411
Methadone, 91
Methimazole, 183, 201E
Methotrexate
  breastfeeding and, 467E
  for ectopic pregnancy, 347, 347t, 348Q, 350E
  for gestational trophoblastic tumor, 206–207, 210E, 471E
  for *Trichomonas vaginalis* vaginitis, 294–295
α-Methyldopa, 171, 178Q, 179E, 439
Methyldopa, 393, 402E

Methylergonovine, 28, 33E
Methyltestosterone, 466E
Metronidazole
  for bacterial vaginosis, 45E, 292, 298Q, 300E, 305
  for gastric fluid aspiration, 149, 153E
  for pelvic inflammatory disease, 323
  for trichomoniasis, 313
Metrorrhagia, 233, 236, 390
Microadenomas, 223, 227, 436, 460Q, 471E
Microcephaly, 75, 79, 80, 81, 83
Micronor (*see* Minipill)
Microphthalmia, 80, 83
Microphthalmia encephalitis, 81
Midforceps, 136
Mifeprex (*see* Mifepristone)
Mifepristone, 6, 139, 276, 280E
Migraines, 433
β-Mimetics
  for abruptio placentae, 101
  action of, 106
  for preterm labor, 90, 107t, 163
Minerals, prenatal, 40–41
Minipill, 271, 280E
Minoxidil, 261
Mirena IUD, 421
Miscarriage (*see* Spontaneous abortion)
Mittelschmerz, 329, 334E
Mixed germ cell tumors, 413
Mixed gonadal dysgenesis, 254
Molar pregnancy (*see* Hydatiform mole)
Molluscum contagiosum, 312, 317E
Mondor's disease, 284, 286E
Monilia, 246
Moniliasis, 246, 293–294
Mons pubis, 287
Morning-after pill, 276, 280E, 364
Morning sickness, 20
Morphine, 147
Mortality
  fetal, 46, 47, 52
  maternal (*see* Maternal mortality)
  perinatal/neonatal (*see* Perinatal mortality)
Motherhood, surrogate, 424–425, 429Q, 430E
MSAFP (*see* Maternal serum α-fetoprotein)
Mucoid degeneration, 353
Mucolipidoses, 62
Mucopolysaccharidoses, 62
Müllerian malformations, 160, 224, 253
Multigravida, 35
Multiparity, 35, 48, 176
Multiple gestation
  cesarean section for, 130
  hCG levels and, 2
  placenta previa and, 97
  preterm labor and, 161
  progesterone production and, 5
  risks of, 47
  ultrasonography for, 64

Multiple marker screening, 3, 35t, 39, 62, 64, 422
Mumps, 83, 85Q, 86E
Muscular dystrophy, Duchenne, 34, 68
Muscularis, 289
Mycobacterim tuberculosis, 191, 455Q, 467E
Mycoplasma, 305
Mycoplasma hominis, 268, 291, 319
Mycoplasma pneumoniae, 191
Myocardial infarction, 273
Myolysis, 357
Myomas (*see* Leiomyomas)
Myomectomy, 51, 356–357
Myometritis, 318
Myometrium
  endometrial cancer and, 409
  labor and, 106
  postterm pregnancy and, 154–155
  progesterone levels and, 5–6
Myosin, 106
Myosin light-chain kinase, 106

Nägele's rule, 22, 35, 159E
Nalbuphine, 147
Naloxone, 147, 463Q, 472E
Naproxen, 342E
Narcotic antagonists, 147
National Center for Injury Prevention and Control (NCIPC), 361
National Domestic Violence Hotline, 362
Nausea of pregnancy, 20, 41
NCIPC (National Center for Injury Prevention and Control), 361
Necrosis, 353
Negligence, 420, 425, 426, 428Q, 430E
Neimann-Pick disease, 62
Neisseria gonorrhoeae, 184, 268, 301, 302, 319, 323
Neonatal mortality (*see* Perinatal mortality)
Neonates
  circulatory adjustments of, 14
  depressed, 463Q, 472E
  forceps delivery and, 136–137
  hepatitis B immunization of, 56
  hyperbilirubinemia in, 15, 201E
  large size, 49
  low birth weight, 47, 80, 95E, 130
  maternal diabetes and, 52, 181, 201E
  respiratory distress syndrome in, 23
  vacuum-extractor delivery and, 136–137
  vitamin K for, 462Q, 472E
Neovagina, 228
Nerve block
  paracervical, 140, 149
  pudendal, 148–149, 153E
Neural tube defects
  diabetes and, 79
  folic acid for, 41
  prenatal diagnosis of, 39, 55, 62, 68, 72E, 181, 422